Lecture Notes in Bioengineering

Lecture Notes in Bioengineering (LNBE) publishes the latest developments in bioengineering. It covers a wide range of topics, including (but not limited to):

- Bio-inspired Technology & Biomimetics
- Biosensors
- Bionanomaterials
- Biomedical Instrumentation
- Biological Signal Processing
- Medical Robotics and Assistive Technology
- Computational Medicine, Computational Pharmacology and Computational Biology
- Personalized Medicine
- Data Analysis in Bioengineering
- Neuroengineering
- Bioengineering Ethics

Original research reported in proceedings and edited books are at the core of LNBE. Monographs presenting cutting-edge findings, new perspectives on classical fields or reviewing the state-of-the art in a certain subfield of bioengineering may exceptionally be considered for publication. Alternatively, they may be redirected to more specific book series. The series' target audience includes advanced level students, researchers, and industry professionals working at the forefront of their fields.

Indexed by SCOPUS, INSPEC, zbMATH, SCImago.

Aakash Gupta · Tarun Kumar Singh · Ekta Singla
Editors

Application of Robotics in Dentistry

Springer

Editors
Aakash Gupta
Conservative Dentistry and Endodontics
All India Institute of Medical Sciences
Bathinda, Punjab, India

Tarun Kumar Singh
Conservative Dentistry and Endodontics
All India Institute of Medical Sciences
Bathinda, Punjab, India

Ekta Singla
Department of Mechanical Engineering
Indian Institute of Technology Ropar
Rupnagar, Punjab, India

ISSN 2195-271X ISSN 2195-2728 (electronic)
Lecture Notes in Bioengineering
ISBN 978-981-95-1469-4 ISBN 978-981-95-1470-0 (eBook)
https://doi.org/10.1007/978-981-95-1470-0

This Springer imprint is published by the registered company Springer Nature Singapore Pte Ltd.
The registered company address is: 152 Beach Road, #21-01/04 Gateway East, Singapore 189721, Singapore

Dedicated to God Almighty, my spiritual master H. H.Sant Rajinder Singh Ji Maharaj, my parents, and my teachers for their unending support and love.

—Dr. Aakash Gupta

Dedicated to God Almighty, my family, and my respected teachers.

—Dr. Tarun Kumar Singh

Dedicated to God Almighty, my family members, and my students.

—Dr. Ekta Singla

Foreword

In recent years, the fields of robotics and artificial intelligence (AI) have revolutionized countless industries, and dentistry is no exception. The integration of these advanced technologies into dental practice has transformed the way oral healthcare is delivered, improving precision, enhancing patient care, and expanding the possibilities for diagnosis, treatment, and patient management. This book, *Applications of Robotics in Dentistry*, explores the profound impact these innovations have had on modern dentistry and highlights the potential they hold for the future.

From robotic-assisted surgery and automated orthodontic procedures to AI-driven diagnostics and personalized treatment planning, the synergy between robotics and AI is reshaping the landscape of dental care. The ability to analyze vast amounts of patient data with machine learning algorithms enables early detection of dental diseases, while robotic systems enhance surgical accuracy and minimize human error. These advancements not only improve clinical outcomes but also enhance the patient experience through minimally invasive techniques and shorter recovery times.

This book serves as a comprehensive guide for dental professionals, researchers, and students seeking to understand and harness the potential of robotics and AI in their practice. By combining theoretical insights with practical applications, it offers valuable knowledge on how these technologies can be integrated into everyday dental procedures. The authors have meticulously compiled evidence-based research, case studies, and expert perspectives to provide a well-rounded understanding of this rapidly evolving field.

As you embark on this exploration of robotics and AI in dentistry, I am confident that you will gain a deeper appreciation for the technological innovations shaping modern oral healthcare. May this book inspire you to embrace these advancements and contribute to the future of dentistry with creativity, precision, and a commitment to excellence.

September 2025

Dr. Rajiv Kumar Gupta, M.S., M.Ch.
Professor and Head, CTVS
All India Institute of Medical Sciences
Bathinda, Punjab, India

Preface

The rapid advancements in robotics and artificial intelligence (AI) have ushered in a new era in healthcare, and dentistry stands at the forefront of this technological transformation. Over the past decade, the integration of robotics and AI into dental practice has not only enhanced clinical precision and efficiency but also redefined patient care and treatment outcomes. This book, *Applications of Robotics in Dentistry*, aims to provide a comprehensive exploration of these groundbreaking technologies and their impact on modern dental practice.

The motivation behind writing this book stems from the growing need for dental professionals to understand and adapt to the evolving technological landscape. As robotic systems become more sophisticated and AI algorithms more accurate, the potential for improved diagnostics, automated treatment planning, and enhanced surgical precision becomes increasingly evident. The ability to harness these technologies effectively will undoubtedly define the future of dentistry.

This book covers a wide range of topics, including the fundamentals of robotics and AI, their current applications in dentistry, and the challenges and opportunities they present. Through detailed case studies, expert insights, and evidence-based analysis, we seek to offer readers a balanced and practical understanding of how these technologies can be integrated into clinical practice.

We have designed this book to serve as a valuable resource for dental professionals, researchers, students, and technology enthusiasts. Whether you are exploring the field for the first time or looking to deepen your expertise, this book will provide you with the knowledge and tools necessary to navigate the intersection of robotics, AI, and dentistry with confidence.

We would like to express our gratitude to the contributors and experts whose insights have enriched this work. We hope that this book will not only inform but also inspire innovation and progress in the field of dental care.

We invite you to explore the pages ahead with curiosity and an open mind. The future of dentistry is being shaped by robotics and artificial intelligence, and that future is already here.

Bathinda, India	Dr. Aakash Gupta
Bathinda, India	Dr. Tarun Kumar Singh
Rupnagar, India	Dr. Ekta Singla

Acknowledgments The completion of this book, *Applications of Robotics and Artificial Intelligence in Dentistry*, would not have been possible without the invaluable support, guidance, and contributions of many individuals and institutions. We are deeply grateful to everyone who played a part in bringing this work to life.

First and foremost, we extend our sincere gratitude to the researchers, clinicians, and experts in the fields of robotics, artificial intelligence, and dentistry whose groundbreaking work and insights have laid the foundation for this book. Their dedication to advancing dental science and technology has been instrumental in shaping the content and direction of this work.

We would like to thank our colleagues and mentors who offered their expertise and thoughtful feedback throughout the development of this book. Their insights and encouragement have enriched the quality and depth of the material presented.

A special thanks to the contributors who shared their knowledge, case studies, and experiences, adding practical value to the theoretical framework of this book. Their willingness to collaborate and provide detailed information has made this work more comprehensive and relevant.

We are also grateful to the editorial and publishing teams for their professionalism, patience, and attention to detail throughout the writing and production process. Their support ensured that this book meets the highest standards of clarity and accuracy.

Lastly, we extend our heartfelt appreciation to our families and friends for their unwavering support and understanding. Their encouragement and belief in this project have been a source of motivation and strength.

It is our hope that this book will serve as a valuable resource for dental professionals, researchers, and students, inspiring further exploration and innovation at the intersection of dentistry, robotics, and artificial intelligence.

Dr. Aakash Gupta
Dr. Tarun Kumar Singh
Dr. Ekta Singla

Competing Interests The authors have no competing interests to declare that are relevant to the content of this manuscript.

Contents

About the Editors

Dr. Aakash Gupta is a renowned endodontist and aesthetic dentist whose expertise is in micro endodontic surgeries, retreatment cases and regenerative procedures. He is a social worker, innovator and experienced teacher. He was a university topper during his graduation final examination and was awarded best paper and poster award during post-graduation (M.D.S.) in Conservative Dentistry and Endodontics. He is an associate editor of several reputed journals. He has also served as chairperson at different state conferences. He has numerous national and international publications to his credit and is presently working in the Department of Dentistry at All India Institute of Medical Sciences, Bathinda (Punjab).

Dr. Tarun Kumar Singh is an associate professor in the Division of Conservative Dentistry and Endodontics at All India Institute of Medical Sciences (AIIMS) Bathinda. With a robust academic and clinical background, Dr. Singh has established himself as a leading expert in his field. He has extensive experience in performing complex root canal treatments and is committed to advancing dental education and research. Dr. Singh's work focuses on integrating innovative techniques and technologies to enhance patient care, including the use of AI-driven Clinical Decision Support Systems (CDSSs) for improving diagnostic accuracy and treatment outcomes. His dedication to his profession is evident in his numerous publications and presentations at national and international conferences. As an educator, Dr. Singh is passionate about mentoring the next generation of dental professionals, fostering a culture of excellence and continuous learning at AIIMS Bathinda.

Dr. Ekta Singla is serving as an associate professor and head of the Mechanical Engineering Department at IIT Ropar. With her research interests in modular robotics, service robots, customized optimal designs, evolutionary robotics and hybrid morphologies, she has more than 15 years of experience in robotics and in applied optimization fields. She is a recipient of the institute gold medal during her master's program, the national doctoral fellowship during her doctoral program at IIT Kanpur, the CNRS postdoctoral fellowship for UPMC Paris and a recent national award from the Institute of Engineers. Her current research projects are in maintenance and service robotics and in rehabilitation robotics, progressing through industrial partnerships, two UK—India collaborations and active association with the University of Stony Brook, New York—for the robotic applications in medical and defense fields.

Introduction

Aakash Gupta and Tarun Kumar Singh

Instead of adorning yourself with diamonds, consider safeguarding natural ones within your oral cavity–Aakash Gupta

1 History Overview

The origins of dentistry can be traced back to the earliest days of human civilization, as evidenced by archaeological findings tracing its roots back to the Indus Valley Civilization around 7000 BC to 5500 BC and stands as one of the most ancient medical professions in existence (Daugherty 2023). The history of dentistry is deeply intertwined with the development of humanity, reflecting the importance placed on oral health and the recognition of dental issues even in ancient times. These early discoveries provide valuable insights into the practices and techniques employed by our ancestors to maintain dental hygiene and address dental problems.

Dentistry usually encompasses practices related to the oral cavity. Pierre Fauchard, born on 2 January 1679 and passing away on 21 March 1761, was a renowned French physician who holds the esteemed title of the "Father of Modern Dentistry." His significant contribution lies in his authorship of the pioneering and comprehensive scientific account of dentistry, titled "*Le Chirurgien Dentiste*" or "The Surgeon Dentist" (Fauchard 1728), which was published in the year 1728 (Fig. 1). In India (Bharat), Dr. Rafiuddin Ahmed is widely recognized as the "Father of Modern Dentistry." Although in 1530, the "*Artzney Buchlein*" emerged as the inaugural book that exclusively delved into the realm of dentistry. Subsequently, in 1685, Charles Allen authored the pioneering dental textbook in English, titled "*Operator for the Teeth.*" Significant progress in scientific research occurred during the nineteenth century, leading to the transformation of dentistry from a mere trade to a recognized

A. Gupta (✉) · T. K. Singh
Division of Conservative Dentistry and Endodontics, Department of Dentistry, All India Institute of Medical Sciences, Bathinda, India
e-mail: guptaaakash95@gmail.com

A. Gupta et al. (eds.), *Application of Robotics in Dentistry*, Lecture Notes in Bioengineering, https://doi.org/10.1007/978-981-95-1470-0_1

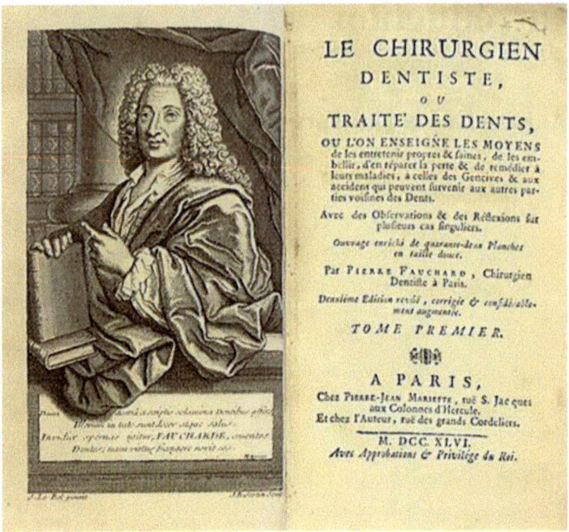

Fig. 1 *Le Chirurgien Dentiste* published in 1728

profession. Toward the end of the nineteenth century, the dental profession underwent government regulation. In the United Kingdom, the Dentists Act was enacted in 1878, followed by the establishment of the British Dental Association in 1879 (Mahant et al. 2017). Notably, in that same year, Francis Brodie Imlach achieved a remarkable milestone by becoming the first dentist ever to be elected as the President of the Royal College of Surgeons (Edinburgh). This achievement marked a significant turning point, as it elevated dentistry to the same level of importance as clinical surgery for the first time.

In the year 1840, the inaugural dental college, known as the Baltimore College of Dental Surgery, commenced its operations, thereby highlighting the necessity for enhanced supervision and regulation in the field of dentistry. In 1867, the Harvard University Dental School was established as the inaugural dental institution affiliated with a university.

Modern dentistry was introduced in India by Dr. Ahmed with the establishment of the first dental college in India in 1920, Dr. R. Ahmed Dental College and Hospital (Fig. 2), located in Sealdah, Kolkata (West Bengal) and is still operational. In 1925, the *Indian Dental Journal* was founded by him. In 1946, he founded the Bengal Dental Association, subsequently rebranded as the Indian Dental Association (IDA). In recognition of his immeasurable contribution, the Indian Dental Association (IDA) designated 24 December as National Dentists' Day in 2016, as a tribute to his remarkable achievements (Kerkhof 2024).

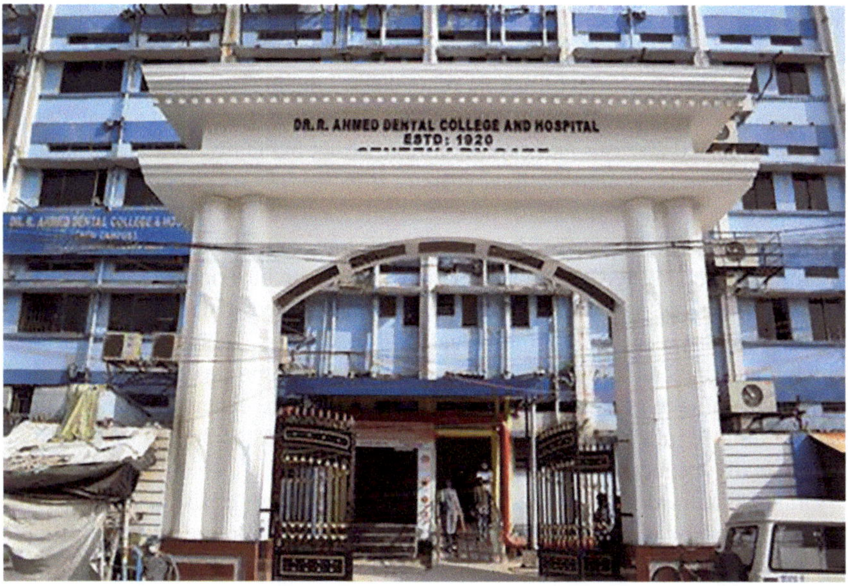

Fig. 2 Dr. R. Ahmed Dental College and Hospital

2 Dentistry as a Profession

Dentistry is widely regarded as the initial field of specialization within the medical profession, having subsequently evolved to establish its own recognized degree program encompassing various specialized areas. Dentistry is unique in its form as it is such a vast topic to be included as a subject in medical field. The contemporary trend in dentistry, known as evidence-based dentistry, emphasizes the utilization of top-notch scientific research and evidence to inform decision-making processes. This approach is particularly relevant in areas such as tooth conservation and the implementation of fluorides. Furthermore, evidence-based dentistry plays a crucial role in effectively addressing oral diseases. The World Health Organization (WHO) provides a definition of oral health as the condition of the mouth, teeth, and orofacial structures that allows individuals to carry out necessary functions like eating, breathing, and speaking. It also includes psychosocial aspects such as self-assurance, overall well-being, and the capacity to engage in social and professional interactions without experiencing pain, discomfort, or embarrassment. Oral health is not static and changes throughout a person's lifespan, from infancy to old age. It is closely connected to overall health and plays a crucial role in enabling individuals to actively participate in society and reach their full potential (Kezian 2020). The WHO pointed that the global problem of the oral disease still persists despite great improvements in the oral health of population in several countries. There are practically no geographic areas in the world whose inhabitants do not exhibit some evidence of oral disease. According to the World Health Organization, oral diseases are major public health problems due to their high incidence and prevalence across the globe. In the last few years, oral diseases have had a significant impact on the global population, affecting approximately 3.5 billion individuals per annum (Hussain and Khan 2014). These oral conditions hold the distinction of being the most prevalent among the vast array of over 300 diseases and conditions that afflict humanity. Oral diseases affect individuals from birth until the final years of life.

Disparities in oral health status persist among various population segments, indicating a notable discrepancy. These inequalities arise from a multifaceted combination of interconnected elements, several of which lie beyond the control of individuals themselves. Specifically, oral ailments tend to affect underprivileged, vulnerable, and socially marginalized individuals within societies. This includes individuals with limited financial resources, those grappling with disabilities, elderly individuals residing in solitude or care facilities, individuals who are either refugees, incarcerated, or situated in remote and rural areas, and individuals belonging to minority or other socially excluded groups.

Oral health professionals promote the avoidance of oral diseases by emphasizing the importance of maintaining proper hygiene and scheduling regular checkups for professional cleaning and evaluation, typically twice or more annually. The oral cavity acts as a doorway for diagnosing and treating diseases affecting other parts of the body. It is worth noting that oral infections and inflammations can have an impact on overall health, and the conditions observed in the oral cavity can serve as indicators of systemic diseases such as osteoporosis, diabetes, celiac disease, or cancer. Numerous studies have also demonstrated a correlation between gum disease and an elevated risk of diabetes, heart disease, and preterm birth. This interrelation between oral health and systemic health is commonly referred to as "oro-systemic health" (Coppa et al. 2006; Guerini 1909).

Dentistry has covered a long path from utilizing ancient tools to contemporary instruments for orodental procedures. Archaeological findings provide evidence indicating that ancient civilizations, including the Egyptians, Greeks, and Romans, made endeavors to address dental issues by employing various tools such as twigs, bone fragments, and even gold wires. These tools were utilized in attempts to alleviate toothaches and combat dental decay. The teeth of the ancient Romans were brightened by employing a toothpaste concocted from a combination of human urine and goat milk. Several remedies were employed to address gum diseases, such as inhaling the essence of wild mint, utilizing hare bones, and rinsing the mouth with the ash derived from deer horns. Nowadays, different tools like burs, discs, wheels, and micro instruments are available for better outcomes while consuming less time (Dabry 1863).

3 Dental Nomenclature

For better understanding of dentition, several numbering systems have been introduced. Specifically, when referencing a particular tooth, utilizing a tooth number proves to be significantly more convenient. There exist numerous types worldwide; however, we will elucidate a few types that are predominantly utilized by dentists:

1. International or FDI Tooth Numbering System

The FDI system, which stands for Federation Dentaire Internationale, is used to number teeth. It is recognized as the international standard for tooth numbering (Alt and Pichler 1998). The teeth are numbered according to this system as follows:

For permanent dentition (Fig. 3): Adults have four quadrants in their mouth, numbered from 1 to 4 in a clockwise direction, starting from the upper right side. The teeth in adults are also numbered from 1 to 8, starting from the central incisor and ending at the third molar or wisdom teeth.

For primary dentition (Fig. 4): Children's mouths are divided into four quadrants, labeled from 5 to 8 in a clockwise direction, starting from the upper right side. Primary teeth are numbered from 1 to 5, starting with the central incisor and going to the second molar, as premolars are absent in primary dentition.

2. Palmer Tooth Numbering System

It is one of the oldest systems proposed in 1861 (Andresen 1936). The teeth numbering system assigns numbers to teeth in the following manner:

For permanent dentition (Fig. 5).

For primary dentition (Fig. 6).

3. Universal System

Fig. 3 Tooth nomenclature for permanent dentition [FDI]

Permanent Teeth	
Upper Right	Upper Left
18 17 16 15 14 13 12 11	21 22 23 24 25 26 27 28
48 47 46 45 44 43 42 41	31 32 33 34 35 36 37 38
Lower Right	Lower Left

Fig. 4 Tooth nomenclature for primary dentition [FDI]

Primary Teeth	
Upper Right	Upper Left
55 54 53 52 51	61 62 63 64 65
85 84 83 82 81	71 72 73 74 75
Lower Right	Lower Left

Fig. 5 Tooth nomenclature for permanent dentition [Palmer]

Permanent Teeth	
Upper Right	Upper Left
8 7 6 5 4 3 2 1	1 2 3 4 5 6 7 8
8 7 6 5 4 3 2 1	1 2 3 4 5 6 7 8
Lower Right	Lower Left

Primary Teeth	
Upper Right	Upper Left
E D C B A	A B C D E
E D C B A	A B C D E
Lower Right	Lower Left

Fig. 6 Tooth nomenclature for primary dentition [Palmer]

Permanent Teeth	
Upper Right	Upper Left
1 2 3 4 5 6 7 8	9 10 11 12 13 14 15 16
32 31 30 29 28 27 26 25	24 23 22 21 20 19 18 17
Lower Right	Lower Left

Fig. 7 Tooth nomenclature for permanent dentition [Universal]

This system is widely utilized in the United States and other Western countries (Armitage 2020).

For permanent dentition (Fig. 7).

For primary dentition (Fig. 8).

4. Haderup System (Artzneybuch (Anonymous) 1546)

For permanent dentition (Fig. 9).

For primary dentition (Fig. 10).

Primary Teeth	
Upper Right	Upper Left
A B C D E	F G H I J
T S R Q P	O N M L K
Lower Right	Lower Left

Fig. 8 Tooth nomenclature for primary dentition [Universal]

Permanent Teeth	
Upper Right	Upper Left
8+ 7+ 6+ 5+ 4+ 3+ 2+ 1+	+1 +2 +3 +4 +5 +6 +7 +8
8- 7- 6- 5- 4- 3- 2- 1-	-1 -2 -3 -4 -5 -6 -7 -8
Lower Right	Lower Left

Fig. 9 Tooth nomenclature for permanent dentition [Haderup]

Primary Teeth	
Upper Right	Upper Left
V+ IV+ III+ II+ I+	+I +II +III +IV +V
V- IV- III- II- I-	-I -II -III -IV -V
Lower Right	Lower Left

Fig. 10 Tooth nomenclature for primary dentition [Haderup]

4 Specialties in the Field of Dentistry

Dentists often pursue additional training following their primary degree to acquire specialization in specific areas of their choice. Different postgraduation specialties are mentioned as follows:

1. Cosmetic dentistry—The main objective is to enhance the aesthetic appeal of the oral cavity, including the mouth, teeth, and smile, by improving their overall appearance and creating a more visually pleasing and attractive look. By addressing dental imperfections and improving the overall appearance of the mouth, teeth, and smile (Askitopoulou et al. 2017), individuals can experience a significant boost in self-esteem and enjoy the benefits of a beautiful and healthy-looking oral cavity.
2. Forensic odontology—The collection and utilization of dental evidence in legal matters can be carried out by any dentist who possesses expertise or training in this particular domain. The primary role of a forensic dentist is to document and authenticate the identity of individuals. During World War II, after the demise of Adolf Hitler, his dental remains were extracted from the soil. The autopsy report of Adolf Hitler, which was made public in 1968, played a crucial role in confirming the authenticity of his dental remains in 1972. Forensic odontologists Reidar F. Sognnaes and Ferdinand Strøm utilized this information to validate Hitler's dental remains (Axelsson and Lindhe 1981). In 2017, French forensic pathologist Philippe Charlier further corroborated the findings by discovering Hitler's dental remains, including teeth attached to a part of a jawbone, in the Soviet archives (Fig. 11). Charlier employed electron microscopy to meticulously examine the tartar present on the dental remains. Interestingly, the tartar solely contained plant fibers, a detail that aligns with Hitler's vegetarian lifestyle. In a collaborative research paper published in 2018, Charlier and his colleagues concluded that these dental remains are unquestionably authentic, citing their significant signs of wear (Axelsson et al. 1991).
3. Anesthesiology—Dental procedures are facilitated through the advanced application of general anesthesia, sedation, and pain management in this specialized field of dentistry (Axelsson et al. 2004). The role of an anesthesiologist begins before the surgery, as they assess the patient's medical history, perform a physical examination, and order any necessary tests to determine the most appropriate anesthesia plan. They collaborate with the surgical team to develop an individualized anesthetic plan that takes into account the patient's specific needs, the type of surgery, and any underlying medical conditions.
4. Dental public health—The examination of epidemiology and social health policies pertaining to oral health involves a comprehensive analysis of the factors that influence the prevalence and distribution of oral diseases within a population, as well as the policies and interventions implemented to address these issues (Badcock 1677). Epidemiological studies help identify risk factors, such as poor oral hygiene, tobacco use, unhealthy diet, and socioeconomic status, that contribute to the development of these diseases.

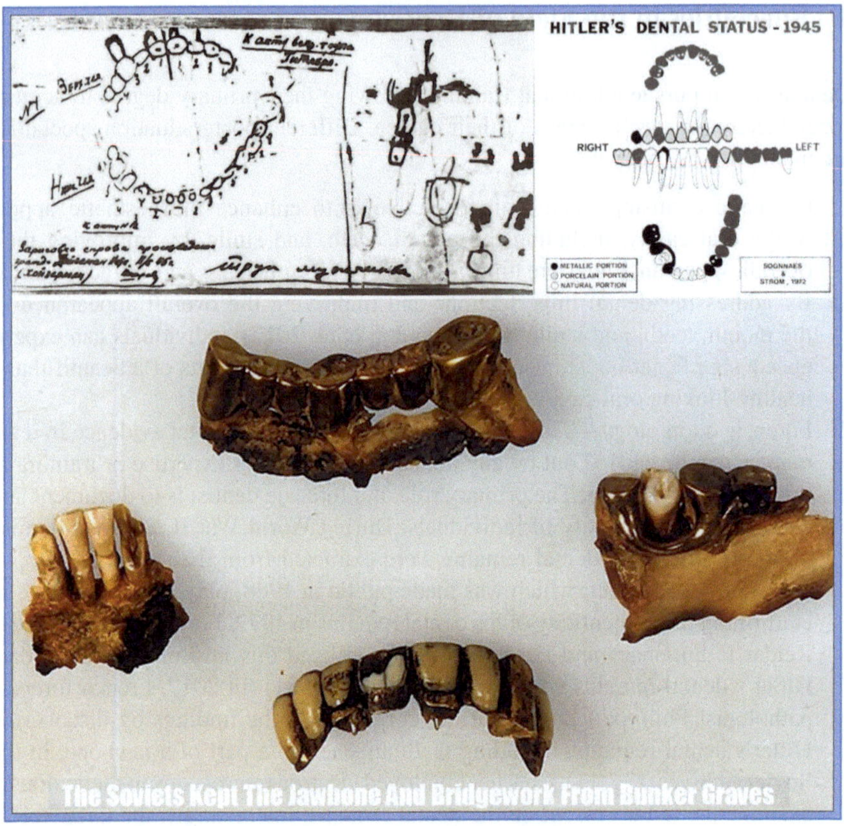

Fig. 11 Dental remains of Hitler present in Soviet archives

Social health policies, on the other hand, are the strategies and interventions implemented by governments, healthcare organizations, and other stakeholders to promote oral health and prevent oral diseases. These policies aim to address the social determinants of oral health, such as access to dental care, education, income, and social support systems. They may include initiatives such as community water fluoridation, school-based oral health programs, public awareness campaigns, and the establishment of dental clinics in underserved areas (Becker 1997).

5. Endodontics (also called endodontology)—Endodontics is a specialized branch of dentistry that focuses on the diagnosis, prevention, and treatment of diseases and injuries affecting the dental pulp and surrounding tissues. It involves procedures such as root canal therapy, which aims to remove infected or damaged pulp from the tooth and seal it to prevent further infection. Endodontists are highly trained dental professionals who possess advanced knowledge and skills

in performing these intricate procedures. By preserving the natural tooth structure, endodontics plays a crucial role in maintaining oral health and preventing the need for tooth extraction (Becker and Turfa 2017).

6. Geriatric dentistry (also called geriodontics)—The provision of dental services to elderly individuals encompasses the identification, prevention, and management of issues related to the natural aging process and age-related ailments. This is carried out in collaboration with a multidisciplinary team consisting of various healthcare practitioners. One aspect of this provision is the identification of dental issues that may arise as a result of the natural aging process. As individuals age, they may experience a range of oral health problems such as tooth decay, gum disease, and tooth loss. Dental professionals specializing in geriatric dentistry are trained to recognize and diagnose these issues early on, allowing for timely intervention and treatment (Bell 1829).
7. Oral and maxillofacial pathology—The field of oral and maxillofacial pathology focuses on the study and diagnosis of diseases and abnormalities that affect the mouth, jaws, and related structures. This specialized branch of pathology examines various conditions such as oral infections, oral cancer, salivary gland disorders, and developmental abnormalities (Bennett 1869). By analyzing tissue samples and conducting thorough examinations, oral and maxillofacial pathologists play a crucial role in identifying and treating these pathological conditions, ultimately contributing to the overall oral health and well-being of patients.
8. Oral and maxillofacial radiology—Oral and maxillofacial radiology is a specialized field within dentistry that focuses on the use of imaging techniques to diagnose and treat diseases and conditions affecting the head, neck, and oral cavity. It involves the interpretation of various imaging modalities such as X-rays, computed tomography (CT), magnetic resonance imaging (MRI), and cone beam computed tomography (CBCT) (Fig. 12) to provide detailed information about the structures and tissues in the maxillofacial region (Bennion 1986).

Maxillofacial radiologists play a crucial role in the diagnosis and treatment planning of various oral and maxillofacial conditions, including dental caries, periodontal diseases, temporomandibular joint disorders, oral and facial tumors, trauma, and congenital abnormalities. They work closely with other dental and medical specialists to provide comprehensive care to patients.

In addition to interpreting imaging studies, maxillofacial radiologists also perform advanced imaging procedures such as sialography, which involves injecting a contrast agent into the salivary glands to evaluate their function and detect any abnormalities. They may also use image-guided procedures to assist in the placement of dental implants, biopsy of oral lesions, and treatment of temporomandibular joint disorders (Berdmore 1768).

9. Oral medicine—Oral medicine is a branch of dentistry that focuses on the diagnosis and management of oral and maxillofacial diseases. Oral medicine specialists, also known as oral medicine physicians, are trained to diagnose and treat a wide range of conditions affecting the oral cavity, including oral mucosal diseases, oral manifestations of systemic diseases, oral infections, and oral cancer

Fig. 12 CBCT machine

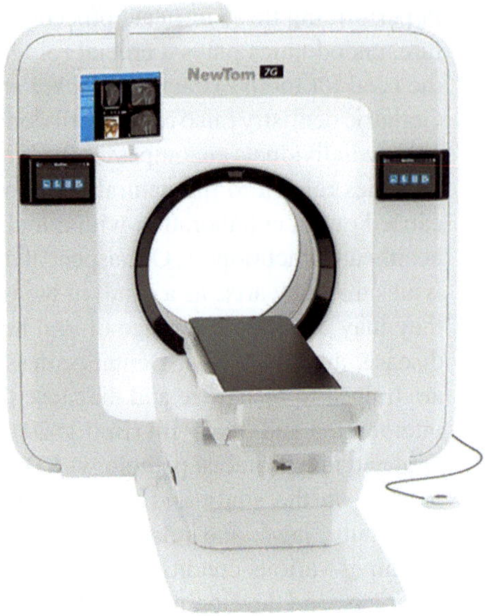

(Bird 1981). Oral medicine specialists are skilled in performing comprehensive oral examinations, taking detailed medical and dental histories, and ordering and interpreting laboratory tests and biopsies. They work closely with other dental and medical specialists to provide multidisciplinary care to patients with complex oral and maxillofacial conditions.

In addition to diagnosing and managing oral diseases, oral medicine specialists also play a crucial role in the prevention and early detection of oral cancer. They perform oral cancer screenings, educate patients about the risk factors and signs of oral cancer, and provide counseling on tobacco cessation and oral hygiene practices.

10. Oral and maxillofacial surgery (also called oral surgery)—Oral and maxillofacial surgery is a specialized field that focuses on treating conditions related to the mouth, jaw, and face. This branch of surgery encompasses a wide range of procedures, including tooth extractions, dental implants, corrective jaw surgery, and treatment of facial trauma. Oral and maxillofacial surgeons undergo extensive training to acquire the necessary skills and knowledge to perform these complex procedures. They work closely with other healthcare professionals, such as dentists, orthodontists, and plastic surgeons, to provide comprehensive care to patients (Bond 1851). The goal of oral and maxillofacial surgery is to improve both the functional and aesthetic aspects of the oral and facial regions, enhancing the overall quality of life for individuals in need of such interventions.
11. Orthodontics and dentofacial orthopaedics—Orthodontics and dentofacial orthopedics is one of the novel fields within the realm of dentistry. Orthodontics primarily focuses on the diagnosis, prevention, and treatment of dental and facial irregularities, such as misaligned teeth and jaws. This branch of dentistry

aims to improve the functionality and aesthetics of a patient's smile by utilizing various orthodontic appliances, such as braces and aligners (Lack 1908).

On the other hand, dentofacial orthopedics encompasses the study and treatment of skeletal and dental irregularities in the face and jaws. It involves the use of orthopedic appliances to guide the growth and development of the facial bones and jaws, ensuring proper alignment and harmony between the teeth, jaws, and facial structures. By addressing issues such as overcrowded teeth, malocclusions, and facial asymmetry, these disciplines contribute to the improvement of a patient's bite function, speech, and self-confidence. Through the expertise of orthodontists and dentofacial orthopedists, individuals can achieve a healthy and harmonious smile.

12. Pediatric dentistry (also called pedodontics)—Pediatric dentistry, also known as pediatric oral health, focuses on providing dental care to children and adolescents. It is a specialized field within dentistry that caters to the unique dental needs of young patients. Pediatric dentists undergo additional training to understand the growth and development of children's teeth, as well as the specific oral health issues that may arise during childhood (Black and McKay 1916). By offering preventive and therapeutic dental services, pediatric dentistry aims to promote optimal oral health and ensure a positive dental experience for children.
13. Periodontology (also called periodontics)—Periodontics is a specialized branch of dentistry that focuses on the prevention, diagnosis, and treatment of diseases and conditions affecting the supporting structures of the teeth, including the gums, periodontal ligament, and alveolar bone. It involves the study and management of periodontal diseases, such as gingivitis and periodontitis, as well as the placement of dental implants and the treatment of gum recession. Periodontists are dental professionals who have undergone additional training and education in this field to provide comprehensive care for patients with periodontal issues. By addressing these conditions, periodontics plays a crucial role in maintaining oral health and preventing tooth loss (Brown 1842).
14. Prosthodontics (also called prosthetic dentistry)—Prosthodontics is a specialized branch of dentistry that focuses on the restoration and replacement of missing teeth and oral structures. It involves the diagnosis, treatment planning, and fabrication of dental prostheses, such as dentures, dental implants, and dental bridges. Prosthodontists are highly skilled dental professionals who have undergone extensive training to provide comprehensive oral rehabilitation to patients with complex dental needs. By utilizing advanced techniques and materials, prosthodontics aims to improve the function, aesthetics, and overall oral health of individuals who have lost teeth or have significant dental impairments (Yadav and Sonkurla 2013).

Certain prosthodontists possess expertise in the field of maxillofacial prosthetics, focusing specifically on the restoration of individuals with congenital facial and oral abnormalities such as cleft lip and palate, as well as those born with an underdeveloped ear (microtia). In contemporary times, the primary role of maxillofacial prosthodontists is to restore both functionality and aesthetics to patients who have acquired defects due to the surgical removal of head and neck tumors or as a result of trauma caused by war or road traffic accidents (Grover et al. 2020).

15. Oral implantology—Oral implantology refers to the field of dentistry that focuses on the placement and restoration of dental implants. Dental implants are artificial tooth roots that are surgically placed into the jawbone to support replacement teeth or dental prostheses. This branch of dentistry combines the principles of oral surgery, prosthodontics, and periodontics to provide patients with functional and aesthetically pleasing dental restorations. Oral implantology plays a crucial role in restoring oral health and improving the quality of life for individuals who have lost their natural teeth (Hans et al. 2014).
16. Special needs dentistry (also called special care dentistry)—Special care dentistry refers to a specialized branch of dentistry that focuses on providing oral healthcare to individuals with special needs. This field of dentistry caters to patients who may have physical, intellectual, or emotional disabilities, as well as those who require additional support due to medical conditions or advanced age. The aim of special care dentistry is to ensure that these individuals receive the necessary dental treatment in a safe and comfortable environment, taking into consideration their unique needs and challenges. This may include interdisciplinary approach from different medical specialties for treating specific cases requiring greater consideration (Gambhir and Gupta 2016).
17. Sports dentistry—Sports dentistry is a specialized branch of dentistry that focuses on the prevention and treatment of dental injuries and oral health issues related to sports activities. It involves the application of dental knowledge and techniques to address the unique dental needs and challenges faced by athletes. Sports dentists work closely with athletes, coaches, and trainers to provide customized dental care and preventive measures to minimize the risk of dental injuries during sports participation (Andrews 2017). They also play a crucial role in the management and treatment of dental trauma, such as fractured teeth, jaw fractures, and soft tissue injuries, that may occur during sports events. By promoting oral health and providing appropriate dental care, sports dentistry aims to enhance athletes' performance, overall well-being, and long-term oral health. The sports dentist operates either as an independent consultant or as a part of the Sports Medicine Team (Atchison et al. 2018).

Recently, Maharashtra University of Health Sciences (MUHS) has approved a **one-year fellowship course in sports dentistry** at the Government Dental College and Hospital (GDCH) in Nagpur, India (Greenberg et al. 2010). The course is designed to educate dental professionals about the importance of protecting athletes' oral health, especially those with malocclusion or other risk factors. The fellowship will cover topics such as prevention, diagnosis, management, education, and research of sport-related orofacial injuries. The course will also incorporate activities not only for adults but also for toddlers, children, and even senior citizens.

18. Veterinary dentistry—The field of veterinary dentistry focuses on the oral health and dental care of animals. It involves the diagnosis, treatment, and prevention

of dental diseases and conditions in various animal species. Veterinary dentists are trained professionals who specialize in providing dental care to animals, including routine dental cleanings, tooth extractions, and oral surgeries. They play a crucial role in maintaining the overall health and well-being of animals by ensuring proper dental hygiene and addressing any dental issues that may arise. Veterinary dentistry is an important aspect of veterinary medicine, as dental problems can have a significant impact on an animal's quality of life (Joshi et al. 2021).

5 Paradigm Shift

When the majority of individuals envision a dentist, they typically imagine themselves reclining in a chair with a dentist examining their wide-open mouth and wielding a drill. Although this will continue to be a component of the dental experience, it will gradually diminish in significance as technology progresses.

In ancient times, due to lack of resources and technology, dental health professionals used to do each and every work during the procedure individually, but due to sterilization issues, time consumption, fatigue of clinician, etc., the concept of "four-handed dentistry" was introduced at the conference on "training dental students to utilize chairside assistants" in 1960 for exchange of knowledge and insights among dental professionals (Alabdullah and Daniel 2018). The proceedings of this significant event shed light on the strategies and techniques employed to equip dental students with the necessary skills to effectively collaborate with chairside assistants. Nowadays, six-handed dentistry (Fig. 13) is practiced due to introduction of magnification and sedation in dentistry (Petersen 2004).

Moreover, in previous times, people used to think that every person doing dental treatment was a doctor, and they were not aware of specializations of these persons and their expertise in the field of dentistry, and the drastic difference in dental clinician-to-population ratio in urban and rural landscapes gave rise to "street

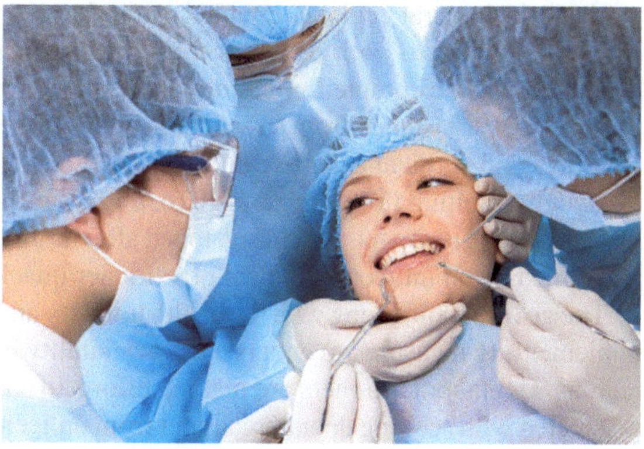

Fig. 13 Six-handed dentistry

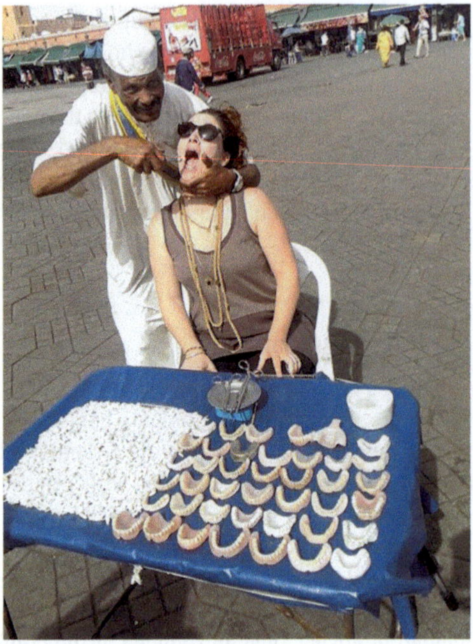

Fig. 14 Street dentistry being practiced

dentistry" (Kumari et al. 2022). Street dentistry, in its truest sense, refers to the act of practicing dentistry in public spaces (Fig. 14). However, for some, it remains a clandestine practice, conducted discreetly behind closed doors, within the confines of a patient's home, or in makeshift offices. This alternative option, although less expensive, carries significant risks and is often resorted to by individuals who cannot afford regulated dental care. Despite the prevalence of licensed dentistry in numerous regions worldwide, street dentistry continues to persist (Manohar 2021). The concept of tooth extraction was prevalent at that time, even though the tooth could have been saved.

The scarcity of skilled practitioners and limited availability of dental facilities, particularly in rural regions, coupled with elevated levels of illiteracy, exorbitant expenses associated with dental procedures, and inadequate awareness about oral healthcare, have prompted numerous individuals in different countries around the globe to seek assistance from street dentists. The absence of proper infection control measures and surgical expertise undoubtedly gives rise to numerous complications, ultimately resulting in fatalities. In 2016, a 12-year-old boy from Morocco tragically lost his life due to sepsis, which developed after he underwent an extraction procedure performed by an unlicensed dental practitioner/quack (Britton and Bradley 2021).

The government, along with the health ministry and dental associations, is actively implementing measures to enhance the availability of affordable healthcare in rural regions. Dental practitioners are making efforts to educate the public about the risks associated with seeking dental treatment from unlicensed practitioners on the streets,

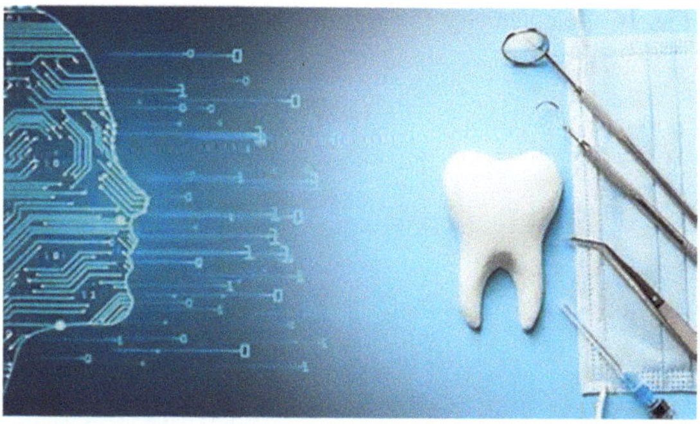

Fig. 15 Artificial intelligence and digitalization in the field of dentistry

and they are urging the government to establish and enforce stringent laws against fraudulent dental practices (Schulein 2005).

Dental health professionals have dedicated extensive years of their lives to acquire the necessary knowledge and skills to meet and uphold the educational standards essential for practicing dentistry. Our training encompasses a wide range of areas, including infection control, oral and systemic disease processes, and proficient utilization of dental instruments, among various other aspects.

Nowadays, most of the patients are aware of maintaining oral health and the various specializations in the field. With the advancements of various technologies, aseptic methods, and strict government guidelines, the era of evidence-based dentistry has now come into picture, which is evidence driven, utilizing various advancements like artificial intelligence (AI), digitalization (Fig. 15), magnification, 3-D imaging modalities, etc., in routine dental procedures for better efficacy and safety (Singh et al. 2024). At present, the concept of "six-handed" dentistry is in focus.

In certain complex procedures, the need of a secondary assistant is mandatory. The dentist focuses on performing the surgery while relying on the assistant to provide support and assistance. One of the key responsibilities of the assistant is to retract and prepare materials, which is particularly challenging when working with a microscope. Operating with microscope requires the joint effort of both the dentist and the primary assistant to maximize its benefits.

While the primary assistant remains actively involved in the treatment at the surgical site, the second clinical assistant takes on the responsibility of preparing additional materials, ensuring that everything is readily available when needed. This includes anticipating the need for specific instruments, materials, or medications and having them ready for immediate use. The second clinical assistant also assists in maintaining a sterile environment by handling instruments and materials in a controlled and organized manner. This helps to minimize the risk of contamination and ensures that the surgery proceeds smoothly (Alvitez-Temoche et al. 2024).

We now have the capability to harness the power of the technological revolution and leverage novel advancements like artificial intelligence, data mining, gene editing technology, and even augmented reality to proactively address and manage oral health issues before they escalate into more severe conditions.

Fig. 16 Teledentistry

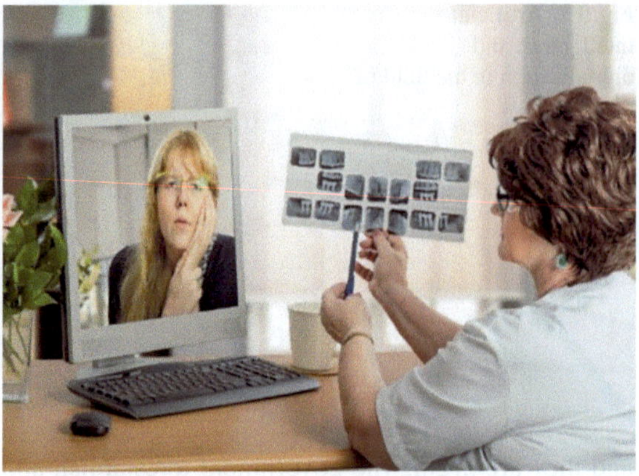

Recent global health crisis like COVID-19, which led to less aerosol-generating procedures (Dev et al. 2024) and changing patient preferences, nevertheless, have contributed to stimulating the advancement of innovative dental technology solutions in order to enhance the quality of care provided by dentists and establish stronger relationships with their clientele. Teledentistry, which involves utilizing digital tools like synchronous or asynchronous video for dental consulting or basic examinations, presents an opportunity to address the existing divide. Teledentistry (Fig. 16) is a concept that involves the amalgamation of telecommunications and dentistry. It entails the transmission of clinical data, reports, and pictures across vast distances in order to aid in dental diagnosis, management, and treatment planning (Chen et al. 2020). Teledentistry tools can also assist in assessing the presence of a genuine dental emergency, thereby determining whether an immediate visit to the dentist is necessary or if the patient can wait until their routine checkup.

Nowadays, virtual reality (VR) is employed as a means to induce relaxation in patients and alleviate their pain, while simultaneously fostering a sense of empathy toward the dentist. Furthermore, VR finds application in the realm of dental education, enabling dentistry students to virtually immerse themselves in dental procedures and gain valuable hands-on experience (Fahim et al. 2022).

AI serves as an additional set of eyes, verifying the accuracy of the findings. AI algorithms undergo training using vast amounts of data to make informed decisions by analyzing the available evidence, granting them a distinct advantage over humans in the realm of identifying particular circumstances. New advancements in dental technology provide numerous advantages, including enhanced accessibility, decreased patient anxiety, enhanced precision in diagnosis, and reduced expenses related to materials.

6 Oral Health and Its Significance

Oral health refers to the condition of the mouth, teeth, and orofacial structures, which allows individuals to carry out vital functions like mastication, swallowing, and speaking. It also includes psychological and social aspects such as self-assurance, overall well-being, and the capacity to interact and work without experiencing pain, discomfort, or embarrassment. Oral health changes throughout a person's lifespan, from infancy to old age, and is closely connected to overall health. It plays a crucial role in enabling individuals to actively engage in society and reach their full potential (Srinivasan et al. 2020).

Oral health is not just limited to the absence of oral diseases or conditions, but also encompasses the maintenance of healthy teeth and gums, proper functioning of the jaw and facial muscles, and the overall well-being of an individual. It is a fundamental aspect of overall health and has a significant impact on an individual's quality of life (Gupta et al. 2021).

Significance

Starting from infancy, oral health is crucial for the development of a child's teeth and jaw. Proper oral hygiene practices, such as regular brushing and flossing, help prevent tooth decay and gum diseases. It also promotes the healthy growth of permanent teeth and ensures proper alignment, which can have long-term effects on speech development and self-esteem.

As individuals grow older, maintaining good oral health becomes even more important. Poor oral health can lead to various oral diseases, such as tooth loss, gum diseases, and oral cancers. These conditions not only cause pain and discomfort but can also have a negative impact on an individual's ability to eat, speak, and socialize. Moreover, oral health issues have been linked to systemic diseases like diabetes, cardiovascular diseases, and respiratory infections, highlighting the interconnectedness between oral health and overall health (Barranca-Enríquez and Romo-González 2022).

In addition to physical well-being, oral health also has psychological and social implications. A healthy and attractive smile can boost self-confidence and improve one's overall appearance. On the other hand, oral health problems, such as missing teeth or bad breath, can lead to embarrassment, social isolation, and even affect professional opportunities. Therefore, maintaining good oral health is essential for individuals to feel confident, interact with others, and perform well in their personal and professional lives.

Promoting oral health requires a comprehensive approach that includes regular dental checkups, preventive measures, and education on proper oral hygiene practices. Dental professionals play a crucial role in diagnosing and treating oral diseases, as well as providing guidance on maintaining good oral health. Additionally, public health initiatives, community programs, and policies that prioritize oral health promotion can contribute to improving the overall oral health of populations (Fiorillo 2019).

7 Conclusion

In conclusion, oral health is not just about having a healthy mouth, but it encompasses various aspects of an individual's well-being. It is closely linked to overall health and plays a vital role in enabling individuals to lead a fulfilling life. By prioritizing oral health, individuals can maintain their ability to eat, speak, and interact without pain or discomfort, while also enhancing their self-confidence and overall quality of life.

References

Alabdullah JH, Daniel SJ (2018) A systematic review on the validity of teledentistry. Telemed J E Health 24(8):639–648

Alt KW, Pichler SL (1998) Artificial modifications of human teeth. In: Alt KW, Rösing FW, Teschler-Nicola M (eds) Dental anthropology. Fundamentals, limits and prospects. Springer Wien New York, p 387–415. (Intentional Dental Modifications, dental mutilations jade decoration of upper incisors in the Tlaxala skull, Mexico 500–900 A.D., p 405)

Alvitez-Temoche D, Del Aguila E, Galarza-Valencia D, Calderón I, Espinoza-Carhuancho F, Pacheco-Mendoza J, Mayta-Tovalino F (2024) Current trends and spatial-temporal dynamics of veterinary dentistry research: a scientometric study. Vet World 17(3):666–671. https://doi.org/10.14202/vetworld.2024.666-671

Andresen V (1936) The Norwegian system of functional gnatho-orthopedics. Acta Gnathol 1:5–36. (The Norwegian System of Orthodontics)

Andrews EA (2017) The future of interprofessional education and practice for dentists and dental education. J Dent Educ 81(8):eS186–eS192

Armitage GC (2020) A brief history of periodontics in the United States of America: pioneers and thought-leaders of the past, and current challenges. Periodontology 82:12–25. (History of periodontics)

Artzneybuch (Anonymous) (1546) Artzneybuch. Edited by Melchior Sachse and Introduced by Tarquinius Ocyorus (alias Schellenberg)

Askitopoulou H, Nyktari V, Papaioannou A et al (2017) The origins of oral medicine in the Hippocratic collected works. J Oral Med Path 46:689–694

Atchison KA, Rozier RG, Weintraub JA (2018) Integration of oral health and primary care: communication, coordination, and referral. Washington (DC): National Academy of Medicine. https://doi.org/10.31478/201810e

Axelsson P, Lindhe J (1981) (a). Effect of controlled oral hygiene procedures on caries and periodontal disease in adults—results after 6-years. J Clin Periodontol 8:239–248

Axelsson P, Lindhe J, Nyström B (1991) (b). On the prevention of caries and periodontal disease. Results of a 15-year longitudinal study in adults. J Clin Periodontol 13:182–189

Axelsson P, Nyström B, Lindhe J (2004) (c). The long-term effect of a plaque control program on tooth mortality, caries and periodontal disease in adults: results after 30 years of maintenance. J Clin Periodontol 31:740–757

Badcock W (1677) A touchstone for gold and silverwares or a manual for goldsmiths. John Bellinger, London, p 1 (instruments and goldsmith's workshop illustration). https://babel.hathitrust.org/cgi/pt?id=gri.ark:/13960/t0vq6wf90&view=1up&seq=7&skin=2021

Barranca-Enríquez A, Romo-González T (2022) Your health is in your mouth: a comprehensive view to promote general wellness. Front Oral Health 14(3):971223. https://doi.org/10.3389/froh.2022.971223

Becker MJ (1997) Early dental appliances in the Eastern Mediterranean. Berytus 42:71–102. (Egyptian, Greek, and Roman wiring of loose mandibular teeth)
Becker MJ, Turfa JM (2017) The etruscans and the history of dentistry. The Golden Smile Through the Ages. Taylor and Francis (General reference for Etruscan dental appliances)
Bell T (1829) The anatomy, physiology and diseases of the teeth. S. Highley, London, pp 93–103. (Improved arch bar and a gold crown on permanent molars to move vestibularly malpositioned teeth)
Bennett HD (1869) Partial sets of teeth without plate, clasp, or pivot. Dental Cosmos 11(10):509–510. (First description of a bridge done by B.J. Bing in Paris)
Bennion HD (1986) Antique dental instruments. Sotheby's Publications. P 137 (General reference)
Berdmore T (1768) A treatise on the disorders and deformities of the teeth and gums, p 259
Bird PD (1981) The development of dental radiology. Brit Dent J 151:28–31
Black GV, McKay SF (1916) Mottled teeth: an endemic developmental imperfection of the enamel of the teeth heretofore unknown in the literature of dentistry 58(2):129–156
Bond TE (1851) A practical treatise on dental medicine as connected with the study of dental surgery. Lindsey and Blakiston, Philadelphia. (first oral medicine and pathology text)
Britton J, Bradley N (2021) Why should everybody care about special care dentistry? Br Dent J 231(6):331–333. https://doi.org/10.1038/s41415-021-3465-2
Brown S (1842) Of the insertion of entire sets of artificial teeth, both upper and lower, on plates of gold, without clasps or springs. American J Dental Sci II(4):265–279
Chen YW, Stanley K, Att W (2020) Artificial intelligence in dentistry: current applications and future perspectives. Quintessence Int 51(3):248–257. https://doi.org/10.3290/j.qi.a43952. Erratum in: Quintessence Int. 51(5):430
Coppa A, Bondioli L, Cucina A, Frayer DW, Jarrige C, Jarrige JF et al (2006) Palaeontology: Early neolithic tradition of dentistry Nature, 755–6
Dabry PP (1863) Medicine among the Chinese consul of France in china. Member of the League Asian Paris
Daugherty G (2023) How humans took care of their teeth through history. History; A&E Television Networks
Dev A K, Gupta A, Dalai S (2024) A comparative investigation of aerosol generation and exposure risk during access cavity preparation with or without rubber dam application. Cureus 16(6):e61758. https://doi.org/10.7759/cureus.61758
Fahim S, Maqsood A, Das G, Ahmed N, Saquib S, Lal A, Khan AAG, Alam MK (2022) Augmented reality and virtual reality in dentistry: highlights from the current research. Appl Sci 12:3719. https://doi.org/10.3390/app12083719
Fauchard P (1728) Le Chirurgien Dentiste ou Traité des dents. Odontologie Jean Mariette
Fiorillo L (2019) Oral health: the first step to well-being. Medicina (Kaunas) 55(10):676. https://doi.org/10.3390/medicina55100676
Gambhir RS, Gupta T (2016) Need for oral health policy in India. Ann Med Health Sci Res 6(1):50–5. https://doi.org/10.4103/2141-9248.180274. PMID: 27144077; PMCID: PMC4849117
Greenberg BL, Glick M, Frantsve-Hawley J, Kantor ML (2010) Dentist's attitudes toward chairside screening for medical conditions. J Am Dent Assoc 141(1):52–62
Grover S, Pahuja M, Pradhan S et al (2020) Rural oral health: challenges and pit falls: time to recover and rebuild the pathway: a review article. Indian J Public Health Res Dev 11(6):893–897
Guerini V (n.d.) National dental association. [from old catalog]. A history of dentistry from the most ancient times until the end of the eighteenth century 1909 Philadelphia and New York: Lea & Febiger
Gupta A et al (2021) Dental cariology- concepts and trends in India. IJDSR 1(1):30–37
Hans MK, Hans R, Nagpal A (2014) Quackery: a major loophole in dental practice in India. J Clin Diagn Res 8(2):283
Hussain A, Khan FA (2014) History of dentistry. Arch Med Health Sci 2(1):106–110. https://doi.org/10.4103/2321-4848.133850

Joshi V, Bhardwaj P, Joshi NK, Singh K, Bajaj K, Suthar P (2021) A scoping review of challenges, scope and assessment approaches of teledentistry: an Indian perspective. Indian J Comm Health 33(4):559–567.https://doi.org/10.47203/IJCH.2021.v33i04.004

Kerkhof M (2024) The history of dentistry from ancient to modern times; health, science, technology

Kezian SA (2020) The history of the dental profession—from ancient origins to modern day. Pacific J Health 3(1):Article 2. https://doi.org/10.56031/2576-215X.1006

Kumari A, Kundra R, Kumar R, Thomas AM (2022) Sports dentistry: an ounce of prevention is worth a pound of cure. Indian J Dental Sci 14(1):40–44. https://doi.org/10.4103/IJDS.IJDS_209_20

Lack GV (1908) A work on operative dentistry, Chicago 2:105–210

Mahant R, Agrawal SV, Kapoor S, Agrawal I (2017) Milestones of dental history. CHRISMED J Health Res 4:229–234

Manohar B (2021) Special care dentistry in India. Saint Int Dent J 5:3. https://doi.org/10.4103/sidj.sidj_6_21

Petersen P (2004) Challenges to improvement of oral health in the 21st century—the approach of the WHO Global Oral Health Programme. Int Dent J 54(S6):329–343

Schulein TM (2005) Significant events in the history of operative dentistry. J Hist Dent 53:63–72; Indramohan J, Karthika B, Mohiddin G (2012) Myth of endodontics in oral focal infection. Indian J Multidiscip Dent 2:380–2

Singh R, Gupta A, Pradhan GS, Kataria A (2024) Unravelling the unique case of congenital infiltrating lipomatosis of face with its rare associations—a case report. J Oral Biol Craniofacial Res 14(6):767–772, ISSN: 2212-4268. https://doi.org/10.1016/j.jobcr.2024.10.006

Srinivasan M, Dhanavel C, Rayapudi J (2020) Evolution of magnifications in endodontics: a review. J Sci Den 10(1):21–24

Yadav SS, Sonkurla S (2013) Sarjeev's supernumerary tooth notation system: a universally compatible add-on to the Two-Digit system. Indian J Dent Res 24:395–396

Dental Terminologies

Aakash Gupta and Tarun Kumar Singh

Terminologies

- **Abscess**–Localized inflammation, whether acute or chronic, is often accompanied by the accumulation of pus and the destruction of surrounding tissues. This condition is commonly associated with infection and is often characterized by swelling.
- **Abutment**–In various clinical scenarios, the term for "implant case" refers to the fixture positioned between the implant body, also known as the implant post, and the restorative prosthesis, such as a single crown or denture. On the other hand, in the context of a "natural tooth case," it pertains to the tooth utilized as the foundation for one end of a denture.
- **Accession**–The process includes adding a test sample obtained by a healthcare professional to a collection of laboratory specimens. The specimen's essential information is recorded in a file maintained by the laboratory, organized chronologically. An identification code is then assigned for tracking and identification.
- **Actuators**–In order for a device to qualify as a robot, it must possess a frame or body that is capable of movement. The actuators within the device are the key components that enable this mobility.
- **Adhesion**–Adhesion occurs when two surfaces are joined together by chemical or physical forces, with or without adhesive. It is a key part of bonding.
- **Adhesive**–any material that promotes the close adhesion of two or more surfaces; a material that facilitates the bonding of two materials to each other.
- **Alloplastic**–synthetic material frequently utilized for tissue augmentation or replacement.

A. Gupta (✉) · T. K. Singh
Division of Conservative Dentistry and Endodontics, Department of Dentistry, All India Institute of Medical Sciences, Bathinda, India
e-mail: guptaaakash95@gmail.com

A. Gupta et al. (eds.), *Application of Robotics in Dentistry*, Lecture Notes in Bioengineering, https://doi.org/10.1007/978-981-95-1470-0_2

- **Alloy**–a compound formed by the combination of two or more elements, exhibiting unique properties that are not present in any of the individual elements.
- **Alveolar bone**–The bone to which a tooth is affixed is referred to as the alveolar bone.
- **Ancillary**–acting in a subordinate or auxiliary capacity to another entity or individual; providing additional support or assistance.
- **Analgesia**–the reduction or eradication of pain.
- **Anxiolysis**–the reduction or eradication of anxiety.
- **Anomaly**–An anomaly refers to a departure from the typical anatomical arrangement, growth, progression, or operation; a deviation from the norm.
- **Apex**–the terminal point of the tooth's root.
- **Apicoectomy/apex amputation**–The removal of the tip of a tooth through surgical intervention is referred to as apex amputation/apicoectomy.
- **Arthrogram**–an imaging method involving X-rays that is utilized to visualize bone structures subsequent to the introduction of a contrast agent into a specific joint.
- **Artificial intelligence**–Artificial intelligence refers to the intelligence exhibited by machines, and it is a field within computer science that strives to develop and replicate this intelligence.
- **Augmenting robots**–Augmenting robots, also referred to as virtual reality (VR) robots, serve the purpose of either enhancing the existing capabilities of humans or substituting the capabilities that a human might have lost.
- **Avulsion**–the dislodgement of a tooth from its socket as a result of physical injury.
- **Behavior management**–methods or interventions employed to modify or regulate the behaviors of a patient undergoing dental care.
- **Bilateral**–referring to both the right and left sides, or taking place on both sides.
- **Bionics**–The field of biomimetics, also referred to as biognosis, biomimicry, or bionical creativity engineering, involves the utilization of biological techniques and systems discovered in nature for the examination and development of engineering systems and contemporary technology.
- **Biopsy**–the procedure of extracting tissue for histological examination.
- **Clenching**–Clenching refers to the act of bringing the jaws and teeth together by clamping and pressing them. This action is often linked to psychological stress or physical exertion.
- **Cobots**–Cobots, or collaborative robots, are robots designed to work alongside humans. These robots prioritize safety by using sensors to remain aware of their surroundings, executing slow movements and ceasing actions when their movements are obstructed.
- **Coronal**–The term "coronal" pertains to the anatomical structure of the crown of a tooth.
- **Cone beam computed tomography (CBCT)**–also known as C-arm CT, cone beam volume CT, flat panel CT, or digital volume tomography (DVT), is a medical imaging method that utilizes X-ray computed tomography. In this technique, the X-rays are emitted in a divergent manner, creating a cone-shaped beam.

- **CAD/CAM systems**–which stand for computer-aided design and computer-aided manufacturing, have the capability to be seamlessly incorporated into robotic processes.

- **Control system**–The control system of a robot, commonly known as its central processing unit, encompasses all the elements involved in computation.

- **Curettage**–scraping and purifying the surfaces of an actual or potential area, such as a gingival pocket or bone, with the intention of eliminating pathological substances.
- **Cyborg**–A cyborg, alternatively referred to as a cybernetic organism, is an entity that combines elements of both biology and artificiality, such as electronic, mechanical, or robotic components.
- **Cyst**–a pathological void, commonly lined with epithelial tissue, that encloses either fluid or soft substance.
- **Dental arch**–the arched combination of the original teeth and the ridge that remains following the extraction of some or all of the natural teeth.
- **Dental cavity**–Tooth structure loss can result from various factors such as decay, erosion, or abrasion. When tooth decay is the culprit, it is commonly known as a carious lesion.
- **Dentin**–The dental hard tissue, originating from the dental papilla and dental pulp, constitutes the majority of the tooth structure and becomes mineralized as it matures.
- **Degree of freedom**–The degrees of freedom refer to the level of mobility that a robot possesses, which is measured in terms of its ability to move in Cartesian coordinates (x, y, and z) and perform angular movements (yaw, pitch, and roll).
- **Digital dentistry**–involves the utilization of dental technologies or devices equipped with digital or computer-controlled elements for the execution of dental procedures, as opposed to traditional mechanical or electrical tools.
- **Diagnostic imaging**–an exhibition of structural or functional arrangements intended for diagnostic assessment, which can take the form of photographs or radiographs.
- **Enamel**–the calcified tissue that encases the dentin of the tooth's crown.
- **End effectors**–End effectors are the tangible components, usually situated externally, which enable robots to successfully complete their assigned operations.
- **Ergonomics**–alternatively referred to as human factors or human factors engineering (HFE), involves the utilization of psychological and physiological principles in the engineering and design of products, processes, and systems.
- **Evidence-based dentistry**–aligns with the broader trend toward evidence-based medicine and other evidence-based approaches within healthcare.
- **Envelope**–The envelope refers to the spatial capacity that accommodates the full range of motion intended for all components of a robot, such as the end effector, workpiece, and any additional attachments.

- **Exudate**–a substance typically formed as a consequence of inflammation or necrosis, consisting of fluid, cells, and/or other remnants.
- **Fracture**–Fracture refers to the disruption or breakage of a component, particularly a bone structure, or the breaking of a tooth.
- **Furcation**–the region within a multirooted tooth where the roots separate and branch out anatomically.
- **Graft**–a fragment of tissue or synthetic material positioned in proximity to tissue in order to rectify a flaw or enhance a shortage.
- **Humanoid robots**–Humanoid robots are machines that mimic human appearance and behavior, performing tasks like running, jumping, and handling objects. Some even have human-like facial features and expressions.
- **Hydraulics**–The manipulation of mechanical power and motion through the utilization of pressurized liquid is known as hydraulics.
- **Inhalation**–an approach to management involving the introduction of a gaseous or volatile substance into the lungs, with its main impact resulting from absorption through the gas/blood interface.
- **Industrial robots**–Industrial robots are utilized to mechanize various tasks within manufacturing settings such as factories and warehouses.
- **Intraoral cameras**–also known as IOCs, are utilized by dental professionals or physicians to provide patients with a visual representation of the inside of their oral cavity, serving as a substitute for traditional mirrors.
- **Intraoral scanner**–In dentistry, intraoral scanners (IOSs) are utilized as tools for obtaining direct optical impressions.
- **Kinematics**–The field of kinematics focuses on analyzing the motion of robots, encompassing aspects like designing linkages for movement, ensuring power, control, and stability, as well as strategizing movement sequences to accomplish larger objectives.
- **Local anesthesia**–the suppression of sensation, notably pain, in a particular body region via the topical application or regional injection of a pharmaceutical substance.
- **Locus**–a site or place.
- **Microrobotics**–encompasses the examination and advancement of robots at a diminutive scale. Frequently measuring no more than a millimeter, the size of microrobots can fluctuate depending on the circumstances.
- **Medical robots**–play a crucial role in aiding healthcare practitioners across a range of situations, effectively contributing to the overall well-being of individuals. These advanced machines heavily depend on artificial intelligence and sensors to efficiently maneuver within healthcare settings, seamlessly engage with humans, and carry out intricate tasks with utmost precision.
- **Minimally invasive dentistry**–Minimal intervention dentistry is a contemporary approach to dental care that prioritizes the preservation of the natural tooth structure. Its primary objective is to minimize the amount of dental intervention required, ensuring that as much of the original tooth is conserved as possible.

- **Navigation dentistry**–Dentistry navigation, or guided dentistry, is the integration of digital technology with surgical procedures, resulting in enhanced safety, predictability, and reduced invasiveness.
- **Occlusion**–the contact between the biting or chewing surfaces of the upper (maxillary) and lower (mandibular) teeth.
- **Optical magnification**–the technique employed to increase the apparent size of an object, without altering its physical dimensions. The extent of this enlargement is measured using a size ratio known as optical magnification.
- **Periapical**–the vicinity adjacent to the termination of the tooth root.
- **Pulp**–The pulp cavity of a tooth is filled with connective tissue that includes blood vessels and nerve tissue.
- **Power supply**–Just as the human body needs food to operate, robots need power to function. Power can be in the form of compressed gases, solar power, hydraulic power, or flywheel energy.
- **Quadrant**–one of the four equivalent divisions that can be made in the dental arches, starting from the midline of the arch and extending toward the back to the last tooth.
- **Radiograph**–a visual representation captured on a radiation-sensitive medium such as film, plate, emulsion, or sensor through the interaction with ionizing radiation.
- **Robotics**–encompasses a wide range of disciplines that involve the design, creation, functionality, and application of robots.
- **Robot**–A robot is an automated device that is capable of executing a predefined set of instructions to accomplish a specific task.
- **Root canal**–a comparatively slender tubular conduit or passageway.
- **Sensors**–Sensors furnish a robot with stimuli via electrical signals that are interpreted by the controller, facilitating the robot's interaction with the external surroundings.
- **Software bots**–or simply "bots," are computer programs which carry out tasks autonomously. They are not technically considered robots.
- **Succedaneous tooth**–a mature tooth that takes the place of a primary tooth.
- **Surgical excision**–Surgical excision of bone or tissue involves the deliberate and precise removal of either bone or tissue through a surgical procedure.
- **Suture**–stitches employed to mend a laceration or injury.
- **Temporomandibular joint** (TMJ)–the articulation joint linking the cranial base (temporal bone) and the mandible (lower jaw).
- **Tissue conditioning**–material designed for short-term use in direct contact with tissues to help facilitate the recovery of a healthy state.
- **Tooth hemisection**–the surgical separation of a multirooted tooth dividing the tooth into separate parts.
- **Tool center point (TCP)**–the origin of the tool coordinate system.
- **Tooth transplantation**–relocation of a tooth from one socket to another, whether within the same individual or between different individuals.
- **Torus**–a skeletal prominence or protrusion of osseous tissue.

- **Transitional dentition**–denotes the mixed dentition phase; it commences with the eruption of the permanent first molars and concludes with the shedding of the deciduous teeth.
- **Trismus**–limited mouth opening, typically caused by inflammation or fibrosis of the masticatory muscles.
- **Treatment plan**–the step-by-step plan outlining the patient's treatment as prescribed by the dentist's evaluation, which is employed by the dentist to achieve the best possible oral health through restoration and/or maintenance.
- **Unerupted**–tooth or teeth that have not emerged through the gumline in oral cavity.
- **Unilateral**–relating to or impacting only one side.
- **Xerostomia**–diminished salivary output resulting in a parched and, at times, stinging sensation in the oral mucosa and/or decay around the neck of the teeth.
- **3D printing**–or additive manufacturing, creates 3D objects using a computer model. It involves precise control of material placement, fusion, or solidification. Various materials like plastics, liquids, or powder grains are added layer by layer.

Need for Robotics

Aakash Gupta, Tarun Kumar Singh, and Ekta Singla

1 Current Challenges in Medical Field

The practice of medicine today faces numerous challenges, ranging from an ageing population with increasingly complex healthcare needs to a shortage of skilled healthcare professionals. These challenges underscore the urgency for innovative solutions that can augment human capabilities and improve efficiency without compromising patient safety. Traditional surgical techniques, while effective, can be limited by the dexterity and precision of human hands, particularly in complex and delicate surgeries. Moreover, the rising burden of chronic diseases and conditions requiring long-term management underscores the need for efficient and cost-effective healthcare solutions (Yang et al. 2020; Deo and Anjankar 2023). The global shortage and maldistribution of healthcare professionals pose significant challenges to healthcare delivery.

2 Machine Revolution

A machine is a tangible mechanism that utilizes energy to exert forces and regulates motion in order to carry out a specific task. There are several reasons for the radical shift of mankind towards machines, which are as follows:

A. Gupta · T. K. Singh (✉)
Division of Conservative Dentistry and Endodontics, Department of Dentistry, All India Institute of Medical Sciences, Bathinda, India
e-mail: drtarunkumarsingh@gmail.com

E. Singla
Department of Mechanical Engineering, Indian Institute of Technology, Ropar, Punjab, India
e-mail: ekta@iitrpr.ac.in

A. Gupta et al. (eds.), *Application of Robotics in Dentistry*, Lecture Notes in Bioengineering, https://doi.org/10.1007/978-981-95-1470-0_3

First, machines offer consistent and reliable performance in tasks that are repetitive or require high precision, which can lead to increased productivity and reduced error rates. In manufacturing, for example, automated machines can operate 24/7 without the need for breaks, thereby optimizing production timelines and lowering costs per unit (Sarbadhikari 2017).

Second, machines are capable of performing tasks that are hazardous or physically demanding for humans. This not only enhances workplace safety but also reduces the risk of injury or accidents. In environments such as mining, construction, or even medical surgeries, machines can take on tasks that pose risks to human health and safety (Liu et al. 2020).

Third, advancements in technology have enabled machines to handle increasingly complex operations with greater efficiency and accuracy than ever before. This includes tasks that require intricate calculations, rapid data processing, or real-time decision-making, all of which machines can execute at a speed and scale far beyond human capabilities (Ajmera and Jain 2019; George et al. 2018).

Moreover, the adoption of machines is often driven by economic factors, including the potential for cost savings through reduced labour costs, improved operational efficiency, and the ability to scale production or services more flexibly in response to market demands.

While the shift towards machines raises concerns about job displacement or the potential for reduced human interaction in certain roles, it also opens up opportunities for upskilling/reskilling the workforce in areas such as machine maintenance, programming, and supervision. Ultimately, the shift towards machines reflects a broader trend towards leveraging technological advancements to improve productivity, safety, and innovation across various industries (Bora et al. 2020; Ng and Tam 2014).

3 Enter Robotics—Paradigm Shift

The origins of robotics extend beyond three millennia. Throughout this extensive timeline, inventors and artisans have conceptualized and created prototypes of robots that mimic the traits of animals or humans. Nevertheless, these inventions can merely be categorized as mechanical apparatuses that predominantly accomplished automated tasks through mechanical and physical principles, lacking the intelligence and autonomy characteristic of contemporary robots (Archibald and Barnard 2018). These innovations exemplify the advancements in engineering technology and mechanical production during ancient periods, establishing a groundwork for subsequent studies in robotics.

Joseph Engelberger, often referred to as the Father of Robotics, established Unimation Corporation in 1958, which was the first factory dedicated to robot manufacturing globally, thereby initiating the industrialization of robotics. In 1978, Unimation Corporation introduced the Programmable Universal Machine for Assembly

(PUMA), a pivotal advancement in the evolution of industrial robotics on an international scale (Bhandari et al. 2020; Abdi et al. 2018).

Robotics in medicine promises to address these challenges by introducing precision, efficiency, and reliability into various aspects of healthcare delivery. Unlike traditional methods, where human error and limitations can sometimes affect outcomes, robotics offers a controlled, predictable approach that enhances both diagnostic and therapeutic procedures (Wada et al. 2003).

The creation of robots, with their own unique intelligence, is a testament to the ingenuity and capabilities of mankind. Robots are increasingly preferred over humans in certain tasks and industries for several compelling reasons:

1. **Precision and consistency**: Robots can perform tasks with a high degree of precision and consistency, which is crucial in medical fields such as surgeries, endodontic therapies, where uniformity and quality control are paramount. They can repeat the same motion or operation without variation, leading to fewer errors and higher product reliability (Nelivigi 2007).
2. **Speed and efficiency**: Robots operate at speeds that often exceed human capabilities, particularly in tasks that require rapid and repetitive actions. This leads to increased production rates and faster turnaround times, which are advantageous in industries striving for efficiency and competitive advantage.
3. **Safety**: Robots excel in performing tasks that are hazardous or pose risks to human safety. Whether it is handling toxic materials, working in extreme temperatures, or executing tasks in environments with high physical risks, robots can operate without risking human health or well-being.
4. **24/7 operation**: Unlike humans, robots can operate continuously without the need for breaks, rest, or shifts. This capability allows for continuous therapy or service delivery, thereby maximizing uptime and operational efficiency.
5. **Cost efficiency**: Over the long term, robots can be more cost effective than humans, especially when considering factors such as wages, benefits, and training costs. While initial investment in robotics can be substantial, ongoing operational costs can be lower, particularly in tasks where robots can replace multiple human workers (Pugin et al. 2011).
6. **Complexity and adaptability**: Robots are increasingly capable of handling complex tasks that require advanced technical skills or specialized knowledge. With advancements in artificial intelligence (AI) and machine learning, robots can adapt to changing conditions and perform tasks that require cognitive abilities, decision-making, and learning from data (Barbash and Glied 2010).
7. **Reduced human error**: By automating tasks, robots can significantly reduce the potential for human error, which can be costly or even dangerous in industries such as healthcare, aerospace, and manufacturing.
8. **Scalability**: Robots offer scalability in production or service delivery, allowing businesses to quickly adjust output or operations in response to market demand fluctuations without the constraints of hiring and training additional human workers.

While robots offer numerous advantages, there are also considerations such as initial investment costs, maintenance requirements, and the need for skilled technicians to operate and maintain robotic systems. Additionally, in many industries, there remains a need for human oversight, decision-making, creativity, and interpersonal skills that robots cannot fully replicate. Therefore, the preference for robots over humans often depends on the specific task requirements, industry dynamics, and overall business objectives (Parekattil and Gudeloglu 2013).

4 Robotics in Medical Field

The groundbreaking research undertaken by the National Aeronautics and Space Administration (NASA) signifies the inception of robot-assisted surgical procedures. During the mid-1980s, NASA engineered a remotely operated robotic system designed for surgical interventions on soldiers in combat zones and astronauts in extraterrestrial environments. In the year 2000, the U.S. Food and Drug Administration (FDA) granted approval for the first robotic system intended for laparoscopic surgery, facilitating a doctor–robot collaborative approach, and Yomi was the first FDA-approved dental robot (O'Malley et al. 2006) (Fig. 1).

Robotics has emerged as a transformative force in the medical field, addressing critical needs and revolutionizing healthcare delivery. One of its primary roles lies in enhancing surgical procedures, where robots offer unparalleled precision, dexterity, and minimally invasive capabilities. These advancements translate into reduced trauma, faster recovery times, and improved patient outcomes. Moreover, robotics aids in complex surgeries that demand high levels of accuracy, such as neurosurgery

Fig. 1 Yomi dental robot

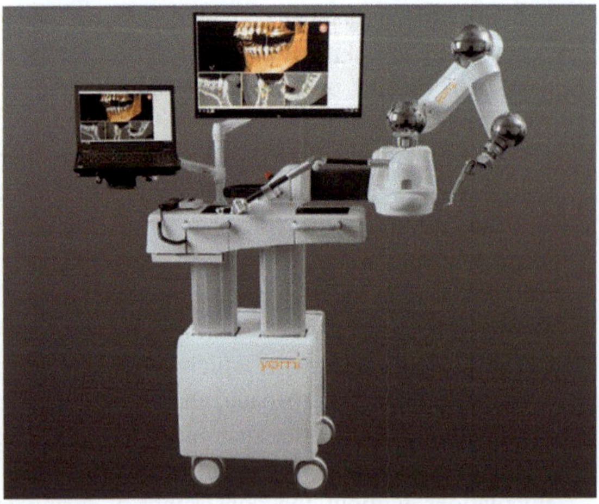

and cardiac procedures. Beyond surgery, robots support healthcare providers in diagnostics and therapy, enabling more accurate imaging, targeted drug delivery, and precise rehabilitation techniques (Hans et al. 2012; Abel and Moore 2012).

Robots also serve as indispensable tools in telemedicine and remote surgery, bridging geographical gaps and bringing specialized care to underserved areas. As the healthcare landscape evolves, robotics continues to play a pivotal role in advancing medical practices, fostering innovation, and ultimately improving the quality of life for patients worldwide.

5 Robotics in Dentistry

The latest generation of robots designed for human safety is now capable of collaborating directly with human colleagues, providing assistance, and alleviating them from monotonous and labour-intensive routine activities. Concurrently, these entities demonstrate a significant level of efficiency and are increasingly gaining economic importance. In the foreseeable future, this trend is expected to result in the deployment of robots across a variety of new applications, particularly as collaborators not only within the industrial sector but also in the public sphere as intelligent assistants. One particularly promising field is dentistry, as it offers numerous opportunities for assistive technologies and the automation of straightforward routine tasks, thereby enhancing the efficiency of dental personnel and elevating the overall quality of care provided (Autorino et al. 2013; Morgan et al. 2022a).

In the field of dentistry, several manual robotic systems are utilized, which are operated through a computer control interface. These manual robots offer enhanced safety and precision in drilling procedures compared to conventional dental practices. Scholars and professionals are progressively endorsing digital process redesign as an effective strategy to minimize variations in practice and enhance the overall quality of healthcare delivery (Summerfield et al. 2011). The integration of advanced robotic technology within dental practices, particularly as support for dental professionals, has the potential to significantly enhance the existing technological framework. A key motivating aspect of this integration may stem from human considerations, such as the mental and physical strain experienced by human assistants during prolonged periods of work that demand sustained concentration, as well as the absence of ergonomically designed workspaces (Astrid et al. 2021).

Recently, a start-up located in Boston has achieved a groundbreaking milestone in dental care by executing the first fully automated dental procedure utilizing AI-driven robotic technology. The dental robot developed by the Boston-based firm Perceptive has received approval from the U.S. Food and Drug Administration (FDA). This innovative device utilizes artificial intelligence (AI) in conjunction with 3D imaging software to control a robotic arm, enabling it to carry out various dental procedures (Abdi et al. 2018).

The robot developed by Perceptive employs three-dimensional volumetric data to facilitate the planning of diagnostics and therapeutic interventions. It conducts an optical coherence tomography (OCT) scan of a patient's oral cavity utilizing a portable intraoral scanning device (The Future of Surgery 2023).

The scanner produces intricate three-dimensional images, encompassing areas beneath the gum line, thereby offering a comprehensive overview of oral health. Patients are able to examine these images, which aids in their comprehension of necessary treatment options. In addition to this, artificial intelligence algorithms evaluate the data to devise treatment plans, allowing the robotic arm, fitted with dental instruments, to execute procedures autonomously (Morgan et al. 2022b).

The field of high-precision human-controlled robotic surgery is experiencing significant advancements, effectively diminishing the reliance on an exceptionally steady hand. Furthermore, as evidenced in the development of humanoid robotics, the initiation of teleoperation may lead to the training of these robots to eventually execute the same tasks autonomously. Consequently, this concept is likely to become increasingly familiar in the years ahead.

Nonetheless, significant opportunities remain for enhancing the simplification and adaptability of robotic surgical techniques and comprehensive education. By harnessing the capabilities of machine learning and artificial intelligence, future clinical practice will benefit from more accurate diagnostic and therapeutic alternatives, advanced medical decision support systems, and adaptable, precise surgical interventions (Burdea et al. 1999; Chang et al. 2018).

With each evolving era, technological advancements lead to societal upliftment—how to utilize the discoveries and developments in the service of mankind. Robotics has come into existence nearly five decades ago, but the associated advancements have entered the human routine in recent times only. Robotic manipulators were reported during the era of Industry 3.0 and were exploited to a large extent in manufacturing and automotive industries. To possess robotic assistance in our routines and in the service of humankind was considered a fiction for a long time. It is with the technological developments in Industry 4.0 and 5.0—involving Internet of Things (IoT), cloud-based analysis, smart manufacturing systems, virtual and augmented reality, etc.—that the current robotics revolution has gained multiple facets (Goh and Ali 2022; Laut et al. 2016).

6 Evolution of Robotic Manipulators

Robotic manipulators, the human-arm-like mechanisms consisting of a series of links usually connected with revolute or prismatic joints, play important roles in industrial automation. The conventional manipulators may cover a significant range of tasks, such as material handling, welding, inspection and monitoring, operations in hazardous environments, maintenance, and assembly (Sridhar et al. 2017). During the 1980s, many standard robotic configurations were reported, which included conventional configurations, such as Programmable Universal Machine for Assembly (PUMA) (Fig. 2a) and Selective Compliance Assembly Robot Arm (SCARA)

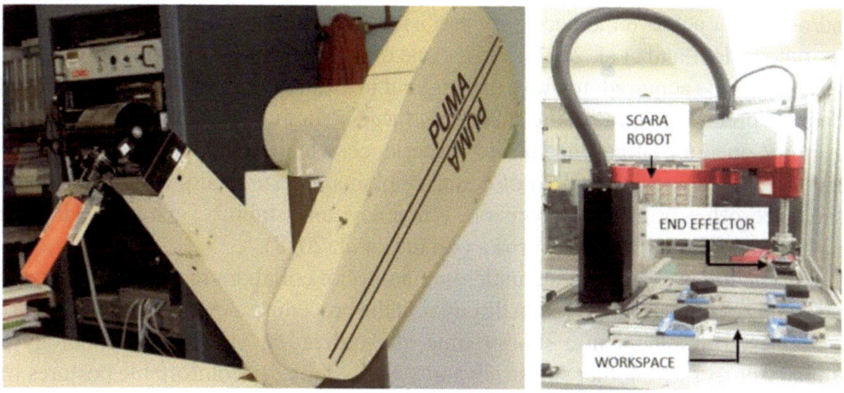

(a) (b)

Fig. 2 PUMA **a** and SCARA **b** robotic systems

(Fig. 2b), and these configurations have been well exploited through various industrial applications for decades.

A large number of manufacturers have developed their robotic manipulators, based upon these configurations, and their applications have evolved from unconstrained environments to constrained work cells and from pick-and-place applications to the complicated tasks of assembly operation. How to screw a nut? How to insert a small peg in a hole? How to increase the working speeds in each operation with improvements in accuracy and precision had remained the objectives of advanced studies during the 1990s. With the closing of the twentieth century, developments in robotic manipulators had witnessed further complex configurations such as snake-like manipulators, control of flexible links, parallel manipulators, and complexities of modular systems (Carpenter and Sundaram 2017). Replicating natural motions associated with animals, insects, birds, and even aquatic creatures had followed the trends of robotic research in the past two decades. All these advancements are majorly aimed at the development of artificial structures and mechanisms, which can be utilized for assisting mankind—in health sector, safety and defence sector, agriculture and food sector, and in more effective industrial practices (Gomez et al. 2016; Bezerra Junior et al. 2018).

7 Why Robotic Assistance in Medical Applications?

Precision and Accuracy

Precisely placing the tools and surgical instruments at the target locations is one of the major challenges for doctors while utilizing minimally invasive surgical procedures. The doctors face the difficulty in guiding the instruments to the desired positions because they do not have enough visual information about the target location and/or cannot achieve the necessary precision without the support of any technical equipment (Holland et al. 2021). This is one of the prime reasons why robotic assistance should be acquired: to move the surgical instrument to the target locations with adequate precision. Some of the challenges faced by human operators include limited visibility, operator fatigue, and limited experience, which are doctor specific and may lead to errors. Even in the field of dental implants and surgical procedures, robotic assistance offers improved precision, efficiency, and stability, enhancing implant accuracy and reducing surgical risks (Adams et al. 2018).

The robotic systems operate under human–robot collaboration, with the surgeon maintaining control and oversight throughout the procedure. Apart from the provision of improved treatment in a shorter time, the utilization of robotic technology in dentistry possesses another strong advantage of avoiding uncomfortable postures for doctors.

Automating Repetitive Tasks: Avoid Human Error

Maintaining consistency in work abilities throughout the long hours of surgery and other medical procedures is another challenge faced by the medical practitioners. Even with the best experience, it is highly unlikely to achieve a level of repeatability by the human operators. This may be associated with rehabilitation exercises, continuous monitoring of vitals for long hours or even days, repetitive tasks in monitoring the same vitals for a large number of patients, etc., which are the basic requirements where robotic assistance shows promising significance (Niravkumar et al. 2021; Son et al. 2017).

An automated system with appropriate feedback strategies serves efficiently at any hour of the day, for continuous hours without fatigue. One such concept is referred to as robotic process automation (RPA), which plays the role of human behaviour and helps mitigate repetitive activities in processes whose variation in each iteration is little or nil. The potential of RPA is numerous as much as it has a high impact: rationalization of daily tasks, cost reduction, performance, and productivity gains, but also enhancement of human know-how and expertise within the company (Masamune and Hong 2014). Beyond the productivity benefit, the elimination of repetitive tasks contributes to better employee satisfaction and fulfilment, allowing them to focus on value-added activities within the work environment and take breaks without disturbing the work schedule. Humans are not replaced; rather, their own work-life balance gets improved with robotic assistance.

Traits of Security and Flexibility

Human safety in robotic assistance can be viewed from two distinct perspectives. The first perspective emphasizes the reduction of human error, which is linked to enhanced precision and consistency in medical procedures. The second perspective focuses on safeguarding humans from potential risks posed by the robots themselves. Effective human–robot collaboration is essential for the successful integration of robotic assistance in medical settings, with ensuring human safety being a paramount concern (Kyrarini et al. 2021b). This area of research falls under the broader domain of human–robot interaction (HRI), which introduces various challenges, including safety, autonomy, and acceptance. It is evident that the future of robotics is anticipated to move towards a more integrated approach, where humans and machines work together seamlessly, emphasizing the reliability of robotic assistance (Gorpas et al. 2019; Wang et al. 2021).

One notable advancement in the safety features of robotic applications is the implementation of force–torque sensors, which allow for immediate cessation or redirection of robotic operations upon detecting a human or obstacle nearby. These systems, known as collaborative robots (cobots), have garnered significant interest from researchers, users, and manufacturers alike (Qian et al. 2020). Recently, there has been a development of flexible robotic systems aimed at improving minimally invasive procedures on internal organs situated in confined areas of the human body. These surgical instruments are engineered to navigate anatomical pathways through single-port access, utilizing natural openings or minimal incisions for intraluminal interventions (Krebs and Hogan 2006). With enhanced precision, spatial adaptability, and dexterity, robotic technology can significantly improve surgical outcomes, making minimally invasive flexible access a quicker, safer, and more efficient approach for internal interventions without the need for extensive incisions. Flexible robots empower surgeons to visualize and manipulate anatomical structures that would otherwise be challenging to access (Shoushtari et al. 2016).

Data Analytics and Advanced Attributes

Robots integrated with advanced sensors and AI systems collect and process vast amounts of data in real time. This capability enhances decision-making and optimizes performance in complex environments. The robots can serve patients through customized services—based on patients' data, medical histories, genetic profiles, and lab results. Integrating robotic systems with AI provides a huge support to any medical organization, as it is highly unlikely to refer to all aspects at any point in time while managing each and every patient (Mohammad 2013).

Guidance in Emergencies and Crisis Situations

Robots are crucial in dangerous and unsafe settings. They have significantly improved efficiency in crisis situations, particularly evident during the COVID-19 pandemic (Fig. 3). The use of robotic assistance emerged as a vital strategy to minimize infection risks during sample collection, facilitate contactless delivery of food and medicine, reduce exposure, and maintain public safety in healthcare facilities and other institutions (Grischke et al. 2020; Palagi and Fischer 2018).

Bridging Skill Gaps and Enhancing Human Lifestyle

It is observed as a general mindset that robotic assistance may replace human workers and take away human jobs. In fact, in practice, the robotic utilization helps in managing manpower and compensates for labour shortages and skill management, as the human help can be inclined more towards specialized expertise (Lanfranco et al. 2004a; Haleem et al. 2022).

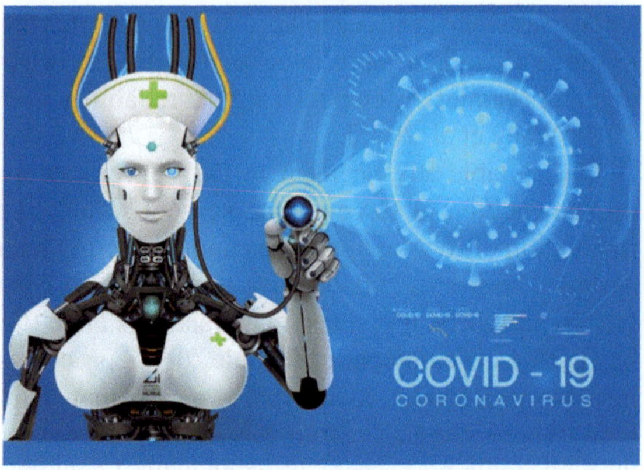

Fig. 3 AI robot medic explaining COVID-19

8 Economic Aspects in Adopting Robotic Assistance

Investing in robotics results in long-term cost savings by minimizing operational costs and maximizing the utilization of resources (Lanfranco et al. 2004b). For example, automated packaging systems reduce the need for manual labour, cutting payroll costs while improving throughput.

Optimization of Resources

Robots ensure optimal use of resources, including raw materials and energy. Advanced algorithms help minimize waste during production processes. For instance, robotic material handling systems optimize inventory flow, reducing spoilage and excess stock.

Enhanced Return on Investment (ROI)

Though the initial investment in robotic systems is high, the return on investment (ROI) is significant due to increased efficiency and reduced operational costs. Many businesses report break-even points within a few years, with substantial long-term profitability.

Competitive Advantage

Companies adopting robotics gain a competitive edge by delivering superior products and services more efficiently. This advantage is particularly critical in industries with high customer expectations for quality and speed, such as e-commerce.

Economic Scalability

Robotic systems scale effortlessly to meet increased demand. Modular designs allow businesses to expand or modify operations without significant downtime, ensuring they remain competitive in fluctuating markets.

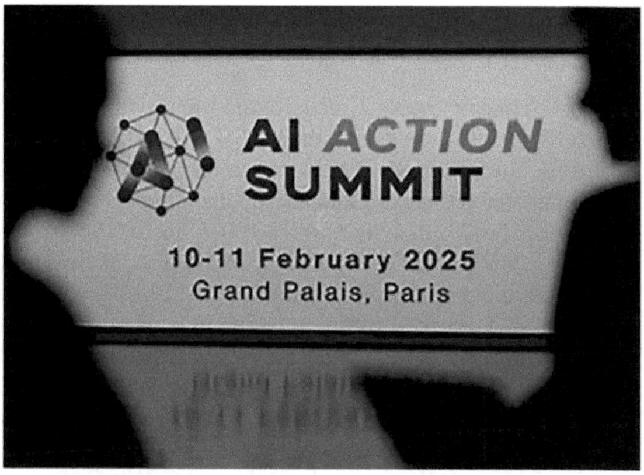
AI ACTION
SUMMIT
10-11 February 2025
Grand Palais, Paris

Fig. 4 Global AI summit in Paris

Scalability Helps in Fast Adoption of Changing Business Needs

Robotic systems are inherently scalable, enabling businesses to adapt quickly to changes in demand. Adding more robotic units to a production line can exponentially increase output without major infrastructural overhauls.

Reduction in Waste and Rework Costs

- Minimizing Halts and downtime.

9 Global AI Summit

In contemporary society, governments across various nations are convening global AI conferences aimed at fostering innovation, promoting technology-friendly environments, and prioritizing human-centric workplaces. These initiatives are designed to position AI as a valuable asset in streamlining daily tasks (Mohr et al. 2001).

A notable illustration of AI's advantages was presented by Indian Prime Minister Narendra Modi at the AI summit held in Paris 2025 (Fig. 4), who noted that when individuals upload their medical reports to an AI application, it can interpret the information in straightforward terms, devoid of complex jargon, thereby enhancing understanding of one's health. However, if the same application is tasked with generating an image of a person writing with their left hand, it is likely to produce an image of someone using their right hand, reflecting the predominance of right-handed data in its training set. This example underscores the remarkable potential of AI while simultaneously highlighting the significant biases that warrant careful consideration (Spehar et al. 2025).

The advancement of artificial intelligence is occurring at an extraordinary rate and magnitude, with its adoption and implementation taking place at an even more accelerated pace.

References

Abdi J, Al-Hindawi A, Ng T, Vizcaychipi MP (2018) Scoping review on the use of socially assistive robot technology in elderly care. BMJ Open 8(2):e018815

Adams SJ, Burbridge BE, Badea A, Kanigan N, Bustamante L, Babyn P et al (2018) A crossover comparison of standard and telerobotic approaches to prenatal sonography. J Ultrasound Med 37:2603–2612. https://doi.org/10.1002/jum.14619

Ajmera P, Jain V (2019) Modelling the barriers of health 4.0—the fourth healthcare industrial revolution in India. Oper Manag Res 12:129–145

Archibald MM, Barnard A (2018) Futurism in nursing: technology, robotics and the fundamentals of care. J Clin Nurs 27:2473–2480. https://doi.org/10.1111/jocn.14081

Astrid F, Beata Z, Van den Nest M, Julia E, Elisabeth P, Magda DE (2021) The use of a UV-C disinfection robot in the routine cleaning process: a field study in an Academic hospital. Antimicrob Resist Infect Control 10(1):84

Autorino R, Kaouk JH, Stolzenburg JU et al (2013) Current status and future directions of robotic single-site surgery: a systematic review. Eur Urol 63:266–280

Barbash GI, Glied SA (2010) New technology and health care costs—the case of robot-assisted surgery. N Engl J Med 363:701–704

Bezerra Junior JE, Queiroz PGG, de Lima RW (2018) A study of the publications of educational robotics: a systematic review of literature. IEEE Lat Am Trans 16(4):1193–1199. https://doi.org/10.1109/TLA.2018.8362156

Bhandari M, Zeffiro T, Reddiboina M (2020) Artificial intelligence and robotic surgery: current perspective and future directions. Curr Opin Urol 30:48–54. https://doi.org/10.1097/MOU.0000000000000692

Bora GS, Narain TA, Sharma AP, Mavuduru RS, Devana SK, Singh SK, Mandal AK (2020) Robot-assisted surgery in India: a SWOT analysis. Indian J Urol 36:1–3. https://doi.org/10.4103/iju.IJU_220_19

Brunete A et al (2020) Smart assistive architecture for the integration of IoT devices, robotic systems, and multimodal interfaces in healthcare environments. Sensors 21(6):2212. https://doi.org/10.3390/s21062212

Burdea GC, Dunn SM, Levy G (1999) Evaluation of robot-based registration for subtraction radiography. Med Image Anal 3:265–274

Carpenter BT, Sundaram CP (2017) Training the next generation of surgeons in robotic surgery. Robot Surg 4:39–44. https://doi.org/10.2147/RSRR/S70552

Chang KD, Raheem AA, Rha KH (2018) Novel robotic systems and future directions. Indian Journal of Urology 34(2):110–114. https://doi.org/10.4103/iju.IJU_316_17

Deo N, Anjankar A (2023) Artificial intelligence with robotics in healthcare: a narrative review of its viability in India. Cureus. 15(5):e39416. https://doi.org/10.7759/cureus.39416

George EI, Brand TC, LaPorta A, Marescaux J, Satava RM (2018) Origins of robotic surgery: from skepticism to standard of care. JSLS 22. https://doi.org/10.4293/JSLS.2018.00039

Goh EZ, Ali T (2022) Robotic surgery: an evolution in practice. J Surg Protoc Res Methodol (1):snac003. https://doi.org/10.1093/jsprm/snac003

Gomez ED, Aggarwal R, McMahanW BK, Kuchenbecker KJ (2016) Objective assessment of robotic surgical skill using instrument contact vibrations. Surg Endosc 30:1419–1431. https://doi.org/10.1007/s00464-015-4346-z

Gorpas D, Phipps J, Bec J et al (2019) Autofluorescence lifetime augmented reality as a means for real-time robotic surgery guidance in human patients. Sci Rep 9:1187. https://doi.org/10.1038/s41598-018-37237-8

Grischke J, Johannsmeier L, Eich L, Griga L, Haddadin S (2020) Dentronics: Towards robotics and artificial intelligence in dentistry. Dent Mater 36(6):765–778. https://doi.org/10.1016/j.dental.2020.03.021

Halder Roy A, Ghosh S, Gupta B (2023) Robotics in medical domain: the future of surgery, healthcare and imaging. Wireless Pers Commun 132:2885–2903. https://doi.org/10.1007/s11277-023-10747-z

Haleem A, Javaid M, Pratap Singh R et al (2022) Medical 4.0 technologies for healthcare: features, capabilities, and applications. Internet Things Cyber Phys Syst 2:12–30. https://doi.org/10.1016/j.iotcps.2022.04.001

Hans S, Delas B, Gorphe P, Ménard M, Brasnu D (2012) Transoral robotic surgery in head and neck cancer. Eur Ann Otorhinolaryngol Head Neck Dis 129:32–37

Holland J, Kingston L, McCarthy C, Armstrong E, O'Dwyer P, Merz F, McConnell M (2021) Service robots in the healthcare sector. Robotics 10(1):47. https://doi.org/10.3390/robotics10010047

Krebs HI, Hogan N (2006) Therapeutic robotics: a technology push. Proc IEEE 94(9):1727–1738. https://doi.org/10.1109/JPROC.2006.880721

Kyrarini M et al (2021a) A survey of robots in healthcare. Technologies 9(1):8. https://doi.org/10.3390/technologies9010008

Kyrarini M, Lygerakis F, Rajavenkatanarayanan A et al (2021b) A survey of robots in healthcare. Technologies 9:8. https://doi.org/10.3390/technologies9010008

Lanfranco AR, Castellanos AE, Desai JP, Meyers WC (2004a) Robotic surgery: a current perspective. Ann Surg 239(1):14–21. https://doi.org/10.1097/01.sla.0000103020.19595.7d

Lanfranco AR, Castellanos AE, Desai JP et al (2004b) Robotic surgery. Ann Surg 239(1):14–21. https://doi.org/10.1097/01.sla.0000103020.19595.7d

Laut J, Porfiri M, Raghavan P (2016) The present and future of robotic technology in rehabilitation. Curr Phys Med Rehabil Rep 4(4):312

Liu Z, Liu Q, Xu W, Wang L, Zhou Z (2020) Robot learning towards smart robotic manufacturing: a review. Robot Comput Integr Manuf 77:102360

Masamune K, Hong J (2014) Advanced imaging and robotics technologies for medical applications. Int J Optomechatronics 4(5):299–321. https://doi.org/10.1080/15599612.2011.633210

Mohammad S (2013) Robotic surgery. J Oral Biol Craniofacial Res 3(1):2. https://doi.org/10.1016/j.jobcr.2013.03.002

Mohr FW, Falk V, Diegeler A et al (2001) Computer-enhanced "robotic" cardiac surgery: experience in 148 patients. J Thorac Cardiovasc Surg 121(5):842–853. https://doi.org/10.1067/mtc.2001.112625

Morgan AA, Abdi J, Syed MAQ et al (2022a) Robots in healthcare: a scoping review. Curr Robot Rep 3:271–280. https://doi.org/10.1007/s43154-022-00095-4

Morgan AA, Abdi J, Syed MAQ et al (2022b) Robots in healthcare: a scoping review. Current Robotics Reports 3:271–280. https://doi.org/10.1007/s43154-022-00095-4

Nelivigi GG (2007) Robotic surgery: India is not ready yet. Ind J Urol 23:240–244. https://doi.org/10.4103/0970-1591.33443

Ng AT, Tam PC (2014) Current status of robot-assisted surgery. Hong Kong Med J 20:241–250. https://doi.org/10.12809/hkmj134167.DOI:10.12809/hkmj134167

Niravkumar P, Jiawen Y, Gang L, Reza M, Lukasz P, Helen D-S, Joyce J, Andrew D, Andreas M, Karun S, Iulian I, Kevin C (2021) Body-mounted robotic system for MRI-guided shoulder arthrography: cadaver and clinical workflow studies. Front Robot AI. https://doi.org/10.3389/frobt.2021.667121

O'Malley BW Jr, Weinstein GS, Snyder W, Hockstein NG (2006) Transoral robotic surgery (TORS) for base of tongue neoplasms. Laryngoscope 116:1465–1472

Palagi S, Fischer P (2018) Bioinspired microrobots. Nat Rev Mater 3:113–124. https://doi.org/10.1038/s41578-018-0016-9

Parekattil SJ, Gudeloglu A (2013) Robotic assisted andrological surgery. Asian J Androl 15:67–74

Pugin F, Bucher P, Morel P (2011) History of robotic surgery: from AESOP® and ZEUS® to da Vinci®. J Visc Surg 148(5 Suppl):e3–e8

Qian L, Wu JY, DiMaio SP, Navab N, Kazanzides P (2020) A review of augmented reality in robotic-assisted surgery. IEEE Trans Med Robot Bionics 2(1):1–16. https://doi.org/10.1109/TMRB.2019.2957061

Sarbadhikari S (2017) Digital health in India—as envisaged by the national health policy. BLDE Univ J Health Sci 4:1–6

Shoushtari AL, Dario P, Mazzoleni S (2016) A review on the evolvement trend of robotic interaction control. Ind Robot Int J 43(5):535

Son D, Dogan MD, Sitti M (2017) In IEEE International Conference on Robotics and Automation, 2017 (p. 1132). IEEE

Spehar D (2023) Paris AI summit 2025: 5 critical themes shaping global AI policy. Forbes, Feb 10, 2025, 11:23am EST

Sridhar AN, Briggs TP, Kelly JD et al (2017) Training in robotic surgery—an overview. Curr Urol Rep 18:58. https://doi.org/10.1007/s11934-017-0710-y

Summerfield MR, Seagull FJ, Vaidya N, Xiao Y (2011) Use of pharmacy delivery robots in intensive care units. Am J Health Syst Pharm 68(1):77–83

Van Abel KM, Moore EJ (2012) The rise of transoral robotic surgery in the head and neck: emerging applications. Expert Rev Anticancer Ther 12:373–380

Wada K, Shibata T, Saito T, Tanie K (2003) Effects of robot assisted activity to elderly people who stay at a health service facility for the aged. IEEE Int Conf Intell Robots Syst 3:2847–2852

Wang G, Zeng Y, Sheng X (2021) Instructions for use of Da Vinci surgical robots. In: Wang G, Zeng Y, Sheng X (eds) Robotic surgery and nursing. Springer. https://doi.org/10.1007/978-981-16-0510-9_2

Yang G et al (2020) Homecare robotic systems for healthcare 4.0: visions and enabling technologies. IEEE J Biomed Health Inf 24(9):2535–2549. https://doi.org/10.1109/jbhi.2020.2990529

Technical Aspects of Robotics

Ekta Singla, Aakash Gupta, and Tarun Kumar Singh

1 Definition

The International Organization for Standardization (ISO) defines a robot as a programmable, multifunctional manipulator that operates automatically and is controlled by position across multiple axes. This device is capable of handling a range of materials, components, tools, and specialized equipment through programmable automation to execute designated functions (Denecke and Baudoin 2022).

2 Classification of Robotics

A. Based on Application

- Welding robot
- Assembly robot
- Heavy-duty robot
- Medical robot

B. Based on Coordinate System

- Cartesian
- Cylindrical
- Spherical

E. Singla (✉)
Department of Mechanical Engineering, Indian Institute of Technology, Ropar, Punjab, India
e-mail: ekta@iitrpr.ac.in

A. Gupta · T. K. Singh
Division of Conservative Dentistry and Endodontics, Department of Dentistry, All India Institute of Medical Sciences, Bathinda, India

A. Gupta et al. (eds.), *Application of Robotics in Dentistry*, Lecture Notes in Bioengineering, https://doi.org/10.1007/978-981-95-1470-0_4

- Anthropomorphic
- Gantry
- Selective compliance assembly robot arm (SCARA)

C. Based on Actuation System

- Pneumatic
- Hydraulic
- Electric

D. Based on Control Method

- Servo/non-servo control
- Path control

E. Based on Programming Method

- Online programming
- Offline programming

3 Asimov's Laws of Robotics

Asimov's laws of robotics were established in 1942 (Habuza et al. 2021; Badash et al. 2016):

1. A robot is prohibited from causing harm to a human being or, by failing to act, permitting a human being to suffer injury.
2. A robot is required to follow commands issued by humans, unless such commands would contradict the First Law.
3. A robot is obligated to ensure its own survival, provided that this self-preservation does not interfere with the First or Second Law.

4 Concept and Design of Robots

The evolution of medical robotics represents an extensive journey of investigation. Following substantial validation within the realm of industrial robotics, this technology has gained global prominence and has become a crucial component of contemporary manufacturing and daily living. A robot's structure typically consists of four parts (Fig. 1):

The actuation system
The drive transmission system
The control system
The intelligent system.

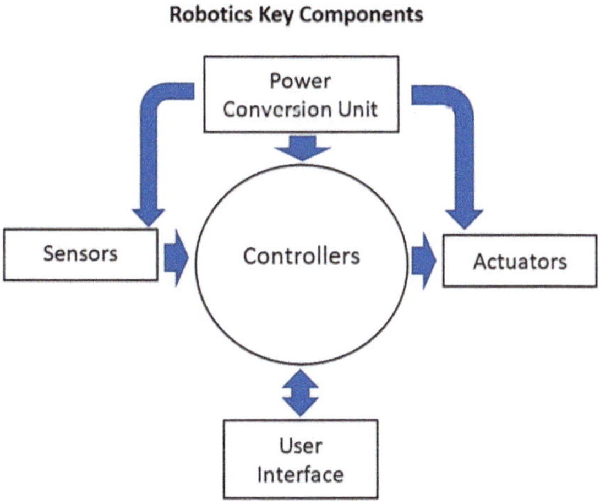

Fig. 1 Key components of robotics

The actuation system functions as the component of the robot that executes tasks, analogous to the role of a human hand. The drive transmission system conveys force and motion to the actuator via a power source. The manipulation of the robot's body, arm, motion, and wrist necessitates precise control over the movements of its individual joints. This control is facilitated by the drive system that powers the robot. The joints are actuated by specific types of drive systems that provide the necessary movement (Ajoudani et al. 2017). The control system consists of a control computer, control software, and servo controllers, paralleling the functions of a human brain. Additionally, the intelligent system generally encompasses a perception system along with an analytical decision-making component.

Robots can typically do three things:

1. Sense
2. Compute
3. Act

The variation among these three components is significant across different robotic systems. Certain robots utilize basic sensing mechanisms, such as sonar for obstacle detection, whereas others employ a more complex array of sensors, which may include cameras, gyroscopes, and laser range finders.

Coordinate System

A. World Coordinate System (WCS) (Fig. 2)

The origin and axis of the robot manipulator are defined relative to the robot base.

B. Tool Coordinate System (TCS) (Fig. 3)

The alignment of the axis system is defined relative to the orientation of the wrist faceplate (to which the end effector is attached).

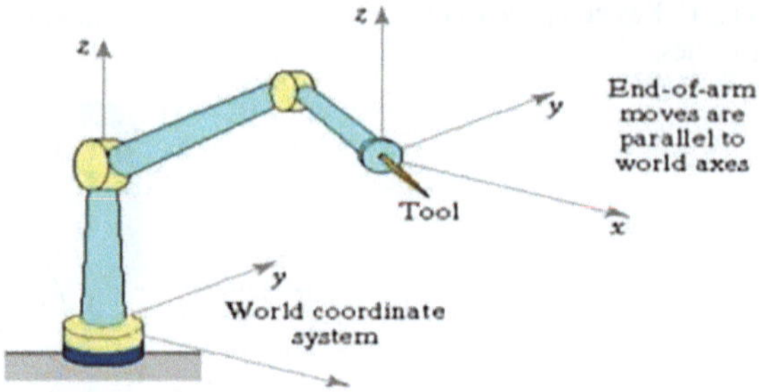

Fig. 2 World coordinate system

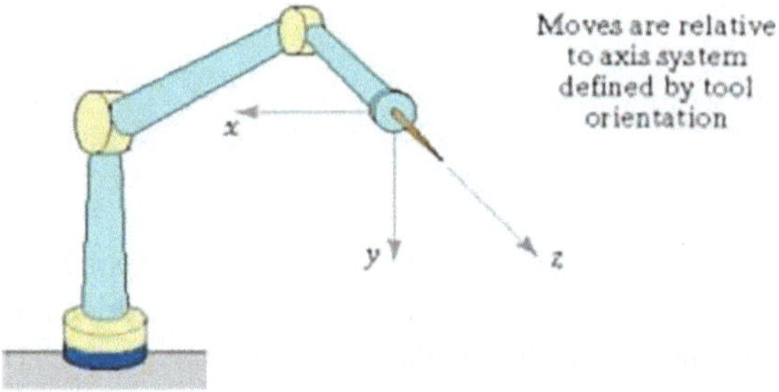

Fig. 3 Tool coordinate system

Technical Aspects of Robotics Integration of AI and IoT

1. Advances in Control Systems

Modern robotics relies on sophisticated control systems that ensure precision and adaptability. Real-time feedback loops allow robots to adjust their operations dynamically, accommodating variability in tasks or environments (Madhavi et al. 2024).

2. Sustainable Robotics

Technological advancements are making robotics more sustainable, with energy-efficient designs and the use of eco-friendly materials. Solar-powered robots, for example, operate in remote locations without dependence on conventional power sources.

3. Human–Robot Interaction (HRI)

Collaborative robots emphasize safe and effective human–robot interactions. Enhanced HRI technologies ensure that robots can work alongside humans without compromising safety, such as through force sensors and adaptive behavior algorithms.

5 Applications of AI, ML, and DL in Advanced Industrial Robotics

Quality assurance: Artificial intelligence (AI), machine learning (ML), and deep learning (DL) technologies can continuously oversee production lines, detecting defects or inconsistencies in real time. This enhances product quality and minimizes the need for human oversight during inspections (Ahmidi et al. 2017; Artificial intelligence, machine learning and deep learning in advanced robotics 2024).

Maintenance prediction: AI and ML enable predictive maintenance by identifying potential equipment failures before they occur. This proactive approach reduces unexpected downtimes and enhances operational efficiency.

Self-operating robots: With the integration of AI and ML, robots in manufacturing can function independently, especially in hazardous or precision-demanding environments where human access is limited or unsafe (Dalvand et al. 2014).

Robotic assembly: Smart technologies allow assembly robots to become more responsive and efficient. AI facilitates adaptation to new tasks, collaboration with humans, and continuous improvement through experiential learning. Additionally, it enhances safety by tracking robot movements and flagging risks, while also streamlining production workflows (Kwoh et al. 1988; Hamet and Tremblay 2017).

Process efficiency: These technologies help design optimal production methods, reducing resource wastage and improving throughput.

Supply chain efficiency: AI and ML forecast demand and manage inventory dynamically, helping ensure materials are available as needed while reducing excess stock.

Collaborative robotics: These tools enable robots to safely and effectively work alongside humans, taking over repetitive or hazardous tasks while human workers focus on complex problem-solving.

6 Advantages of AI, ML, and DL Applications in Advanced Robotic Systems

Object identification: Deep learning, particularly through neural networks trained on extensive datasets, enables robots to accurately recognize and classify objects in their surroundings (Kim et al. 2019).

Anticipatory maintenance: Utilizing sensor data, predictive models forecast component wear and potential failures, allowing for timely maintenance and minimizing downtime.

Interaction recognition: Robots can interpret and respond to gestures and speech, exemplified by service robots like Pepper, enhancing their usability in customer service and healthcare (Fig. 4).

AI-assisted surgery: AI-powered surgical robots support clinicians in performing delicate procedures with improved precision, lowering risks, and improving patient results (Fig. 5).

Defense applications: Robotics in military contexts benefit from AI in tasks such as reconnaissance, surveillance, and bomb disposal, using intelligent systems to assess and act on data.

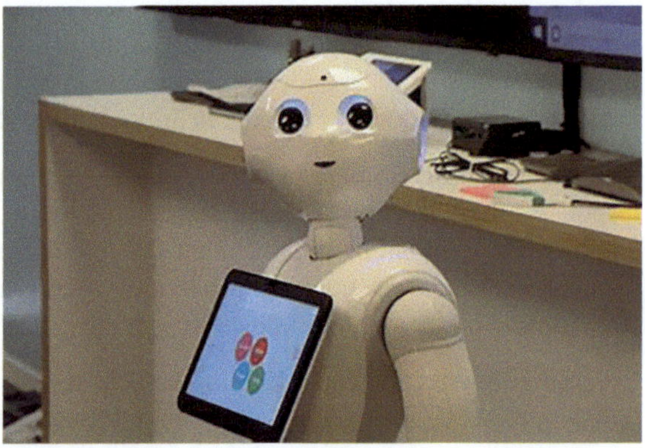

Fig. 4 Pepper—semi-humanoid robot with ability to read emotions

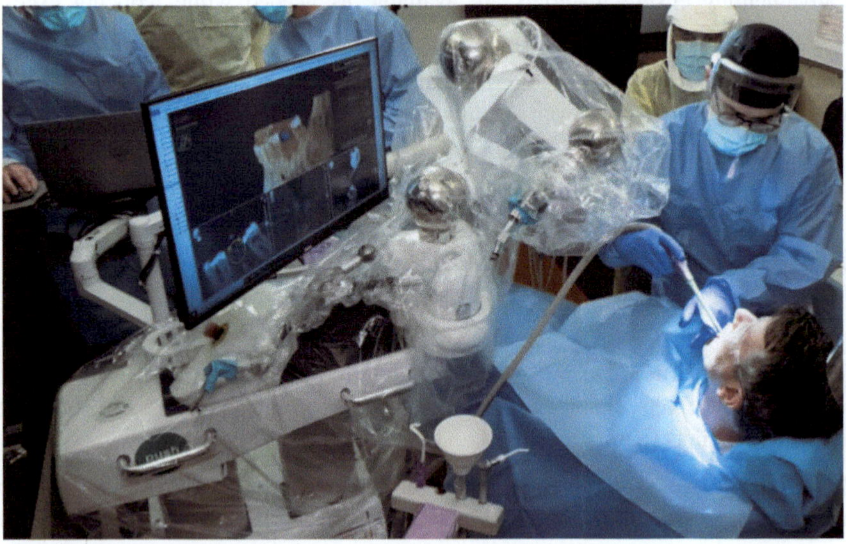

Fig. 5 Surgical robots as an aid to dental surgical procedures

Smart farming: Agricultural robots use AI and ML to autonomously manage crops and optimize farming operations—predicting weather, conserving water, and monitoring plant health.

Medical imaging and drug delivery: DL excels at identifying patterns in complex medical imagery, aiding in early disease detection (Olshannikova et al. 2015). ML models, such as decision trees and neural networks, improve targeted drug delivery for infectious diseases (Fig. 6).

Service automation: Service robots use AI to understand human needs, supporting tasks like cleaning, delivery, and hospitality (Montani and Striani 2019).

Self-driving technology: Autonomous vehicles utilize AI for object detection and real-time decision-making, adapting to varying road conditions and improving navigation.

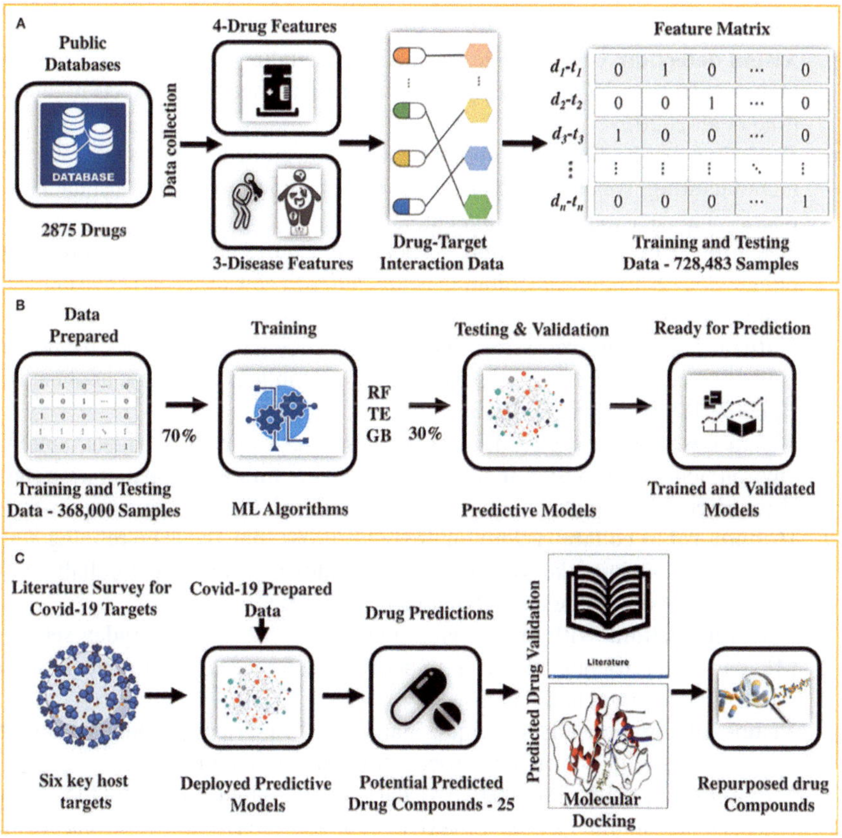

Fig. 6 Machine learning model for drug discovery, its application, and delivery systems

Industrial automation: In factories, AI enhances robotic systems involved in tasks like welding, painting, and assembly by increasing their precision and reducing human involvement (Bitterman et al. 2020).

AI in Robotics Research and Development

1. **Visual perception**: Advanced algorithms like convolutional neural networks (CNNs) are revolutionizing how robots perceive their environment through object recognition.
2. **Motion strategy**: Techniques such as reinforcement learning, including deep deterministic policy gradient (DDPG), have greatly enhanced robotic motion planning.
3. **Precision control**: Deep reinforcement learning algorithms, like proximal policy optimization (PPO), allow robotic systems to perform complex tasks such as object manipulation with high accuracy (Carriere et al. 2019).
4. **Position tracking**: Technologies like support vector machines (SVM) and random forests have significantly improved how robots determine their location within a space.
5. **Visual detection**: Cutting-edge DL models, including Faster R-CNN and You Only Look Once (YOLO), excel at identifying and localizing objects in images (Tao et al. 2020).
6. **Real-time navigation**: AI supports automated guided vehicles (AGVs) and manufacturing robots by processing sensor input to make instantaneous operational decisions (Tavakoli et al. 2020).
7. **Learning from demonstration**: Robots can acquire new skills by observing human demonstrations, facilitating adaptability to new tasks and environments (Ahn et al. 2019).
8. **Natural language processing (NLP)**: NLP allows robots to understand and engage in human dialogue, expanding their role in human-centric applications (Lane 2018; Mezger et al. 2013).
9. **Vision-based movement**: ML and DL empower robots to navigate complex environments using visual inputs for object recognition and spatial awareness (Luxton et al. 2016).
10. **Human–robot collaboration**: Future innovations may focus on refining algorithms that enhance the synergy between human workers and collaborative robots (cobots) (Casilari and Oviedo-Jiménez 2015).
11. **User interaction**: With the growing presence of robots in everyday settings, ML can tailor robotic behavior to human preferences, improving intuitive interactions (Sriram and Palaniswamy 2019).
12. **Visual intelligence**: DL techniques enable real-time identification of objects and activities, vital for effective robot–environment interaction.
13. **Manipulation skills**: Progress in visual recognition enables robots to handle objects more naturally and accurately, a promising area for future enhancements (Nibras et al. 2021).

14. **Swarm robotics**: This field explores coordination among multiple robots to perform complex tasks, using ML to facilitate communication, cooperation, and adaptability in dynamic environments.

7 Sensors Used in Dental Robotics

Force Sensors

Detect contact forces between tools and the patient's tissues, providing feedback to ensure safe and precise operations, especially during drilling or tooth preparation. Enable haptic feedback for surgeons in master–slave robotic systems.

Imaging Sensors

3D imaging: uses intraoral scanners or cameras for accurate mapping of the oral cavity. These sensors help in planning and navigation.

Optical localization: tracks instrument positions in real time, crucial in maxillofacial surgery and implant placement (Maciejasz et al. 2014).

X-ray and computed tomography (CT)-based sensors: used for detailed internal imaging, aiding in diagnosis and preoperative planning.

Tactile Sensors

Provide dentists with a sense of touch when using robotic systems, aiding in precise manipulation during delicate procedures.

Augmented Reality (AR) Sensors

Combine real-world views with virtual overlays, assisting in surgical guidance and improving procedural accuracy (Akbari et al. 2021).

8 Actuators Used in Dental Robotics

1. Electromagnetic actuators: found in robotic arms and drills to deliver controlled motion during surgeries, such as maxillofacial or implant procedures.
2. Piezoelectric actuators: used for micromovements in tools like ultrasonic scalers and laser positioning systems.
3. Soft robotics actuators: enable flexibility and adaptability in confined spaces, such as navigating the oral cavity during minimally invasive procedures (Howard 2017).
4. Voice coil motors: precise, small-scale actuators employed in laser-based tooth preparation systems, allowing detailed control over scanning and ablation.

5. Hydraulic and pneumatic actuators: provide the force required for certain manipulations, such as bending orthodontic wires or operating dental implant tools.

These technologies, combined with advanced control systems, ensure the high precision and safety required for dental robotics, paving the way for more effective and efficient patient care.

Key technologies in dental robotics focus on precision, adaptability, and efficiency in dental care. Here is a summary of the main technologies highlighted:

1. Mechanical Design and Modular Integration

Robots are designed with modular components to allow for flexibility in performing diverse dental procedures. Features include multi-degree-of-freedom (DoF) arms for intricate movements and adaptable end effectors that mimic the dexterity of a dentist's hand (Gorman and Gustafsson 2020; Li et al. 2011). Modular integration includes swappable tools and imaging devices for varied tasks like drilling, implant placement, and tooth preparation.

2. Manipulation Planning and Control

Algorithms support precise motion planning within the confined oral cavity. Control systems coordinate sensory data and actuator outputs to execute accurate drilling, filling, or other manipulations. Emergence of soft robotics allows safe navigation in complex oral structures, reducing the risk of tissue damage.

3. State Monitoring and Exception Handling

Real-time monitoring systems detect anomalies and maintain safety during operations. Multisensory fusion strategies integrate diverse data for stable and reliable robotic performance. Exception handling technologies, such as collision detection and predictive models, ensure robust error management in complex procedures.

4. Integration with AI and Machine Learning

AI-driven diagnostic tools and predictive analytics enable personalized treatment plans. Learning algorithms enhance robotic autonomy, allowing the execution of tasks like drilling and implant placement with minimal human intervention (Tulu et al. 2005).

5. End Effectors and Actuators

Advanced actuators, including piezoelectric, electromagnetic, and voice coil motors, support precise tool control. Specialized end effectors are designed for specific tasks such as tooth cleaning, implant positioning, and crown preparation (Lai et al. 2020).

These technologies collectively improve the precision, safety, and efficiency of dental robotics, advancing patient care and enabling innovations in digital dentistry.

9 Robotic Dental Applications

The application of robotics in different fields of dentistry leverages cutting-edge technologies to improve precision, efficiency, and patient outcomes. Here is an overview of robotics applications across various dental specialties:

1. Oral and Maxillofacial Surgery

Robots are used in surgeries involving the face, mouth, and jaws, such as oral cancer resection, trauma repair, and reconstructive surgeries.

Key technologies: Robots like the da Vinci system and master–slave surgical robots offer enhanced visualization and precision for minimally invasive procedures.

Benefits: shorter recovery times, fewer complications, and improved surgical accuracy (Valtolina and Marchionna 2021).

2. Dental Implants

Robots assist in placing dental implants with high precision and stability.

Examples: The Yomi robotic system, the first FDA-cleared robotic dental surgery system, provides preoperative and intraoperative guidance.

Technologies: Real-time imaging, optical navigation, and robotic drilling systems ensure precise implant positioning and reduce errors (Falck et al. 2020).

3. Prosthodontics

Robotics aids in the design and fabrication of dental prosthetics, such as crowns and dentures.

Key applications: laser-assisted tooth preparation robots for accurate shaping; mastication simulators to test the performance of prosthetics under realistic chewing forces.

Advantages: enhanced fit, function, and efficiency in prosthetic creation.

4. Orthodontics

Robots automate wire bending and appliance customization for braces and aligners.

Examples: SureSmile robots for precision wire bending (Fig. 7); computer numerical control (CNC)-based systems for orthodontic archwire preparation.

Impact: reduced treatment time and increased precision in orthodontic procedures.

5. Endodontics

Robotic systems improve root canal treatments through precision drilling and canal cleaning.

Technologies: microrobots for shaping and cleaning canals; automated tool changers for various endodontic instruments.

Benefits: increased treatment accuracy and less invasive procedures (Fig. 8).

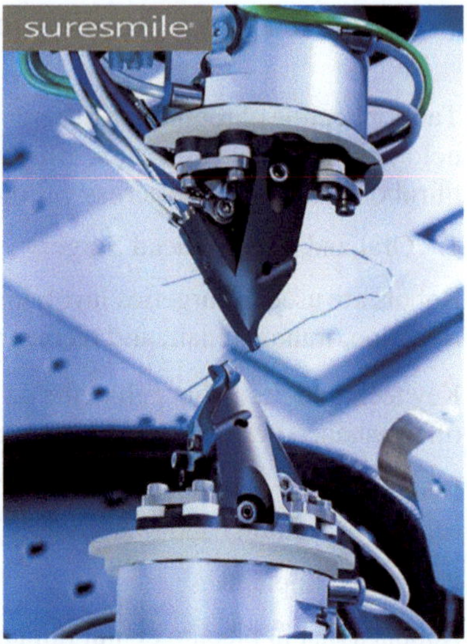

Fig. 7 SureSmile robot doing wire bending exercises for orthodontic treatment

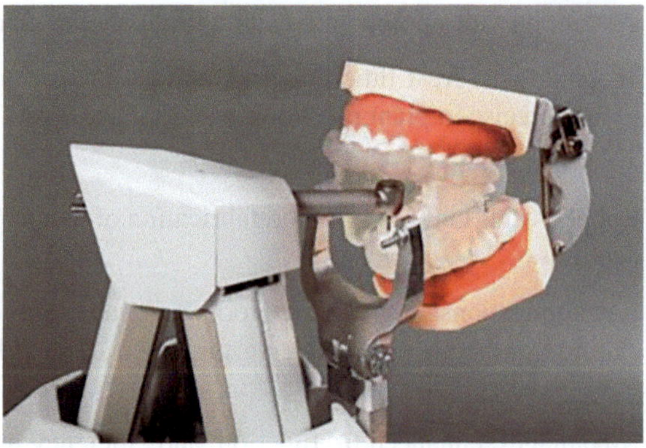

Fig. 8 Robotic system doing precise tooth cutting for less invasive procedures

6. Dental Education and Training

Simulation robots mimic patient conditions, providing a risk-free environment for training dental students.

Examples: Simroid and Dentaroid robots simulate patient reactions and dental conditions.

Advantages: bridging the gap between theoretical knowledge and practical skills (Bohr Memarzadeh 2020).

7. Dental Cleaning and Hygiene

Autonomous robots perform tasks like plaque removal and oral cleaning with precision.

Examples: automated toothbrushes and microrobots for biofilm disruption.

Key benefits: consistent cleaning, particularly useful for individuals with limited dexterity.

Robotics in dentistry continues to evolve, with advancements in AI, AR, and machine learning driving more personalized and effective patient care. Each field benefits uniquely from these technologies, making dentistry more efficient and accessible (Sutton et al. 2020; Saddler et al. 2020).

9.1 *Robotic Assistance in Dentistry: Revolutionizing the Dental Field*

1. Enhancing Dental Procedures

Robots have introduced precision, consistency, and efficiency in dental practices. From automated implant placement to endodontic treatments, robotics ensures less invasive and more accurate procedures.

2. Patient-Oriented Specific Solutions

Robotic systems offer personalized solutions tailored to individual dental anatomies. Real-time data analysis ensures that each intervention is accurate and minimally invasive, reducing recovery times and enhancing patient satisfaction (Deng et al. 2014).

3. Maintenance and Scalability in Clinics

Robotic systems designed for dental clinics are scalable, allowing for easy integration into existing workflows. Their maintenance is straightforward, with modular components enabling quick replacements and upgrades.

9.2 *Importance of Robot Operating System (ROS)*

The Robot Operating System (ROS) provides a flexible and standardized framework for robotic software development. Its modularity allows developers to build, test, and implement robotics solutions efficiently.

Application Examples

ROS has been pivotal in various robotic applications, from autonomous robots to industrial automation. Its extensive libraries and community support make it an invaluable tool for researchers and engineers.

1. Collaboration

ROS fosters collaboration by enabling different robotic systems to communicate seamlessly. This capability is critical in environments requiring coordinated multirobot operations, such as warehouse automation.

2. Streamlined Development

ROS simplifies robotic development with its open-source framework, providing tools for simulation, testing, and deployment. Developers can leverage its modularity to create custom solutions for diverse applications.

How ROS Supports Dental Robotics

1. Integration of Multiple Components

ROS enables seamless integration of sensors, actuators, imaging systems, and AI modules in robotic dental systems. This integration ensures synchronized operation during complex procedures like dental surgery or implant placement (Leventhal 2017; Gu et al. 2020).

2. Simulation and Testing

ROS provides simulation tools (e.g., Gazebo) that allow developers to test robotic systems in virtual environments before real-world implementation. For dental robotics, this ensures safe and precise operation without risking patient safety during development stages.

3. Navigation and Control

In robotic-assisted dental surgery, ROS-based navigation systems guide the robot with submillimeter accuracy. These systems use data from imaging modalities (e.g., cone beam computed tomography [CBCT]) to map the patient's oral anatomy and ensure precise tool positioning.

4. Adaptive Algorithms for Real-Time Adjustments

ROS allows the implementation of AI-driven algorithms that adapt to real-time feedback from sensors. For instance, during robotic drilling, the system can adjust speed and pressure based on bone density to prevent damage.

5. Remote Assistance and Teleoperation

ROS supports teleoperation, enabling specialists to assist or perform procedures remotely. This capability is especially useful in underserved regions where access to expert dental care is limited.

6. Customizable Interfaces

ROS allows developers to design user-friendly interfaces for dentists, enhancing control and monitoring of robotic systems. Such interfaces provide visual feedback, procedural guidance, and customization options tailored to individual patient needs.

7. Scalability for Future Enhancements

ROS's modular design ensures scalability, allowing integration of future advancements in robotics, AI, or imaging technology without overhauling the entire system. This adaptability supports long-term use in rapidly evolving dental practices (Jain et al. 2020).

9.3 Quick Points for Robotic Assistance in Dental Healthcare

1. Enhanced Precision and Accuracy

Robots can perform dental procedures with exceptional precision, reducing human errors. This is ideal for procedures like dental implant placement, cavity filling, and crown placement. The use of robotic arms for steady and controlled movements ensures optimal outcomes (Awad et al. 2017).

2. Minimally Invasive Procedures

Robots can navigate complex oral structures with minimal tissue damage. This ensures faster recovery for patients and reduces postoperative pain. Robots also help in targeted drug delivery or microsurgery within the oral cavity.

3. Real-Time Imaging and Diagnostics

Robots equipped with advanced imaging systems provide real-time 3D visualization. They facilitate early detection of oral diseases like cavities, periodontal diseases, and oral cancers. Integration with AI can suggest treatment plans based on diagnostic data (Mahajan et al. 2020).

4. Assistance in Orthodontics

Robotic systems assist in designing and manufacturing custom braces and aligners. Robots can help position brackets or adjust aligners with higher precision. They reduce the overall duration of orthodontic treatment.

5. Training and Simulation for Dental Students

Robotic simulators provide hands-on training on models for student education (Fig. 9).

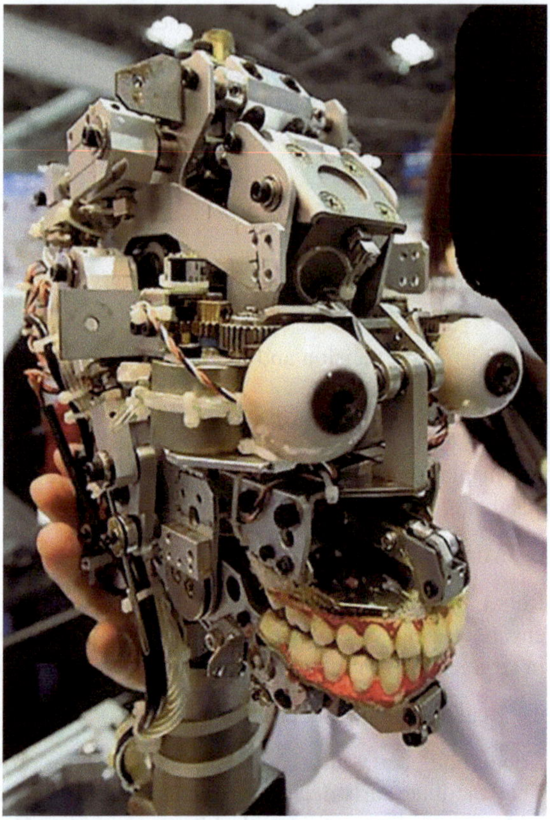

Fig. 9 Dental robot used for educational purposes

References

Ahmidi N et al (2017) A dataset and benchmarks for segmentation and recognition of gestures in robotic surgery. IEEE Trans Biomed Eng 64(9):2025–2041

Ahn HS, Yep W, Lim J, Ahn BK, Johanson DL, Hwang EJ et al (2019) Hospital receptionist robot v2: design for enhancing verbal interaction with social skills. In: 2019 28th IEEE international conference on robot and human interactive communication (RO-MAN). IEEE, New Delhi, pp 1–6. https://doi.org/10.1109/RO-MAN46459.2019.8956300

Ajoudani A, Zanchettin AM, Ivaldi S et al (2017) Progress and prospects of the human–robot collaboration. Auton Robot 42(5):957–975. https://doi.org/10.1007/s10514-017-9677-2

Akbari A, Haghverd F, Behbahani S (2021) Robotic home-based rehabilitation systems design: from a literature review to a conceptual framework for community-based remote therapy during COVID-19 pandemic. Front Robot AI 8:612331. https://doi.org/10.3389/frobt.2021.612331

Artificial intelligence, machine learning and deep learning in advanced robotics—Indian Minerology. https://indianminerology.blogspot.com/2024/01/artificial-intelligence-machine.html

Awad A, Bader–El–Den M, McNicholas J (2017) Patient length of stay and mortality prediction: a survey. Health Serv Manage Res 30:105–120. https://doi.org/10.1177/0951484817696212

Badash I, Burtt K, Solorzano CA et al (2016) Innovations in surgery simulation: a review of past, current and future techniques. Ann Transl Med 4(23):453–453. https://doi.org/10.21037/atm.2016.12.24

Bitterman DS, Aerts HJWL, Mak RH (2020) Approaching autonomy in medical artificial intelligence. Lancet Digit Health 2:e447–e449. https://doi.org/10.1016/S2589-7500(20)30187-4

Bohr A, Memarzadeh K (eds) (2020) The rise of artificial intelligence in healthcare applications. In: Artificial intelligence in healthcare. Elsevier, Oxford, pp 25–60. https://doi.org/10.1016/B978-0-12-818438-7.00002-2

Carriere J, Fong J, Meyer T, Sloboda R, Husain S, Usmani N et al (2019) An admittance-controlled robotic assistant for semi-autonomous breast ultrasound scanning. In: 2019 International symposium on medical robotics (ISMR). IEEE, Atlanta, GA, pp 1–7. https://doi.org/10.1109/ISMR.2019.8710206

Casilari E, Oviedo-Jiménez MA (2015) Automatic fall detection system based on the combined use of a smartphone and a smartwatch. PLoS ONE 10:e0140929. https://doi.org/10.1371/journal.pone.0140929

Dalvand MM, Shirinzadeh B, Shamdani AH, Smith J, Zhong Y (2014) An actuated force feedback-enabled laparoscopic instrument for robotic-assisted surgery. Int J Med Robot Comput Assist Surg 10(1):11–21

Denecke K, Baudoin CR (2022) A review of artificial intelligence and robotics in transformed health ecosystems. Front Med (Lausanne) 9:795957. https://doi.org/10.3389/fmed.2022.795957

Deng H, Wu Q, Qin B, Chow SSM, Domingo-Ferrer J, Shi W (2014) Tracing and revoking leaked credentials: accountability in leaking sensitive outsourced data. In: Proceedings of the 9th ACM symposium on information, computer and communications security. Association for Computing Machinery, New York, NY, pp 425–434. (ASIA CCS'14). https://doi.org/10.1145/2590296.2590342

Falck F, Doshi S, Tormento M, Nersisyan G, Smuts N, Lingi J et al (2020) Robot DE NIRO: a human-centered, autonomous, mobile research platform for cognitively-enhanced manipulation. Front Robot AI 7:66. https://doi.org/10.3389/frobt.2020.00066

Gorman C, Gustafsson L (2020) The use of augmented reality for rehabilitation after stroke: a narrative review. Disabil Rehabil Assist Technol 17:409–417. https://doi.org/10.1080/17483107.2020.1791264

Gu Q, Nie C, Zou R, Chen W, Zheng C, Zhu D et al (2020) Automatic generation of electromyogram diagnosis report. In: 2020 IEEE international conference on bioinformatics and biomedicine (BIBM). IEEE, Seoul, pp 1645–1650

Habuza T, Navaz AN, Hashim F et al (2021) AI applications in robotics, diagnostic image analysis and precision medicine: current limitations, future trends, guidelines on CAD systems for medicine. Inform Med Unlocked 24:100596. https://doi.org/10.1016/j.imu.2021.100596

Hamet P, Tremblay J (2017) Artificial intelligence in medicine. Metabolism 69:S36-40. https://doi.org/10.1016/j.metabol.2017.01.011

Howard MC (2017) A meta-analysis and systematic literature review of virtual reality rehabilitation programs. Comput Hum Behav 70:317–327. https://doi.org/10.1016/j.chb.2017.01.013

Jain V, Wason R, Chatterjee JM, Le D-N (eds) (2020) Ontology-based information retrieval for healthcare systems, 1st ed. Wiley-Scrivener. https://doi.org/10.1002/9781119641391

Kim J, Campbell AS, de Ávila BE-F, Wang J (2019) Wearable biosensors for healthcare monitoring. Nat Biotechnol 37:389–406. https://doi.org/10.1038/s41587-019-0045-y

Kwoh YS, Hou J, Jonckheere EA, Hayati S (1988) A robot with improved absolute positioning accuracy for CT guided stereotactic brain surgery. IEEE Trans Biomed Eng 35(2):153–160

Lai L, Wittbold KA, Dadabhoy FZ, Sato R, Landman AB, Schwamm LH et al (2020) Digital triage: novel strategies for population health management in response to the COVID-19 pandemic. Healthc Amst Neth 8:100493. https://doi.org/10.1016/j.hjdsi.2020.100493

Lane T (2018) A short history of robotic surgery. Ann R Coll Surg Engl 100:5–7. https://doi.org/10.1308/rcsann.supp1.5

Leventhal R (2017) How natural language processing is helping to revitalize physician documentation, vol 34. Healthc Inform, Cleveland, OH, pp 8–13
Li A, Montaño Z, Chen VJ, Gold JI (2011) Virtual reality and pain management: current trends and future directions. Pain Manag 1:147–157. https://doi.org/10.2217/pmt.10.15
Luxton DD, June JD, Sano A, Bickmore T (2016) Intelligent mobile, wearable, and ambient technologies for behavioral health care. In: Artificial intelligence in behavioral and mental health care. Elsevier, pp 137–162. Available online at: https://linkinghub.elsevier.com/retrieve/pii/B9780124202481000064. Google Scholar
Maciejasz P, Eschweiler J, Gerlach-Hahn K, Jansen-Troy A, Leonhardt S (2014) A survey on robotic devices for upper limb rehabilitation. J Neuro Eng Rehab 11:3. https://doi.org/10.1186/1743-0003-11-3
Madhavi CR, Vidhya MJ, Padmaja KV (2024) Synergism of medicine and robotic applications for the future—a review. In: 2024 8th international conference on computational system and information technology for sustainable solutions (CSITSS), Bengaluru, India, pp 1–6. https://doi.org/10.1109/CSITSS64042.2024.10817040
Mahajan SM, Mahajan A, Nguyen C, Bui J, Abbott BT, Osborne TF (2020) Predictive models for identifying risk of readmission after index hospitalization for hip arthroplasty: a systematic review. J Orthop 22:73–85. https://doi.org/10.1016/j.jor.2020.03.045
Mezger U, Jendrewski C, Bartels M (2013) Navigation in surgery. Langenbecks Arch Surg 398:501–514. https://doi.org/10.1007/s00423-013-1059-4
Montani S, Striani M (2019) Artificial intelligence in clinical decision support: a focused literature survey. Yearb Med Inform 28:120–127. https://doi.org/10.1055/s-0039-1677911
Nibras N, Liu C, Mottet D, Wang C, Reinkensmeyer D, Remy-Neris O et al (2021) Dissociating sensorimotor recovery and compensation during exoskeleton training following stroke. Front Hum Neurosci 15:645021. https://doi.org/10.3389/fnhum.2021.645021
Olshannikova E, Ometov A, Koucheryavy Y, Olsson T (2015) Visualizing big data with augmented and virtual reality: challenges and research agenda. J Big Data 2:22. https://doi.org/10.1186/s40537-015-0031-2
Saddler N, Harvey G, Jessa K, Rosenfield D (2020) Clinical decision support systems: opportunities in pediatric patient safety. Curr Treat Options Pediatr 6:325–335. https://doi.org/10.1007/s40746-020-00206-3
Sriram KNV, Palaniswamy S (2019) Mobile robot assistance for disabled and senior citizens using hand gestures. In: 2019 international conference on power electronics applications and technology in present energy scenario (PETPES). IEEE, Mangalore, pp 1–6. https://doi.org/10.1109/PETPES47060.2019.9003821
Sutton RT, Pincock D, Baumgart DC, Sadowski DC, Fedorak RN, Kroeker KI (2020) An overview of clinical decision support systems: benefits, risks, and strategies for success. NPJ Digit Med 3:17. https://doi.org/10.1038/s41746-020-0221-y
Tao R, Ocampo R, Fong J, Soleymani A, Tavakoli M (2020) Modeling and emulating a physiotherapist's role in robot-assisted rehabilitation. Adv Intell Syst 2:1900181. https://doi.org/10.1002/aisy.201900181
Tavakoli M, Carriere J, Torabi A (2020) Robotics, smart wearable technologies, and autonomous intelligent systems for healthcare during the COVID-19 pandemic: an analysis of the state of the art and future vision. Adv Intell Syst 2:2000071. https://doi.org/10.1002/aisy.202000071
Tulu B, Chatterjee S, Laxminarayan S (2005) A taxonomy of telemedicine efforts with respect to applications, infrastructure, delivery tools, type of setting and purpose. In: Proceedings of the 38th annual Hawaii international conference on system sciences. IEEE, Big Island, HI, p 147
Valtolina S, Marchionna M (2021) Design of a chatbot to assist the elderly. In: Fogli D, Tetteroo D, Barricelli BR, Borsci S, Markopoulos P, Papadopoulos GA (eds) End-user development. Lecture notes in computer science; Bd. 12724. Springer International Publishing, Cham, pp 153–168
Zhang W, Su C, He C (2020) Rehabilitation exercise recognition and evaluation based on smart sensors with deep learning framework. IEEE Access 8:77561–77571. https://doi.org/10.1109/ACCESS.2020.2989128

Diagnostic Imaging Modalities

Shagun Gill, Aakash Gupta, Ramandeep Singh, and Tarun Kumar Singh

Diagnosis is not the end, but the beginning of practice
—Martin Fischer

1 Introduction

It was on November 8, 1895, when Wilhelm Conrad Röntgen accidentally discovered an image formed by a cathode ray generator which was projected well beyond the cathode rays' potential range. When Röntgen took an image of his wife's hand on a photographic plate created by an unidentified radiation that he called X-rays, a week after the discovery, he realized its potential medicinal applications. The image showcased her bones and her wedding band clearly. In January 1896, Dr. Otto Walkhoff took the first original dental roentgenogram from a section of a glass imaging plate in his own mouth during a 25-min exposure period. Since then, there have been significant advancements in dental imaging and its use in different specialties. Intraoral and extraoral, analog and digital, ionizing and nonionizing, and two-dimensional (2D) and three-dimensional (3D) imaging are the general categories into which imaging techniques used in dentistry can be divided (Shah et al. 2014).

Three significant advancements have dominated the imaging field in recent years: First, the end users do not want a "better diagnosis alone" if it has no bearing on the therapeutic process; second, interventional treatments are becoming more significant

S. Gill (✉)
Department of Conservative Dentistry and Endodontics, Gian Sagar Dental College and Hospital, Ramnagar, Rajpura, Patiala, Punjab, India
e-mail: shagungill3008@gmail.com

A. Gupta · T. K. Singh
Division of Conservative Dentistry and Endodontics, Department of Dentistry, All Indian Institute of Medical Sciences, Bathinda, Punjab, India

R. Singh
Department of Radiodiagnosis and Imaging, All India Institute of Medical Sciences, Bathinda, Punjab, India

A. Gupta et al. (eds.), *Application of Robotics in Dentistry*, Lecture Notes in Bioengineering, https://doi.org/10.1007/978-981-95-1470-0_5

than diagnostics alone; and third, a general transition of organs from 2D slices to 3D models has been noted. Every imaging modality now in use is impacted by these trends (Sakas 2002).

Since its invention, radiology has undergone a revolutionary journey, with its tremendous influence resonating throughout modern medicine. From the discovery of X-rays to the latest incorporation of deep learning (DL) and artificial intelligence (AI), this diverse field is always evolving, both internally and in relation to the healthcare environment it supports. The use of various diagnostic modalities, along with the recent advancements, has been reviewed in this chapter.

2 Diagnostic Tools

Radiographic Methods

A. Analog Radiography
    a. Intraoral: Periapical radiograph
        - Bitewing radiograph
        - Occlusal radiograph
    b. Extraoral: Panoramic radiograph
        - Cephalometric radiograph

B. Digital Radiography
    a. Radiovisiography (RVG)
    b. Xeroradiography
    c. Modified radiographic techniques
        i. Computer image analysis (COMENDEX)
        ii. Digital subtraction radiography
        iii. Cone beam computed tomography (CBCT)
        iv. Computed tomography (CT)
            • Microcomputed tomography (micro-CT)
            • Spiral coherence tomography
            • Tuned-aperture coherence tomography (TACT)
            • Optical coherence tomography (OCT)
        v. C-arm imaging.

Optical Detection

a. Digital imaging fiber-optic transillumination (DIFOTI)
b. Transillumination with near-infrared light
c. Quantitative light-induced fluorescence (QLF)

d. DIAGNOdent
e. Infrared fluorescence

Endoscopy/Videoscopy

Recent Advances/Newer Techniques

a. Terahertz imaging (THz)
b. Multiphoton imaging
c. Optical coherence tomography (OCT)
d. Infrared thermography
e. Frequency domain infrared photothermal radiometry (PTR) and modulated luminescence (LUM)
f. Magnetic resonance imaging (MRI)
g. Ultrasonic imaging (UI)
h. LASER optical disc storage
i. Deep learning (DL) and artificial intelligence (AI)
j. Robotics.

Radiographic Methods

Analog Radiography

(a) Intraoral radiographs
(b) Extraoral radiographs

The techniques used in conventional radiography are:

Paralleling cone technique/long cone technique: Gordon M. Fitzgerald created the paralleling or long cone technique, a unique periapical radiography method in which the central X-ray beam is aimed at a right angle to both the film and the teeth and the film is positioned parallel to the tooth's long axis for radiography. The focal spot becomes smaller as a result of the tube's long cone, lengthening the distance between the source and the object. By avoiding the overlapping of other anatomical components, which could overshadow the teeth, this procedure lessens geometric deformation. The X-ray image must be standardized so as to maintain the same horizontal and vertical angulations at each follow-up visit in order to track the healing of the periapical lesion. There are a number of film-holding mechanisms that make it possible to replicate the same angulation for subsequent radiographs (White and Pharoah 2018).

Bisecting angle technique/short cone technique: This method is predicated on the "Cieszeynski's Rule of Isometry," a straightforward geometric theorem. This method involves placing the film in the palate or on the floor of the mouth as close to the lingual surface of the concerned tooth as possible. The cone is then adjusted such that the central ray is oriented perpendicular to the bisector of the angle formed between the tooth and the film (White and Pharoah 2018).

(b) **Intraoral Radiographs**

Periapical radiograph: The periapical radiograph offers comprehensive information on the teeth and surrounding tissues. Its primary applications include evaluating the morphology of the pulp and root canals, detecting crown/root fractures and supporting the alveolar bone health in the interdental area. It helps in pretreatment assessment of calcifications, curvatures, periapical lesions, working length determination, quality of root canal obturation, and monitoring of posttherapy healing.

Bitewing radiograph: The primary purpose of these interproximal radiographs is to assess alterations in the coronal tooth structure of three to four upper and lower teeth at the same time. The cone gives an image of the crown and alveolar crest when it is held parallel to the film. The method is helpful for determining the coronal pulp's shape, interproximal caries, and secondary caries beneath restorations and assessing the state of the interproximal bone. The bitewing X-ray gets its name from the flap on the film, which the patient bites to hold it in place against the crowns of the concerned teeth.

Occlusal radiograph: A cyst or other significant area of a dental arch that is not seen on a periapical radiograph can be seen on an occlusal radiograph. It assists in identifying extra or impacted teeth, foreign objects in the jaws, and stones in the submandibular gland ducts (Rotstein and Ingle 2023).

(c) **Extraoral Radiographs**

Panoramic radiograph: It is a specialized tomographic technique that creates a flat image of the 3D surfaces of the jaws. It is based on the "curved surface tomography" concept. It provides a panoramic or bird's-eye view of the jaws by visualizing the whole craniofacial skeleton, maxilla, mandible, temporomandibular joints (TMJ), impacted teeth, dental implant locations, pathological lesions, and maxillary and mandibular fractures. Despite its advantages, it has a comparatively limited spatial resolution and is susceptible to significant and unpredictable geometric distortion.

Cephalometric radiographs: The entire side of the head can be visualized on cephalometric radiographs, which aid in assessing the spatial relationships between the dental and cranial structures. They are useful in assessing how the dental and skeletal structures, including the soft tissue profile (with less exposure to X-rays), have changed in growth and development before, during, and after orthodontic treatment (Shah et al. 2014).

Digital Radiography

a. **Radiovisiography (RVG)**

The first digital radiography system for dentistry was introduced by Trophy in 1987 in France with radio-visio-graphy (RVG, formerly Trex-Trophy Radiology Inc., Marietta, GA). Digital radiography is the process of taking a radiograph with a solid-state

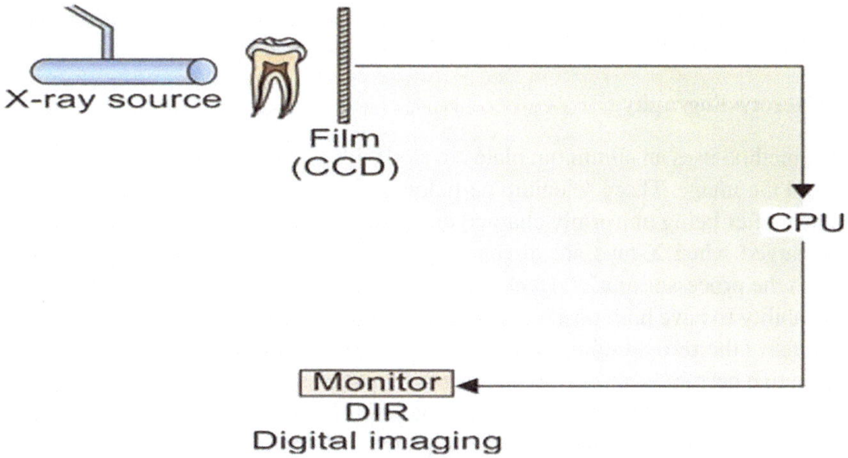

Fig. 1 Diagrammatic representation of digital imaging (Sakas 2002)

sensor, dividing it into electronic parts, and then using a computer to display and save the image. Ionizing radiation is digitalized by radiovisiography, producing an immediate image on a video monitor (Fig. 1).

Three parts make up direct digital radiography systems:

1. **"Radio" component**: It consists of a high-resolution sensor plate which has an active surface area and dimensions comparable to those of a radiography film. A fiber-optic coating shields the sensor's active surface from X-ray deterioration, and a cable connects this sensor to the computer. The sensor is made from any of the following components:

    (a) Charge-coupled device (CCD)
    (b) Complementary metal oxide semiconductor (CMOS)
    (c) Photostimulable phosphor detectors (PSP).

    The active surface area of the sensor plate becomes sensitized when exposed to X-rays, and radio waves carry the image straight to the computer. This reduces the amount of time needed to process a traditional film.

2. **"Visio" component**: This includes a digital processing unit and a visual monitor. After analysis, the data collected by the sensor plate is shown as an image. A software that incorporates digital enhancement, contrast, magnification, colorizing, and reversal can be used to modify it in several dimensions.
3. **"Graphy" component**: A high-resolution video printer is used to create a duplicate of the screen image. In indirect digital radiography, the traditional film is digitalized. A laser scan is used to transfer the radiography image to a reusable plate that resembles a film. The digital processing unit processes the image on the plate and displays it on the monitor (Udoye and Jafarzadeh 2010).

Analog and digital radiography differ from one another in several ways, which are depicted in Table 1.

b. **Xeroradiography**

This method uses an aluminum plate covered with a coating of selenium particles to record the image. These selenium particles are kept in a device known as a "conditioner" after being uniformly charged electrostatically. The particles are selectively discharged when X-rays are directed upon the film. This creates a latent image, which the processor unit's "development" process transforms into a positive image. The ability to have both positive and negative prints combined is one of the primary features of the xeroradiography process. Positive particles are drawn to the film when a negative current is applied, while negative particles are drawn to the film when a positive current is applied (Udoye and Jafarzadeh 2010). The various advantages and disadvantages of xeroradiography are depicted in Table 2.

c. **Modified Radiographic Techniques**

i. **Computer Image Analysis (COMENDEX)**

In order to overcome the differences in radiographic interpretation done by different observers, the computers enabled the use of automated processes that potentially

Table 1 Differences between analog and digital radiography

Aspect	Analog radiography	Digital radiography
Image capture	Uses X-ray film to capture the image	Uses digital sensors (e.g., CCD or flat-panel detectors)
Image processing	Requires physical development in a darkroom	Processes images instantly on a computer screen
Image quality	Lower resolution; can degrade over time	Higher resolution; clearer images, adjustable for enhancement
Radiation exposure	Generally requires higher radiation doses	80% reduction in radiation dose
Storage	Requires physical storage (film archives)	Digital storage, easily saved, shared, and retrieved
Image manipulation	Limited ability to adjust image after development	Can be digitally manipulated (contrast, brightness, etc.)
Speed	Slower; requires time for film development	Faster; results available immediately
Cost	Lower initial cost for equipment, but higher ongoing costs (film, chemicals)	Higher initial cost for equipment, but lower ongoing costs (no film or chemicals)
Durability	Film can degrade with time, handling, and improper storage	Digital images are more durable and can be backed up
Environmental impact	More chemicals and waste associated with film development	Less waste; more eco-friendly overall

Table 2 Advantages and disadvantages of xeroradiography

Advantages	Disadvantages
• High contrast and improved resolution • Both positive and negative displays are available • Twice as sensitive as traditional D-speed films • Allows for "edge enhancement," which is the differentiation of areas with varying densities, particularly at the edges or borders	• High probability for artifacts • Since the oral cavity's humid environment serves as a conduit for the flow of current, the electric charge over the film frequently causes discomfort for the patient • Thickness of the plate remains unknown, so exposure times may vary • The development process must be finished in 15 min

compensate for the limitations of the human vision. A software for automatic interpretation, the "Expert System," was developed which includes information on pathologic diseases. When the clinician enters the patient's data in the software, the algorithm compares it with the fundamental understanding of the disease. This application shows the potential diagnosis and also suggests other conditions that might be present. Applications have also been created to quantify carious lesions and assist in the interpretation of angular periodontal bone abnormalities (Sikri 2019a). The advantages and disadvantages of this system are mentioned in Table 3.

ii. **Digital Subtraction Radiography**

A high-quality video camera is used to capture an image of the radiograph in order to digitize it. This is fed into a device called a digitizer, which is used for computer imaging. Two standardized radiographs are created using the same exposure geometry. The first image serves as the "reference image," while the following images are for comparison. The screen displays the reference image, and the following images are then superimposed. An image of the differences between the two radiographs is produced by subtracting the gray-level values of one radiograph from the equivalent gray levels of another radiograph (Hekmatian et al. 2025).

Both photographic and electronic techniques can be used to create subtraction images. The various advantages and disadvantages of this technique are depicted in Table 4.

Table 3 Advantages and disadvantages of computer image analysis

Advantages	Disadvantages
• Sensitive and objective observation of small lesions that may otherwise be invisible to the human eye is possible with automated analysis • Possible to quantify small lesions	• Standardization of exposure geometry is always required • Specificity is lower while sensitivity is higher • Time consuming • Expensive equipment

Table 4 Advantages and disadvantages of digital subtraction radiography

Advantages	Disadvantages
• Ability to remove structured noise • Detects proximal caries, recurrent caries • Detects progress of remineralization and demineralization patterns of dentinal caries • Can detect 5% mineral loss in contrast to 30–60% for conventional radiographs	• No geographic repeatability of X-ray source-to-object relationship (intraoral stent to X-ray source) • Expensive • Difficult to improve sensitivity

iii. **Cone Beam Computed Tomography (CBCT)**

Cone beam computed tomography can create three-dimensional (3D) scans of the maxillofacial skeleton using an imaging scanner intended for head and neck imaging. The size of the cone beam computed tomography machine is comparable to that of panoramic radiography equipment.

CBCT machinery consists of a revolving gantry with a fixed fulcrum that holds the X-ray source and a digital detector. Through the anatomy of interest, a diverging X-ray beam in the shape of a cone or pyramid is projected. When the source and detector revolve in an arc of 180° to 360°, the ionizing radiation travels through the desired field of view (FOV) so as to produce hundreds of planar images (Fig. 2). A computer is then used to rebuild these images into tomographic images.

CBCT provides three-dimensional view of teeth (Fig. 3) and its surrounding structures like temporomandibular joint (Fig. 4), thus providing a complete picture for better diagnosis and treatment planning over two-dimensional imaging modalities.

Exposure dose: Tube voltage between 60 and 120 kV and current between 1 and 10 mA are used. Each imaging session can last anything from 5 to 40 s. Voxels of length 0.08 to 0.4 mm are used in CBCT imaging. The breadth and height of the field of view (FOV) can vary from 4 to 20 cm and 3 to 20 cm, respectively. Patients may lie on a table, stand, or sit, depending on the CBCT machine (Bromberg and Brizuela 2025). The various advantages and disadvantages of CBCT are depicted in Table 5.

iv. **Computed Tomography (CT)**

A 3D image of an object with a slice thickness of 1.0–2.0 mm can be obtained and evaluated by computed tomography (CT). Earlier CT scanners captured X-rays using a single detector. Later, arc-shaped and circular detectors helped make multiple detectors (64) more widely used in modern CT scanners (Fig. 5) (Berman and Hargreaves 2020).

Though CT helps in providing accurate 3D images by removing anatomical noise, high radiation dose, inadequate geometric resolution, and expensive equipment limit its use for routine cases.

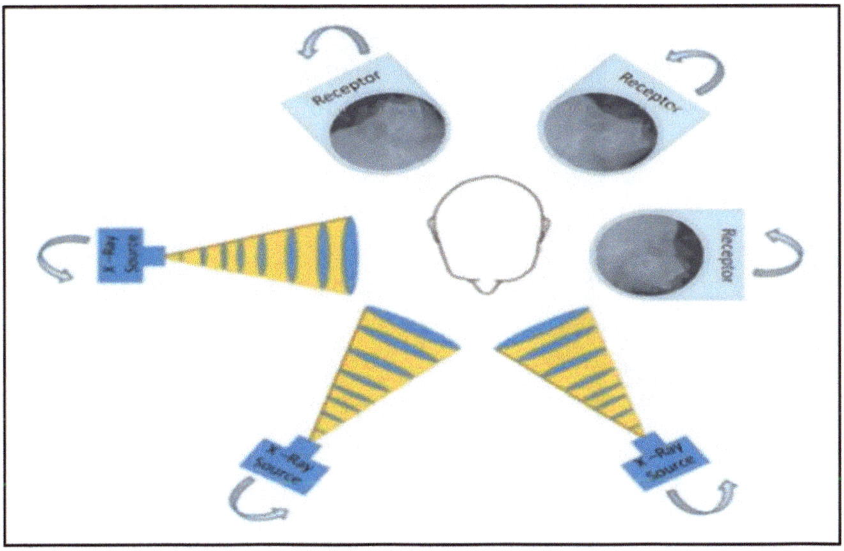

Fig. 2 Principle of basic image acquisition, wherein X-ray source and image receptor reciprocate around patient 180–360° to acquire 180–1024 2D cephalometric images (Venkatesh and Elluru 2017)

Microcomputed tomography (micro-CT): In micro-CT, the X-rays converge over a sample and are picked up by a sensor. Digital images are created from the projected rays. Micro-CT provides volumetric pixels (voxels) with a range of 5–50 µm. It is advantageous for root canal instrumentation, retreatment of failed root canals, in vitro investigation of the internal architecture of teeth, etc. Also, the same sample can be used for multiple examinations. However, this imaging modality can examine only a limited number of in vitro specimens (Sikri 2019a).

Spiral computed tomography: Spiral sampling with 3D reconstruction is used to obtain projection data. This method improves the ability to resolve small objects by reconstructing overlapping structures at random intervals. Applications of this approach in endodontics specifically include assessing root fractures, analyzing root resorption, locating additional or aberrant root canals, and identifying other irregularities in the pulp space (Sikri 2019a).

Tuned-aperture computed tomography (TACT): It produces images that are free of artifacts and have reduced anatomical noise. This method is used to detect anomalies in root canal anatomy as well as vertical fractures (Sikri 2019a).

Optical coherence tomography (OCT): This imaging method can produce 2D or 3D images of subsurface tissues. It uses laser light with wavelengths between 840 and 1310 nm. The scattering of this light can be used to distinguish between sound and carious enamel.

When the laser light enters the tissue, the light that emerges is measured with respect to its phase, which indicates how far it has traveled. Demineralization causes the tooth tissue's reflectance to drop. Superluminescent diodes are used as the light

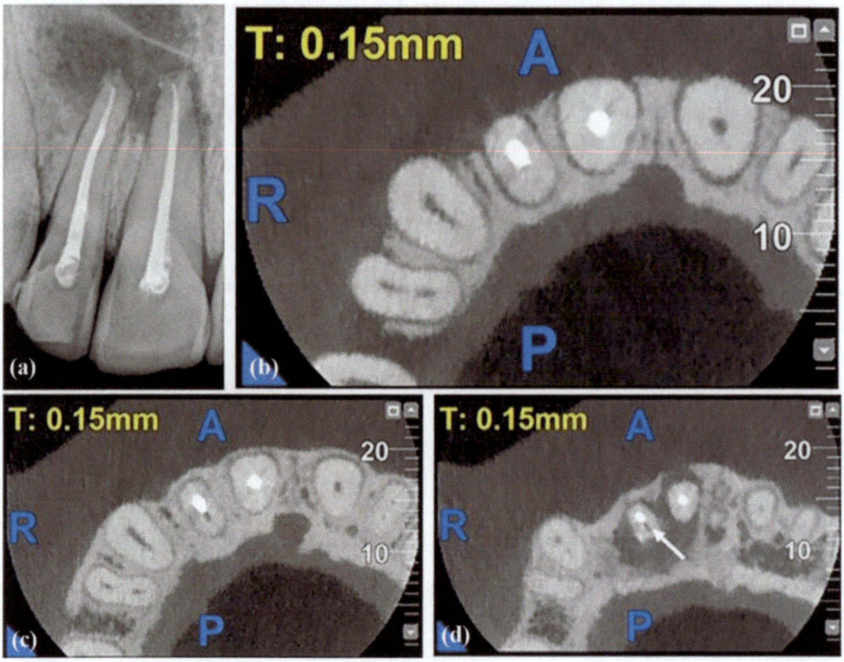

Fig. 3 (From left to right) RVG revealing perfect obturation in relation to 11, 12 (**A**), CBCT axial view revealing proper obturation in relation to 11, 12 at coronal third (**B**), CBCT axial view revealing dead space in canal lumen in relation to 12 (**C**), and CBCT axial view revealing untouched part of canal lumen shown by arrow (**D**)

source in OCT devices. The degree of dispersion of light and the degree of mineralization are related to the signal alterations. OCT has also been utilized to evaluate the contact between the tooth and the restoration (Berman and Hargreaves 2020).

v. **C-arm Imaging**

C-arm CBCT is an advanced imaging technique that uses flat-panel fluoroscopy systems to acquire and display 3D images, providing high- and low-contrast soft tissue (CT-like) images in multiple viewing planes. Unlike the stationary conventional dental radiography, this is a new, dynamic, innovative, and mobile real-time imaging technique which allows clinicians to observe live imaging events.

The flat-panel detector, X-ray tube, and collimator are connected to a C-arm, which is a part of the stand used for capturing 3D images. It maintains a precise alignment of the apparatus at different viewing angles (Fig. 6). X-ray exposure parameters, including detector entrance dose (the X-ray dosage measured behind the antiscatter grid) and system dose (detector entrance dose evaluated at a reference detector zoom format), are adjusted by the C-arm imaging systems with automatic exposure control. When using analog image intensifiers, the X-ray is attenuated to varying degrees across the patient's body before striking a fluorescent surface. The intensity of the radiation will determine how brilliant the surface glows. The glow is

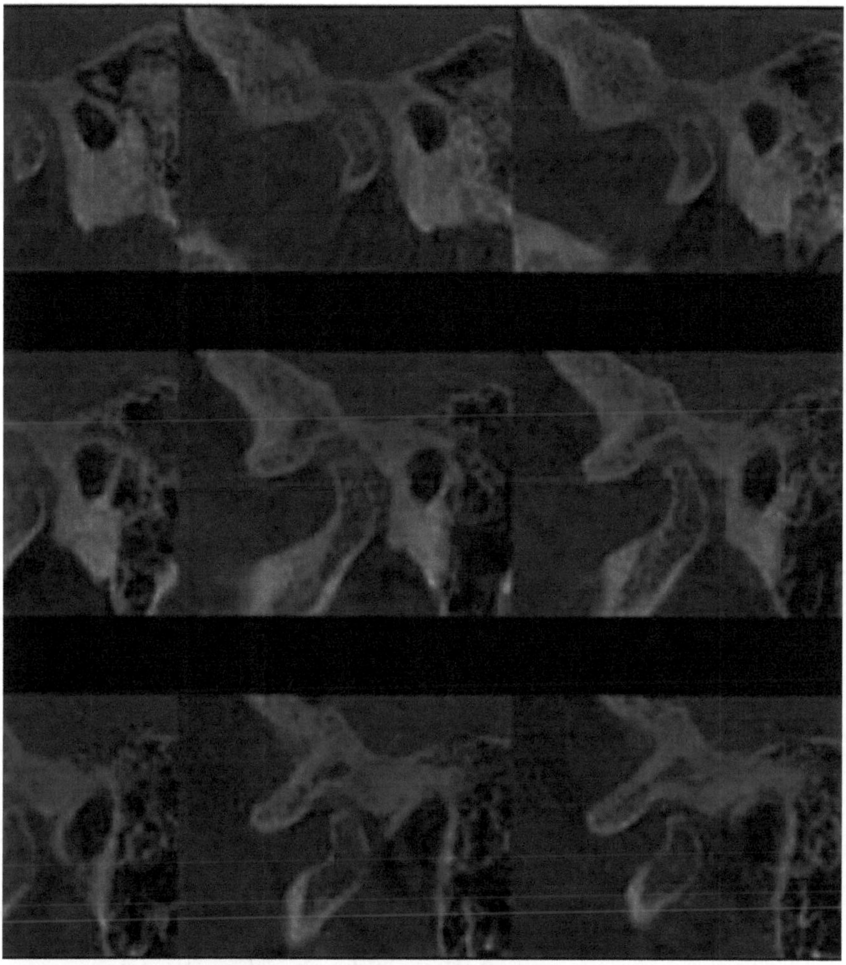

Fig. 4 Sagittal slices of the left TMJ taken on a dedicated head and neck CBCT scanner

captured by a vacuum tube and shown on the monitor. The incident X-rays' intensity is immediately transformed into a digital value (Rajkumar 2014). The various advantages and disadvantages of this imaging technique are enlisted in Table 6.

Optical Detection

(a) Digital Imaging Fiber-Optic Transillumination (DIFOTI)

By integrating fiber-optic transillumination (FOTI) with a digital CCD camera, DIFOTI was created in an effort to lessen the apparent drawbacks of FOTI. A digital electronic CCD camera takes images of the tooth after the light from the DIFOTI probe is positioned on it. Several images are then instantaneously projected onto a computer and compared for clinical changes (Astvaldsdóttir 2012).

Commercially available product: DIAGNOcam (KaVo, Germany).

Table 5 Advantages and disadvantages of cone beam computed tomography

Advantages	Disadvantages
• High-resolution images obtained with a maximum spatial resolution of 0.076 mm • Feasible to reconstruct projection data that shows accurate spatial relationships in the axial, sagittal, and coronal planes • Window/level changes, text or arrow annotations, and zoom magnification possible • Cursor-driven measuring algorithms provide real-time dimensional assessment No geometric inaccuracies in the measurements taken on-screen	• Inferior spatial resolution as compared to 2D film-based or digital intraoral radiography • Scattered radiation causes image noise • "Heel effect" seen due to anode's variable X-ray emission intensity • Beam hardening can cause cupping artifacts, streaks, and dark bands • Patient's movement during radiation exposure may result in patient-related artifacts, such as reduced sharpness • Circular or ring-shaped flaws may occur as a consequence of scanner-related artifacts • Partial volume averaging, sampling, and cone-beam effect cause cone beam-related errors • Insufficient soft tissue contrast

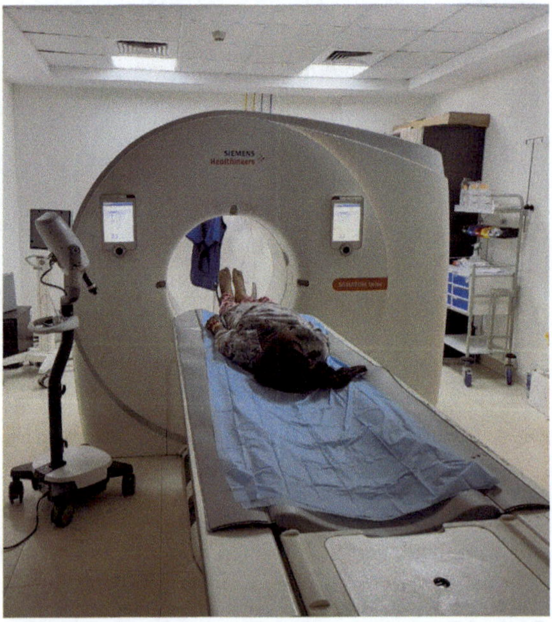

Fig. 5 Computed tomography scanner

The various advantages and disadvantages of this imaging modality are enlisted in Table 7.

(b) **Transillumination with Near-Infrared Light**

Near-infrared light transillumination of tooth enamel is a promising nonionizing imaging technique for early caries detection. At 1300 nm, the enamel is extremely

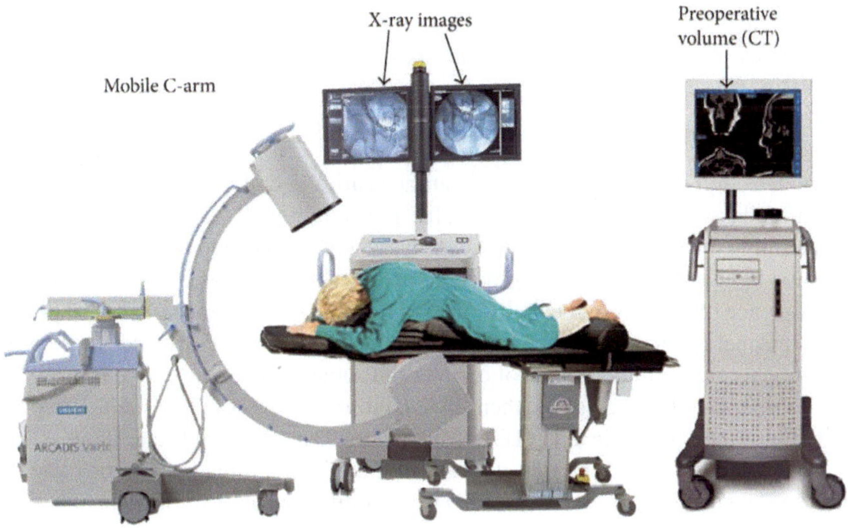

Fig. 6 C-arm imaging setup (Shao et al. 2014)

Table 6 Advantages and disadvantages of C-arm imaging

Advantages	Disadvantages
• High-quality 3D imaging • Minimally invasive • Real-time imaging • Reduced need for multiple images • Enhanced precision in surgical planning • Less distortion • Low radiation exposure (maximum—0.25 mSv for a 5-s exposure)	• Limited field of view • Expensive equipment • Requires trained personnel • Space requirement: C-arm units can be bulky and require a significant amount of space in the dental office • Patient discomfort

Table 7 Advantages and disadvantages of DIFOTI

Advantages	Disadvantages
• Noninvasive • Instant high-resolution image projection • Shows surface changes associated with early demineralization • Can detect even incipient, frank, and recurring caries • Operator can capture a full-mouth DIFOTI image in just 3 s	• Cannot measure depth of carious lesions • Cannot differentiate dental caries from stained fissures • Expensive

transparent in near-infrared spectrum. Scattering and absorption increase with greater mineral loss. Since less light reaches the detector, cavities appear as dark areas (Sikri 2019a).

(c) **Quantitative Light-Induced Fluorescence (QLF)**

Early detection of fissure and smooth surface caries is done using visible light. An argon ion laser emits a broad beam of blue-green light with wavelength of 488 nm, illuminating the tooth, while fluorescence is seen in the 540-nm range. To block out the blue light scattered by the tooth, a yellow high-pass filter is used to monitor the fluorescence of enamel in the yellow area (540 nm). The presence of chromophores in the enamel is what causes the fluorescence of the tooth structure. Due to a loss of chromophores, the fluorescence of carious and sound enamel differs.

Demineralized tissues glow intensely and absorb colors such as sodium fluorescein, Fluorol thioglycolic acid (TGA), and others. Dye-enhanced laser fluorescence is the term used to describe this. The actual image is captured using a tiny camera and displayed on a computer screen. Demineralization or early lesions appear as dark areas, while bacterial presence is indicated by the red color of caries and plaque (Sikri 2019a). The schematic setup of the QLF system is shown in Fig. 7.

Commercially available products: SOPROLIFE (Acteon Group, France); Inspektor Pro (Inspektor Dental Care, Amsterdam, the Netherlands).

The various advantages and disadvantages of QLF are enlisted in Table 8.

(d) **DIAGNOdent**

Principle of working: This gadget uses laser autofluorescence technology, except it uses red light with a wavelength of 655 nm rather than blue light. Caries is highlighted by the QLF system's output as having less fluorescence than a tooth that is in good condition. The light source is a diode laser that shines light onto a tooth's occlusal

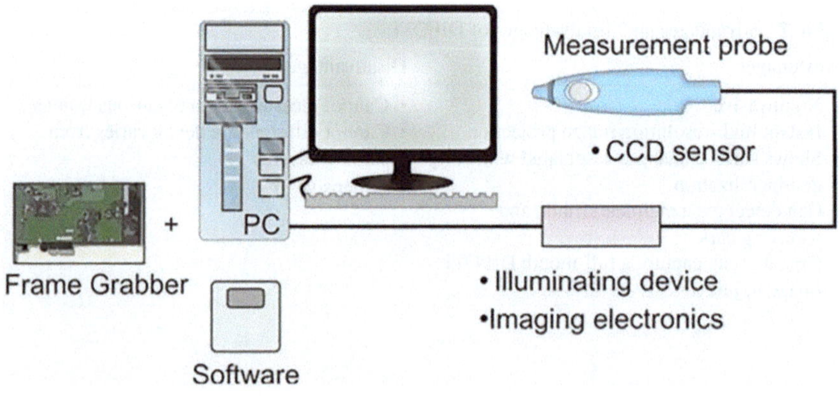

Fig. 7 Schematic setup of QLF system (Sikri 2019a)

Table 8 Advantages and disadvantages of QLF

Advantages	Disadvantages
• Quick and convenient to use • Identifies carious lesions and quantifies the mineral loss they cause • Detects early caries or mineral loss adjacent to orthodontic brackets and restorations • Identifies and measures natural lesions that are less than 1.0 mm in diameter and 5–10-mm deep; assesses preventive interventions • High sensitivity of laser excitation • Nondestructive technique • High spatial resolution • Selectively target specific compounds that exhibit fluorescence, making it useful for specific analytical applications • Can be used for both quantitative measurements (e.g., concentration determination) and qualitative analyses (e.g., identifying molecular structures) Minimal sample volume is sufficient	• Expensive • Cannot differentiate between caries and calculus • Interference from background fluorescence • Samples require specific preparation or conditioning to be suitable for fluorescence analysis • Some molecules may experience quenching (loss of fluorescence) under certain conditions • Environmental sensitivity to temperature, pH, or ionic strength • Not all compounds exhibit fluorescence, which limits the scope of analysis to only those that do • Photobleaching due to prolonged exposure to laser

surface at a wavelength of 655 nm via a fiber-optic bundle. Within a central fiber, the light is delivered to the angulated tip. To gather fluorescent light from oral hard tissues, several fibers are concentrically placed around the primary fiber. A filter removes the ambient and reflected light. The amount of fluorescence light that passes through the filter is measured by a photodiode (Sikri 2019a). After processing, this signal is shown on the screen as an integer between 0 and 99 accompanied by an audio beep (Fig. 8). The various advantages and disadvantages of this modality are enlisted in Table 9.

(e) **Infrared Fluorescence**

This method involves exposing the teeth to light (irradiation) that has a wavelength of 700–15,000 nm. Any ensuing fluorescence is observed using barrier filters. The

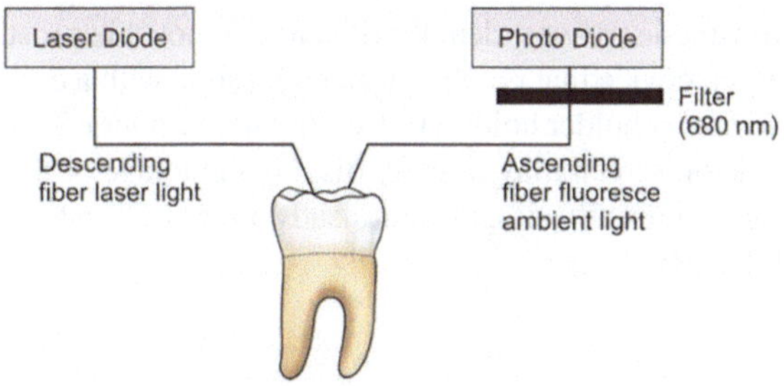

Fig. 8 Working principle of DIAGNOdent

Table 9 Advantages and disadvantages of DIAGNOdent

Advantages	Disadvantages
• Pit and fissure caries can be diagnosed with 90% accuracy • Sensitivity (0.92) is higher than that of an electronic caries monitor • Excellent dependability and reproducibility • Quick and simple to use • Easily transportable • Painless and noninvasive • Not subject to operator bias • Safe; no exposure to X-rays • Patient is involved in the examination process through interaction • Stored images can be reanalyzed and compared with newly acquired images	• Inaccurate results due to debris and plaque • Inability to differentiate between carious and hypomineralized structure • Quantity of dentinal deterioration has no bearing on the readings • Unsuitable for persistent dental cavities • Insufficient scientific proof that the severity of the disease and the numerical diagnostic reading are directly correlated • QLF gadget provides information on fluorescence loss rather than just the arbitrary value characteristic of DIAGNOdent

technique's ability to distinguish between carious and sound enamel and dentin has been proved. It has been somewhat challenging to identify a specific coherent source of this type of radiation. The identification relies on the use of infrared-sensitive detectors such as charge-coupled devices (CCDs) or film. Given the higher penetration and decreased dispersion of the longer wavelength, the heating effects of infrared irradiation absorption may have potentially harmful consequences on the dental pulp (Sikri 2019a).

Endoscopy/Videoscopy

The foundation of the endoscopic technique is the observation of the fluorescence that happens when a tooth is exposed to blue light with a wavelength between 400 and 500 nm. The fluorescence of carious and sound enamel differs from one another. White spot lesions appear darker than enamel when viewed using a particular broad-band gelatin filter on the fluoresced tooth. To observe the teeth without a filter, a fiber-optic connection can be used to link a white light source to an endoscope. "White light endoscopy" is the name given to this procedure.

It has been demonstrated that this method makes it possible to see tiny carious lesions in the enamel that are hard to see with the unaided eye. It also aids in the diagnosis of accidentally ingested tools such as rubber dam clamps, files and reamers, metallic cores, prosthetic crowns, dental drills, and removable prostheses.

A videoscope is a device that combines an endoscope with a camera. A specially designed metallic mirror holder holds a tiny color video camera. This is made in such a way that a television screen may directly display the image of the enamel surface (Silva 2015). The various advantages and disadvantages of endoscopy/videoscopy are enlisted in Table 10.

Table 10 Advantages and disadvantages of endoscopy/videoscopy

Advantages	Disadvantages
• Magnified image provided • Clinically feasible • Possible to store images on a camera	• Requires meticulous drying and isolation • Time consuming • Costly • Invasive procedure

Recent Advances/Newer Techniques

(a) Terahertz Imaging (THz)

Terahertz waves (THz), which have a wavelength of about 30 μm or a frequency of 1012 Hz, are used in this imaging technique. This waveform is long enough to avoid significant signal loss from scattering yet short enough to offer a respectable resolution. THz images can also be captured with a CCD detector (Fig. 9). This approach has shown promising results in dentistry (Cong, et al. 2023). The various advantages and disadvantages of THz imaging are mentioned in Table 11.

(b) Multiphoton Imaging

Tooth multiphoton imaging has been performed using infrared light ($\lambda = 850$ nm). A fluorescent chemical in the tooth is excited by a single "blue" photon in the traditional fluorescence imaging (QLF). However, the multiphoton approach involves the simultaneous absorption of two infrared photons, each of which has half the energy of a blue photon. At 200 MHz, 850-nm laser light is produced in ultrashort pulses (100 fs). Beam power is often in the multiwatt range. The fluorescence caused by two-photon excitation can be recorded from the focal plane by scanning a focused beam. A sequence of optical sections can be produced by altering the focal plane and then passing through the enamel and into the dentin.

Using this method, carious tooth tissue fluoresces far less than sound tooth tissue, which fluoresces robustly. Caries will show up as a dark shape inside a tooth that fluoresces strongly. The image may be shown in a negative form to draw attention to the diseased tissue, making caries in a dark tooth appear bright (Lin 2010). The advantages and disadvantages of multiphoton imaging are enlisted in Table 12.

Table 11 Advantages and disadvantages of terahertz imaging

Advantages	Disadvantages
• Human tissues are relatively sensitive to terahertz radiation • Imaging powers are low (~1 μW) • Nonionizing radiation is used • Tissues under examination do not change electrically, therefore there is little chance of harmful thermal repercussions	• Laser source has a complex nature • Precise manipulation required • Since water absorbs terahertz waves strongly, there is a risk of complications in the oral cavity while interpreting images • Expensive setup

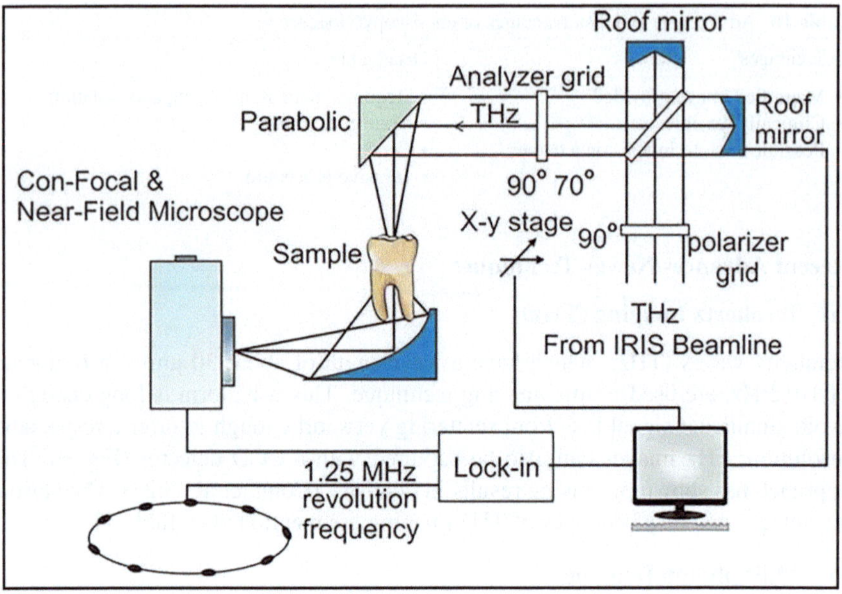

Fig. 9 Schematic diagram of THz scanning (Sikri 2019a)

Table 12 Advantages and disadvantages of multiphoton imaging

Advantages	Disadvantages
• Provides a 3D image • Noninvasive method • Greater depth of penetration (500 microns) because of the longer incident wavelength • Minimal risk of phototoxicity to the pulp because of the low average speed of laser power used Potential for assessment of mineral loss from a carious lesion in three dimensions as a function of fluorescence loss	• Currently, the procedure has only been used on extracted teeth Extensive research is still required in this less explored technique to create an image that can evolve into a form that can be used in clinical settings

(c) **Optical Coherence Tomography (OCT)**

It is an imaging method that can produce 2D or 3D images of subsurface tissue. It is possible to take advantage of the variations in polarization or dispersion between carious and sound enamel. It uses laser light with wavelengths between 840 and 1310 nm. As it enters the tissue, the light that emerges is measured with respect to its phase, which indicates how far it has traveled. Demineralization causes the tooth tissue's reflectance to drop. One way to quantify the change in the tissue's mineral status after demineralization is to look at the percentage change in reflectance. Superluminescent diodes are used as the light source in OCT devices. The degree of dispersion and potentially the degree of mineralization are related to the signal alterations. OCT has also been utilized to evaluate the contact between the tooth and the restoration. The noninvasive diagnosis of secondary caries may be affected by this (Hsieh 2013).

(d) Infrared Thermography

Kaneko et al. (1999) developed a technique based on water evaporation from the tooth surface to measure the extent of mineral loss and lesion depth on the flat surfaces of incisors with artificial lesions.

Technique: The tooth in question is dried, and thermal sensors (indium/antimony, which can detect temperature changes of up to 0.025 °C) are used to collect data on temperature variations. The demineralized areas or cavitated surfaces contain fluid that evaporates upon drying. A temperature drop proportional to the extent of the lesion is anticipated since the amount of water held inside the tooth will depend on the degree of enamel porosity and the length of dentin cavitation. The temperature change of the lesion is contrasted with that of the surrounding healthy tooth structure, while air is continuously flowing over the tooth's surface (Fig. 10).

Since there is little to no water collection at sound surfaces and fissures, thermodynamic effects are minimal or nonexistent. On the other hand, regions experiencing early demineralization will exhibit a longer evaporation period and a lower temperature across the entire surface (Zakian 2010).

(e) Frequency Domain Infrared Photothermal Radiometry (PTR) and Modulated Luminescence (LUM), Canary System

It is a dual-probe method that combines the benefits of modulated luminescence (LUM) and photothermal radiometry (PTR). Four signal channels are simultaneously produced by the PTR and LUM combined technique. The amplitudes and phases of photothermal and luminescence waves are produced in response to excitation from a harmonic laser source.

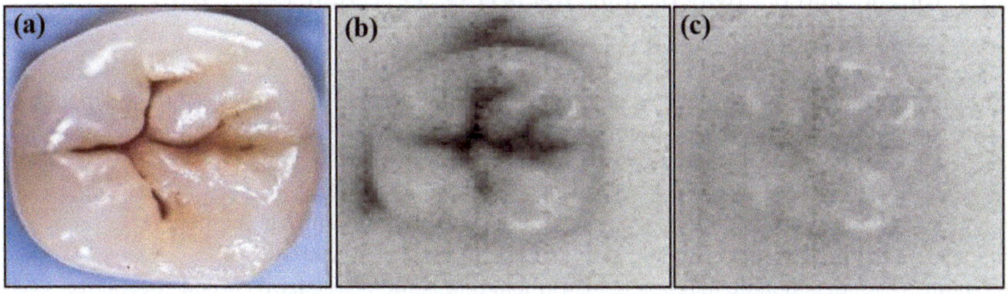

Fig. 10 **a** Depicts a colored image taken before the drying period (without forced drying), **b** thermal image taken during the drying period, where darkened regions correspond to areas with lower temperature, and **c** thermal image taken immediately after the drying period (without forced drying) (Zakian 2010)

When a lesion is developing, there is a corresponding change in the signal because the heat (PTR) is concentrated in the demineralized area, which lowers the luminosity (LUM). The tooth's thermal and LUM characteristics will progressively revert to those found in healthy tooth structure as the remineralization process proceeds.

The intensity, amplitude, and temporal difference or phase of the converted thermal energy and released light are all measured by the system. The Canary Number, which ranges from 0 to 100, is produced by processing the signals using an algorithm.

An explanation of the Canary Numbers:

0–20: Sound and healthy tooth structure.

21–70: Initial decay.

71–100: Advanced decay (Al Saffan 2023).

The various advantages of this technique are mentioned in Table 13.

(f) **Magnetic Resonance Imaging (MRI)**

Operating principle of MRI: MRI relies on the behavior of hydrogen protons within the magnetic field to generate high-quality cross-sectional images of the body using nonionizing electromagnetic radiation. The hydrogen protons in the patient spin on their axis normally. The nuclei of numerous atoms in the body, including hydrogen, align with the magnetic field's action when the patient is exposed to a strong magnetic field. The alignment of this magnetization is routinely changed from a longitudinal to a transverse plane by a radio frequency (RF) radiation that is directed toward the body structures and knocks the hydrogen protons. This causes the body to produce a revolving magnetic field that a scanner can detect (Fig. 11), which a computer then uses to create the MR image (Rotstein and Ingle 2023).

MRI in dentistry: After being utilized for medical diagnostics in humans for the first time in 1977, MR imaging gained interest for possible use in dentistry in the 1980s. In dentistry, MRI is typically utilized to diagnose conditions involving the temporomandibular joint, inflammatory conditions of the facial skeleton, salivary glands, maxillary sinuses, early bone changes like neoplasms, osteomyelitis, fractures, changes to the tongue and mouth floor, some cases of squamous cell carcinoma of the tongue, and pathway of sinus tracts (Fig. 12) (Niraj, et al. 2016).

Table 13 Advantages of frequency domain infrared photothermal radiometry (PTR) and modulated luminescence (LUM) imaging modality

Advantages
• Unlike previous photonic-based systems, it uses a depth profilometric method • Sensitive to changes in the sample's optical and thermal characteristics • Noninvasive, dependable diagnostic instrument that combines sensitivity and specificity • Can detect early lesions as tiny as 50 microns and up to 5 mm beneath the surface of the tooth • Can detect root caries, acid erosion lesions, occlusal pit and fissure caries, smooth surface caries, and interproximal carious lesions • Allows evaluation of demineralization and remineralization in early carious lesions (Al Saffan 2023)

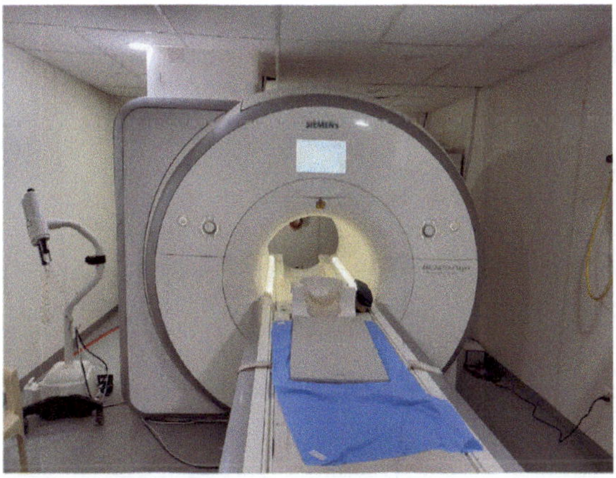

Fig. 11 Magnetic resonance imaging scanner

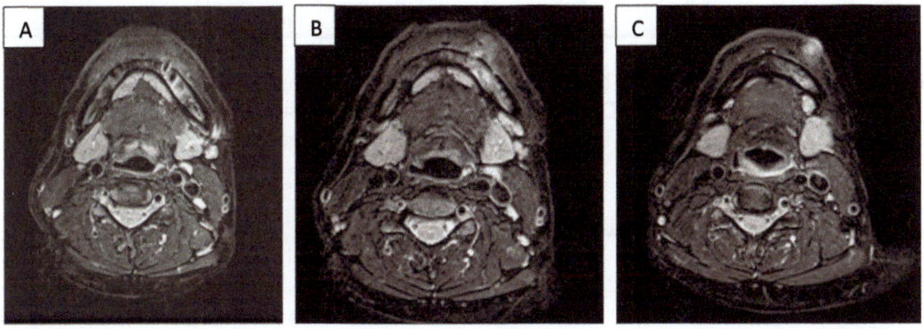

Fig. 12 MRI images (A, B, and C) showing oblique path of extraoral sinus tract arising from offending tooth in relation to 34, going till cutaneous surface of that region

With the advancement of techniques that enable imaging of hard tooth tissues including enamel, dentin, cementum, and bone, the potential applications of MRI in dentistry have grown. It is possible to successfully identify the number of roots in multirooted teeth, the thickness of the cortical bone, the degree of periapical lesions, and the smaller branches of the neurovascular bundle entering the apical foramina. Additionally, it can be applied to periodontal structures, dental implant planning (Fig. 13), and periapical surgery (Flügge 2023).

Sweep imaging with Fourier transformation (SWIFT), a newly developed MRI technique, solves many of the challenges associated with identifying quick relaxing signals. Without exposing patients to ionizing radiation, the method provides 3D study of both soft and hard tissues. Similar to MRI, this method is based on nuclear magnetic resonance (NMR) and uses a regulated magnetic field. Histological investigations have proven that the approach can create extremely precise 3D reconstructions of teeth and carious lesions in the lab. However, there is currently no clinical applicability for this technology (Rotstein and Ingle 2023). The various advantages and disadvantages of this imaging modality are enlisted in Table 14.

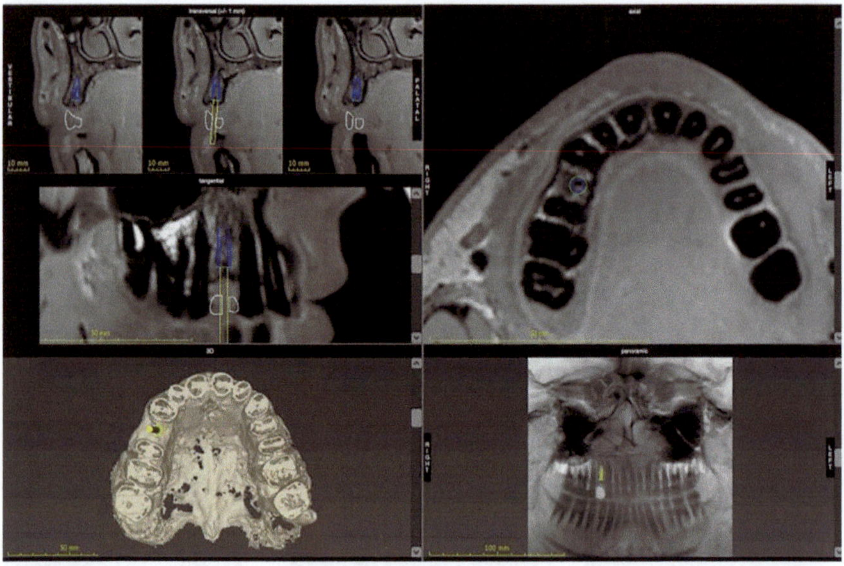

Fig. 13 Dental implant planning based on MRI with transversal, tangential, and axial cross sections, panoramic reconstruction, and 3D rendering. The missing dental surfaces in the 3D image, based on grey values, are also reversed in comparison with CBCT (Flügge 2023)

Table 14 Advantages and disadvantages of MRI

Advantages	Disadvantages
• No ionizing radiation used • A direct multiplane image can be obtained without the patient having to be reoriented • Good soft tissue spatial resolution • Safe for expectant mothers and infants • Image can be manipulated • Unaffected by artifacts from metallic restorations • Provide valuable information about pulp tissue vitality	• Requires excessive time • Metal present in the vicinity of the imaging magnet can be hazardous • Contraindicated in patients with pacemakers, cochlear implants, neurostimulators, and infusion pumps • Expensive • Not useful for assessing bony structures • Reduced patient comfort • Hard tissues such as enamel and dentin cannot be differentiated from one another or from metallic objects, since all appear radiolucent • Claustrophobia may affect patient's motion • Contrast materials can cause allergic tissue reactions

(g) **Ultrasonic Imaging (UI)**

Ultrasound (US) imaging, or ultrasonography, is being used to overcome computed tomography's drawbacks (high cost and higher radiation dose). It is based on the principle of reflection of sound waves, having a frequency higher than what humans

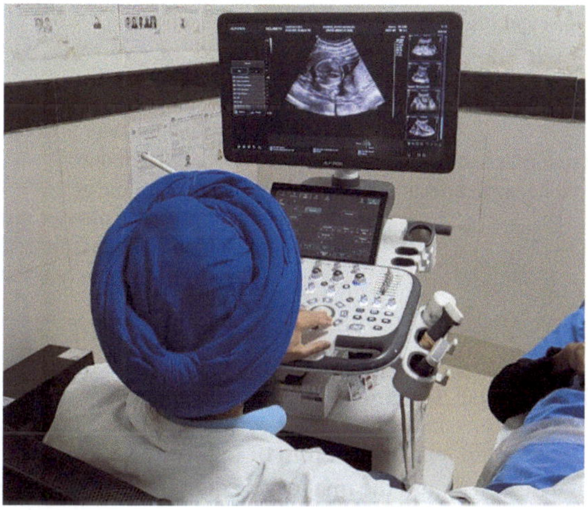

Fig. 14 Operator performing ultrasound examination

can perceive (1–20 kHz), due to the varying acoustic characteristics of tissue interfaces (Fig. 14). The transducer transforms the echoes into an electrical signal, which causes the screen to display white and gray tones.

- Low echo signal: dark spots
- High echo signal: bright/white spots
- Hypoechoic/transonic: low echo intensity
- Anechoic: no reflection of echoes; appears black (soft tissues, fluid-filled area)
- Hyperechoic: High echo intensity; appears white (bone).

US imaging was developed to identify early carious lesions on smooth surfaces. The ultrasonic pulse echo technique is used to measure the demineralization of natural enamel. It is found that the relative echo amplitude variations and the mineral content of the lesion body are correlated. In addition to sending longitudinal waves to the tooth's surface, the ultrasonic probe also has the ability to receive the waves. Surface echoes are either nonexistent or very feeble in the early stages of white spot lesions that only reach the enamel. The amplitude of the echoes produced by the sites with visible cavitation is significantly higher. This highly sensitive technique could serve as a substitute for radiographic caries detection on proximal surfaces (Reda 2021). Table 15 enlists various advantages and disadvantages of this imaging modality.

US imaging is successful in differentiating between a cyst and a granuloma by revealing the nature of bony lesion content:

- Cystic lesion: hypoechoic, well-contoured cavity surrounded by bony walls, filled with fluids (does not exhibit vascular supply in color Doppler examination)
- Granulomas: poorly defined lesion, can be hypo- or hyperechoic (exhibits vascular supply in color Doppler examination).

Table 15 Advantages and disadvantages of ultrasound imaging

Advantages	Disadvantages
• Identifies the underlying disease process accurately • Does not cause superimposition of structures • US waves have no negative effects	• US imaging cannot evaluate periapical lesions unless there is discontinuity in the buccal cortical bone • Provides a 2D image • Not feasible in posterior region because of thick cortical plate (thick cortical plate prevents US waves from traversing those areas)

(h) **LASER Optical Disc Storage**

A concentrated laser beam heats a thin film of tellurium suboxide at particular locations on the optical disc to record the image. The diagnostic advantage of laser optical disk storage is superior since it has a display and retrieval time of 0.5 s. It can store 10,000 photos on an 8-inch optical disk (Sikri 2019b).

(i) **Deep Learning (DL) and Artificial Intelligence (AI)**

One computer technology that has spurred the creation of artificial intelligence (AI) applications is deep learning (DL). DL is a type of neural network-based machine learning technique. Since the twentieth century, a neural network, which is a collection of algorithms with mathematical models that resemble the networks of neurons in the brain, has been the subject of extensive research. DL has proven to be beneficial in machine system control, natural language processing, predictive analytics, image analysis, and processing.

Since DL demands a high level of computer performance, it becomes difficult to provide accurate and thorough diagnoses in images that span a larger region. Consequently, a method for performing classification and cropping to a region of interest (ROI) from a larger X-ray image is preferred. This technique has been used to study DL categorization for a variety of anatomical features and diseases. Pathologies such as maxillary sinusitis, molar tooth root morphology, temporomandibular joint morphological abnormalities, and aspirated food and drinks in videofluorographic (VF) analysis of swallowing images are some among them (Fig. 15) (Katsumata 2023).

3 Classification Task

In dental practice, taking several intraoral periapical radiographs may occasionally make identification of the left and right sides, maxilla, and mandible quite challenging. Artificial intelligence can help with these tasks by utilizing well-known DL networks like LeNet and ResNet, which can recognize handwritten characters and numbers with a reasonable degree of accuracy (Fig. 16).

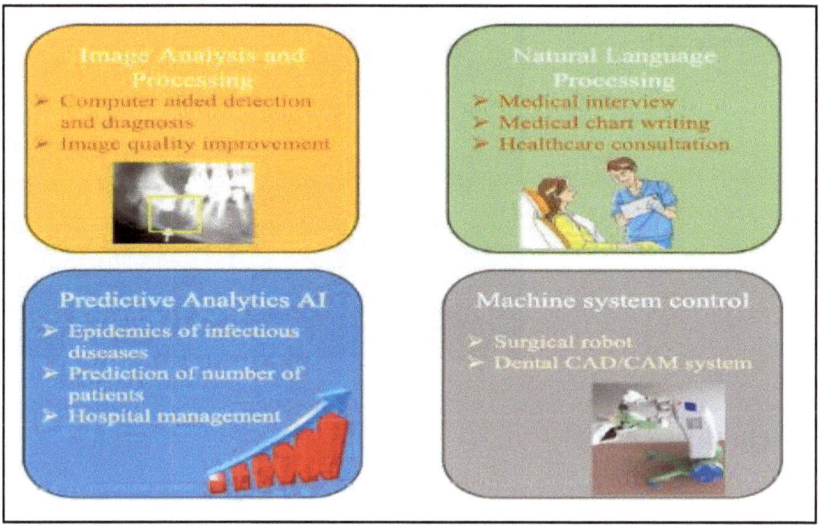

Fig. 15 Potential clinical applications of deep learning in dentistry (Katsumata 2023)

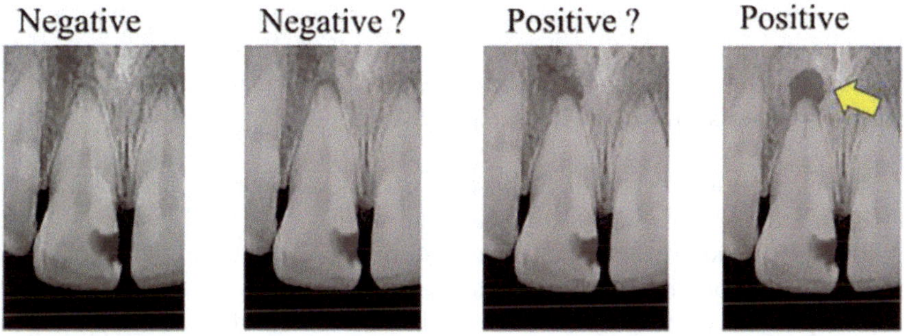

Fig. 16 Classification task showing development of periapical lesion (Katsumata 2023)

Region detection task: AI can automatically define a rectangular ROI in the objective images under DL after learning from a large number of manually annotated ROIs by experts (Fig. 17).

Segmentation task: It is a method that separates an image into objective segments. Semantic segmentation uses distinct colors to identify the objects to be chosen from the backdrop and other objects (Fig. 18).

The region detection or segmentation DL tasks are necessary to categorize positive and negative radiographic findings and develop relevant ROIs in every X-ray image. Every identified tooth is categorized based on its pathological and therapeutic condition, including the existence of dental implants, restorative, prosthetic, or endodontic therapies, eruption disorders, and tooth decay. This method is helpful for automatically gathering comprehensive data about a patient's dentition in addition to identifying dental diseases (Katsumata 2023).

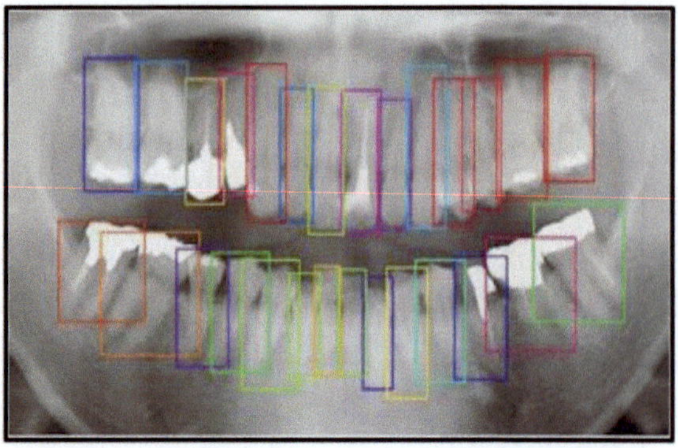

Fig. 17 Region detection task (Katsumata 2023)

4 Generative AI

DL models are used by generative AI to identify intricate patterns and produce new images that closely mirror the training data. Generative adversarial networks (GANs) can learn the underlying structures and properties from image datasets.

According to the reports, GANs can help reduce obstructive elements in dental CBCT images, which can impede accurate diagnosis and image interpretation. Artifacts from the oral prosthesis and image noise from the half-circle scan are examples of these obstructive variables. There have also been reports of using GANs to improve the blurry images that show up in the incisor region of panoramic radiography (Fig. 19).

Recent generative AI methods make it possible to organize training datasets, although their potential applications in dentistry have not yet been investigated. Deep learning and artificial intelligence still have potential to improve for use in dentistry. Therefore, it is crucial that the dental profession pursues the most recent technological developments in addition to basic clinical and research applications (Najjar 2023).

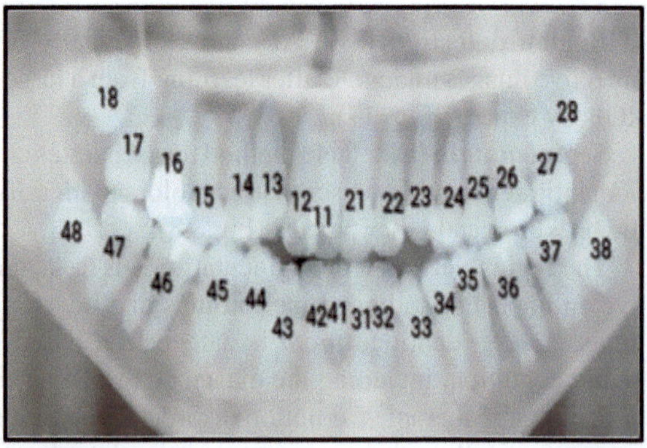

Fig. 18 Segmentation task (Katsumata 2023)

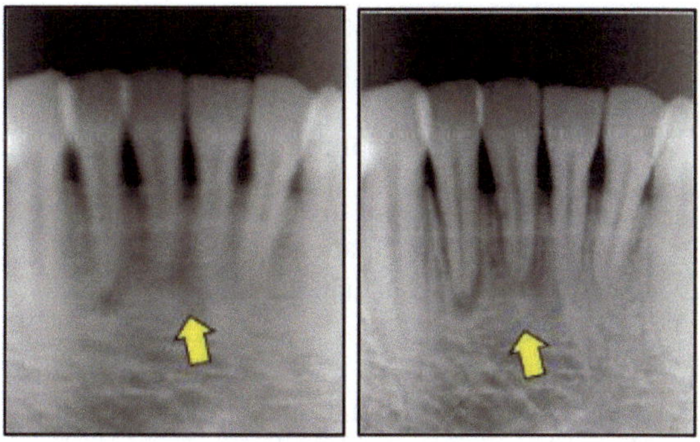

Fig. 19 Image processing by generative AI showing refinement of blurred images in a panoramic radiograph (Katsumata 2023)

5 Robotics

The twentieth century saw the introduction of the term "robot." In 1920, the Czech author Karel Čapek released *Rossum's Omnipotent Robots*, a science fiction script in which the word "robot" was originally derived from the Czech word "*robota*," which means "labor" or "drudgery." According to the American National Standards Institute, a "robot" is a "mechanical device that can be programmed and can perform certain operations and mobile tasks under automatic control" (Liu et al. 2023).

Each grayscale pixel in a 2D radiograph has an intensity or brightness that indicates the object's density. An AI algorithm may identify patterns and make predictions based on these features. A study on the detection and diagnosis of dental caries using a deep learning-based convolutional neural network (CNN) algorithm demonstrated remarkably high performance in detecting carious lesions in periapical radiographs (Lee et al. 2018).

Intelligent robots have now found usage in oral implantology in the following ways:

(1) Preoperative digital 3D scanning of the implant site and imaging data collection/ diagnosis analysis
(2) Digital implant surgery plan design
(3) Real-time navigation and automatic drilling during the operation to improve the accuracy of dental implant surgery, reduce surgical trauma, and shorten the operation time (Liu et al. 2023).

Most often, surgical resection is necessary for malignant lesions. Early diagnosis and detection of mucosal lesions are crucial for preventing surgery. Sometimes lesions with similar appearances need to be definitively diagnosed by biopsy or radiography. A study was conducted in which a CNN algorithm was applied to identify oral squamous cell carcinoma (OSCC) from confocal laser endomicroscopy images of patients who had been diagnosed with OSCC. The findings indicated that the CNN algorithm was effective for early SCC diagnosis (Aubreville et al. 2017) The CNN algorithm was also found to be successful in diagnosing cases of ameloblastoma and keratocystic odontogenic tumor (KCOT) (Poedjiastoeti and Suebnukarn 2018).

Furthermore, the CNN algorithm was also used to detect periodontal disorders such as periodontal bone loss (PBL), teeth with reduced periodontal health, etc. (Krois et al. 2019).

Despite the varied applications of robotics in dental diagnosis, it has certain disadvantages such as:

1. Potential risk for the patient
2. Lack of research data and guidelines
3. Trust issues
4. High cost
5. Security or privacy issues and ethical dilemmas
6. Unemployment in the dental sector
7. Responsibility, accountability, and liability
8. Inappropriate data quality (Kaur 2024).

6 Conclusion

Dental diagnoses and treatment planning have been transformed by recent developments in the imaging technologies. With proper use and interpretation of the right imaging technology, adherence to as low as reasonably achievable (ALARA) principles, and cost-effectiveness, newer radiographic techniques can help detect pathologies at earlier stages, ultimately reducing morbidity and mortality and improving the quality of life of the patients.

References

Al Saffan AD (2023) Current approaches to diagnosis of early proximal carious lesion: a literature review. Cureus (Preprint). https://doi.org/10.7759/cureus.43489

Astvaldsdóttir A et al (2012) Approximal caries detection by DIFOTI: In vitro comparison of diagnostic accuracy/efficacy with film and digital radiography. Int J Dent 326401. https://doi.org/10.1155/2012/326401

Aubreville M, Knipfer C, Oetter N, Jaremenko C, Rodner E, Denzler J (2017) Automatic classification of cancerous tissue in laser endomicroscopy images of the oral cavity using deep learning. Sci Rep 7:11979

Berman LH, Hargreaves KM (2020) Cohen's pathways of the pulp, 12th edn. Elsevier—Health Sciences Division, Philadelphia, PA

Bromberg N, Brizuela M (2025) Dental cone beam computed tomography. In: StatPearls. Treasure Island (FL): StatPearls Publishing

Cong M et al (2023) Biomedical application of terahertz imaging technology: a narrative review. Quant Imaging Med Surg 13(12):8768–8786. https://doi.org/10.21037/qims-23-526

Flügge T et al (2023) Dental MRI—only a future vision or standard of care? A literature review on current indications and applications of MRI in dentistry. Dentomaxillofacial Radiol 52(4):20220333. https://doi.org/10.1259/dmfr.20220333

Hekmatian E, Sharif S, Khodaian N (2025) Literature review: digital subtraction radiography in dentistry. https://www.emro.who.int/imemrf/drj_2005_2_2_106.pdf. Accessed 25 Jan 2025

Hsieh Y-S et al (2013) Dental optical coherence tomography. Sensors (Basel, Switzerland), 13(7): 8928–8949. https://doi.org/10.3390/s130708928
Kaneko K, Matsuyama K, Nakashima S (1999) Quantification of early carious enamel lesions by using an infrared camera in vitro. In: Stookey GK (ed) 4th Annual Indiana conference, pp 83–100
Katsumata A (2023) Deep learning and artificial intelligence in dental diagnostic imaging. Jpn Dent Sci Rev 59:329–333. https://doi.org/10.1016/j.jdsr.2023.09.004
Kaur K (2024) Artificial intelligence in robo dentistry: a double-edged sword. J Oral Med Oral Surg Oral Pathol Oral Radiol 10(2):88–92. https://doi.org/10.18231/j.jooo.2024.016
Krois J, Ekert T, Meinhold L, Golla T, Kharbot B, Wittemeier A (2019) Deep learning for the radiographic detection of periodontal bone loss. Sci Rep 9:116
Lee JH, Kim H, Jeong SN, Choi SH (2018) Detection and diagnosis of dental caries using a deep learning-based convolutional neural network algorithm. J Dent 77:106–111
Lin P-Y et al (2010) Imaging carious dental tissues with multiphoton fluorescence lifetime imaging microscopy. Biomed Opt Express 2(1):149–158. https://doi.org/10.1364/BOE.2.000149
Liu L, Watanabe M, Ichikawa T (2023) Robotics in dentistry: a narrative review. Dent J 11(3). https://doi.org/10.3390/dj11030062
Najjar R (2023) Redefining radiology: a review of artificial intelligence integration in medical imaging. Diagnostics (Basel, Switzerland) 13(17):2760. https://doi.org/10.3390/diagnostics13172760
Niraj LK et al (2016) MRI in dentistry—a future towards radiation-free imaging: systematic review. J Clin Diagn Res JCDR 10(10):ZE14–ZE19. https://doi.org/10.7860/JCDR/2016/19435.8658
Poedjiastoeti W, Suebnukarn S (2018) Application of convolutional neural network in the diagnosis of jaw tumors. Healthc Inf Res 24(3):236–241
Rajkumar B et al (2014) Dental implant placement using C-arm CT real-time imaging system: a case report. J Indian Prosthodont Soc 14(Suppl 1):308–312. https://doi.org/10.1007/s13191-014-0366-y
Reda R et al (2021) Ultrasound imaging in dentistry: a literature overview. J Imaging 7(11):238. https://doi.org/10.3390/jimaging7110238
Rotstein I, Ingle JI (eds) (2023) Ingle's endodontics, 7th edn. PMPH, Shelton, CT
Sakas G (2002) Trends in medical imaging: from 2D to 3D. Comput Graph 26(4):577–587. https://doi.org/10.1016/s0097-8493(02)00103-6
Shah N, Bansal N, Logani A (2014) Recent advances in imaging technologies in dentistry. World J Radiol 6(10):794–807. https://doi.org/10.4329/wjr.v6.i10.794
Shao Z, Guan Y, Tan J (2014) Virtual reality-aided positioning of mobile C-arms for image-guided surgery. Adv Mech Eng 6:943025. https://doi.org/10.1155/2014/943025
Sikri VK (2019a) Essentials of endodontics, 2nd edn. CBS Publishers & Distributors, New Delhi, India
Sikri VK (2019b) Textbook of conservative and restorative dentistry. CBS Publishers & Distributors, New Delhi, India
Silva RF (2015) Retrieving dental instruments through endoscopy: a literature review. World J Stomatol 4(4):137. https://doi.org/10.5321/wjs.v4.i4.137
Udoye CI, Jafarzadeh H (2010) Xeroradiography: Stagnated after a promising beginning? A historical review. Eur J Dent 4(1):95–99
Venkatesh E, Elluru SV (2017) Cone beam computed tomography: Basics and applications in dentistry. J Istanb Univ Fac Dent 51(3 Suppl 1):S102–S121. https://doi.org/10.17096/jiufd.00289
White SC, Pharoah MJ (2018) White and Pharoah's oral radiology: principles and interpretation, 8th edn. Mosby, London, England
Zakian CM et al (2010) Occlusal caries detection by using thermal imaging. J Dent 38(10):788–795. https://doi.org/10.1016/j.jdent.2010.06.010

Digital Dentistry

Amanurrahman Zubair Ahemad, Hariram Sankar, Sabah Zaheer, and Mohammad Muneeb Mubashir

1 Introduction

The applications of digital dentistry span various specialities, including prosthodontics, orthodontics, implantology, periodontics, and endodontics. These advancements have improved diagnostic accuracy, streamlined treatment processes, and optimised patient outcomes. The integration of intraoral scanners, cone beam computed tomography (CBCT), and artificial intelligence (AI)-driven analysis has further contributed to clinical efficiency and enhanced patient communication. However, despite its increasing adoption, digital dentistry remains underutilised in certain clinical settings due to financial barriers, steep learning curves, and varying levels of acceptance among practitioners. Additional concerns, such as data security, regulatory challenges, and the need for evidence-based validation of digital workflows, further complicate widespread implementation (Suganna et al. 2023).

Although existing research has explored specific aspects of digital dentistry such as computer-aided design/computer-aided manufacturing (CAD/CAM) applications, digital imaging, and AI-driven diagnostics, a comprehensive evaluation of its broader impact on accessibility, patient care, and clinical efficacy remains necessary. Furthermore, the role of emerging technologies, including cloud-based digital storage, AI-assisted diagnostics, and teledentistry, warrants further investigation as they continue to reshape modern dental practice. As the demand for minimally invasive and patient-centred treatments grows, understanding the implications of digital technology on

A. Z. Ahemad (✉) · H. Sankar
Department of Dentistry, All India Institute of Medical Sciences, Bathinda, India
e-mail: amanurrahman02@gmail.com

S. Zaheer
Department of Oral and Maxillofacial Surgery, Government Autonomous College of Dentistry, Indore, India

M. M. Mubashir
Department of Dentistry, Government Medical College Handwara, Kupwara, India

A. Gupta et al. (eds.), *Application of Robotics in Dentistry*, Lecture Notes in Bioengineering, https://doi.org/10.1007/978-981-95-1470-0_6

clinical decision-making, patient satisfaction, and treatment efficiency is essential (Umer et al. 2025).

2 Principle and Scope of Digital Dentistry

Digital dentistry is based on precision, efficiency, patient-centred care, and the integration of advanced technologies to enhance treatment outcomes. The domain of digital dentistry not only encompasses diagnostics and treatment but also impacts education, research, and interdisciplinary collaboration. This encompasses multiple disciplines, such as prosthodontics, orthodontics, periodontics, endodontics, and implantology, transforming clinical workflows and enhancing patient experiences.

Fundamental Principles of Digital Dentistry

- Digital imaging and scanning technologies, such as cone beam computed tomography (CBCT), intraoral scanners, and digital radiography, yield high-resolution three-dimensional (3D) images that enhance diagnostics and treatment planning.
- Computer-aided design/computer-aided manufacturing (CAD/CAM) facilitates digital impressions, prosthetics, and restorations, allowing for expedited chairside fabrication (Suganna et al. 2023).
- Advancements in additive and subtractive manufacturing techniques, such as 3D printing and milling, facilitate the customisation of prosthetic and orthodontic appliances (Rakhshan et al. 2018).
- Artificial intelligence (AI) in diagnostics employs machine learning algorithms to facilitate early disease detection, automate treatment planning, and enhance clinical decision-making.
- Teledentistry and digital communication enable remote diagnosis, consultation, and patient monitoring, thereby enhancing healthcare accessibility.

Benefits of Digital Dentistry

1. **Precision and accuracy**: Digital tools, including intraoral scanners, cone beam computed tomography (CBCT), and digital radiography, yield highly detailed images of dental structures. These technologies facilitate precise diagnoses and treatment planning, thereby enhancing the quality of patient care.
2. **Streamlined workflow and chairside dentistry**: Digital workflows enhance dental procedures by minimising the time needed for impressions, restoration fabrication, and orthodontic treatment planning. CAD/CAM technology facilitates same-day restorations, permitting patients to obtain crowns, veneers, or bridges within a single appointment.
3. **Improved patient experience**: Digital imaging and virtual simulations enhance patient education by facilitating visualisation of treatment plans. This enhances patient engagement and satisfaction by improving their understanding of dental conditions and treatment options.

4. **Advanced treatment modalities**: Technologies such as 3D printing and digital orthodontics facilitate the creation of highly tailored dental restorations and aligners. This has revolutionised prosthodontics and orthodontics, resulting in enhanced treatment outcomes and increased aesthetic appeal.

Challenges in Digital Dentistry

- **Higher expenses**: The implementation of CBCT, CAD/CAM systems, and 3D printing technologies requires substantial financial investment, which restricts accessibility for small dental practices (1).
- **Training and learning curve analysis**: Specialised training is necessary for clinicians to effectively integrate digital workflows, presenting a challenge for traditional practitioners.
- **Concerns regarding data security and storage**: The growing dependence on cloud-based records and AI-assisted diagnostics has heightened cybersecurity risks, which continue to be a significant concern.

3 Applications of Digital Dentistry

1. **Digital Smile Design**

The efficacy of aesthetic dental treatments is significantly influenced by smile aesthetics. The primary objective is to perform a thorough facial and dental evaluation that effectively addresses patient concerns by assessing both the smile and facial structure. An aesthetic analysis should include three primary components: dental, dentogingival, and facial aesthetics. Both manual and digital methods can be employed to design a smile. In recent years, a variety of Digital Smile Design (DSD) software programs have been incorporated into clinical practice and research, thereby improving communication, increasing treatment predictability, and augmenting diagnostic accuracy (Alharkan 2024; Jafri et al. 2020).

An innovative approach to modern dentistry, DSD incorporates digital technology into the aesthetic planning of dental treatments. It allows clinicians to utilise sophisticated imaging, software modelling, and digital simulations to devise, predict, and communicate treatment outcomes prior to performing any irreversible procedures (Jain et al. 2024). This patient-centred approach improves patient engagement and satisfaction, facilitates interdisciplinary collaboration among dental specialists, and enhances diagnostic precision (Thomas et al. 2022).

The demand for aesthetic outcomes that are predictable and personalised has increased as a result of the increasing number of patients who are interested in advanced treatment options. By utilising technology, interdisciplinary collaboration, and patient engagement, DSD fulfils these expectations. The subsequent sections investigate the applications, advantages, and potential future advancements of DSD in the field of modern dentistry.

Historical Evolution and Pioneers in the Field

Smile design as a concept has evolved considerably over the past few decades, transitioning from analogue techniques to advanced digital workflows. In the past, dentists would manually draw concepts on printed photographs to illustrate potential outcomes. The accuracy of this analogue approach was inadequate, and it was difficult to establish a connection with genuine dental models (Jafri et al. 2020). The first digital two-dimensional (2D) smile design attempts were made possible by the emergence of accessible digital photography and software in the early 2000s. For instance, programs such as Microsoft PowerPoint or Photoshop were employed to redraw dental enhancements on photographs. A significant advancement was made when these 2D designs were able to be correlated with physical models and subsequently with 3D digital models, thereby bridging the distance between a flat image and actual dentition. Dentists are now able to design smiles in three dimensions with facial movement in mind, as DSD has evolved into fully integrated 3D operations and even exploratory '4D' conceptions that incorporate motion.

Dr Christian Coachman, a Brazilian dentist, is largely acknowledged as the originator of the Digital Smile Design idea, which he presented and popularised in 2007. Coachman, together with others like Marcelo Calamita, established DSD as a systematic methodology for aesthetic treatment planning in the late 2000s and early 2010s. Their 2012 study highlighted DSD as a novel multifunctional tool for diagnostic and visual communication in aesthetic dentistry. Coachman classified the progression of grin design into 'generations', ranging from entirely analogue procedures to the advanced digital and multidisciplinary methodologies now employed. These innovators showed that the utilisation of digital pictures, films, and CAD/CAM technology enables dentists to attain an enhanced level of accuracy in smile makeovers. Today, DSD advances its mission by integrating artistic dental concepts with advanced imaging technology, a legacy that continues to influence contemporary cosmetic and restorative dentistry (Thomas et al. 2022).

Principles of DSD: DSD is based on aesthetics and usefulness. It ensures that any smile augmentation matches the patient's facial features and oral health needs, not just the teeth. Visual appeal, symmetry, and functional elements including occlusal alignment, phonetics, and long-term health are fundamental. A DSD plan must consider the patient's smile, speech, and mastication, as well as teeth, gums, lips, and face. Digital Smile Design combines aesthetics and biology to create a grin that is appealing, fits the person, and works well.

Key smile design parameters: In Digital Smile Design, dentists evaluate several levels of aesthetics, often categorised as facial, gingival, macro, and micro aspects of the smile. These parameters help ensure a comprehensive analysis: from the broadest view of the face down to the finest tooth details.

- **Facial aesthetics**: This includes the patient's face and smile integration. Dentists consider face shape, symmetry, and proportions while creating smiles (Fig. 1). The facial midline, interpupillary line, and lip line determine tooth location and angulation. The smile is evaluated for facial features such as the dental midline aligning with the face midline and the grin arc matching the lower lip curvature.

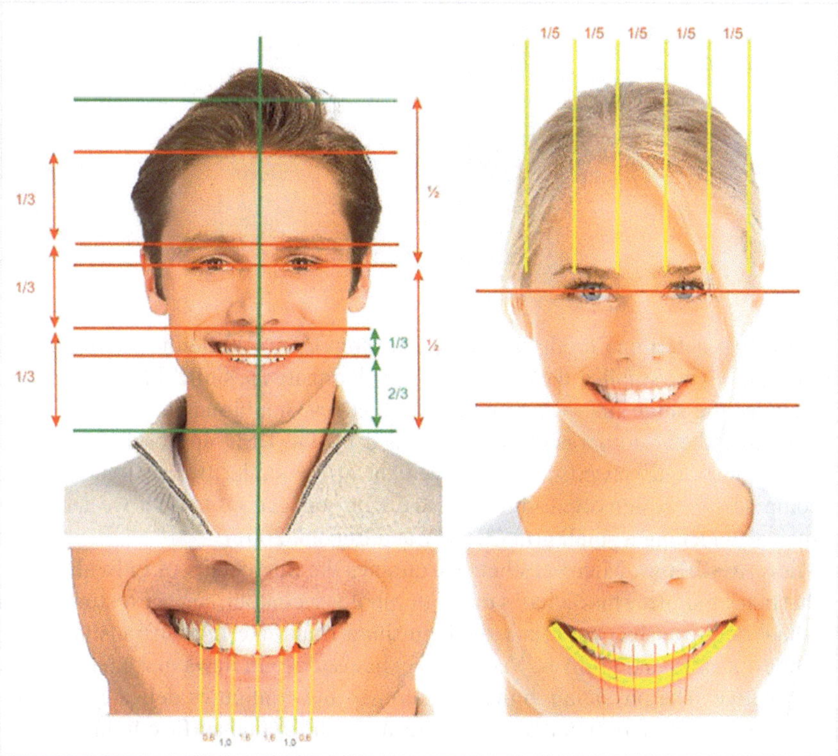

Fig. 1 Illustration depicts facial and dental proportions, highlighting symmetry, golden ratio divisions, and optimal aesthetic measures for a harmonious smile and facial balance

Misalignment with the face or lips makes teeth seem bad. Thus, facial aesthetics provide a thorough foundation for DSD, emphasising that teeth must match the individual's facial shape.

- **Gingival aesthetics**: Since gums support teeth, their shape and health affect grin aesthetics. This metric measures gum visibility when smiling as well as the gingival line, the upper gum contour. The best gingival presentation is balanced and symmetrical; a 'gummy smile', or uneven gum heights, may damage attractiveness (Fig. 2). In DSD, doctors check if the gingival borders of linked teeth, such as anterior incisors or canines, are aligned and if the tissue matches the smile. To create an attractive gingival framework, the DSD plan may include gum contouring or crown lengthening if gum visibility or irregular shapes are severe. An attractive smile requires healthy, pink, and well-shaped gums (Impellizzeri et al. 2023).
- **Macro-aesthetics**: Macro-aesthetics emphasises the smile's size, shape, and location of the teeth, lips, and gums. Arch form, tooth size ratios, and neighbouring tooth relationships are included. Grin breadth, buccal corridors, and tooth-to-tooth proportions like the golden proportion or recurrent aesthetic dental (RED)

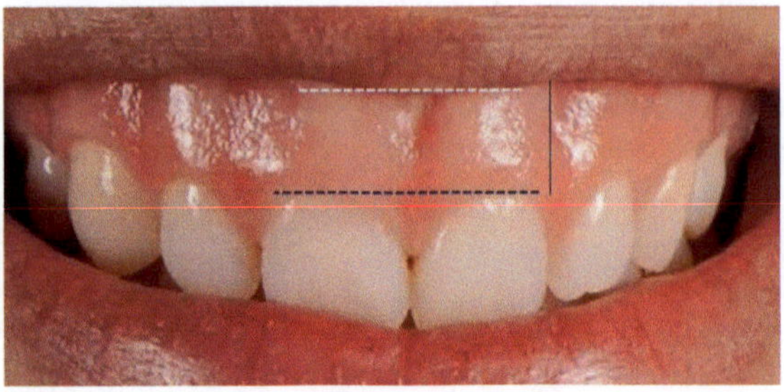

Fig. 2 Gingival exposure while smiling. Courtesy: Impellizzeri et al. (2023)

ratios that determine tooth dimensions are important. While the lateral incisors and canines are smaller, the central incisors dominate the smile. Macro-aesthetics includes the smile line, where upper tooth edges should match lower lip curve. Macro-aesthetic components are examined by the DSD approach to ensure a harmonious and natural tooth arrangement in the smile. Before treatment, the computerised design often adjusts these bigger connections to improve aesthetics, such as widening a small grin (Morley and Eubank 2001).

- **Micro-aesthetics**: Micro-aesthetics examines the tiny details of individual teeth that make a smile. This includes tooth morphology, contour, surface texture, colour (shade and translucency), and distinguishing traits like incisal translucency or white speckles and grooves. Variations in hue and slight flaws make natural teeth distinctive. The physician digitally examines and configures delicate properties such as incisal margin curvature, embrasures, and dental surface light reflection in DSD. Micro-aesthetic planning may need a restoration to have a certain margin translucency or line angle to match adjacent teeth or mimic youthfulness. DSD provides mathematically precise and lifelike results by emphasising on micro-aesthetics. Veneers, crowns, and restorations should match the patient's natural dentition and facial features down to the last detail (Lekha et al. 2019).

Each case is assessed for facial, gingival, macro, and micro-aesthetic parameters by Digital Smile Design to create a harmonious smile. A comprehensive aesthetic vision guides all treatments (veneers, braces, gum surgery, etc.), ensuring the end is attractive, natural, and consistent with the patient's face traits and personality. In addition, DSD's concentration on visualisation ensures that functional features like occlusion and phonetics are considered alongside aesthetics, resulting in smile designs that are both attractive and long-lasting.

4 DSD Workflow and Technology

Modern Digital Smile Design employs a step-by-step digital workflow that integrates photography, 3D imaging, and computer-aided design/computer-aided manufacturing (CAD/CAM) technology. The process is highly visual and data-driven, ensuring that the envisioned smile can be turned into reality with precision. Below is a breakdown of a typical DSD workflow and the technologies involved:

Step 1: Acquisition of digital records—The DSD procedure commences with the collection of exhaustive patient records in digital format. It is imperative to obtain high-quality digital photographs of the patient's teeth and visage, as these images serve as the foundation for smile design. Standard photographs consist of full-face views (both smiling and at repose), close-up smile views, and retracted intraoral photographs of the teeth from a variety of angles. In addition, numerous DSD practitioners record brief videos of the patient speaking and beaming, which offer dynamic information. This aids in the evaluation of the patient's overall facial expressions, lip mobility, and dental display during speech. A digital intraoral scan of the teeth is obtained using an intraoral scanner (if available) in conjunction with photographs to generate a precise 3D model of the patient's dentition. Traditional plaster models and impressions are supplanted by this 3D scan. In certain instances, a 3D CBCT scan or facial scan may be employed to capture the bone structure or a 3D representation of the patient's face, particularly in complex cases such as orthognathic planning or implants. The foundation for digital smile planning is comprised of all of these documents, including photographs, videos, 3D tooth models, and any radiographic data. It is essential that the records are taken in a standardised manner and are accurate, as any distortion in the design can result from an error in the scan or photo angle. The data is imported into specialised DSD software for analysis after it has been collected.

Step 2: Analysis of smile and digital design—Upon loading the patient's images and models digitally, the dentist or a digital lab specialist conducts a smile analysis and initiates the design of the new smile. Initially, reference lines are established on the photographs, such as a horizontal line through the pupils or lips for orientation and a vertical midline through the face. The alignment of the teeth is guided by these factors in the design. The present smile is assessed in relation to aesthetic standards. Are the teeth misaligned or asymmetrical? Is the curvature of the smile line appropriate? What is the extent of gingival display? The clinician utilises DSD software to create guidelines and shapes on photographs for the purpose of visualising corrections. Digital measurements commonly encompass the dimensions of teeth, the positioning of the incisal edge in relation to the lip, and the symmetry of gingival contours. Following this analysis, the dentist modifies the smile digitally, such as by adjusting the length of teeth, spacing, or gingival contour in the image. Numerous DSD software tools include libraries of tooth shapes, enabling dentists to superimpose a proposed set of digital teeth onto the patient's photograph or 3D model (Fig. 3). This process functions as a digital wax-up conducted via computer software. The practitioner chooses optimal tooth shapes, such as slightly rounded incisors for a softer appearance, organises them to address misalignment or gaps, and verifies that the arrangement aligns with the facial context. This stage involves consideration of both aesthetic and functional factors, such as ensuring that the occlusion remains effective following the proposed changes. The capacity to manipulate a virtual model allows for rapid exploration of various design alternatives. Certain systems facilitate a two-dimensional smile simulation on photographs, whereas more sophisticated systems combine the two-dimensional design with three-dimensional tooth models, enabling two-and-a-half-dimensional or three-dimensional simulations. The outcome of this phase is a proposed smile design, comprising digital plans that include photographic mock-ups, measurements, and 3D designs to depict the potential appearance of the patient's new smile (Sanchez-Lara et al. 2019).

Step 3: Digital mock-up and visualisation—Upon completion of the preliminary design, the subsequent step involves creating a mock-up to facilitate a more concrete visualisation. Several approaches exist in this context. The dentist frequently generates a two-dimensional digital mock-up by modifying the patient's photograph, thereby illustrating a before-and-after comparison of the smile (Fig. 4). Numerous DSD systems produce a realistic image of the patient smiling with the suggested dental arrangement, which can be displayed on a screen or tablet. The experience of observing one's own face with a new smile serves as a significant moment for patients, as it renders the potential outcome tangible. In addition to 2D images, DSD may also encompass the creation of a 3D mock-up. The digital design, represented as a 3D model of ideal teeth, can be converted into a physical form through CAD/

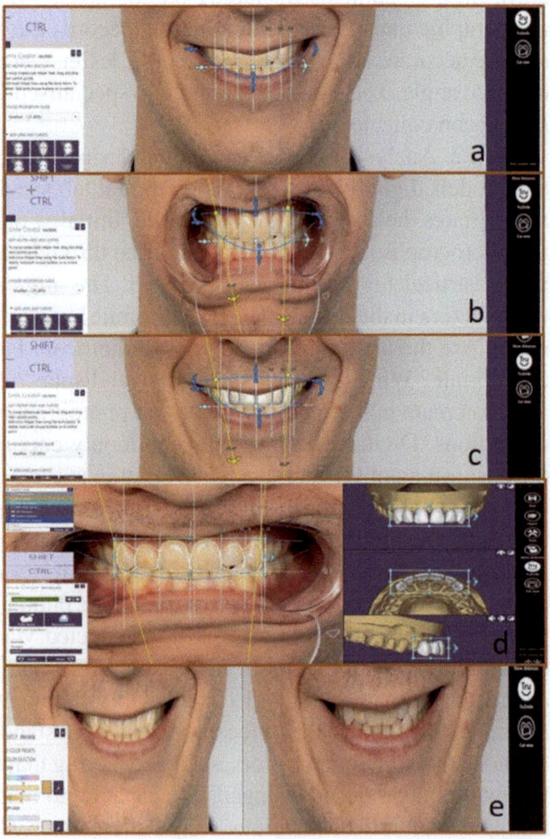

Fig. 3 Exocad 3D smiling design: **a** and **b** illustrate face and intraoral reference lines, **c** combines face and dental analysis, **d** shows 3D optimal dental outlines, and e compares digital smile to original

CAM technology. The dentist can utilise 3D printing or milling techniques to create a model or a set of temporary overlay veneers, commonly referred to as a 'trial smile' or wax-up, according to the specified design. The 3D printed resin mock-up can be temporarily placed in the patient's mouth using a clear stent to transfer composite resin, allowing the patient to evaluate the new smile. The mock-up stage is essential for visual communication, allowing the patient to visualise and experience the proposed outcome prior to committing to the treatment. This also enables the dentist to confirm that the design is functionally effective in practical applications. At this stage, modifications remain straightforward; for example, if a tooth appears excessively elongated or the patient perceives the shape as incorrect, the design can be adjusted in the software, and a new mock-up can be produced.

Step 4: **Patient presentation and feedback**—DSD is highly patient-centric. The dentist will present the Digital Smile Design to the patient, often using a slide show, simulation video, or mirror with the mock-up in place. This is usually done in a consultation appointment dedicated to reviewing the planned smile. Because the patient sees a clear visualisation of the outcome, it opens a two-way dialogue: The patient can express likes or concerns, and the dentist can educate the patient on the treatment needed to achieve that result. Patients are encouraged to give feedback—for example, a patient might say 'I love the shape of these teeth, but can we make them a shade whiter?' or 'I feel the canines are too pointy', etc. This collaboration ensures the final plan aligns with the patient's aesthetic preferences and expectations. Involving patients at this stage greatly increases case acceptance and

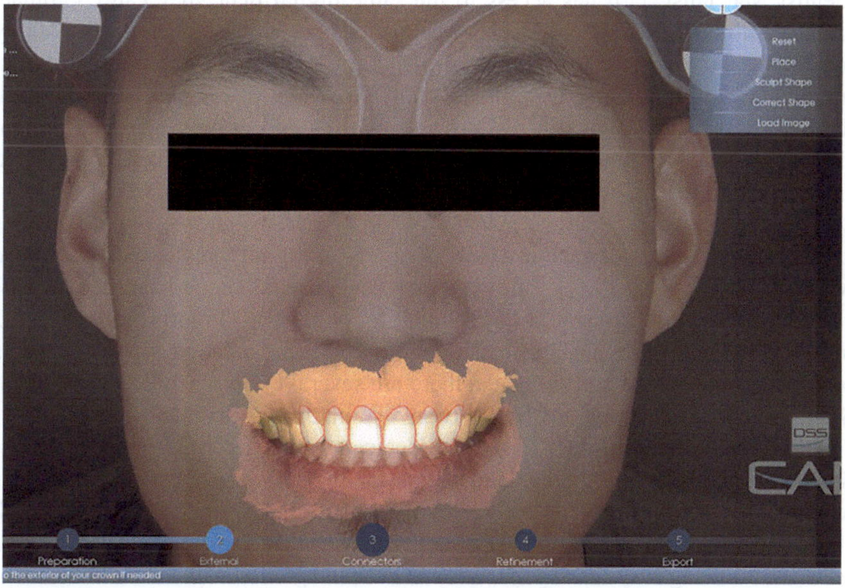

Fig. 4 Overlay of pretreatment scan and facial image. Proposed digital waxing is based on scans and correlated with smile photographs. Courtesy: Sanchez-Lara et al. (2019)

satisfaction, because they have a voice in designing their own smile. It also manages expectations: the dentist can clarify what's realistic and adjust the plan accordingly, thereby avoiding misunderstandings (since purely digital images can sometimes set unrealistically high hopes if not tempered with clinical context). Many clinicians report that once patients see the potential result through DSD, they become more motivated and confident to proceed with the necessary treatments, since the end goal is clear and personalised to them. Essentially, this step turns treatment planning into a collaborative and engaging experience, rather than a dentist-directed monologue.

Step 5: **Treatment planning and execution**—After the patient approves the proposed design, the DSD plan is translated into a concrete treatment plan. This often involves an interdisciplinary approach—for example, orthodontic alignment first, then restorative work, or gum surgery followed by veneers, etc., depending on what the design requires. The digital design acts as a blueprint for all these procedures. With the final smile design data, the dentist and lab technician can proceed to fabricate the actual restorations using CAD/CAM technology (Fig. 5). For instance, if porcelain veneers or crowns are part of the plan, the lab can use the digital tooth shapes to mill or 3D-print restorations that match the design exactly. If orthodontics is needed, the orthodontist can use the target tooth positions from the DSD plan to guide bracket placement or clear aligner set-up. In surgical cases (like implants or periodontal surgery), surgical guides can be designed and printed in accordance with the DSD outcomes (for example, a guide to ensure an implant is placed such that the final crown will emerge at the right spot defined in the smile design). Throughout execution, DSD also introduces quality control—since every practitioner involved (dentist, specialist, lab) has access to the same digital plan, they can coordinate more seamlessly. Adjustments during treatment can be checked against the plan by overlaying intraoral scans or photos of preparatory work onto the original design for comparison. In the end, because the entire workflow was digitally orchestrated, the delivered result (final veneers, crowns, etc.) should closely match the initial simulation, barring minor fine-tuning. The patient then gets to see the predicted smile become reality, which is a rewarding finale to the DSD process (Alharkan 2024).

Technology and software in DSD: A variety of digital tools support the above workflow at each stage. Key hardware includes a digital single-lens reflex (SLR) camera (or high-quality smartphone camera) for photos, an intraoral scanner for 3D impressions, and often a 3D printer or milling unit for creating physical models or restorations. On the software side, there are several options available for Digital Smile Design. Some popular DSD software and platforms include:

DSD App (Coachman's DSD App): A dedicated application developed by Christian Coachman's team to guide dentists through the smile design steps. It provides templates for facial analysis, automatic alignment guides, and a library of tooth shapes, making the process more standardised. The DSD App integrates with cloud services, allowing easy sharing of cases and even integration with the DSD Planning Center for expert input (Fig. 6). The program, available just for iPad and MacBook (M1 series or later), allows users to model realistic and attainable grin alterations, hence improving patient communication and clinical results. It supports treatment

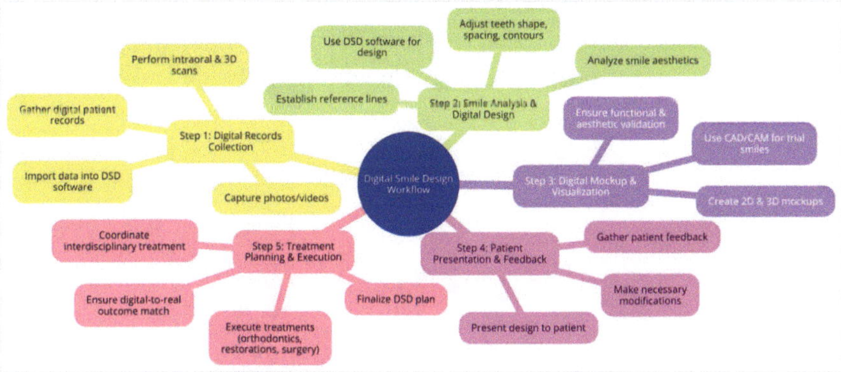

Fig. 5 Workflow of digital smile designing

planning, helps create unique smile designs in two dimensions with only ten simple steps, assists in the planning of both aesthetic and practical restorations based on the dimensions of the face, and encourages the practice of orthodontics, prosthodontics, and cosmetic dentistry (Thomas et al. 2022).

- **Adobe Photoshop (with Smile Design add-ons)**: Many practitioners use graphic design software like Photoshop to perform 2D smile editing on patient photos. Photoshop allows layering of images (for example, overlaying an image of ideal teeth onto the patient's smile) and precise control of colours and shapes (Fig. 7). While it requires more manual work and skill, it has been a go-to tool especially before specialised dental software became common. Dentists can import a patient's portrait and use lines and shapes to simulate changes (for example, using the lasso tool to widen a smile or the clone tool to adjust gumlines). It is very flexible, though not dental-specific (Sundar 2018; McLaren 2018).
- **Planmeca Romexis® Smile Design**: This is a module within Planmeca's Romexis dental software suite. It allows 2D smile design on photographs and can integrate with Planmeca's 3D scanners and CAD/CAM systems for a seamless flow from design to fabrication (Fig. 8). Romexis Smile Design is more user-friendly for dentists than generic software, offering guided steps to mark facial reference lines and automatically suggest tooth proportions.
- **Smile Designer Pro (SDP)**: A standalone smile design software (by Tasty Tech Ltd) that provides an intuitive interface for importing patient photos and designing smiles digitally. It has tools for drawing guidelines, adjusting tooth outlines, and creating before/after presentations. Smile Designer Pro focuses on 2D design but can also integrate with 3D data to some extent. It is known for being relatively easy to learn and effective for patient presentations (Fig. 9).
- **Digital Smile System (DSS)**: Italian dentists created the Digital Smile System (DSS) to improve Digital Smile Design (DSD). DSS simplifies and professionalises smile design for dental practitioners by integrating and developing DSD tools like Keynote (Fig. 10). DSS gives dentists exact smile aesthetic control

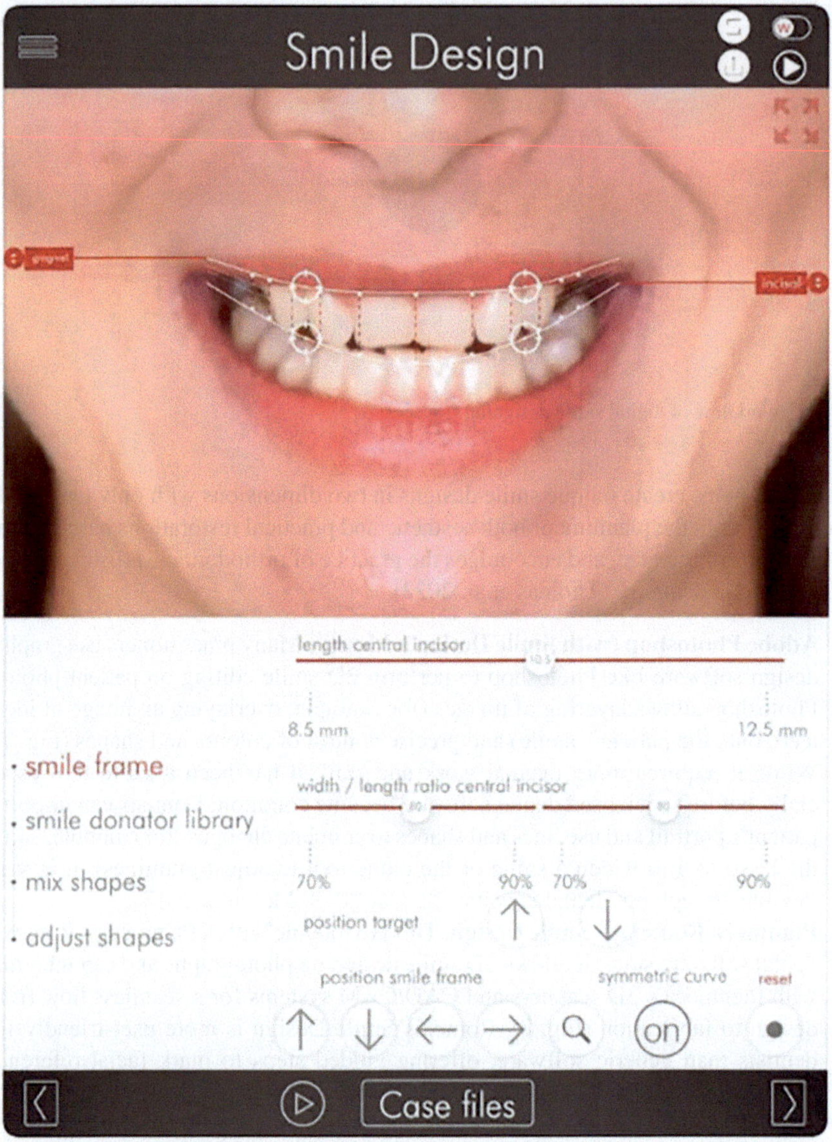

Fig. 6 Screenshot of DSD App by Christian Coachman

with enhanced features beyond traditional presentation software. DSS automatically creates a detailed report on smile design parameters after completion. This report helps dental technicians make restorations that match the design. DSS's clinician-focused interface makes smile design easy even for digital design novices.

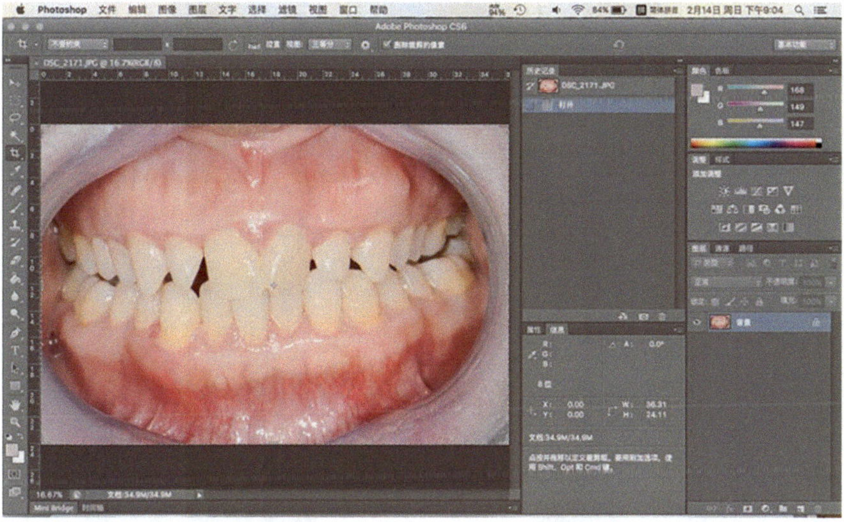

Fig. 7 Interface of photoshop software. Courtesy: Liu et al. (2012)

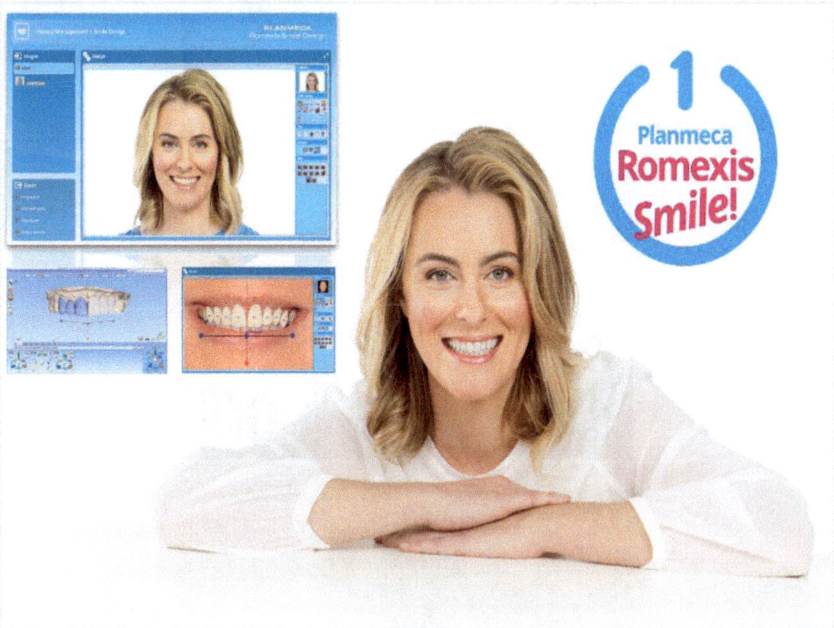

Fig. 8 Interface of Planmeca Romexis®

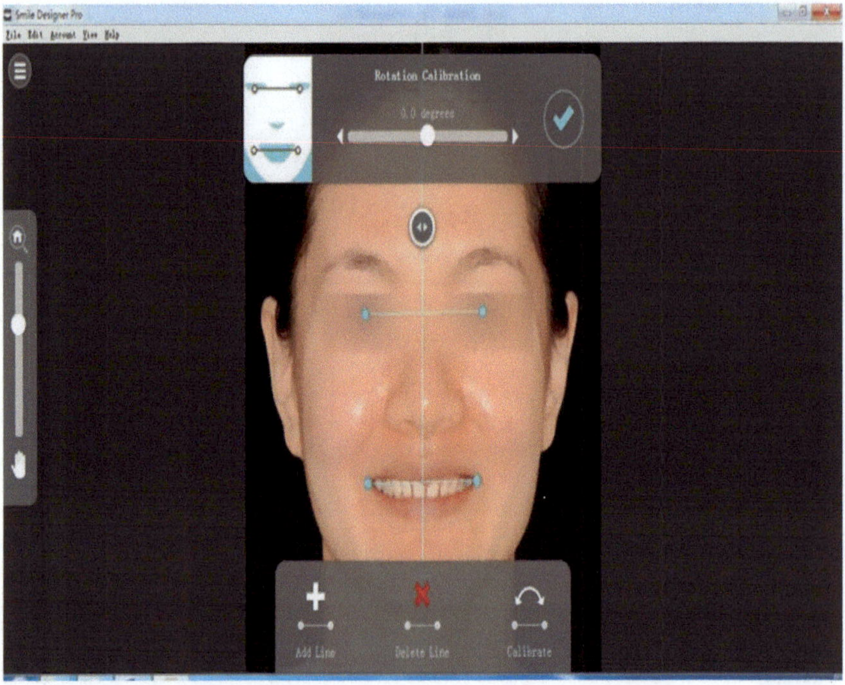

Fig. 9 Workflow of smile design software. Courtesy: Liu et al. (2012)

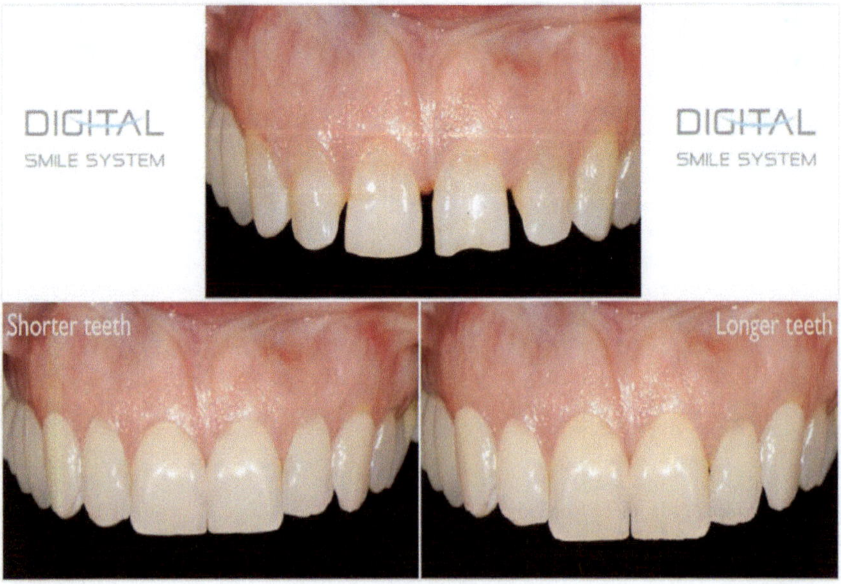

Fig. 10 Interface of Digital Smile System (DSS). Courtesy: Liu et al. (2012)

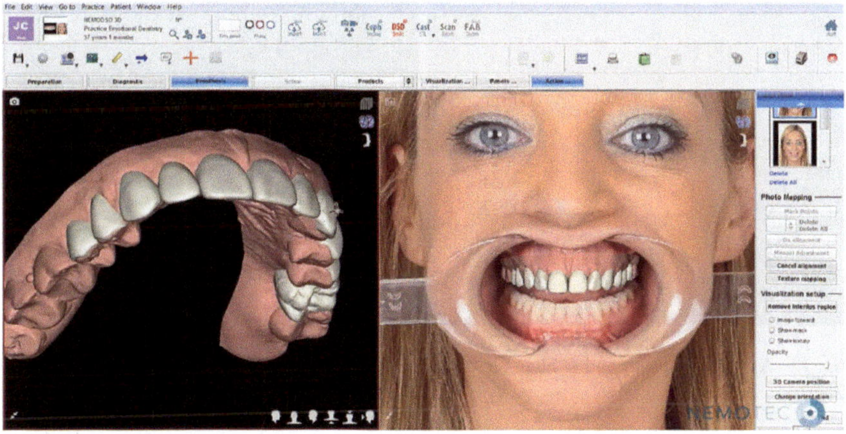

Fig. 11 Interface of Nemo DSD 3D®

- **Other tools**: There are numerous other programs and systems in the market. For example, **Keynote or PowerPoint** have been creatively repurposed for smile design by some (using shapes over slides). Specialised 3D software like **exocad DentalCAD** or **3Shape Smile Composer** allow full 3D smile design and link directly to CAD/CAM production. **Nemo DSD** is another platform that offers 3D facial integration (Fig. 11). Many of these tools offer similar capabilities—the choice often comes down to what integrates best with a dentist's existing equipment or what they find most comfortable. The trend is towards integrated ecosystems (for example, scanning the mouth, designing the smile, and fabricating restorations all within one software suite). Regardless of the software used, the objective is the same: to create a digital plan of the smile that can be communicated and executed predictably. DSD technology, therefore, is a combination of imaging, design software, and fabrication tools working in concert to deliver a precise outcome.

5 Applications of DSD in Dentistry

Digital Smile Design began in the realm of cosmetic dentistry, but its applications now span across various dental disciplines. By providing a clear visualisation of the intended result, DSD serves as a unifying framework for **interdisciplinary treatment planning.** Below are some of the key areas in dentistry where DSD is effectively applied:

- **Restorative dentistry and prosthodontics**: Perhaps the most common use of DSD is in planning restorative cases such as veneers, crowns, bridges, and full-mouth reconstructions. In prosthodontics, DSD guides the design of restorations to ensure they meet aesthetic goals and functional requirements before any tooth is

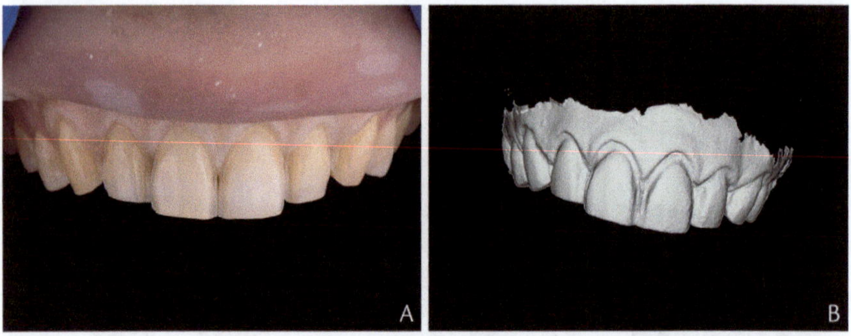

Fig. 12 **A** Prepared tooth and **B** STL file obtained by digital scan. Courtesy: Sanchez-Lara et al. (2019)

prepped. For example, when designing porcelain veneers, DSD allows the dentist to determine the ideal tooth shape and alignment digitally and then use that as a blueprint for tooth preparation and ceramic fabrication (Fig. 12). This results in restorations that *blend seamlessly* with the patient's smile and facial features. Because everything is planned virtually, adjustments (like altering the length of a crown or the curvature of an incisal edge) are made in the software rather than by drilling additional tooth structure. DSD also helps in matching restorative materials to the patient's natural dentition: By analysing shade and translucency digitally, the final crowns or veneers can be fabricated to closely mimic natural teeth. Moreover, complex cases such as full-mouth rehabilitations benefit from DSD's interdisciplinary insight: the vertical dimension, occlusion, and aesthetics can be tested in a digital mock-up, involving the prosthodontist and laboratory technician in collaborative planning. The end result is a restoration that restores not just individual teeth but the natural smile as a whole, often with minimal adjustments needed chairside due to the high level of pre-planning.

- **Orthodontic treatment planning**: Orthodontics is not just about straightening teeth for function; it often has a huge aesthetic component. DSD can be used to simulate the outcome of orthodontic treatment, helping both the orthodontist and the patient to see the expected alignment and smile arc after braces or clear aligners. For instance, by digitally 'straightening' the teeth on a patient's photo and adjusting the tooth display, the orthodontist can set clear goals and communicate the need for certain movements. This is particularly useful in adult orthodontic cases where cosmetic concerns are paramount. DSD also plays a role in interdisciplinary ortho-restorative cases: Sometimes, the ideal smile involves not just moving teeth, but also restorations after orthodontics (or vice versa). Using DSD, the dentist and orthodontist can together decide which spaces to close with braces and which to restore with bonding or veneers, all based on the visualised final result. It essentially serves as a virtual set-up tool. Research and case reports have shown DSD to be valuable in complex ortho cases; for example, in planning the smile for patients with missing teeth or jaw discrepancies, DSD helps decide if

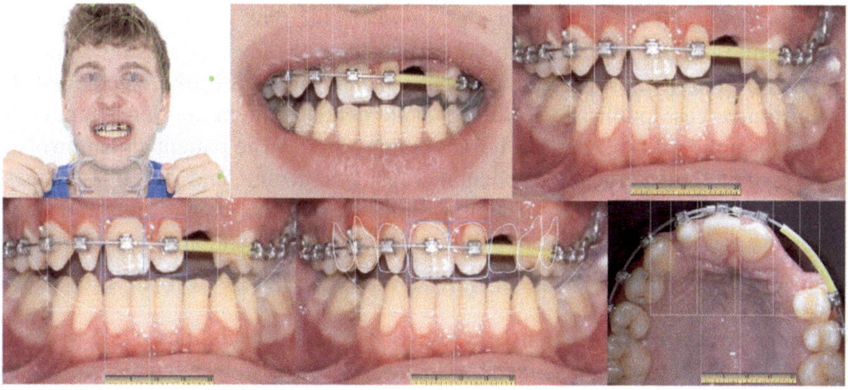

Fig. 13 DSD planning for orthodontic treatment. Courtesy: Charavet et al. (2019)

tooth movement alone will suffice or if additional prosthetic or surgical steps are needed. Furthermore, DSD improves patient acceptance of orthodontic treatment by showing them *why* it is needed for a better smile. Seeing a before-and-after simulation can motivate a patient to undergo orthodontics as part of a larger smile makeover, since they understand how it contributes to the final aesthetics (Fig. 13). In summary, DSD in orthodontics ensures that aligning the teeth is done with the *facial smile outcome* in mind, not just a correct bite—it aligns the goals of the orthodontist with the cosmetic vision.

- **Periodontal applications and gingival contouring**: Achieving an ideal smile often requires attention to the gums and underlying bone—this is where periodontics intersects with DSD. A common example is planning a case of excessive gingival display (a 'gummy smile'). Using DSD, a dentist can digitally alter a photo to show less gum and more tooth (simulating a gingivectomy or crown lengthening) and include this in the smile design plan. This allows both patient and periodontist to see the envisioned gumline before any surgery. In practice, periodontists can use DSD plans to guide crown lengthening surgeries with high precision. As one report notes, crown lengthening supported by digital smile planning lets the surgeon know exactly how much gum to remove and where, to match the ideal tooth proportions outlined in the DSD project. The use of digitally designed surgical guides (for example, 3D-printed templates) based on the DSD can translate the virtual gum line into the patient's mouth during surgery, improving accuracy. Aside from gummy smile corrections, DSD is useful in any periodontal recontouring—even minor adjustments of uneven gingival margins can be planned and tested on a photo first. Another periodontal aspect is implant dentistry in the aesthetic zone: When replacing a front tooth, DSD can help plan the implant positioning and any soft tissue grafting by visualising where the final crown should appear through the gum. Essentially, DSD encourages interdisciplinary coordination: The periodontist (or oral surgeon) works in tandem with the restorative dentist, both following the same digital plan. The result is more predictable gum aesthetics and a smile where the pink (gingiva) complements the white (teeth). Patients also appreciate this, as they can see the combined effect of gum and tooth treatments beforehand, setting proper expectations. An illustrative case published in the cosmetic dentistry literature demonstrated an interdisciplinary DSD approach for a gummy smile: The patient's plan involved lip repositioning surgery, periodontal crown lengthening, and veneers—all these steps coordinated through a Digital Smile Design that ensured the final gum heights and tooth shapes were balanced (Fig. 14). The outcome was an aesthetically pleasing smile and a satisfied patient, highlighting DSD's power in complex cases.

- **Cosmetic and aesthetic dentistry**: Beyond specific specialities, DSD is fundamentally a tool for *cosmetic dentistry*—any case where improving the appearance of the smile is the goal. This can range from a simple case of resin bonding on a chipped tooth to a complete smile makeover. Cosmetic dentists use DSD to design whiter, well-proportioned smiles tailored to patient wishes. For example, if a patient wants a Hollywood smile, the dentist can digitally show what a set of porcelain veneers in a brighter shade and ideal shape would look like. If a patient has old composites or discolourations, a DSD preview can illustrate the effect of replacements or teeth whitening in context. Even for treatments like tooth recontouring or minor adjustments, having a digital plan ensures that the changes enhance the smile's overall harmony. One of the advantages in cosmetic cases is increased patient engagement: The patient can effectively co-design their smile (choosing, for example, how rounded or square they want their incisor corners) which adds a level of customisation beyond standard cosmetic practice. DSD is also invaluable when multiple cosmetic procedures are combined—for instance, aligning teeth (orthodontics or Invisalign), bleaching, and then veneering the teeth. The DSD process orchestrates these steps by first defining the final look. By visualising the *final shade and shape* of teeth, the dentist can decide how much whitening is needed or what veneer colour to use. In summary, for any aesthetic-driven case, DSD provides a road map that ensures all cosmetic enhancements are pulling towards the same final vision. It takes into account the patient's desires (perhaps gleaned from reference photos or smile libraries) and blends them with professional design principles. This results in highly individualised smile makeovers—whether subtle or dramatic—with a higher likelihood of meeting or exceeding patient expectations. Cosmetic dentistry is as much art as science, and DSD supplies the artist (dentist) with a digital canvas and tools to preview the art before committing it to reality.

In all these applications, **Digital Smile Design facilitates team collaboration**. A restorative dentist, orthodontist, periodontist, and laboratory technician can all be literally on the same page by referring to the DSD project of the patient's case. It aligns their efforts towards a unified aesthetic and functional goal. The holistic view that DSD provides ensures that whether it is moving teeth, sculpting gums, or crafting porcelain, each action is contributing to the *ideal smile design* that was

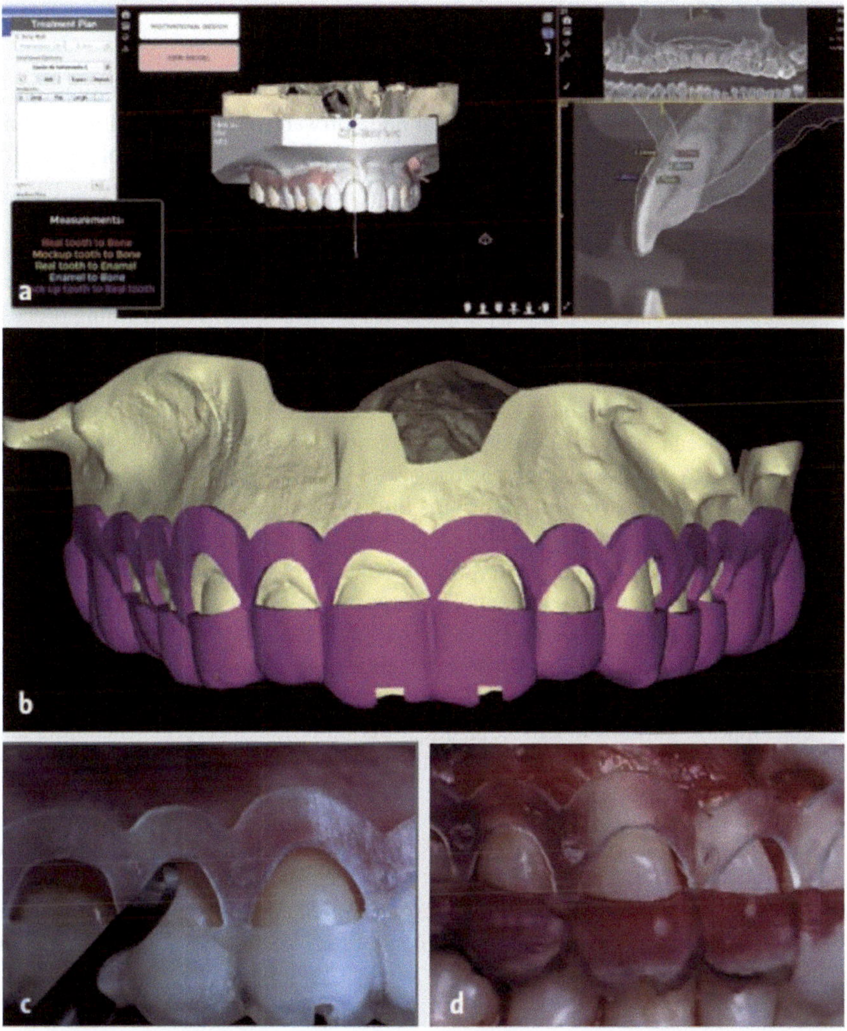

Fig. 14 CBCT image for periodontal treatment planning overlaid on virtual model with tooth #8 wax-up, gingivectomy, and osteotomy measurements (demarcation levels on lower and upper guides). The initial intraoral picture after crown lengthening surgery and the result. Courtesy: Pocztaruk et al. (2019)

agreed upon at the start. This interdisciplinary utility is one of the reasons DSD has gained worldwide adoption in comprehensive dental care.

6 Limitations and Challenges of DSD

1. **Financial investment and accessibility**: Adopting DSD necessitates substantial expenditure on specialised equipment and software, including digital imaging tools, intraoral scanners, and 3D printers. These costs can be prohibitive for smaller practices or those in underserved regions, potentially limiting patient access to DSD-enhanced treatments.
2. **Learning curve and expertise development**: Integrating DSD into clinical practice requires dental professionals to acquire new skills in digital imaging, software manipulation, and comprehensive smile design principles. This learning process demands time and dedication, which may be challenging for busy practitioners.
3. **Technical sensitivity and data quality**: The precision of DSD outcomes is heavily reliant on the quality of input data. Inaccurate or substandard photographs and scans can lead to flawed designs, emphasising the need for meticulous adherence to data acquisition protocols.
4. **Discrepancies between digital plans and clinical results**: Despite meticulous digital planning, translating virtual designs into clinical reality can result in subtle differences due to material properties, biological variations, and technical constraints. These potential discrepancies necessitate effective patient communication to manage expectations appropriately.
5. **Integration into clinical workflow and time management**: Incorporating DSD into existing practice workflows can initially extend treatment planning and consultation durations. This adjustment period requires careful scheduling and may impact practice efficiency until the team becomes proficient with the new processes.

Addressing these challenges involves strategic investment in technology and training, strict adherence to data collection standards, and clear communication with patients regarding potential outcomes. As digital dentistry continues to evolve, these obstacles may diminish, making DSD more accessible and efficient for dental professionals and patients alike.

7 Teledentistry and Digital Patient Management

The use of digital technology in healthcare has revolutionised several sectors, including dentistry. Teledentistry is a pioneering application in digital dentistry that enables remote consultation, diagnosis, treatment planning, and follow-up care using digital communication tools. Teledentistry is a branch of telehealth that employs synchronous (real-time video conversations) and asynchronous (store-and-forward) communication methods for patient treatment (Gurgel-Juarez et al. 2022).

The importance of teledentistry became particularly evident during the COVID-19 pandemic, which required social distancing and reduced physical encounters in hospital environments (Wallace et al. 2021). During this period, teledentistry facilitated remote patient monitoring, emergency triage, and sustained access to dental consultations, illustrating its feasibility as a long-term option for enhancing access to oral healthcare services. Notwithstanding its benefits, the use of teledentistry is inconsistent throughout various areas and healthcare systems, attributable to technological obstacles, insufficient legislative clarity, and apprehensions surrounding diagnostic precision.

Fernández et al. (2021) assert that teledentistry includes a range of virtual communication technologies:

- Synchronous interactions: real-time consultations via video calls or live chats between dentists and patients
- Asynchronous interactions: pre-recorded communications, mobile applications, and online instructional resources accessible to patients at their discretion
- Remote monitoring: digital instruments like intraoral cameras and mobile applications for longitudinal surveillance of oral health issues
- Mobile health (mHealth): the use of mobile applications and text message reminders to promote oral hygiene practices and enhance adherence to dental procedures

Applications

Remote consultations and diagnosis in teledentistry: Teledentistry facilitates remote consultations and diagnoses through the transmission of clinical information, images, and diagnostic data across distances, enabling specialist consultations, treatment planning, and follow-up care. This method is advantageous for rural areas, underserved populations, and emergency situations, facilitating timely and cost-effective dental care without requiring physical visits to a specialist. Teledentistry facilitates early identification of oral diseases, enables remote patient monitoring, and enhances access to specialists, thereby improving healthcare efficiency and outcomes.

Remote consultations in teledentistry primarily use **two major methods**, along with an additional method of remote monitoring (Jampani et al. 2011).

(a) **Real-Time Consultation (Synchronous Mode)**

Definition: Engages in real-time, interactive video consultations between dental professionals and patients, or between general dentists and specialists.

Technological Applications

- Software for videoconferencing
- Intraoral cameras with high resolution
- Internet connections that are secure

Utilisations

- Real-time assessment of dental conditions (for example, dental infections, orthodontic concerns)
- Consultations for trauma cases in emergency settings
- Referrals to specialists that do not necessitate physical transportation

Benefits

- Prompt feedback from experts
- Beneficial for real-time second opinions and treatment modifications
- Minimises travel time for patients

Challenges

- Requires high-speed Internet and satisfactory video quality
- Challenges related to time zones and scheduling for specialists and patients

(b) **Store-and-Forward Technique (Asynchronous Mode)**

This method entails the electronic transmission of patient data, images, and clinical records to specialists for subsequent review.

Technological Applications

- Digital radiographs (X-rays) are a form of imaging technology that utilises digital sensors to capture and display images of internal structures.
- Photographs are taken intraorally.
- Electronic patient records are digital versions of patients' paper charts, designed to streamline the management of patient information and enhance healthcare delivery.

Utilisations

- Diagnosis of oral lesions and dental caries utilising digital imaging
- Assessment of orthodontic treatment progress through remote evaluation
- Planning for prosthetic and restorative treatments

Benefits

- Does not necessitate simultaneous online presence of both parties
- Specialists can conduct thorough case reviews prior to offering recommendations
- Reduces unnecessary referrals through improved pre-screening

Challenges

- Delay in response time relative to real-time consultations
- Accuracy—contingent upon the quality of the captured images

Specialist Referrals

Teledentistry specialist referrals involve the transmission of patient data, images, radiographs, and case details to specialists who offer expert opinions and treatment recommendations remotely. This process improves access to specialised care, especially for patients in rural or underserved regions.

a. **Maxillofacial Surgery**: Digital imaging of impacted third molars reduces referrals. Teleconsultation pre-surgery examinations reduce in-person appointments. Teleconsultation lets specialists advise general dentists on dental emergencies. Teledentistry reduces travel time and expenses by enabling precise remote diagnosis and planning for oral procedures, according to studies.
b. **Orthodontics**: Orthodontic screening with digital photographs and radiographs. Initial malocclusion assessments before in-person visits. Remote orthodontic treatment monitoring reduces clinic visits for minor modifications. Reduces improper referrals, allowing general dentists to manage some conditions with specialised supervision. UK studies revealed that teledentistry decreased needless orthodontic referrals, allowing professionals to focus on complex cases.
c. **Periodontics**: Remote gum disease evaluation utilising digital periodontal charts and photos. Remote examinations let experts decide if periodontal surgery is needed. Post-surgery monitoring allows patients to transmit photos of recovering tissues, reducing clinic visits. U.S. military research found that remote periodontal procedures were efficient, with only one patient needing a follow-up.
d. **Endodontics**: Remote radiography for root canal infection diagnosis. General dentists get complicated endodontic guidance to improve case management. Avoids needless travel by determining if a condition needs a specialist referral. Remote specialists can properly detect periapical diseases and help general dentists in endodontics, according to studies.
e. **Prosthodontics**: Digital consultations for prosthetic treatment planning before specialist visits. Denture and crown adjustments may be examined remotely. Planning for long-distance rehabilitation, particularly for nursing home or rural patients. Videoconferencing for prosthetic consultations improves treatment outcomes in remote places, according to research.
f. **Paediatric Dentistry**: Digital photographs for early childhood caries testing. Behaviour management and prevention advice from experts. Remotely triaging emergencies like infant dental trauma. Research shows that teledentistry is equally successful as in-person exams in diagnosing dental caries in youngsters, making it a helpful referral tool.

8 Education and Training in Teledentistry

1. **Internet's Role in Dental Education**

By creating Internet-based learning platforms that enable professionals and students to study remotely, communicate with teachers, and advance their abilities without having to be physically present in a classroom, teledentistry has had a big impact on dental education.

- With web-based teledentistry instruction, students may select the time, location, and learning style that works best for them.
- Students may see operations, treatments, and expert consultations from any location, thanks to videoconferencing and live streaming.
- Platforms for distance learning are utilised for ongoing professional development, specialised education for dentists working in remote regions, and practical instruction through live demonstrations and online video courses.

2. **Professional Dental Training Through Teledentistry**
    - Many dental schools use online training courses.
    - According to Correa et al.'s evaluation of a web-based practical course on the fundamentals of oral surgery, distance learning and hands-on training worked well together.
    - Long-distance learning in dentistry is feasible, according to Ignatius et al.'s study on the use of videoconferencing in dental speciality education in Finland.
    - A web-based teledentistry consultation system (TME 3/347) was created by the U.S. Department of Defence to offer military dental clinics virtual consultations and continuing education.

Public Health Initiatives

Teledentistry is an affordable technique to alleviate inequities in oral health treatment between urban and rural populations. It plays an important function in:

- Offering remote dental consultations to bridge the rural–urban healthcare divide
- Eliminating needless visits to reduce expenses for both individuals and healthcare systems
- Providing oral healthcare to underprivileged populations, such as the elderly, children, and those with impairments

Addressing the Dental Workforce Shortage

- The report emphasises the expected lack of dentists in the next decades.
- Teledentistry can assist to alleviate this shortage by allowing professionals to diagnose and arrange treatments remotely.
- Teledentistry allows patients in places with few dental specialists to obtain expert views without having to travel vast distances.

Role in Prevention and Early Diagnosis

- Teledentistry-based public health programs prioritise prevention over treatment of dental disorders.
- Remote screenings can help spot dental problems early on, avoiding more serious disorders like periodontal disease and tooth loss.

- Digital reminders (SMS or app notifications) have proven useful in motivating patients to practise good dental hygiene.

Effective Public Health Teledentistry Projects

School-Based Teledental Programs

- Case study (USA): A teledentistry experiment in Rochester, NY, screened 173 youngsters from inner-city primary schools and day care centres. Forty per cent of children aged 12 to 48 months had untreated dental caries. The initiative enabled early diagnosis and referral to dental experts. The key benefit includes improved access to preventative dental treatment for children in underprivileged communities.
- **Rural Community Health Initiatives**: Case study (Taiwan): A feasibility study in Chin-Shan Township (17,000 people) utilised teledentistry to offer remote dental consultations. Digital radiography analysis and expert referrals were provided as needed. The experiment demonstrated that, even with limited resources, teledentistry may be utilised to provide dental treatment in remote places.
- **Teledentistry in Paediatric and Preventive Care**: Case study (Finland): A remote orthodontic consultation system was utilised. Remote dental monitoring was equally beneficial as in-person check-ups. Reduced the number of needless orthodontic referrals. Improved access to child care in rural regions.
- **Teledentistry in Oral Medicine and Surgery**: Case study (Northern Ireland): A teledentistry prototype was evaluated for oral medicine referrals. The study concluded that remote diagnosis of oral disorders is possible and reliable. Helped to shorten wait times for specialised consultations.

9 Teledentistry Benefits Specialist Referrals

Teledentistry makes expert consultations more accessible, quick, and cost-effective, improving referrals. The key benefits include:

- **Greater access**: Remote or underprivileged patients can get speciality treatment without travelling far. This reduces hospital and speciality clinic workload by remotely handling mild cases.
- **Faster diagnosis/treatment planning**: Store-and-forward technology lets professionals analyse cases at their convenience, speeding diagnosis. Wait times for expert visits decrease.
- **Cost savings**: Patient transportation expenses are decreased. Unnecessary specialist appointments and healthcare costs are reduced. Optimising the process saves patients and specialist's time. It also improves dentist–specialist communication, allowing easier sharing of case facts, radiographs, and treatment plans. With specialist advice, general dentists can manage more patients independently, improving cross-speciality teamwork and patient outcomes.

Role of teledentistry in endodontics: To succeed, endodontic operations, especially root canals, require accurate diagnosis and treatment planning. Teledentistry helps identify root canal orifices remotely using high-resolution photographs of endodontically accessible teeth. Specialists may advise distant dentists, minimising the need for endodontists and enhancing treatment accuracy, according to studies. Teledentistry can also identify root-tip infections and periapical lesions (Popovic et al. 2020). General dentists can get expert views on whether a lesion needs root canal therapy or surgery by exchanging X-rays or digital radiographs, speeding up treatment choices and decreasing patient travel. Remote radiographic image interpretation, which is as accurate as in-person analysis, is another benefit of teledentistry. Teledentistry is trustworthy for distant endodontic examinations because digital pictures seen via videoconferencing were as accurate as conventional radiography (Bakeriii et al. 2000).

Teledentistry allows remote consultations for complex endodontic situations. General dentists may struggle with curved root canals, calcified canals, and retreatment situations, which require specialised care. General practitioners can contact endodontic specialists before starting treatment via real-time video consultations or store-and-forward systems, which provide case information and X-rays electronically (Bhuyan et al. 2023). This coordinated approach guarantees patients receive the best treatment regimens even in places without endodontists. In endodontic instances, teledentistry provides for second opinions, especially when deciding whether to extract a tooth or perform root canal therapy. By electronically exchanging radiographs and patient data with experts, dentists can make more confident diagnoses and avoid needless operations. Hence, teledentistry improves patient outcomes, lowers treatment costs, and boosts dental care efficiency.

Role of teledentistry in oral medicine and diagnosis: Digital consultation significantly enhances diagnostic capabilities in dentistry by facilitating remote assessments and diagnoses of oral diseases. Telediagnosis enables dentists to assess digital images, radiographs, and patient records transmitted through secure platforms, thereby enhancing the timeliness and accuracy of evaluations. Research indicates the reliability of this approach, as Torres-Pereira et al. (Torres-Pereira et al. 2008) have confirmed that oral lesions can be accurately diagnosed through image transmission via email. Bradley et al. (Bradley et al. 2010) effectively implemented teledentistry in oral medicine within a community dental service in Northern Ireland, employing a prototype system for remote diagnosis. This advancement enhances accessibility to dental care and improves efficiency in the diagnosis and management of oral conditions. The early detection of oral diseases, including oral cancer, precancerous lesions, and periodontal conditions, represents a key advantage of digital consultation. Digital tools facilitate the early identification of abnormal lesions, enabling timely intervention and markedly enhancing treatment success rates. Leao and Porter (Leao and Porter 1999) demonstrated the feasibility and effectiveness of telediagnosis for orofacial diseases using Internet-based platforms. Utilising digital technologies in dentistry facilitates timely and accurate diagnoses, thereby minimising disease progression and improving overall patient outcomes (Summerfelt 2011).

Role of teledentistry in paediatric dentistry: Digital intraoral cameras provide thorough imaging of a child's dentition, allowing dentists to detect cavities at an early stage and execute prompt therapies prior to their progression. Research has shown that teledentistry serves as a dependable substitute for in-person evaluations, with similar precision in identifying caries in children. Research by Kopycka-Kedzierawski and Billings (Kopycka-Kedzierawski and Billings 2011) showed that remote caries assessments utilising teledentistry techniques were equally successful as conventional visual and tactile tests. A community-based teledentistry effort in Rochester, NY, effectively diagnosed early childhood caries in children in urban childcare centres, ensuring that individuals in underprivileged regions got essential dental treatment. The integration of digital technologies in paediatric dentistry enhances access to early diagnosis and treatment, hence improving children's oral health results (Kopycka-Kedzierawski et al. 2007, 2008; Amável et al. 2009).

Role of teledentistry in oral and maxillofacial surgery: Digital technology has markedly enhanced preoperative examinations in oral and maxillofacial surgery by facilitating remote evaluations. Utilising sophisticated imaging and communications technologies, doctors may evaluate patients prior to surgery without necessitating in-person consultations (Rollert et al. 1999). Research has shown that teledentistry is useful in identifying issues like impacted wisdom teeth (Duka et al. 2009), with accuracy equivalent to traditional in-person assessments. Research corroborates the efficacy of virtual consultations for surgical evaluations, rendering them a significant option for patients in rural or disadvantaged areas. This method improves access to specialised treatment and increases efficiency by minimising the necessity for numerous appointments while preserving diagnostic accuracy (Brickley 2000; Aziz and Ziccardi 2009).

Remote consultations for prosthodontics and periodontics: Remote consultations have emerged as an invaluable resource in prosthodontics and periodontics, improving access to specialised treatment. Patients seeking prosthodontic procedures, including dentures and implants, can visit professionals electronically, which is especially advantageous for those in distant or underserved regions. Research by Ignatius et al. (Ignatius et al. 2006) showed that video consultations for prosthetic treatment planning markedly enhanced access to specialised care in remote areas. In periodontics, digital evaluations enable patients to obtain professional assessments and subsequent therapy without the necessity of regular in-person appointments. This method reduces superfluous travel while guaranteeing ongoing surveillance of periodontal health. The U.S. Department of Defence Teledentistry System successfully implemented remote periodontal care, facilitating follow-ups for patients situated 150 miles from the primary healthcare facility, thereby demonstrating its efficiency and effectiveness (Ignatius et al. 2010).

10 Efficacy of Teledentistry Interventions

(1) **Effects on oral hygiene and plaque management**: A notable finding was the decrease in plaque levels among patients who underwent teledentistry procedures. The standardised mean difference (SMD) of −1.18 demonstrated a clinically significant enhancement in plaque management among individuals who received reminders through mobile applications, text messages, or interactive digital learning resources. This phenomenon can be ascribed to the behavioural reinforcement facilitated by mobile health devices. Patients were regularly reminded about toothbrushing procedures, flossing practices, and oral hygiene maintenance. The self-monitoring feature of mobile applications, enabling patients to assess their progress, certainly enhanced adherence to oral hygiene practices. Gamification and interactive elements in certain mobile applications may have contributed to heightened engagement, especially among younger demographics.

(2) **Diminution of gingival inflammation**: The gingival index (GI) was markedly reduced in the intervention group (SMD: −2.17). Teledentistry treatments resulted in a significant decrease in gum inflammation. Multiple plausible reasons exist for this. Regular reminders facilitated increased and more efficient plaque clearance. Certain treatments comprised educational movies demonstrating correct brushing methods, potentially enhancing the efficacy of plaque removal efforts. The habit formation process enhanced by digital instruments certainly facilitated enduring advancements in oral hygiene over time.

(3) **Prevention of white spot lesions (WSLs)**: White spot lesions (WSLs) are first indicators of enamel demineralisation, frequently observed in orthodontic patients. The meta-analysis indicated that patients utilising teledentistry procedures saw a 52% reduced chance of acquiring white spot lesions (chance ratio: 0.48). This indicates that teledentistry was essential in early identification and prevention. This further emphasises that consistent involvement and education can improve preventative dental care, hence diminishing the necessity for more invasive procedures.

(4) **Enduring impacts and sustainability**: The study revealed that teledentistry therapies maintained a lasting effect, demonstrating improvement at 6–12 months in contrast to early assessments at 1–3 months. This implies that the efficacy of teledentistry improves with extended utilisation. Consistent engagement with instructional material and prompts facilitates enduring behavioural changes. Reinforcement is essential, and patients who received reminders more consistently had superior long-term results.

11 Digital Storage Systems

- **PACS Server**

Picture archiving and communication systems (PACS) are essential for optimising digital workflows, improving diagnostic efficiency, and facilitating uninterrupted access to patient imaging records. PACS functions as a comprehensive system that securely stores, transmits, and retrieves medical images and reports, thereby removing the necessity for physical files and enhancing accessibility for patients and healthcare providers (Choplin et al. 1992). The significance transcends convenience, as it improves collaborative care by enabling dental specialists and general practitioners to access, analyse, and interpret diagnostic images remotely. This is especially beneficial in oral and maxillofacial radiology, where high-resolution digital images are crucial for diagnosing complex conditions and planning detailed dental procedures (Bluemke and Liu 2012; Nair et al. 2009).

PACS comprises four fundamental components

- Imaging hardware—comprises X-ray devices, intraoral cameras, and CBCT scanners for image capture
- Secure network—enables the secure dissemination and exchange of patient photos
- Workstation or mobile device—allows dental practitioners to remotely examine, analyse, and interpret pictures
- Electronic archives—preserve photographs, reports, and associated documents, guaranteeing accessibility for future consultation

Importance of PACS in Digital Dentistry

The integration of PACS into teledentistry is significant due to its capacity for real-time image access, facilitation of remote consultations, and enhancement of patient outcomes via efficient data management. PACS facilitates the availability of diagnostic records to specialists, addressing the issue of limited access to specialised dental care for patients in remote areas. Research demonstrates its efficacy in enhancing clinical workflows, minimising redundancies, and facilitating evidence-based decision-making (Fig. 15). In oral emergency care (OEC) settings, PACS plays a crucial role in monitoring disease progression, enabling physicians to compare historical and current imaging for the evaluation of treatment efficacy. The integration with electronic medical records (EMR) enhances interoperability, streamlining patient management and facilitating comprehensive, long-term care planning (Delantoni and Orhan 2024).

The successful implementation of PACS in teledentistry, despite its advantages, necessitates the resolution of critical infrastructural challenges. A key factor is the necessity for cloud-based solutions that provide scalable storage, remote accessibility, and improved security. Cloud-based PACS facilitate data exchange and ensure compliance with regulatory frameworks, such as Health Insurance Portability and Accountability Act (HIPAA), thereby safeguarding patient confidentiality. Reliable

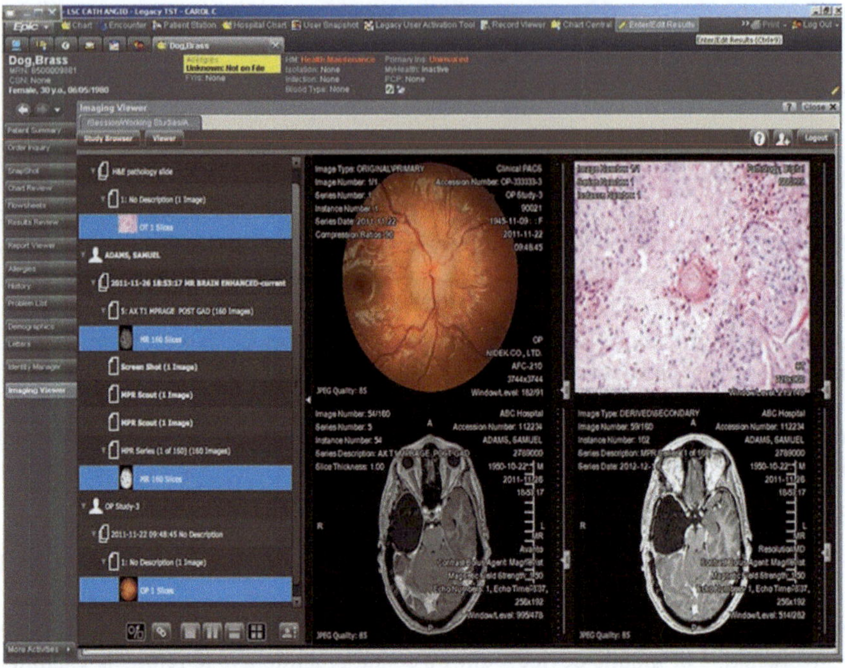

Fig. 15 PACS server serves as the storage solution for the database containing these DICOM files. Courtesy: FUJIFILM Turkey

high-speed Internet connectivity is essential for the efficient operation of cloud-based PACS, especially in geographically isolated areas where digital infrastructure may be lacking. Additionally, it is essential to ensure seamless integration among C-ARM imaging systems, ultrasound machines, and electronic medical records (EMR). Few studies investigate the integration of PACS in teledentistry, assessing its effects on diagnostic accuracy, patient management, and overall healthcare delivery (Hirschorn et al. 2002).

The increasing integration of artificial intelligence (AI), machine learning algorithms, and telecommunication technologies positions PACS as a fundamental component of contemporary teledentistry, facilitating efficient data sharing, accurate diagnostics, and improved patient-centred care. Furthermore, as the field progresses, the integration of automated image analysis and AI-driven decision support systems within PACS is expected to increase, thereby enhancing diagnostic workflows and clinical efficiency (Spangler et al. 2021).

12 Cloud Computing in Dentistry

Cloud computing allows users to access servers, applications, and storage online without the need for physical infrastructure. This technology significantly improves productivity, flexibility, and accessibility, thereby facilitating the seamless administration of remote data (Devasena 2014).

How Cloud Computing Works

Cloud computing employs a **virtual network** to connect **front-end (user interface) and back-end (server-side infrastructure) components.** The three primary **cloud service models** include:

1. **Infrastructure as a Service (IaaS)**—provides **virtualised computing resources** over the Internet
2. **Platform as a Service (PaaS)**—offers a framework for **developers to build and deploy applications**
3. **Software as a Service (SaaS)**—delivers **software applications** over the cloud, such as **teledentistry platforms** (Chow et al. 2014)

Deployment Models in Cloud Computing

Cloud computing can be deployed using different models:

- **Public cloud**—available to multiple users over the Internet
- **Private cloud**—dedicated to a single organisation, offering **enhanced security**
- **Community cloud**—shared among multiple organisations with similar needs
- **Hybrid cloud**—combines features of **public and private clouds**, offering a balanced approach

Cloud-Based PACS in Dentistry

Cloud computing plays a pivotal role in dentistry, particularly for **storing and managing patient records, digital radiographs, and imaging data**. Some of the widely used **cloud-based dental solutions** include:

- **Denticon**: Denticon is a cloud-based dental practice management software created by Planet DDS, aimed at optimising operations for dental practices of various sizes, including those with multiple locations and specialities. Denticon improves efficiency, data security, and patient care through the centralisation of diverse administrative and clinical functions.

Essential Characteristics and Advantages

- Denticon's cloud infrastructure enables dental professionals to securely access patient data and practice information from any location with Internet connectivity. This flexibility enables remote work, enhances collaboration across various offices, and guarantees continuity of care.

- The software provides a customisable scheduler that facilitates efficient appointment management across one or multiple locations. Features encompass rapid access to patient records, real-time updates, and tools for identifying available appointment slots, thereby improving staff productivity and patient convenience.
- Denticon features integrated patient communication through online portals and two-way texting, enabling patients to schedule appointments, fill out registration forms, update insurance details, and interact with the practice efficiently. This integration enhances patient engagement and decreases administrative workload.
- The platform enhances revenue cycle management and insurance processing by incorporating features such as integrated insurance verification, automated claims processing, and accurate treatment cost estimations. These tools assist practices in minimising errors, accelerating reimbursements, and improving financial transparency.
- Denticon offers enterprise-level reporting and real-time data insights, allowing practices to track performance metrics including daily production, patient acquisition, and accounts receivable. This centralised reporting facilitates informed decision-making and strategic planning.
- Optimised clinical workflows: Clinicians gain advantages from functionalities such as customisable charting, treatment planning, and integrated imaging. The software facilitates a unified patient record system, guaranteeing that precise and current information is available across all practice locations.
- Enhanced data security: Denticon employs advanced security measures, such as hardware and software firewalls, intrusion prevention systems, and continuous monitoring, to safeguard sensitive patient information. Regular data backups and adherence to regulations such as HIPAA enhance data integrity protection.
- Denticon is designed to meet the requirements of expanding dental organisations. It includes features such as centralised administrative functions, customisable user permissions, and seamless integration of new locations, making it an appropriate solution for practices seeking efficient scalability (Fig. 16).
- **Dentisoft Online**: A cloud-based dental practice management tool called Dentisoft Online was created to optimise administrative and clinical processes in dental clinics. It is appropriate for practices of all sizes due to its extensive features and easy-to-use interface.

Key Features and Uses

- Appointment management: Dentisoft simplifies scheduling with a drag-and-drop calendar. Automatic email and SMS reminders decrease patient no-shows by notifying patients promptly.
- Patient records management: The program securely stores and retrieves patient data from digital patient charts. This streamlines healthcare provider information exchange, improving collaboration.
- Billing and invoicing: Dentisoft simplifies billing and invoicing with automated insurance claim filings, customisable invoices, and integrated payment systems. These tools streamline billing and reduce mistakes.

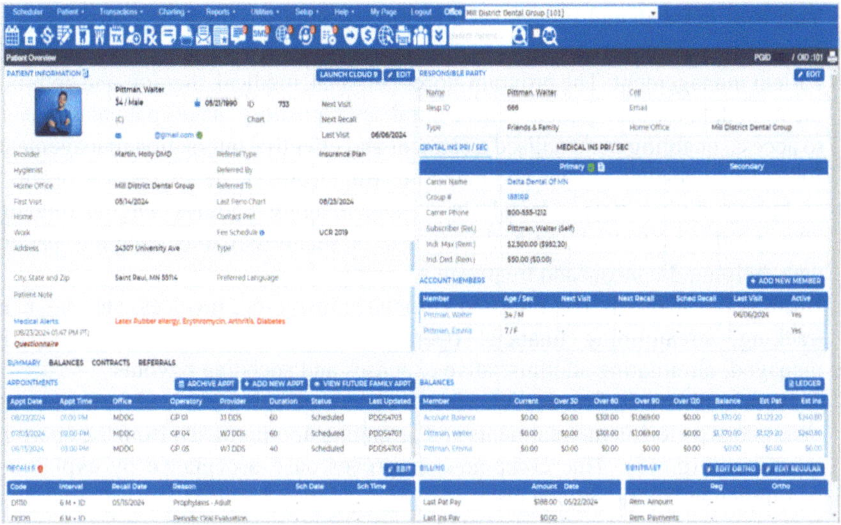

Fig. 16 **Denticon** dental practice management system that displays patient details, medical alerts, appointments, insurance, and invoicing information. Courtesy: Denticon®

- Imaging: The platform interfaces with radiography systems to save and manage dental pictures in patient records. Comprehensive treatment planning and diagnostics are improved by this combination.
- Patient communication and marketing: Dentisoft integrates Facebook and DentistDirectory.com for patient involvement. Online patient forms, secure messaging, automatic reminders, and e-birthday messages improve communication and patient relationships.
- Treatment planning: Dental professionals may develop, maintain, and manage treatment plans using the software's electronic clinical records and treatment planning modules. This involves creating patient handouts and instructional materials for informed decision-making.
- Reporting and analytics: Dentisoft provides over 250 customisable reports to help offices analyse financial performance and patient demographics. Data export to Excel, Word, or PDF aids analysis and record-keeping (Lin et al. 2014).

Practice-Web: Practice-Web is an all-encompassing dental practice management software aimed at optimising many administrative and clinical functions inside a dental office. Founded in 1988, it provides a variety of features designed to enhance efficiency, elevate patient care, and augment profitability for dental clinics.

Key Features

- Appointment scheduling: Practice-Web's easy scheduling function streamlines appointment booking, cancellation handling, and daily calendar optimisation.

This tool helps dental clinics keep a full schedule, eliminating downtime and improving patient satisfaction.

- Patient management: The program stores personal, medical, therapy, and communication data for each patient. This centralised repository makes patient data easy to access, enabling personalised treatment and effective interaction management.
- EHR: Practice-Web creates and maintains full electronic health records (EHRs), including clinical notes, dental charts, and imaging findings. Digital imaging allows radiographs and intraoral images to be seamlessly integrated into patient data, helping diagnosis and treatment planning.
- Billing and invoices: The program automates invoicing, invoices, and payment tracking, streamlining financial operations. Insurance claims are properly managed, eliminating administrative expenses and speeding payouts.
- Treatment planning: Practice-Web lets dentists create, present, and manage treatment plans, prioritising treatments and arranging appointments from the charting interface (Fig. 17). This component improves case acceptance by explaining recommended therapies and costs.
- Patient communication: Practice-Web sends appointment confirmations, recalls, and outstanding treatment plans via automated and two-way texting and email to decrease no-shows and promote patient participation.

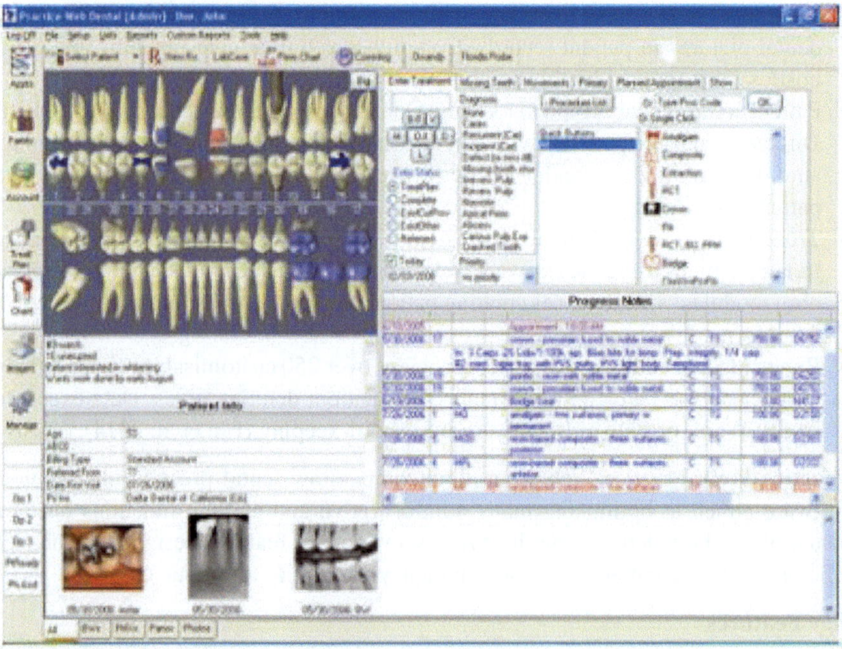

Fig. 17 Practice-web dental®

- Digital forms and signatures: The program allows paperless forms and signatures. Patients can use iPads or other devices to complete registration and permission documents, speeding up check-in and decreasing paperwork.
- Reporting and analytics: Practice-Web offers over 60 thorough reports on productivity, income, daily processes, and more. These insights aid strategic planning and decision-making.
- Integration: The program works with e-prescriptions, electronic claims processing, and digital imaging systems. Interoperability streamlines process and reduces data input.

13 Benefits of Cloud Computing in Dentistry

Cloud computing enhances dental informatics by providing:

- **Financial efficiency**—reduces **infrastructure costs** by eliminating the need for local servers
- **Infinite storage capacity**—enables **scalability** for growing databases of **dental records** and images
- **Remote data accessibility**—allows dental professionals to **retrieve and review images and reports** from any location
- **Automated software updates**—ensures that applications remain **up to date with the latest security patches and features**
- **Optimised data backup and recovery**—provides **redundant storage**, protecting against data loss
- **Real-time collaboration**—enables **multiple specialists** to review and discuss cases remotely (Johnson et al. 2019)

Challenges of Cloud-Based PACS in Dentistry

Despite its advantages, cloud-based PACS in dentistry faces several challenges:

1. **Technological limitations**—Integrating **digital sensors with cloud platforms** can be complex.
2. **Cybersecurity risks**—Data stored in the cloud is vulnerable to **cyber threats and unauthorised access**.
3. **Internet dependency**—Cloud-based systems require a **stable and high-speed Internet connection** for optimal functionality.
4. **Service disruptions**—Cloud outages may lead to **temporary inaccessibility of patient records** (Lightbody et al. 2019).

The future of PACS in teledentistry is expected to be shaped by:

- Artificial intelligence (AI) integration—AI can assist in automated image analysis, early diagnosis, and predictive analytics.
- Blockchain for data security—Blockchain technology can enhance patient data security by preventing unauthorised modifications.

- 5G connectivity—The deployment of 5G networks will improve data transmission speeds, making cloud-based PACS more efficient.

References

Alharkan HM (2024) Integrating digital smile design into restorative dentistry: a narrative review of the applications and benefits. Saudi Dent J. 36(4):561–567

Amável R, Cruz-Correia R, Frias-Bulhosa J (2009) Remote diagnosis of children dental problems based on non-invasive photographs—a valid proceeding? Stud Health Technol Inform 150:458–462

Aziz SR, Ziccardi VB (2009) Telemedicine using smartphones for oral and maxillofacial surgery consultation, communication, and treatment planning. J Oral Maxillofac Surg 67(11):2505–2509

Bakeriii W, Loushine R, West L, Kudryk L, Zadinsky J (2000) Interpretation of artificial and in vivo periapical bone lesions comparing conventional viewing versus a video conferencing system. J Endod 26(1):39–41

Bhuyan L, Mahapatra N, Dhull KS, Doddawad VG, Sahoo N, Panda A (2023) Tele dentistry—its practical applicability, hurdles and future prospects. Bangladesh J Med Sci. 21:52–57

Bluemke DA, Liu S (2012) Imaging in clinical trials. In: Principles and practice of clinical research. Elsevier, p 597–617. https://linkinghub.elsevier.com/retrieve/pii/B9780123821676000412

Bradley M, Black P, Noble S, Thompson R, Lamey PJ (2010) Application of teledentistry in oral medicine in a community dental service. N Ireland Br Dent J 209(8):399–404

Brickley M (2000) Oral surgery: the referral system and telemedicine. Br Dent J 188(7):384–384

Charavet C, Bernard JC, Gaillard C, Le Gall M (2019) Benefits of digital smile design (DSD) in the conception of a complex orthodontic treatment plan: a case report-proof of concept. Int Orthod 17(3):573–579

Choplin RH, Boehme JM, Maynard CD (1992) Picture archiving and communication systems: an overview. Radiographics 12(1):127–129

Chow F, Muftu A, Shorter R (2014) Virtualization and cloud computing in dentistry. J Mass Dent Soc 63(1):14–17

Delantoni A, Orhan K (2024) Digital storage systems PACS servers and cloud dentistry. In: Delantoni A, Orhan K (eds) Digital dentistry. Cham: Springer International Publishing, p 273–84. https://doi.org/10.1007/978-3-031-52826-2_17

Devasena CL (2014) Impact study of cloud computing on business development, vol 1

Duka M, Mihailovic B, Miladinovic M, Jankovic A, Vujicic B (2009) Evaluation of telemedicine systems for impacted third molars diagnosis. Vojnosanit Pregl 66(12):985–991

Eaton KA (2022) The development of digital dentistry in the UK: an overview. Prim Dent J 11(4):94–98

Fernández CE, Maturana CA, Coloma SI, Carrasco-Labra A, Giacaman RA (2021) Teledentistry and mHealth for promotion and prevention of oral health: a systematic review and meta-analysis. J Dent Res 100(9):914–927

Gurgel-Juarez N, Torres-Pereira C, Haddad AE, Sheehy L, Finestone H, Mallet K et al (2022) Accuracy and effectiveness of teledentistry: a systematic review of systematic reviews. Evid Based Dent. https://www.nature.com/articles/s41432-022-0257-8

Hirschorn D, Eber C, Samuels P, Gujrathi S, Baker SR (2002) Filmless in New Jersey: the New Jersey medical school PACS project. J Digit Imaging 15:7–12

Ignatius E, Perälä S, Mäkelä K (2010) Use of videoconferencing for consultation in dental prosthetics and oral rehabilitation. J Telemed Telecare 16(8):467–470

Ignatius E, Mäkelä K, Happonen RP, Perälä S (2006) Teledentistry in dental specialist education in Finland. J Telemed Telecare 12(3_suppl):46–9

Impellizzeri A, Palmigiani R, Horodynski M, D'alfonso T, Polimeni A, De Stefano A et al (2023) Is there a correlation between gingival display and incisal inclination in a gummy smile? Study on cephalometric parameters. Healthcare 11(3):344

Jafri Z, Ahmad N, Sawai M, Sultan N, Bhardwaj A (2020) Digital smile design-an innovative tool in aesthetic dentistry. J Oral Biol Craniofacial Res. 10(2):194–198

Jain A, Bhushan P, Mahato M, Solanki BB, Dutta D, Hota S et al (2024) The recent use, patient satisfaction, and advancement in digital smile designing: a systematic review. Cureus. https://www.cureus.com/articles/258233-the-recent-use-patient-satisfaction-and-advancement-in-digital-smile-designing-a-systematic-review

Jampani N, Nutalapati R, Dontula BSK, Boyapati R (2011) Applications of teledentistry: a literature review and update. J Int Soc Prev Community Dent 1(2):37

Johnson L, Callaghan C, Balasubramanian M, Haq H, Spallek H (2019) Cost comparison of an on-premise IT solution with a cloud-based solution for electronic health records in a dental school clinic. J Dent Educ 83(8):895–903

Kopycka-Kedzierawski DT, Billings RJ (2011) Prevalence of dental caries and dental care utilisation in preschool urban children enrolled in a comparative-effectiveness study. Eur Arch Paediatr Dent 12(3):133–138

Kopycka-Kedzierawski DT, Billings RJ, McConnochie KM (2007) Dental screening of preschool children using teledentistry: a feasibility study. Pediatr Dent 29(3):209–213

Kopycka-Kedzierawski DT, Bell CH, Billings RJ (2008) Prevalence of dental caries in early head start children as diagnosed using teledentistry. Pediatr Dent 30(4):329–333

Leao JC, Porter SR (1999) Telediagnosis of oral disease. Braz Dent J 10(1):47–53

Lekha K, Meshramkar R, Mathur P, Navya N, Gupta M (2019) A study to evaluate the role of macro-, micro-, and miniesthetics in an attractive smile. Int J Prosthodont Restor Dent 9(4):117–123

Lightbody G, Haberland V, Browne F, Taggart L, Zheng H, Parkes E et al (2019) Review of applications of high-throughput sequencing in personalized medicine: barriers and facilitators of future progress in research and clinical application. Brief Bioinform 20(5):1795–1811

Lin CY, Peng KL, Chen J, Tsai JY, Tseng YC, Yang JR et al (2014) Improvements in dental care using a new mobile app with cloud services. J Formos Med Assoc 113(10):742–749

McLaren EA, Goldstein RE (2018) The photoshop smile design technique. Compend Contin Educ Dent Jamesburg NJ 1995 39(5):e17–20

Morley J, Eubank J (2001) Macroesthetic elements of smile design. J Am Dent Assoc 132(1):39–45

Nair MK, Pettigrew JC, Loomis JS, Bates RE, Kostewicz S, Robinson B et al (2009) Enterprise-wide implementation of digital radiography in oral and maxillofacial imaging: the University of Florida Dentistry System. J Digit Imaging 22(3):232–241

Pocztaruk R de L, Sesma N, Amorim KP, Coachman C (2019) Integrating digital smile design and orthodontic aligners 35(3)

Popovic L, Odalovic D, Zivkovic D, Miladinovic M, Lazic Z, Duka M et al (2020) Teledentistry in dental care of children. Vojnosanit Pregl 77(12):1323–1326

Rakhshan V, Sforza C, Vucinic P, Vitalariu AM, De Menezes M (2018) Advanced digital dentistry. Int J Dent 26(2018):1–2

Rollert MK, Strauss RA, Abubaker AO, Hampton C (1999) Telemedicine consultations in oral and maxillofacial surgery. J Oral Maxillofac Surg 57(2):136–138

Sanchez-Lara A, Chochlidakis KM, Lampraki E, Molinelli R, Molinelli F, Ercoli C (2019) Comprehensive digital approach with the digital smile system: a clinical report. J Prosthet Dent 121(6):871–875

Spangler HD, Simancas-Pallares MA, Ginnis J, Ferreira Zandoná AG, Roach J, Divaris K (2021) A web-based rendering application for communicating dental conditions. Healthcare 9(8):960

Suganna M, Kausher H, Tarek Ahmed S, Sultan Alharbi H, Faraj Alsubaie B, DS A et al (2023) Contemporary evidence of CAD-CAM in dentistry: a systematic review. Cureus 14(11):e31687

Summerfelt FF (2011) Teledentistry-assisted, affiliated practice for dental hygienists: an innovative oral health workforce model. J Dent Educ 75(6):733–742

Sundar MK, Chelliah V (2018) Ten steps to create virtual smile design templates with adobe photoshop® CS6. Compend Contin Educ Dent Jamesburg NJ 1995 39(3):e4–8

Thomas PA, Krishnamoorthi D, Mohan J, Raju R, Rajajayam S, Venkatesan S (2022) Digital smile design. J Pharm Bioallied Sci 14(Suppl 1):S43–S49

Torres-Pereira C, Possebon RS, Simões A, Bortoluzzi MC, Leão JC, Giovanini AF et al (2008) Email for distance diagnosis of oral diseases: a preliminary study of teledentistry. J Telemed Telecare 14(8):435–438

Umer MF, Faheemuddin M, Alshehri YA, Algosaibi AA, Alojail AA, Althani AA et al (2025) Assessment of digital dentistry knowledge and practices among dental students at King Faisal University, Saudi Arabia. Med Sci Monit 30. https://www.medscimonit.com/abstract/index/idArt/944692

Wallace CK, Schofield CE, Burbridge LAL, O'Donnell KL (2021) Role of teledentistry in paediatric dentistry. Br Dent J. https://www.nature.com/articles/s41415-021-3015-y

3D-Guided Dentistry

Amanurrahman Zubair Ahemad, Hariram Sankar, Vidya Rattan, and Mohammad Muneeb Mubashir

1 Evolution of 3D-Guided Dentistry

Three-dimensional (3D)-guided dentistry started to develop with the introduction of CAD/CAM technology and digital X-rays in the late 1900s. At first, dentists used two-dimensional (2D) X-rays and traditional techniques to diagnose and plan treatments. However, these old methods had limitations, especially in accuracy and in showing complex body structures (Jacobs et al. 2018).

A major advancement transpired in the 1990s with the advent of cone-beam computed tomography (CBCT), which gave high-resolution three-dimensional images of the maxillofacial area. CBCT helps dentists see bone mass, nerve paths, and other important details in 3D. This improves the accuracy of placing implants and performing surgeries (Sarment 2013). At the same time, new advancements in digital impression technology and intraoral sensors have greatly changed dental care. These tools made patients more comfortable and improved the accuracy of digital models by replacing traditional physical moulds. The rise of 3D printing greatly improved development, making it easier to create custom surgical guides and prosthetic parts with high precision. The use of computer-aided design/computer-aided manufacturing (CAD/CAM) methods made it possible to design and create accurate dental restorations, such as crowns, bridges, and veneers (Mangano et al. 2013).

Recently, directed surgical software has improved the capabilities of 3D-guided dentistry. These tools help doctors repeat surgical procedures, outline where implants

A. Zubair Ahemad (✉) · H. Sankar
Department of Dentistry, All India Institute of Medical Sciences, Bathinda, India
e-mail: amanurrahman02@gmail.com

V. Rattan
Unit of Oral and Maxillofacial Surgery, Oral Health and Sciences Centre (OHSC), Institute of Medical Education and Research (PGIMER), Chandigarh, India

M. M. Mubashir
Department of Dentistry, Government Medical College, Handwara, India

A. Gupta et al. (eds.), *Application of Robotics in Dentistry*, Lecture Notes in Bioengineering, https://doi.org/10.1007/978-981-95-1470-0_7

should be placed, and create standards for the correct position and angle of implants. Three-dimensional (3D) imaging, digital impressions, and guided treatment have made 3D-guided dentistry an important part of modern dental care (Saini et al. 2015).

Traditional Methods in Dentistry Before Modern Digital Tools

Before modern technology, dentists relied on conventional techniques for diagnosing, planning, and performing treatments. While these methods were effective in their time, they were often limited by the tools and technologies available. Early dental procedures were largely manual, depending heavily on the skill and expertise of the dentist. The primary traditional methods included:

1. **Two-Dimensional Radiography**
   - Periapical and panoramic X-rays: These were the most commonly used X-rays for diagnosing dental conditions. Periapical X-rays provided detailed images of individual teeth and their supporting structures, while panoramic X-rays offered a comprehensive view of the entire jaw and dentition.
   - Limitations: Two-dimensional X-rays lacked depth and often resulted in overlapping structures, making it challenging to accurately assess bone density, nerve pathways, and other critical anatomical details.
2. **Physical Impressions**
   - Alginate and polyvinyl siloxane (PVS) impressions: Dentists used impression materials to create physical moulds of a patient's teeth and gums. These moulds were essential for producing study models, crowns, bridges, and other restorations.
   - Limitations: Traditional impressions were often uncomfortable for patients and prone to inaccuracies due to material shrinkage, tearing, or human error. The process was time-consuming and required multiple visits.
3. **Manual Treatment Planning**
   - Diagnostic wax-ups: Dentists crafted wax models to predict the potential outcomes of dental procedures, such as restorations and prosthetic placements. These models helped visualise the intended results but were time-intensive and lacked precision.
   - Limitations: Manual planning was based primarily on the clinician's judgment rather than precise measurements or digital tools, leading to inconsistent results.
4. **Freehand Surgical Techniques**
   - Tooth extractions and implant placements: These procedures were performed using a freehand (FH) approach, guided only by 2D X-rays and the dentist's experience.
   - Limitations: Freehand techniques often resulted in misaligned implants, increased complications, and prolonged healing times. The lack of 3D

visualisation made it difficult to avoid vital structures such as nerves and sinuses.

Limitations of Traditional Dental Methods

Despite their usefulness at the time, traditional dental techniques had several inherent drawbacks that made them less efficient and effective:

1. Lack of precision: The absence of 3D imaging and digital tools made accurate diagnoses and treatment planning difficult, leading to suboptimal outcomes, especially in complex cases.
2. Patient discomfort: Many traditional procedures caused discomfort and anxiety among patients. Additionally, some treatments required longer recovery times due to their invasive nature.
3. Inefficient workflows: Conventional methods involved multiple visits and lengthy lab processes, increasing both treatment time and costs for patients and practitioners.
4. Limited visualisation: With only 2D X-rays and physical models available, dentists had a limited perspective of a patient's anatomy, making precise planning and execution more challenging.
5. Dependence on clinician skill: The success of traditional dental methods relied heavily on the experience and expertise of the dentist, leading to variability in treatment outcomes.

2 Transition to Modern Techniques

The limitations of traditional dental tools and methods highlighted the need for more advanced equipment and improved techniques. The introduction of digital technologies such as 3D imaging, intraoral scanners (IOSs), and CAD/CAM systems has significantly transformed dental practices.

Significance in Modern Dental Practice

The significance of 3D-guided dentistry in modern dental practice cannot be overstated. Its impact is evident in several key areas. Three-dimensional (3D)-guided dentistry greatly impacts today's oral care, leading to important improvements in various areas:

(a) Enhanced diagnostic accuracy: Three-dimensional imaging provides a complete view of a patient's mouth structure. This helps in spotting any problems early, checking bone density accurately, and analysing important anatomical features correctly. Being this specific is important for diagnosing complex situations and creating good treatments.
(b) Improved treatment results: Digital modelling and virtual treatment planning help dentists perform processes accurately, reducing mistakes and significantly improving both the function and appearance of dental work, particularly in implants and restorative dentistry.

(c) Less invasive methods: Three-dimensional guided technology helps doctors perform minimally invasive surgeries more accurately by allowing them to plan and carry out treatments carefully. This reduces stress on nearby tissues, speeds up healing time, and makes patients more comfortable.
(d) Focus on the patient: Using 3D models to explain treatment options helps patients understand better and get more involved in their care. Being open creates trust between the dentist and the patient, leading to greater satisfaction and better following of treatment plans.
(e) Improving efficiency and workflow: Digital processes improve many parts of dental care, including diagnosing problems and creating solutions like tooth restorations. This efficiency reduces the time spent in the chair, lessens the need for many sessions, and boosts total productivity in practice.
(f) Different specialities: Three-dimensional (3D)-guided dentistry is useful in many areas of dentistry, such as implants, braces, root canals, and dentures. Its flexibility makes it a key tool for complete tooth care (Manjunatha et al. 2024).

3 Challenges and Limitations of Adopting 3D-Guided Dentistry

While 3D-guided dentistry offers numerous advantages, its adoption in clinical practice is not without challenges and limitations. These barriers can be categorised into technical, financial, educational, and practical concerns, which may hinder the widespread implementation of this technology.

1. **Technical Challenges**

   - Complexity of technology: Three-dimensional (3D)-guided dentistry involves the integration of multiple technologies, including CBCT imaging, intraoral scanners, CAD/CAM systems, and guided surgery software. Mastering these tools requires a steep learning curve and a deep understanding of digital workflows.
   - Software compatibility issues: Different systems (e.g. imaging devices, scanners, and design software) may not always be compatible, leading to difficulties in data integration and workflow efficiency.
   - Image artefacts and errors: CBCT imaging, while highly detailed, can sometimes produce artefacts due to patient movement, metal restorations, or beam hardening. These artefacts can compromise the accuracy of 3D models and treatment plans.
   - Limited access to advanced equipment: In some regions, especially in developing countries, access to advanced 3D imaging and digital fabrication equipment may be limited, restricting the adoption of 3D-guided dentistry.

2. **Financial Barriers**
   - High initial investment: The cost of acquiring 3D imaging systems (e.g. CBCT scanners), intraoral scanners, and CAD/CAM equipment is substantial. This financial burden can be prohibitive for small- or mid-sized dental practices.
   - Maintenance and upgrades: Beyond the initial investment, ongoing costs for software updates, equipment maintenance, and staff training can add to the financial strain.
   - Return on investment (ROI) concerns: While 3D-guided dentistry can improve efficiency and patient outcomes, the ROI may not be immediate. Practices may need time to build a patient base that justifies the investment.
3. **Educational and Training Gaps**
   - Lack of training programmes: Many dental schools and continuing education programmes have yet to fully incorporate 3D-guided dentistry into their curricula. As a result, clinicians may lack the necessary skills to effectively use these technologies.
   - Resistance to change: Dentists accustomed to traditional methods may be hesitant to adopt new technologies due to a lack of familiarity or confidence in digital workflows.
   - Interdisciplinary collaboration: Three-dimensional (3D)-guided dentistry often requires collaboration between dentists, radiologists, and lab technicians. Miscommunication or a lack of interdisciplinary training can hinder the successful implementation of these technologies.
4. **Practical Limitations**
   - Time-intensive workflows: While 3D-guided dentistry can streamline certain aspects of treatment, the initial set-up and learning phase can be time-consuming. Clinicians may need to dedicate significant time to mastering new tools and workflows.
   - Patient-specific challenges: Not all patients are suitable candidates for 3D-guided procedures. For example, patients with severe anatomical abnormalities or those who cannot remain still during CBCT scans may pose challenges.
   - Data management and security: The use of digital technologies generates large volumes of patient data, which must be stored, managed, and protected in compliance with privacy regulations (e.g. Health Insurance Portability and Accountability Act [HIPAA] in the USA). Ensuring data security can be a significant administrative burden.
5. **Ethical and Legal Considerations**
   - Liability concerns: The use of advanced technologies introduces new potential sources of error, such as software glitches or inaccuracies in digital models. Clinicians must be prepared to address these issues and mitigate liability risks.

- Informed consent: Patients must be adequately informed about the benefits, risks, and limitations of 3D-guided procedures. Ensuring informed consent can be challenging, especially when patients are unfamiliar with the technology.

6. **Limitations in Clinical Applications**
   - Not universally applicable: While 3D-guided dentistry is highly effective for procedures like implant placement and orthodontic planning, it may not be necessary or cost-effective for simpler treatments (e.g. routine fillings or cleanings).
   - Dependence on imaging quality: The accuracy of 3D-guided procedures depends heavily on the quality of the CBCT scan or digital impression. Poor-quality imaging can lead to suboptimal outcomes.
   - Limited accessibility for certain populations: Patients in rural or underserved areas may not have access to practices equipped with 3D-guided technologies, exacerbating disparities in dental care.
7. **Future Directions to Overcome Challenges**
   - Increased training and education: Expanding dental school curricula and continuing education programmes to include 3D-guided dentistry can help bridge the knowledge gap and encourage adoption.
   - Cost reduction and accessibility: As technology advances, the cost of 3D imaging and digital equipment is expected to decrease, making it more accessible to a broader range of practices.
   - Improved interoperability: Developing standardised protocols and software solutions that enhance compatibility between different systems can streamline workflows and reduce technical challenges.
   - Patient education and awareness: Educating patients about the benefits of 3D-guided dentistry can increase demand for these services, encouraging more practices to adopt the technology.

4 History of Dental Technology: Exploration of Advancements Leading to 3D-Guided Methods

Dental technology has significantly evolved throughout the years, leading to the advent of 3D-guided dentistry. Technological developments have evolved from basic tools utilised by early civilisations to the complex digital processes of the present, consistently striving to enhance precision, efficiency, and patient outcomes. This chapter examines the significant advancements in dental technology, specifically highlighting the advances that have contributed to the emergence of 3D-guided techniques.

Early Developments in Dental Technology

1. Ancient and Early Modern Dentistry (Pre-1900s)

The earliest evidence of dental practices dates back to ancient civilisations, such as the Egyptians, Greeks, and Romans. These cultures used basic tools like bow drills and primitive forceps for tooth extraction and rudimentary fillings made from materials like beeswax and gold. During the Middle Ages, dental care was often provided by barbers or general physicians. Tools remained simple, and treatments were largely focused on pain relief and tooth extraction rather than restoration.

2. Birth of Modern Dentistry (Eighteenth and Nineteenth Centuries)—Pierre Fauchard (Father of Modern Dentistry)

In the eighteenth century, Pierre Fauchard introduced systematic approaches to dentistry, including the use of dental fillings, prosthetics, and orthodontic devices. His work laid the foundation for modern dental practices. The nineteenth century saw the invention of the dental chair and the development of specialised hand instruments, such as dental drills and scalers, which improved the precision and comfort of dental procedures. The introduction of anaesthesia (e.g. nitrous oxide and ether) and sterilisation techniques (e.g. autoclaves) in the nineteenth century transformed dentistry by reducing pain and infection risks.

The discovery of X-rays by Wilhelm Roentgen in 1895 revolutionised dental diagnostics. By the early twentieth century, X-rays became a standard tool for visualising teeth, bone, and other oral structures, enabling more accurate diagnoses and treatment planning. Over time, advancements in radiography led to the development of periapical and panoramic X-rays, which provided more detailed views of the oral cavity and surrounding structures.

3. Rise of Digital Dentistry (Late Twentieth Century)

In the 1980s, computer-aided design and computer-aided manufacturing (CAD/CAM) systems were introduced to dentistry. These technologies allowed for the digital design and fabrication of dental restorations, such as crowns, bridges, and veneers, with greater precision and efficiency. The development of intraoral scanners in the 1990s eliminated the need for traditional physical impressions, improving patient comfort and the accuracy of digital models. CBCT imaging, introduced in the late 1990s, provided high-resolution 3D images of the maxillofacial region, enabling detailed visualisation of bone density, nerve pathways, and other anatomical structures. This innovation was a game changer for implantology and surgical planning.

4. Era of 3D-Guided Dentistry (Twenty-First Century)

The twenty-first century has seen the seamless integration of 3D imaging, digital impressions, and CAD/CAM systems into a cohesive digital workflow. This integration has enabled the development of 3D-guided dentistry, where virtual treatment planning and guided surgery are central to clinical practice. Advanced software platforms now allow clinicians to simulate surgical procedures, plan implant placements,

Table 1 Key milestones in dental technology

Year	Milestone description
1957	Introduction of the first air-driven dental handpiece, improving the speed and efficiency of dental procedures
1985	Development of the first commercial CAD/CAM system for dentistry (CEREC) by Dr. Werner Mörmann
1998	Introduction of CBCT imaging, providing 3D visualisation of the maxillofacial region
2000	Widespread adoption of intraoral scanners and digital impression systems
2000	Laser dentistry became mainstream
2010	Integration of 3D printing and guided surgery software into dental practice
2010	3D bioprinting for regenerative dentistry
2017	Exploration of AI-driven diagnostics and treatment planning tools
2021	Robotic-assisted surgery
2021	Smart dental devices and technology
2022	Expansion of teledentistry platforms
2024	Development of AI-powered virtual dental assistants
2025	Nanotechnology and advanced materials

and design surgical guides that ensure optimal positioning and angulation of dental implants.

The advent of 3D printing has further expanded the capabilities of 3D-guided dentistry. Clinicians can now fabricate surgical guides, models, and even custom prosthetics directly from digital designs, reducing turnaround times and costs. Emerging technologies, such as artificial intelligence (AI) and machine learning, are being integrated into dental software to enhance diagnostic accuracy, predict treatment outcomes, and optimise workflows (Table 1).

5 Core Concepts of 3D-Guided Dentistry: Definition, Scope, and Foundational Principles of 3D-Guided Dentistry

Definition of 3D-Guided Dentistry

Three-dimensional (3D)-guided dentistry employs digital technology, including three-dimensional imaging, computer-aided design/computer-aided manufacturing (CAD/CAM), and guided surgery, to improve diagnostic precision, treatment planning, and procedure implementation. Through the integration of these technologies, doctors can deliver personalised patient care and attain enhanced clinical outcomes. This methodology integrates cone beam computed tomography (CBCT), three-dimensional printing, and dynamic navigation technologies to create virtual models, manufacture surgical guides, and develop custom restorations. Three-dimensional (3D)-guided dentistry enhances patient outcomes by minimising human error, lowering procedural invasiveness, and improving precision (Obaid 2020).

Scope of 3D-Guided Dentistry

The scope of 3D-guided dentistry is vast, encompassing a wide range of applications across various dental disciplines. Key areas include:

1. Implantology
   - Precise planning and placement of dental implants using 3D imaging and surgical guides.
   - Evaluation of bone density, nerve pathways, and anatomical structures to ensure optimal implant positioning.
2. Orthodontics
   - Digital models for diagnosis and treatment planning of malocclusions and tooth alignment.
   - Fabrication of custom aligners and appliances using 3D printing.
3. Prosthodontics
   - Design and fabrication of crowns, bridges, veneers, and dentures using CAD/CAM systems.
   - Digital impressions for accurate and comfortable restorations.
4. Endodontics
   - Three-dimensional imaging for diagnosing complex root canal anatomy and planning treatments.
   - Guided access cavity preparation to minimise tooth structure removal.
5. Oral and Maxillofacial Surgery
   - Virtual planning for complex surgical procedures, such as jaw reconstruction and impacted tooth removal.

Foundational Principles of 3D-Guided Dentistry

1. Digital Imaging and Data Acquisition
   - Cone beam computed tomography (CBCT) for three-dimensional anatomical visualisation
   - Intraoral scanners for precise digital impressions
   - Optical and laser scanning technologies for enhanced detail and accuracy
2. Computer-Aided Planning and Design
   - Use of specialised software for virtual treatment simulations
   - Digital workflow integration from diagnosis to final restoration
   - Predictive modelling for treatment success and patient-specific solutions

3. 3D Printing and Guided Surgery
   - Fabrication of custom surgical guides for precise interventions
   - 3D-printed prosthetic components for seamless restoration
   - Reduction of chair time and surgical errors through guided protocols
4. Minimally Invasive and Patient-Centred Approach
   - Precise treatment planning to reduce unnecessary tissue trauma
   - Customisation for better aesthetics and functionality
   - Enhanced communication between dental professionals and patients.
5. Real-Time Feedback
   - Dynamic navigation systems (DNS) (e.g. X-Guide) for live tracking of surgical instruments, enhancing accuracy, and reducing risks.
6. Data-Driven Decision-Making
   - AI algorithms for imaging data analysis to detect pathologies (e.g. cavities, bone loss) early, improving diagnostic accuracy by up to 20%.

6 Systems in 3D Dentistry

1	Equipment and software in 3D dentistry	Detailed discussion on the tools and software essential for 3D-guided dental procedures
2	Imaging systems	Overview of CBCT, intraoral scanners, and other imaging technologies
3	3D printing in dentistry	Applications of 3D printing for models, guides, and prosthetics

Equipment and Software in 3D Dentistry

Three-dimensional (3D)-guided dentistry relies on a combination of advanced hardware and software to achieve precise, efficient, and predictable outcomes. This chapter provides a detailed discussion of the essential tools and technologies used in 3D-guided dental procedures, including imaging systems, 3D printing, and software platforms.

Imaging Systems

Imaging systems are the foundation of 3D-guided dentistry, providing the detailed data needed for diagnosis, treatment planning, and execution. Key imaging technologies include:

1. Cone Beam Computed Tomography (CBCT)

CBCT is a sophisticated imaging technique that is widely used in dentistry, maxillofacial surgery, otolaryngology, and other medical fields. Unlike traditional computed tomography (CT) scans, CBCT produces high-resolution, three-dimensional images with minimal radiation exposure, making it the preferred choice for diagnostic imaging in certain medical applications.

Principle of CBCT

A CBCT system uses fundamental processes to provide high-resolution, three-dimensional imaging with low radiation. Beam generation, X-ray detection, image reconstruction, and image display are essential to image quality and diagnostic accuracy.

The first stage, beam generation, involves controlled X-ray emission from a radiographic-style X-ray tube. CBCT uses a cone-shaped beam instead of a fan-shaped beam like multi-detector computed tomography (MDCT), allowing for a wider data field in one rotation. The X-ray source rotates around the patient, capturing multiple projection images and emitting pulsed X-rays. Pulsed emission reduces radiation while obtaining enough data for image reconstruction. The beam is further collimated to fit the selected field of view (FOV), exposing only the necessary region and reducing radiation to nearby structures. X-ray penetration and intensity are controlled by kilovoltage (kV) and milliamperage (mA), which affect image quality. Kilovoltage affects X-ray penetration and contrast, while milliamperage controls beam intensity and image brightness and clarity. These parameters are adjusted to optimise image contrast and resolution based on patient anatomy and diagnostic needs.

An image receptor captures and converts attenuated X-rays into electrical signals after the beam passes through the patient. Denser tissues like bone absorb more radiation, increasing contrast. Flat-panel detectors (FPDs) and image-intensifier detectors are used in CBCT systems. Most modern CBCT systems use FPDs, which are amorphous silicon panels with a caesium iodide scintillator. Superior image quality is achieved by these detectors' high spatial resolution, signal-to-noise ratio, and image distortion reduction. Earlier systems used image-intensifier detectors, which were effective but prone to geometric distortion, signal degradation, and magnetic field interference. Image-intensifier detectors are being replaced by flat-panel technology due to their frequent calibration.

Data acquisition is followed by mathematical algorithm reconstruction of raw projection images from multiple angles. Reconstruction is needed to turn two-dimensional data into three-dimensional volumetric data. Iterative reconstruction and filtered back projection (FBP) are the main reconstruction methods. The traditional method of filtered back projection uses mathematical filtering to remove noise and sharpen the image for fast reconstruction. Insufficient data may ruin image quality, causing FBP artefacts. The more advanced technique of iterative reconstruction reduces noise and artefacts and lowers radiation doses, improving image quality. After reconstruction, the dataset is aligned along axial, sagittal, and coronal planes. This alignment helps diagnose and treat anatomical structures by allowing precise visualisation. Multiple planar reconstructions (MPR) and secondary reconstructions on CBCT systems allow clinicians to examine the region of interest from multiple angles, improving visualisation.

The final three-dimensional image is displayed using Digital Imaging and Communications in Medicine (DICOM)-compatible software after reconstruction. The software supports multiplanar slices, panoramic reconstructions, cross-sectional views, and three-dimensional volume rendering. For accurate anatomical assessment, multiplanar slices enable detailed visualisation of the scanned area in standard axial, coronal, and sagittal planes. Orthodontic and surgical planning benefit from panoramic reconstructions' wide-field views of dental arches. In implant dentistry, cross-sectional views help measure bone density and implant placement feasibility. Volumetric assessment and virtual manipulation of the scanned region improve diagnostic accuracy and surgical planning with three-dimensional rendering. Dental and maxillofacial applications benefit from advanced image analysis software's segmentation, measurement, and simulation features. Artefact reduction algorithms in modern CBCT software reduce beam hardening and streak artefacts caused by metal restorations or implants.

The sophisticated yet efficient CBCT imaging system uses a structured workflow to provide high-resolution imaging with low radiation. Optimised beam generation, advanced detector technology, refined reconstruction algorithms, and interactive image display software have improved CBCT diagnostics. This technology has become essential in dentistry, maxillofacial surgery, otolaryngology, and radiology, allowing clinicians to gain detailed anatomical insights for better patient care.

Applications

1. Endodontics

Detection of apical periodontitis: CBCT demonstrates superior accuracy compared to conventional X-rays in the early identification of periapical infections. It can detect bone damage prior to its visibility in standard radiographs. Research indicates that CBCT demonstrates a 62% improvement in detecting these issues, particularly in the upper posterior teeth, where overlapping structures may obscure problems.

Comprehending the anatomy of root canals: Identifying the structure of the root canal is essential for effective treatment. CBCT effectively identifies concealed canals that conventional X-rays may overlook. The second mesiobuccal canal (MB2) in maxillary molars is identified in up to 93% of cases via CBCT, whereas traditional radiographs detect it in only 55% of cases. This method is effective for identifying intricate root configurations such as dens invaginatus and fused teeth.

Identifying vertical root fractures: Traditional X-rays are ineffective for the detection of vertical root fractures. CBCT enhances diagnostic capabilities by revealing fractures prior to significant bone loss. This method offers comprehensive images from various perspectives, highlighting fractures that might be overlooked in conventional radiographs. Metal fillings may occasionally produce artefacts resembling fractures.

Detection and evaluation of root resorption: CBCT is essential for the diagnosis of both internal and external root resorption. Standard X-rays frequently have difficulty distinguishing between external cervical resorption (ECR) and internal resorption because of overlapping anatomical structures. CBCT facilitates accurate identification and categorisation of lesions, thereby enhancing treatment planning.

Preparation for endodontic surgery: CBCT is crucial for the planning of surgical procedures such as apicoectomy. It assists in establishing:

- The precise location of roots concerning adjacent structures, such as the maxillary sinus and nerves.
- The magnitude of bone loss.
- The thickness of the bone influences the surgical approach.
- This minimises the likelihood of complications during surgery.
- CBCT demonstrates significant efficacy in the assessment of dental injuries, encompassing root fractures and osseous damage. Conventional X-rays can overlook horizontal fractures, necessitating multiple images taken from various angles. CBCT offers high-resolution three-dimensional images, facilitating the assessment of injury severity and treatment planning.
- Assessment of the proper placement of the root canal filling.
- Should any canals be overlooked or remain untreated?
- The healing process of periapical infections (Kiarudi et al. 2015).

2. Implantology

Planning before implant placement: CBCT's accurate 3D bone images make it popular for dental implant planning. To avoid nerve damage, it measures the alveolar crest–mandibular canal space. CBCT reduces surgery risks by preventing implants from damaging the maxillary sinus and nasopalatine canal.

Checking bone density and quality: CBCT measures bone density, which aids implant success. CBCT does not measure Hounsfield units (HU) as accurately as multi-slice computed tomography (MSCT), but it can help choose implants by assessing bone quality. Checking bone density is crucial for long-lasting implants. Weak bones can fail.

Prevention of nerve and vessel damage: CBCT locates the inferior alveolar nerve and mental foramen to prevent implant nerve damage. It finds bifid mandibular canals and extra openings that panoramic X-rays miss. Recognising these structures reduces pain, numbness, and bleeding.

Lingual undercuts and perforation risk identification: Interior undercuts in the lower jaw can make things difficult. If overlooked, an implant in this area could damage the lingual plate, causing heavy bleeding, blocked airways, or infection. Detailing jaw cross sections with CBCT imaging reduces these risks.

Implant osseointegration assessment: The direct structural and functional connection between living bone and a load-bearing implant is called osseointegration. Dental implant durability and performance depend on osseointegration. The post-surgical examination monitors this process and detects problems.

Monitoring integration with surrounding bone: The main goal is to evaluate the integration between the implant and surrounding bone. Assessments usually involve clinical and radiological examinations. Bone density and implant stability are assessed by periapical radiography, CBCT, and clinical stability tests. No radiolucent patches near the implant–bone interface indicate a solid connection (Salimov et al. 2014).

Early identification of early signs of implant failure: Common symptom is implant movement, which indicates inadequate osseointegration even with light pressure. Radiographic indications of bone resorption around the implant could point to mechanical overload or infection. Symptoms such as redness, swelling, or pus surrounding the implant site point to peri-implantitis, which can cause implant failure should therapy not be received. Routine imaging and follow-ups help to spot these problems early on and apply the required repairs. Successful osseointegration results in an implant able to tolerate functional loads, offering a firm basis for prosthetic restorations (Kochar et al. 2022).

Monitoring implant success and patient recovery:

- Implant position and angle are assessed.
- Proper implant–bone contact is crucial for integration.
- Possible issues include bone loss, edge issues, and misplacement.
- CBCT detects implant issues early and recommends solutions.
- Sinus and nasopalatine canal shape are assessed.
- CBCT is needed to evaluate the maxillary sinus and nasopalatine canal for maxilla implants. It measures sinus floor thickness and detects structural differences that could make implant placement difficult. This reduces sinus and sensory injuries.

Guided implant surgery: Computer-guided implant surgery uses virtual planning software with CBCT data to create personalised surgical guides. These guides improve implant positioning, surgical accuracy, and error reduction (Gupta and Ali 2013).

3. Orthodontics

Evaluation of impacted and ectopic teeth: CBCT offers comprehensive three-dimensional imaging that enables precise identification of the location, angulation, and relationship of impacted and ectopic teeth with respect to adjacent structures. This is particularly beneficial in instances of maxillary canine impaction, as traditional X-rays frequently do not reveal the complete extent of the impaction.

Assessment of root resorption: CBCT facilitates accurate identification of both external and internal root resorption, potentially resulting from orthodontic forces or the presence of impacted teeth. This method offers cross-sectional views that facilitate the assessment of resorption severity and location, enabling clinicians to adjust treatment plans as needed.

Assessment of the pharyngeal airway: CBCT is essential for assessing airway space in orthodontic patients, especially in cases of obstructive sleep apnoea or mouth-breathing tendencies. This assessment facilitates the evaluation of airway volume, soft tissue obstruction, and skeletal relationships, thereby supporting diagnosis and treatment planning.

Evaluation of mini-implant locations: CBCT offers precise measurements of bone density and thickness for orthodontic temporary anchorage devices (TADs), facilitating the accurate placement of mini-implants. This decreases failure rates and enhances treatment outcomes.

Assessment of craniofacial abnormalities: CBCT is advantageous for evaluating skeletal asymmetries, cleft palate, and craniofacial syndromes. The tool offers accurate anatomical measurements, assisting orthodontists in planning both surgical and non-surgical treatment strategies.

Evaluation of sinus and temporomandibular joint: CBCT facilitates a comprehensive analysis of sinus anatomy and pathology, aiding in the diagnosis of sinusitis and orthodontic issues related to the sinuses. It is utilised to evaluate temporomandibular joint (TMJ) conditions, focusing on bone remodelling, joint space, and condylar positioning.

Planning for orthognathic surgery: CBCT facilitates pre-surgical planning and post-surgical assessment in orthognathic procedures. The tool offers precise measurements of skeletal discrepancies, facilitating treatment planning for maxillomandibular advancement, mandibular setback, and various surgical corrections.

Assessment of cortical bone plates: CBCT is utilised to evaluate the thickness of cortical bone, especially in scenarios necessitating tooth movement through cortical bone or expansion procedures. This aids in forecasting treatment stability and associated risks.

4. Oral and Maxillofacial Surgery

Dentoalveolar surgery refers to surgical procedures involving the teeth and surrounding alveolar bone. This field encompasses various interventions aimed at addressing dental pathologies, facilitating tooth extraction, and preparing for prosthetic rehabilitation.

CBCT improves the evaluation of impacted teeth, especially third molars, by offering accurate localisation in relation to nerves, bone, and surrounding structures. It aids in preventing complications like root displacement or nerve injury, which may not be detectable in conventional X-rays.

Disorders of the temporomandibular joint (TMJ): CBCT offers comprehensive imaging of osseous alterations in the TMJ, facilitating the diagnosis of osteoarthritis, condylar resorption, and joint remodelling. Nonetheless, it is suboptimal for soft tissue evaluation, for which magnetic resonance imaging (MRI) is the preferred imaging modality.

Orthognathic surgery refers to surgical procedures aimed at correcting skeletal and dental irregularities, including the alignment of the jaw and teeth. This type of surgery is often performed to improve both function and aesthetics in patients with malocclusion or other jaw-related issues. CBCT is essential for pre-surgical planning and post-operative assessment in orthognathic procedures. This method facilitates accurate measurement of skeletal asymmetries, airway evaluation, and three-dimensional virtual surgical planning, thereby enhancing surgical precision.

Maxillofacial trauma: CBCT is especially effective in assessing fractures of the jaw and facial bones. This tool offers comprehensive 3D reconstructions of intricate fractures, facilitating surgical decision-making and post-operative assessment.

Evaluation of pathology and tumours: CBCT is effective in the detection and evaluation of cysts, tumours, and various bony lesions in the jaw. It offers precise images of lesion boundaries, internal composition, and adjacency to critical structures, enhancing diagnostic accuracy and surgical preparation.

Evaluation of osteomyelitis: CBCT effectively diagnoses osteomyelitis and osteonecrosis by demonstrating alterations in bone density and structure. This method offers enhanced visualisation of sequestra and periosteal reactions relative to traditional radiographs.

5. Otolaryngology (ENT): CBCT is crucial for diagnosing sinus issues, evaluating nasal airway obstructions, and planning ear surgeries. It is especially useful for studying the structure of the middle and inner ear.
6. Oncology: CBCT helps to detect tumours and assess tumour margins in head and neck cancers. It is used for preoperative and post-operative assessments to ensure complete tumour resection and treatment efficacy.
7. Airway and sleep apnoea assessment: CBCT provides precise airway volume measurements to aid in the diagnosis and treatment planning of obstructive sleep apnoea.

Limitations and Risks of CBCT

- Exposure to radiation: CBCT presents a lower radiation dose compared to conventional medical CT; however, it still subjects patients to higher doses than traditional two-dimensional radiography. This presents issues, especially for paediatric patients and those needing numerous scans over an extended period.
- Visual artefacts: CBCT images are susceptible to beam hardening and metal artefacts, leading to structural distortion and diminished image quality. The presence of metal restorations, implants, or orthodontic appliances in patients poses significant challenges during scanning, resulting in potential misinterpretations.
- Inadequate soft tissue contrast: In contrast to medical CT and MRI, CBCT offers restricted soft tissue differentiation. This limits its suitability for evaluating muscles, nerves, and other soft tissues, confining its application mainly to hard tissue imaging.
- Considerations for field of view (FOV): Choosing an unsuitable field of view may result in either excessive or inadequate imaging. An excessively large field of view (FOV) elevates radiation exposure and complicates image interpretation, whereas an insufficiently small FOV risks omitting essential anatomical structures, necessitating further scans.
- Challenges in interpretation: Accurate interpretation of CBCT images necessitates specialised training. Numerous general dentists may not possess the necessary expertise to recognise incidental findings, pathologies, or anatomical anomalies that fall outside their specific area of focus. Misinterpretation may result in incorrect diagnoses or superfluous treatments.

- Cost and accessibility: CBCT machines entail significant acquisition and maintenance costs, resulting in elevated expenses for practitioners and patients alike. The restricted availability of CBCT technology in certain regions may hinder its broader implementation (Friedland and Miles 2014).

2. Intraoral Scanners

Definition and Scope of Intraoral Scanners (IOSs)

Intraoral scanners (IOSs) are digital devices capable of obtaining direct optical impressions of the mouth and constructing three-dimensional (3D) images of the oral cavity and its parts (Fig. 1). Intraoral scanners have integrated some features that, previously, only existed independently, and are digitised in prosthodontics, implantology, orthodontics, and restorative dentistry. Traditionally used impression materials, polyvinyl siloxane and alginate, have a number of drawbacks, such as deformation of the material, inelastic dimensionality, bubbling, and even uncontrolled misfit prosthetic appliances. These and other shortcomings are overcome by IOS with real-time visualisation, precision, and direct incorporation of CAD/CAM technology.

Historical Evolution of IOS

It has been decades since the commencement of intraoral scanners, but their path has only been upward:

- 1984: CEREC-1, the first chairside CAD/CAM system, was developed by Dr Werner Mörmann—the most significant transition from traditional impressions to digital.
- 2000s: Laser and structured-light scanning technologies were introduced to provide better accuracy.

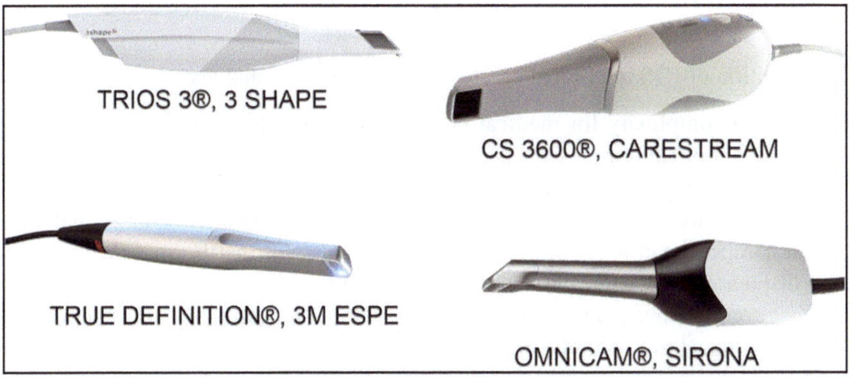

Fig. 1 Four different IOSs (CS 3600®, Carestream, Rochester, NY, USA; TRIOS 3®, 3Shape, Copenhagen, Denmark; CEREC Omnicam®, Sirona Dental System GmbH, Bensheim, Germany; True Definition®, 3 M ESPE, S. Paul, MN, USA) were compared in this study, with the purpose to investigate their trueness and precision in oral implantology (Imburgia et al. 2017)

Table 2 Types of intraoral scanner

Category	Open system intraoral scanners	Closed system intraoral scanners
Definition	Generates output files in standard formats (e.g. STL), compatible with various third-party CAD/CAM software and hardware	Operates within a proprietary ecosystem, producing files only compatible with specific manufacturer-provided software and hardware
Advantages	Flexibility: availability of several milling tools and software at hand Integration: helps cooperation between several labs and partners Upgradability: quickly adopts fresh technology	Seamless integration: every element cooperating effectively Simplified support: technical assistance from a single provider
Considerations	Requires understanding of software compatibility and workflow management May involve coordinating with multiple vendors for support	Limited flexibility: restricted to manufacturer's products Dependence on a single provider for updates and innovations
Ideal for practices	Practices requiring customisation, third-party integration, and future upgradability	Practices preferring an all-in-one solution with direct manufacturer support

- 2010s–present: Sophisticated technologies such as artificial intelligence (AI), machine learning, real-time image stitching, and then wireless connectivity later further refined IOS technologies and eventually paved their path to success in future digital dentistry.

Intraoral scanner types are shown in Table 2.

7 Importance of IOS in Modern Dentistry

The adoption of IOS in clinical practice offers many advantages:

- Reduced complexity for medical professionals: Another advantage afforded by the use of optical impressions is clinical. After completing the learning curve, the use of IOS may give additional clinical benefits by easing impression-making in complex settings, such as those requiring multiple implants or large undercuts that hamper the efficacy of traditional impressions. Furthermore, if the physician is displeased with some parts of the recorded optical impression, they can remove those components and recapture the image without repeating the entire procedure, saving time (Lawson and Burgess 1995; Lee et al. 2013; Lim et al. 2018).
- Decreased discomfort: Traditional impression methods can be uncomfortable for patients because the materials used in the trays can be inconvenient and difficult to handle. The usual method might not work well for everyone, especially for young children or people who easily gag. Using light instead of traditional impression

materials helps these people and makes optical impressions more useful. Using impression trays and other items that may be uncomfortable for patients is no longer needed. Studies show that patients care more about visual appearances than standard aspects (Zimmermann et al. 2015; Muir and Calvert 1988; Wismeijer et al. 2014).

- Time efficiency: Numerous studies have demonstrated that optical impressions save time and money. The latest iOS-compatible intraoral scanners can capture a full-arch scan in less than three minutes. However, the real time savings come from the streamlined digital workflow that follows. In contrast, traditional impressions typically take three to five minutes just for the impression step. With digital optical scans, the dental lab receives the data almost instantly, enabling faster turnaround for prosthetics and other lab work. 3D virtual models (proprietary or Standard Tessellation Language [STL] files) by email rather than courier or postal delivery. This saves significant time and money over the course of a working year. Dental clinics can import optical impression data into CAD software and mill them in CAM software to create chairside prosthetic restorations. Rehabilitation techniques for diverse materials will be defined and applied clinically (Goracci et al. 2016; Burhardt et al. 2016; Sakornwimon and Leevailoj 2017).
- Improved communication with the dental technician: IOS allows clinicians and dental technicians to assess impression quality in real time. Immediately after the scan, the dentist can email it to the laboratory for accurate testing. If the dental technician is dissatisfied with the quality of the optical impression, they can request a new one without losing time or having to reschedule the patient's appointment. This element streamlines and increases the connection between the dentist and dental technician (Marti et al. 2017; Kugel 1995).
- Learning curve: Using IOS in the dental office requires learning and planning. Young dentists who love technology and computing will easily accept IOS. Veteran practitioners with minimal expertise and less passion for technology may find devices and software more challenging. Manufacturers provide little information about their scanning methods, so it is unclear which is best. Multiple machines utilising different scanning methods may produce different results; thus, this feature will be thoroughly tested in the coming years.

Technological Advancements in IOS

- Emerging Technology and Hardware Innovations

The advancements made in IOS hardware contribute towards the improvement of the device's performance and usability in the following ways:

- Aircraft scanners: The Medit i700 has easy mobility and usability features, enhancing the scanner's performance.
- AI-guided scanning with haptic feedback: Some IOSs provide haptic guidance to cover scanning control as user moves to ensure complete scan coverage.
- Automatic calibration: Self-calibrating scanners are competent in measuring and adjusting without frequent manual alterations.

- Compact and lightweight scanners: Ergonomics are designed such that the fatigue experienced by the operator is reduced hence increasing the IOS clinical productivity.
- Software Improvements.

  Software makes the IOS more accurate and efficient by:

- AI scanning: AI software is able to identify and fix scanner problems within a time frame while scanning.
- Continuous capture and easy stitching: Improved algorithms capture, stitch and merge images within the shortest period possible.
- Cloud storage: Cloud enables dentists and labs to have secure instant access for easy collaborations and interactions.
- Augmented and virtual reality: AR/VR is being investigated towards treatment simulations for interactive patient education.

  The features and technologies of key IOS brands are compared in Table 3.

Principles of Intraoral Scanning

Intraoral scanners (IOSs) operate based on optical scanning technologies, capturing high-resolution 3D digital impressions of the oral cavity. These scanners use structured light, laser, or confocal imaging to acquire surface data and generate accurate digital models. The fundamental principles governing their operation include:

1. Optical Triangulation

   - Uses laser beams projected onto the tooth surface.
   - A sensor records the reflection angles, calculating the distance between the scanner and the object.
   - Based on the Pythagorean theorem, this method reconstructs the scanned area in 3D (Fig. 2).

2. Confocal Microscopy

   - Employs multiple focal planes to capture sharp and defocused images.
   - The scanner processes reflected light intensity to generate an accurate depth map of dental surfaces.
   - Allows scanning at various depths with high precision.

3. Structured-Light Projection

   - The scanner projects a known pattern of light (e.g. grids or stripes) onto the teeth.
   - A camera captures the deformed pattern, and software reconstructs the 3D image by analysing distortions.
   - Provides fast and highly accurate digital impressions.

Table 3 Comparison of key IOS brands

Brand	Features	Notable technologies
Primescan (Dentsply Sirona)	High-resolution, full-arch scanning	AI-enhanced trueness and accuracy
TRIOS 4 (3Shape)	Wireless scanning, instant shade detection	AI-driven margin detection
iTero element (Align technology)	Cloud-based storage, Invisalign integration, adaptive anti-fogging technology	Time-lapse progress tracking, Compatible with Invisalign system for orthodontic treatments
Medit i700	Scans up to 70 frames per second for fast data acquisition, cost-effective, ergonomic handpiece design weighing 8.7 oz for comfortable use	Open-source software, wireless capability, 3D in-motion video technology allows for full-colour streaming capture
CS 3600®	Active speed 3D video	High-speed scanning, automatic artefact elimination
CEREC omnicam®	Optical triangulation and confocal microscopy, semi-closed—proprietary files (.CS3, SDT, etc.), convertible to STL via CEREC connect	Small scanner tip for easy access, fully integrated CAD/CAM workflow
True definition®	Active wavefront sampling 3D video technology, semi-closed—proprietary files, convertible to STL via 3 M connection center	Compact design, precise scanning, but requires powder application
ScanRider® (V-GER srl, Bologna, Italy	Equipped with a DLP 600-lm projector and black-and-white 1.3-megapixel cameras, standard resolution between 25–50 μm, an average error (accuracy) of 5–10 μm	Generates detailed scans with up to 2,500,000 triangles per scan and provides outputs in the free STL format
Aoralscan®	Real-time scanning with realistic colour capture, user-friendly motion-sensing for intuitive operation	Data optimisation using artificial intelligence to identify and delete extraneous data
Planmeca Emerald S	Advanced colour and shade detection capabilities	Open system for seamless integration with other CAD/CAM systems

4. Stereophotogrammetry

- Uses multiple images from different angles to determine 3D coordinates of each scanned point
- Relies on passive light recording, reducing dependence on external illumination

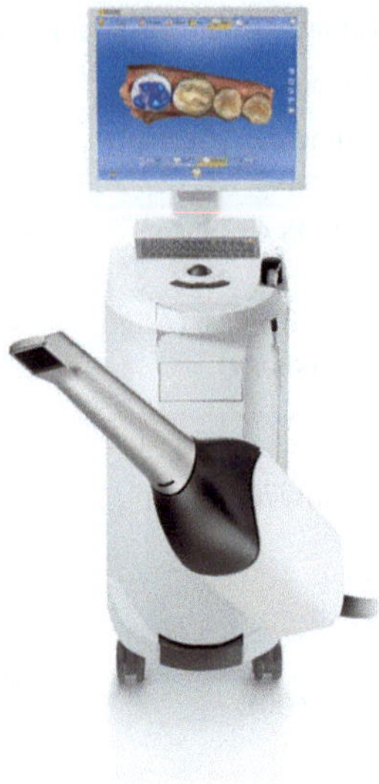

Fig. 2 Sirona Omnicam® intraoral scanner utilises the triangulation approach

- Often used for full-arch scanning in orthodontics and prosthodontics.

5. Active Wavefront Sampling (AWS)
   - Captures surface topography by moving an off-axis aperture in a circular motion
   - Generates depth information through variations in the detected wavefront
   - Improves scanning accuracy for highly reflective surfaces like enamel and metal restorations.

Working Mechanism of an Intraoral Scanner

The working process of intraoral scanners follows a systematic four-step sequence:

Step 1: Data Acquisition

- The handheld scanner wand is placed inside the patient's mouth.
- The scanner emits a light source (laser or structured light) onto the tooth surfaces.
- The sensor records the reflected light, converting it into digital information.

Step 2: Image Processing and Reconstruction

- The captured data undergoes real-time processing using advanced algorithms.
- The system stitches multiple images together to create a continuous digital model.
- Artificial intelligence (AI) assists in error correction and noise reduction.

Step 3: Model Generation and Rendering

- The software converts the scanned data into a polygonal mesh (STL, PLY, OBJ formats).

- High-resolution 3D digital models are rendered for dental restorations, orthodontics, or implant planning.
- The model can be adjusted and viewed from multiple angles for precise evaluation.

Step 4: Data Export and Integration

- The final digital impression is exported to CAD/CAM software.
- The model is used for 3D printing, milling, or treatment simulations.
- The scan can be stored in a cloud-based system for future reference or laboratory collaboration.

Key Features Enhancing IOS Functionality

1. Real-time image stitching: allows seamless merging of multiple images, improving full-arch scanning accuracy
2. AI-assisted error correction: identifies and rectifies scan gaps and artefacts in real time
3. Colour and texture mapping: enables lifelike visualisation of soft tissue, enamel, and restorations
4. Wireless and cloud integration: allows remote access and secure data sharing with dental labs
5. Automated occlusion mapping: analyses and corrects bite relationships digitally.

Challenges in Intraoral Scanning

While IOS has revolutionised digital dentistry, some challenges remain:

- Moisture and saliva interference: Excessive saliva can distort the reflection of structured light, affecting accuracy.
- Metal and highly reflective surfaces: Crowns, fillings, and orthodontic brackets can cause scan distortions.
- Learning curve: Operator skill influences the efficiency and precision of IOS scanning.

Challenges in Full-Arch Scanning

While IOS excels in quadrant scans, full-arch scanning presents challenges:

- Distortion over large areas: Stitching errors can accumulate in longer scans, affecting precision.
- Implant and edentulous cases: Soft tissue scanning remains problematic due to the absence of stable reference points.
- Occlusion capture issues: Accurately recording inter arch relationships requires additional calibration steps.

Factors Influencing IOS Accuracy

Several factors impact the accuracy of IOS:

- Scanning path and technique: A structured scanning approach ensures optimal data acquisition.
- Lighting conditions: Excessive ambient light can interfere with scanner optics, reducing accuracy.
- Operator experience: Training and familiarity with scanner technology improve precision.
- Moisture and saliva interference: Dry-field techniques and retractors minimise scanning errors.

8 Clinical Applications of IOS

1. Restorative and Prosthetic Dentistry

IOS enhances precision in restorative procedures:

- Crown and bridge fabrication: Digital impressions improve marginal adaptation and fit.
- Veneers and inlays/onlays: IOS ensures optimal aesthetics and occlusal function.
- Prosthodontics and full-mouth rehabilitation: Digital workflows streamline complex rehabilitations.

Caries detection: Dental caries is one of the most prevalent chronic diseases worldwide. Accurate diagnosis of caries is crucial for early intervention and minimally invasive treatments. Traditional diagnostic methods include visual examination and bitewing radiography, but these have limitations.

Intraoral scanners (IOSs) now include integrated caries detection tools that use:

- Near-infrared transillumination (NIRI)
- Fluorescence imaging
- Digital image processing.

These technologies eliminate ionising radiation, making them safe for children and pregnant women. However, their reliability in detecting occlusal and proximal carious lesions remains unclear. Intraoral scanners offer a promising radiation-free alternative for detecting early-stage caries.

Schlenz et al (2022) evaluated various caries detection technologies, utilising micro-CT scans as the reference standard for measuring caries depth and severity (Fig. 3). IOS with caries detection technology showed promise for occlusal caries in permanent teeth, but their accuracy was lower than traditional approaches for proximal caries. TRIOS 4 was a good option for occlusal caries detection in primary teeth. Bitewing radiography remains essential for accurate diagnosis of proximal

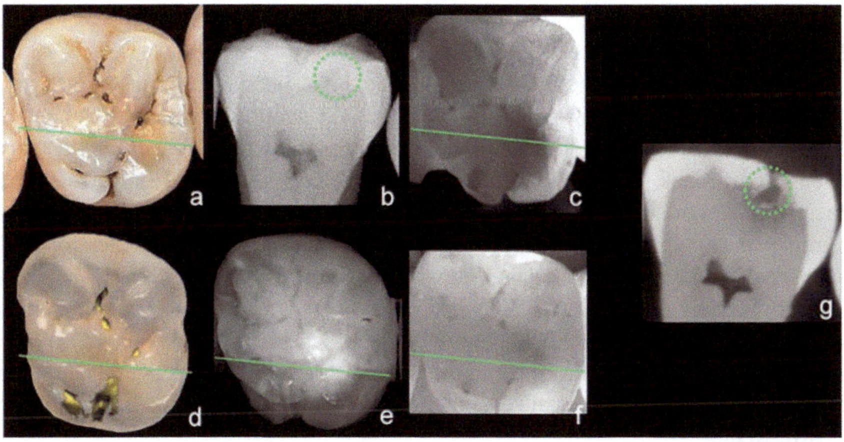

Fig. 3 Methods for diagnosing caries include visual examination (**a**), bitewing radiography (**b**), DIAGNOcam (**c**), TRIOS 4 (**d**), iTero Element 5D (**e**), Planmeca Emerald S (**f**), and μ-CT reference (**g**) (Image courtesy: Schlenz et al. (2022))

Table 4 Accuracy in permanent teeth

Method	Occlusal caries accuracy (kappa value, k)	Proximal caries accuracy (kappa value, k)
Planmeca Emerald S	0.700 (highest accuracy)	0.451
Visual examination	0.512	0.252
DIAGNOcam	0.500	0.318
TRIOS 4	0.431	0.179 (lowest accuracy)
iTero element 5D	0.366	0.379
Bitewing radiography	0.297 (low for occlusal)	0.643 (highest for proximal caries)

Table 5 Accuracy in primary teeth

Method	Occlusal caries accuracy (kappa value, k)	Proximal caries accuracy (kappa value, k)
Visual examination	0.927 (highest accuracy)	0.532
TRIOS 4	0.579	0.400
Bitewing radiography	0.471	0.871 (highest for proximal caries)
DIAGNOcam	0.469	0.212
Planmeca Emerald S	0.402	0.290
iTero element 5D	0.324	0.302

caries. Planmeca Emerald S was the most effective scanner for occlusal caries in permanent teeth (Tables 4 and 5).

A comparison of the accuracy of different caries detection methods is shown in Table 6.

Tooth wear monitoring: Erosive tooth wear is an increasing issue in preventative and restorative dentistry, affecting enamel and dentine structures by chemical dissolution and mechanical forces. Tooth wear is an increasing concern in dentistry, often classified as physiological (normal ageing) or pathological (abnormal wear due to erosion, bruxism, or other factors). Patient-specific factors (e.g. diet, bruxism, acid exposure) significantly impact wear rates. Conventional approaches for evaluating erosive tooth wear include index-based grading systems, such as the Basic Erosive Wear Examination (BEWE), and profilometry (PRO), a non-contact optical scanning tool. Nonetheless, these methodologies possess drawbacks, such as subjectivity, complexity, and time consumption. IOS demonstrated excellent accuracy in detecting even micrometre-scale enamel loss, confirming its potential for monitoring erosive wear.

Table 6 Comparative analysis of caries detection methods

Diagnostic method	Technology used	Best for detecting	Advantages	Limitations
Fluorescence-based IOS (Michou et al. 2020, 2021)	Fluorescence + colour processing	Early enamel lesions	Radiation-free, good for preventive dentistry	Struggles with deep dentine caries
Near-infrared transillumination (Schwendicke et al. 2020)	Infrared light	Occlusal and proximal caries	Good contrast for interproximal caries	Limited depth penetration
Bitewing radiography (Diniz et al. 2012)	X-ray imaging	Deep dentine and proximal caries	Gold standard for detecting hidden caries	Requires radiation exposure
Artificial intelligence (Patil et al. 2019; Schwendicke et al. 2020)	Deep learning models	Pattern recognition for caries activity	Enhances diagnostic accuracy over time	Requires extensive training data
Quantitative light-induced fluorescence (QLF) (Fried 2020)	Laser-induced fluorescence	Monitoring lesion progression	Detects demineralisation changes	Expensive equipment
Optical coherence tomography (OCT), Pretty et al. (2013); de Josselin de Jong et al. (1995)	Cross-sectional imaging using light waves	Subsurface caries and structural defects	High-resolution imaging, no ionising radiation	High cost, limited clinical availability
Teledentistry and remote diagnosis, Estai et al. (2016)	Teledentistry and remote diagnosis	Early caries detection and monitoring in remote areas	Expands access to dental care, enables preventive monitoring	Dependent on image quality, requires AI optimisation

In the research conducted by Witecy et al. (2021), the validity of IOS in detecting erosive tooth wear was assessed in comparison to PRO, and the differences between various IOS devices were also analysed, specifically the TRIOS 3® and Carestream CS 3600®, focusing on their internal and external software analyses. The performance of TRIOS 3® and Carestream CS 3600® was comparable, indicating that differences in scanner brands do not significantly affect measurement precision. The internal IOS software exhibited performance comparable to that of external software (GOM Inspect), establishing IOS as a feasible chairside tool. IOS can be utilised in clinical environments to supplant labour-intensive profilometry methods (Table 7).

Tooth shade selection: Tooth shade selection is an important aspect of prosthetic and restorative dentistry, since it influences the aesthetics of dental restorations. Traditional visual shade-matching approaches are subjective, influenced by lighting conditions, human perception, and amount of experience (Table 8). To solve these limits, IOSs with shade-matching software were created.

Although modern automated shade-matching systems allow for automatic colour assessment, issues persist about their accuracy (proximity to the true shade) and precision (consistency of shade evaluation). IOS does not effectively standardise illumination during scanning, which affects colour perception. Current iOS shade-matching algorithms are less sophisticated than spectrophotometers, resulting in shade discrepancies. IOS cannot yet replace classic spectrophotometers. However, IOS can be used to determine baseline shade levels and track long-term shade changes in patients. Precision is the limiting factor for shade matching. Intraoral scanners are extremely precise, although their shade-matching accuracy is average. They generate reproducible results but frequently misidentify real tooth hues. Spectrophotometers remain the gold standard for precise shade selection in prosthodontics. Unlike spectrophotometers, which are calibrated for exact colour detection, IOS must process numerous optical qualities concurrently (shape, texture, and colour), making shade

Table 7 Comparative analysis: IOS versus other methods for tooth wear

Key studies	Method	Technology	Best use	Advantages	Limitations
Bronkhorst et al. (2023)	Intraoral scanners (IOSs)	Optical 3D scanning	Monitoring long-term wear progression	Non-invasive, high accuracy, real-time visualisation	Limited for detecting very early-stage wear (<10 μm)
Ahmed et al. (2016)	Profilometry (NCLP)	Laser-based scanning	Gold standard for precise wear measurements	Highly accurate	Expensive, requires lab set-up
Diniz et al. (2012)	Bitewing radiography	X-ray	Structural damage assessment	Good for deep lesions	Radiation exposure, not ideal for surface wear
Schwendicke et al. (2020)	AI-based wear detection	Machine learning	Predicting and classifying wear	Self-learning, scalable	Requires large datasets

Table 8 Shade-matching methods

Method	Accuracy	Precision	Advantages	Limitations
Intraoral scanners (IOSs)	Poor	High	Fast, digital workflow, patient education	Inconsistent accuracy, sensitive to lighting
Spectrophotometers	High	High	Gold standard, highly reliable	Expensive, requires training
Colorimeters	Moderate	High	Objective, more reliable than visual methods	Still affected by lighting variations
Visual shade matching	Variable	Low	Widely used, inexpensive	Subjective, observer-dependent

selection more difficult. IOSs are a potential technique for digital shade selection, but they require additional refinement to match the accuracy of spectrophotometers. Until then, a hybrid technique of IOS and traditional shade-matching approaches is recommended (Tabatabaian et al. 2024; Akl et al. 2023).

Importance of Digital Twins in Treatment Planning: The term 'Digital Twins' in dentistry denotes the creation of virtual representations of a patient's dental structure through the integration of various imaging modalities. Digital twins replicate real-world dental structures, facilitating precise diagnosis, treatment planning, and virtual simulations prior to actual procedures. CBCT is the primary tool for 3D imaging of the craniofacial region. However, CBCT has limitations, such as image distortion due to artefacts from metal restorations, orthodontic appliances, and enamel density. To enhance accuracy, CBCT is often combined with additional imaging sources like plaster models, alginate impressions, or recently IOS. Although plaster models are extensively utilised, they pose concerns including fragility, storage difficulties, and retrieval complications (Fig. 4). Recent advancements in digital dentistry have introduced alginate impression scanning and intraoral scanning as substitutes for conventional plaster models (Table 9).

Lee et al. (2023) investigated the feasibility of using IOS and digital imprints as replacements for plaster models in the development of digital twins. They evaluated the precision of various scanning technologies when combined with CBCT. They provided clinical recommendations on selecting the most accurate and effective imaging modality.

2. Implantology

Numerous in vitro studies demonstrate that IOSs serve as a crucial and dependable method for obtaining high-quality impressions, applicable for the fabrication of both simple (onlays, inlays, or single crowns) and complex (fixed partial prostheses) prostheses in dentate patients. IOSs are quite effective in capturing implant impressions, particularly for short-span bridges and partial edentulism (Table 10). The accuracy of full-arch implant instances declines, necessitating additional verification methods or supplementary scanning techniques. Implant-supported restorations need to be

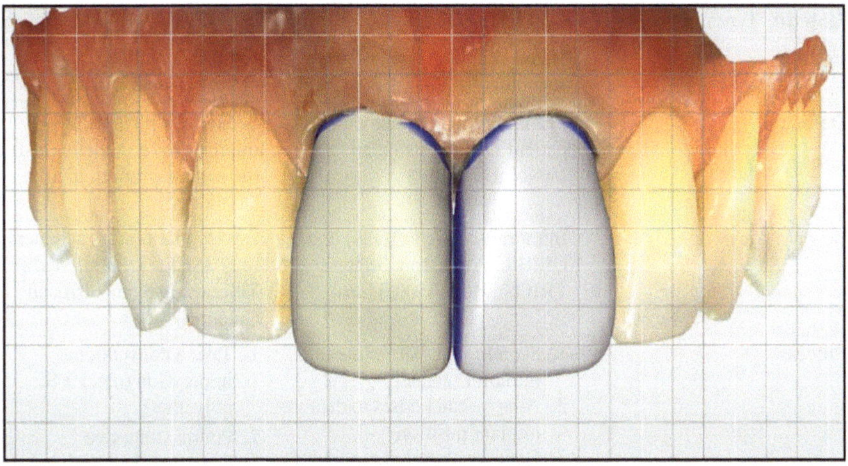

Fig. 4 Digitally created monolithic crowns for maxillary central incisors using an intraoral scanner platform with copy-and-mirror tools and a grid overlay for enhanced alignment and proportion assessment (Image courtesy: Eggman et al. (2024))

Table 9 Comparative analysis: digital dentition models versus traditional methods

Method	Accuracy	Clinical usability	Advantages	Limitations
Plaster models	High	Low	Gold standard for accuracy	Storage issues, fragile, retrieval challenges
Alginate impressions (5 min scan)	High	High	Digital workflow, no physical storage required	Time-sensitive (must scan immediately)
Alginate impressions (2 h scan)	Poor	Low	Easy to acquire	Distortion due to syneresis and imbibition
Intraoral scanners (segmented scan—CS 3600)	Best	Best	Most accurate digital scan, reduces chairside time	Learning curve, requires skilful operator
Intraoral scanners (full-arch scan—i700)	Moderate	High	Fast, efficient for complete digital workflow	Slightly less accurate than segmented scan

very precise to avoid biological (like peri-implantitis) and technical problems (like screws coming loose or implants breaking).

Components of Intraoral Scanning for Implantology

- Intraoral scanner (IOS): captures the 3D structure of implants and soft tissue
- Scan bodies (ISBs): temporary components placed on implants for accurate digital positioning

Table 10 Types of scans in implant dentistry

Feature	Direct scanning (intraoral scanning—IOS)	Indirect scanning (extraoral scanning—lab-based)
Definition	Scanning directly inside the patient's mouth using an intraoral scanner	Scanning a physical impression or model outside the patient's mouth in a laboratory
Scanning devices	Intraoral scanners (IOSs) (e.g. CEREC Primescan, 3Shape TRIOS, Medit i500, iTero)	Desktop/laboratory scanners (e.g. 3Shape D2000, Medit T-Series, Amann Girrbach Ceramill)
Process	1. Scan implant site using an intraoral scanner 2. Attach scan bodies to capture implant position 3. Generate a digital model for CAD/CAM fabrication	1. Take a conventional impression (e.g. PVS, polyether) 2. Pour a stone cast 3. Scan the model using a lab scanner to generate a digital model
Accuracy	Moderate for single/multiple implants, but lower for full-arch implants due to misalignment issues	Higher accuracy due to stable model positioning and scanning in a controlled environment
Errors and limitations	– Errors due to moisture, reflections, or patient movement – Limited accuracy for full-arch cases	– Impression distortions and material shrinkage affecting accuracy – More steps, increasing error accumulation
Best use cases	– Single implants – Multiple-unit cases – Partially edentulous patients	– Full-arch implant restorations – Cases requiring high precision – When intraoral scanning is difficult
Scan body fit	Less reproducible fit compared to lab analogues	More reproducible fit due to controlled scanning conditions
Speed	Faster workflow—digital files available immediately	Slower process—requires additional steps (impression-making, cast pouring, scanning)
Patient comfort	More comfortable—no need for traditional impressions	Less comfortable—requires physical impressions
Cost	Higher initial cost (expensive scanners)	Lower initial cost (but requires physical impression materials)
Clinical workflow suitability	Best for chairside CAD/CAM restorations and digital workflows	Best for complex implant cases requiring high accuracy

- CAD/CAM software: used for prosthetic design and integration with implants
- Digital impression files: typically, in STL or PLY formats, used for fabrication of custom prostheses.

Unlike natural abutments, dental implants are internally designed, making digital recording problematic. As a result, implant manufacturers provide equipment called scan bodies for digitalising them (Table 11). These are screws or clips that are attached to the implants intraorally or to the master cast's laboratory equivalents during scanning (Table 12). To accurately position, angle, and orient dental implants, intraoral digital scanning employs a prosthetic intraoral scan body (Fig. 5a, b). It is required in CAD/CAM processes to mark the placement of implants (Figs. 6 and 7).

Table 11 Types of scan bodies

Type	Description	Usage
Intraoral scan body	Attached to the implant inside the mouth for direct IOS scanning	Best for chairside digital impressions and CAD/CAM workflows
Laboratory scan body	Attached to a lab analogue on a cast model for indirect scanning	Used in traditional impression-based workflows
Radiographic scan body	Visible in CBCT scans to aid in implant planning	Used for implant positioning before surgery

Table 12 Choosing the right scan type for implant cases

Case type	Recommended scan type
Single implant	IOS or CBCT (for bone assessment)
Multiple implants (quadrant)	IOS + scan bodies, CBCT for verification
Full-arch implants	Photogrammetry + CBCT (best for accuracy)
Edentulous patient	Dual CBCT scan + model scan
Compromised visibility (e.g. deep implants)	Lab scanning from physical impressions

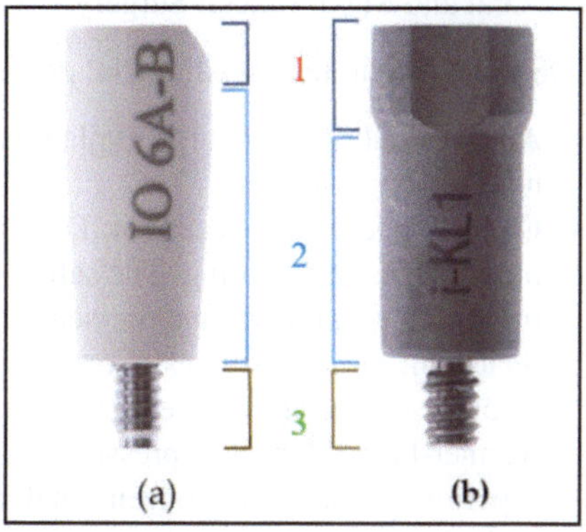

Fig. 5 **a** ISB Elos Accurate® Scan Body, made of PEEK, and **b** Klockner KL-1 (Klockner Implant System, SOADCO, Andorra), made of titanium

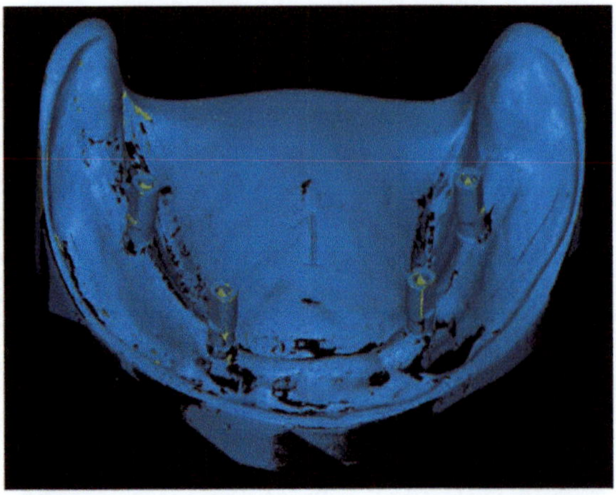

Fig. 6 Original model that was digitised with scan bodies (Image courtesy: Stimmelmayr et al. (2012))

3. Orthodontics

Orthodontic aligners are increasingly used to correct different malocclusions. Virtual treatment planning and IOSs have also become attractive substitutes for conventional procedures at the same time. Still, the data on the accuracy of orthodontic measures taken from digital technology against traditional casts is contradicting. The precise model of IOS used seems to affect the discrepancies (Christopoulou et al. 2022).

- 3D digital study models: eliminates the need for physical impressions.
- Aligner therapy planning: seamless integration with clear aligner systems like Invisalign.
- Treatment monitoring: Time-lapse scanning helps track orthodontic progress.
- Apart from diagnostic and treatment preparation, IOSs help to track root location. Complex 3D dental models can arise by combining pretreatment IOS data with CBCT datasets (Fig. 8). By allowing accurate root position predictions when combined with digital scans taken either before or following treatment, these models help to reduce the need for further CBCT imaging (Benitez et al. 2022).

4. Oral and Maxillofacial Surgery

IOS aids in complex maxillofacial procedures:

- Airway analysis and surgical planning: Scans integrate with CBCT for comprehensive diagnostics.
- Cleft lip and palate treatment: Digital scans facilitate preoperative planning and post-surgical monitoring. The safety, efficiency, and feasibility of IOS for digital impressions in infants and pre-schoolers with cleft lip and palate (CLP) are investigated in various studies. Conventional impressions need extra measures and resources since they pose airway problems. Studies are investigating intraoral scanner-based digital impressions as a safer and more efficient substitute and a superior alternative to conventional impressions for newborns and pre-schoolers with cleft lip and palate (Fig. 9).

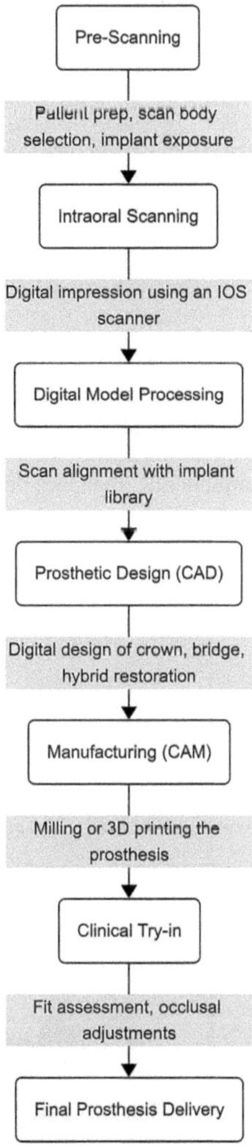

Fig. 7 Steps for fabrication of implant-supported prostheses using intraoral scanning

Shanbhag et al. (2020) proposed creating a pre-surgical nasoalveolar moulding (PNAM) appliance using digital technologies for CLP patients. PNAM historically requires multiple tactile impressions, which can be uncomfortable, time-consuming, and obtrusive for the newborn. This work explores a non-invasive method to create a custom-fitted NAM plate using intraoral scanning, computer-aided design (CAD), and prosthetic milling (Fig. 10).

Ayoub et al. (2021) proposed a new approach for the acquisition and interpretation of 3D images of the nasolabial area in patients of surgically rebuilt unilateral cleft lip and palate (UCLP), and they have evaluated whether post-cleft surgery's residual

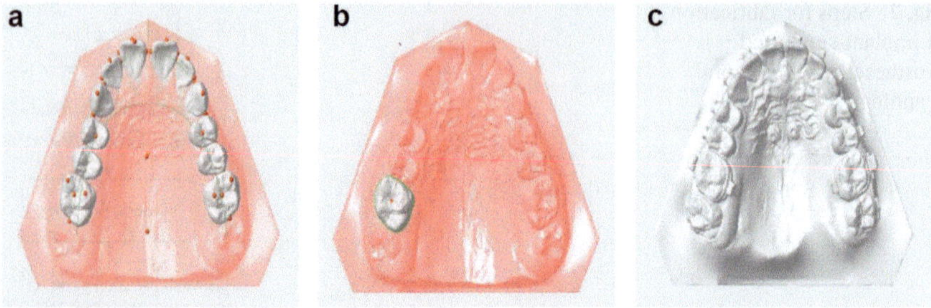

Fig. 8 **a** Maxillary dental arch including marker points on every tooth for model analysis and treatment planning development. Although hand corrections could increase their accuracy, landmarks are automatically detected. **b** First molar focus following segmentation of digital teeth. **c** Intraoral optical impression of a dental arch with an orthodontic palatal implant and a multibracket fixed orthodontic appliance detectable without a scan body (Image courtesy: Eggman et al. (2024))

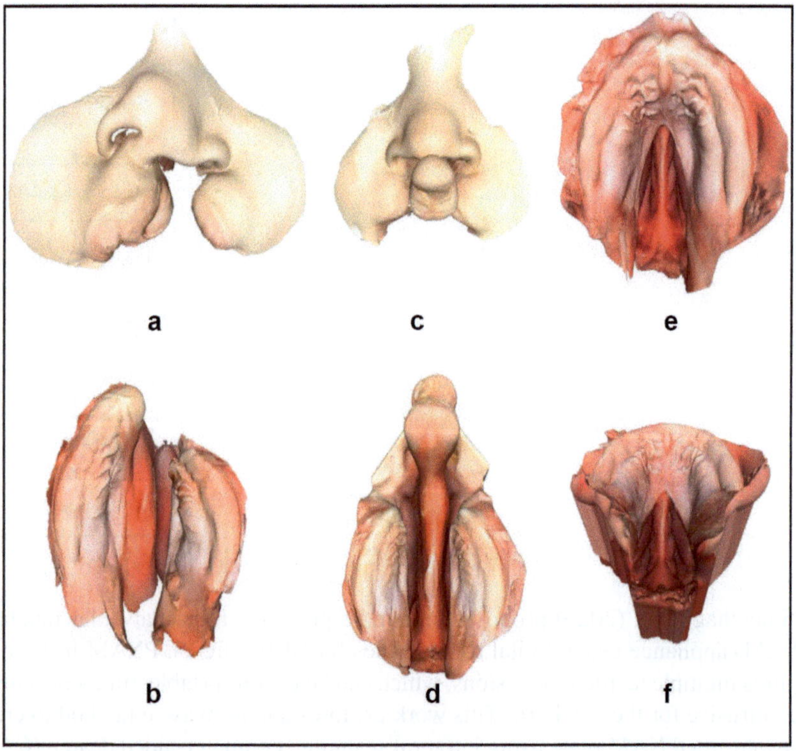

Fig. 9 Examples of digital impressions of the nose and lips, as well as cleft palate scans of babies with **a**, **b** unilateral cleft lip and palate and **b**, **c** bilateral cleft lip and palate scans **c**, **d**, respectively (Image courtesy: Benitez et al. (2022))

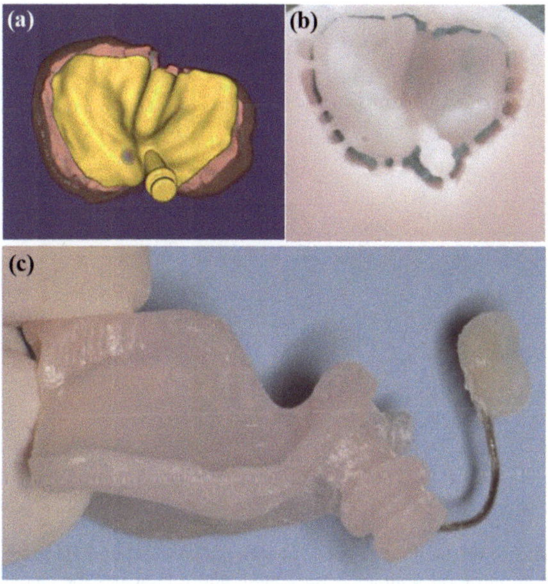

Fig. 10 **a** Nasoalveolar moulding plate created with EXOCAD, **b** plate fabricated from polymethyl methacrylate, and **c** stent attached to plate (Image courtesy: Shanbhag et al. (2020))

scarring and upper lip asymmetry could be consistently measured by IOS (Fig. 11). IOS provides objective, accurate assessment of surgical results, therefore reducing subjective bias in the evaluation of cleft repairs.

5. Endodontics

Root canal treatment for pulp canal obliteration (PCO) represents one of the most arduous treatments in endodontics. PCO is frequently noted in teeth that have experienced trauma, carious development, restorative procedures, or orthodontic treatment. The identification of calcified root canals is difficult and has a significant risk of procedural complications, including root perforation, excessive dentine removal, and instrument fracture.

Guided endodontics (GE) has arisen as a sophisticated approach to address these issues. It integrates CBCT with digital surface images to produce accurate drilling guides for root canal access (Fig. 12). There are two main approaches in guided endodontics:

- Static navigation (template-guided endodontics) employs cutting-edge 3D-printed templates to ensure unparalleled drilling precision, making every procedure a walk in the park for dental professionals (Table 13).
- Dynamic navigation harnesses the power of cutting-edge, real-time computer-assisted navigation (CAN), leveraging the latest in motion-tracking technology to elevate your experience (Connert et al. 2022).

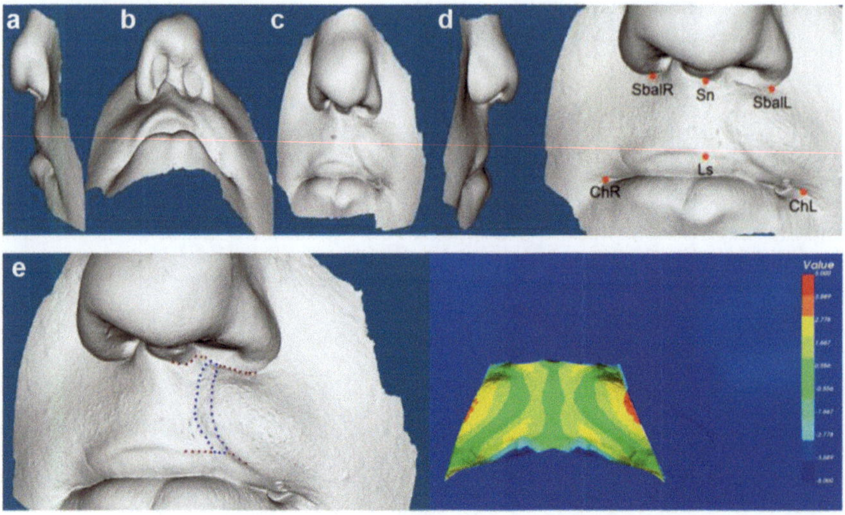

Fig. 11 **a–d** Emphasise the landmarks used for study, a non-textured 3D image of the nasolabial area acquired with an intraoral scanner is presented, and **e** indicates the calculation of the upper lip's scar surface area (left) and asymmetry (right)

Guided endodontics improves accuracy while reducing procedural risks, making it suited for difficult instances such as PCO and post-removal. Dynamic navigation provides intraoperative flexibility, which overcomes some of the constraints of static navigation. Limitations of dynamic navigation systems are their cost and limited availability. The incorporation of AI could enhance automated navigation and real-time guiding. Augmented reality (AR) could be utilised to overlay CBCT images on the actual operational field, removing the need for a monitor (Fig. 13).

6. Teledentistry

Teledentistry is an emerging field that uses digital technologies to provide remote diagnosis and treatment planning. IOSs produce 3D images with near-accurate colours, making it a feasible tool for remote dental examinations (Fig. 14). IOS can precisely identify dental problems including implants, crowns, and filled teeth. Periodontal problems (e.g. gingivitis, periodontitis) are not detected with the same precision since IOS cannot totally replace clinical probing for a thorough periodontal examination. Teledentistry with IOS can help with early diagnosis, treatment planning, and remote consultation in dental offices (Steinmeier et al. 2020).

7. Forensic Dentistry

Although dental records, DNA analysis, and fingerprints are used in forensic identification, each of these methods has inherent limitations, particularly with regard to

Fig. 12 Guided endodontics workflow

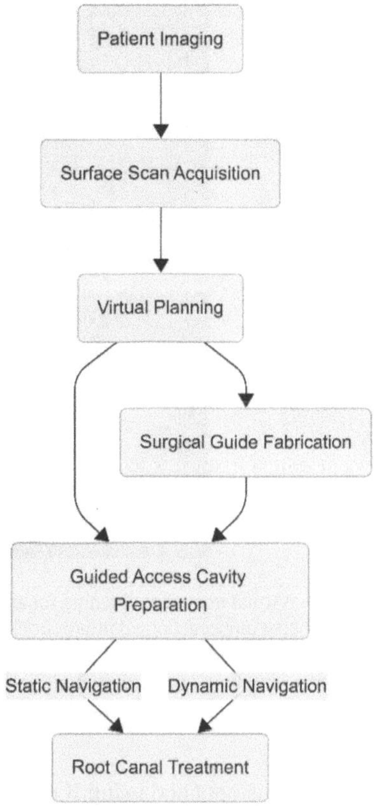

Table 13 Static navigation versus dynamic navigation

Feature	Static navigation (template-guided)	Dynamic navigation
Technology used	Prefabricated 3D-printed surgical guide	Real-time tracking with stereoscopic cameras
Precision	High ($\leq$ 0.34 mm deviation)	Similar to static navigation (1.5°–2.0° angular deviation)
Invasiveness	Minimally invasive	Minimally invasive
Clinical application	PCO, severely calcified canals, post-removal	Flexible for real-time corrections
Set-up complexity	Requires prefabricated template	More complex, requires training
Main limitation	Cannot be adjusted intraoperatively	Learning curve, costly equipment

disaster victim identification (DVI). Palatal rugae patterns are recognised to offer a constant biometric identification because of their temporal stability and heat tolerance as well as trauma, chemical, and pharmacological sensitivity. Digital palatal

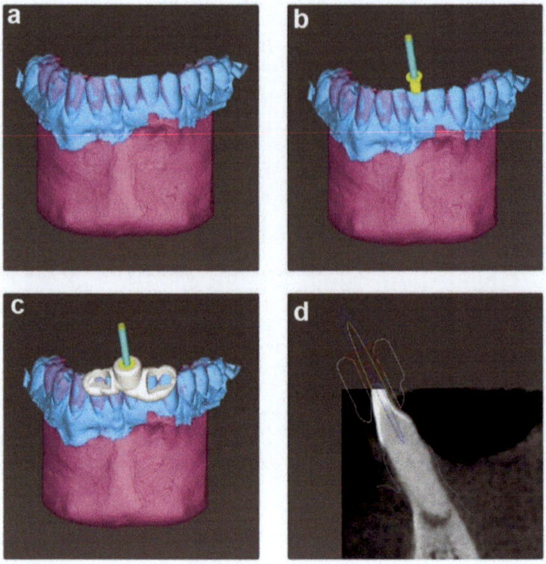

Fig. 13 Virtual treatment planning for an endodontic access cavity in a mandibular incisor: **a** registration of the intraoral optical impression, **b** CBCT imaging used to plan the access cavity for optimal entry, **c** creation of a custom guide to fasten the sleeve system, with inspection windows to ensure proper positioning, and **d** sagittal view of the digital twin's incisor showing detailed access cavity planning and placement of bur, sleeve, and guide (Eggmann and Blatz 2024)

impressions obtained using IOS could offer a consistent and non-invasive approach of forensic identification (Fig. 15). While prior studies have validated the accuracy of IOS, further research is needed into orthodontic procedures, and digitalisation processes evaluate long-term repeatability as well as the impacts of ageing.

8. Oral Hygiene Assessment

Dental plaque forms biofilms that cause gingivitis and periodontitis, making it a major cause of dental cavities and periodontal disorders. Plaque in difficult-to-reach places, like the lingual and interdental surfaces, persists despite regular brushing. For good dental hygiene, plaque build-up must be identified early and managed. The typical plaque evaluation procedures include disclosing agent and intraoral imaging. Plaque Control Plaque is detected using dental pieces during record analysis. These procedures have limitations such as inconsistent monitoring, difficulty in accessing lingual areas, and photography with mirrors or retraction.

IOS offers 3D plaque imaging, making oral hygiene assessments easier for dentists and patients. Compared to standard visual inspection and plaque control record (PCR) analysis, IOS provides a more comprehensive view of plaque build-up, especially on lingual and posterior surfaces that are difficult to detect directly. The study discovered that IOS detected higher PCR values (64%) than optical approaches (57%), implying that traditional methods may underestimate plaque build-up in specific locations.

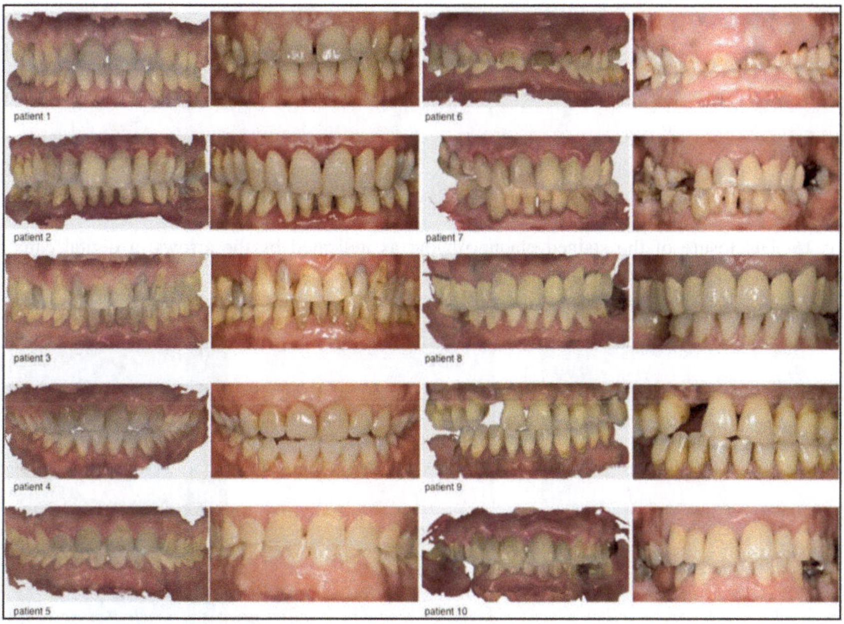

Fig. 14 Patient overview (left: IOS picture; right: intraoral camera) (Image courtesy: Steinmeier et al. (2020))

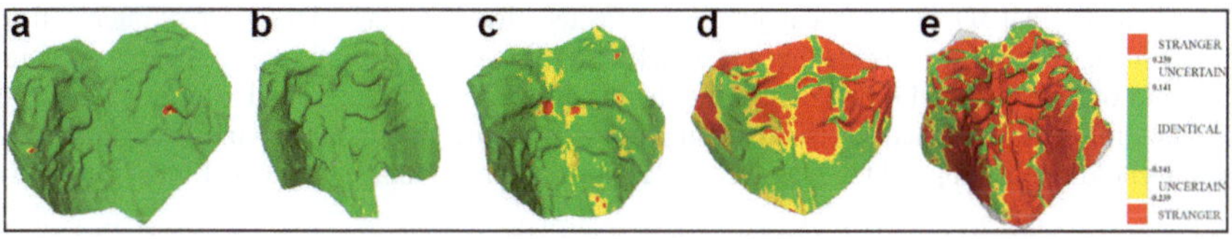

Fig. 15 Colour maps of several chosen cases from each comparison: **a** repeatability (E_E), **b** technical reproducibility (ESA_PS), **c** forensic reproducibility, **d** canine case removed from forensic comparison, and **e** between siblings. Identical (green) and questionable (yellow) ranges were separated at 0.141. Another 0.239 cut-off (red) identified known ranges (Image courtesy: Mikolicz et al. (2023))

Despite the lengthier image processing time (~90 s), IOS simplifies plaque assessment by requiring just one operator, unlike direct inspection, which sometimes takes two professionals (Fig. 16). Future enhancements should concentrate on refining plaque-staining colours to enhance visibility on IOS 3D images (Fig. 17) (Doi et al. 2021).

A study by Jung et al. (2018) shows that intraoral scanners (IOSs) are a reliable and effective method for measuring whole-mouth plaque in contrast to standard visual plaque scoring and intraoral cameras (Table 14).

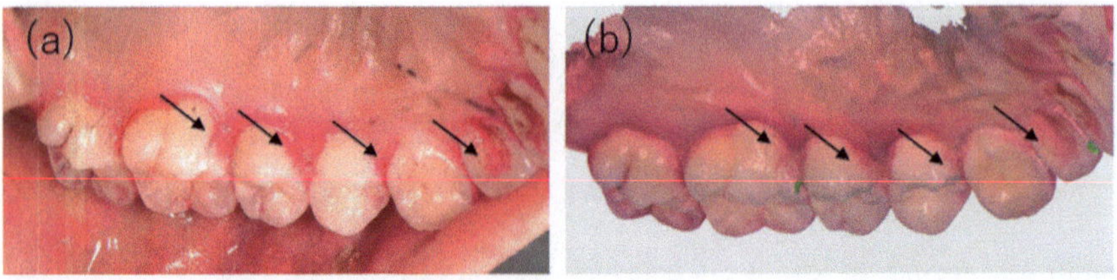

Fig. 16 Disclosure of the stained plaque region, as indicated by the arrows: **a** digital camera photograph and **b** IOS three-dimensional image (Doi et al. 2021)

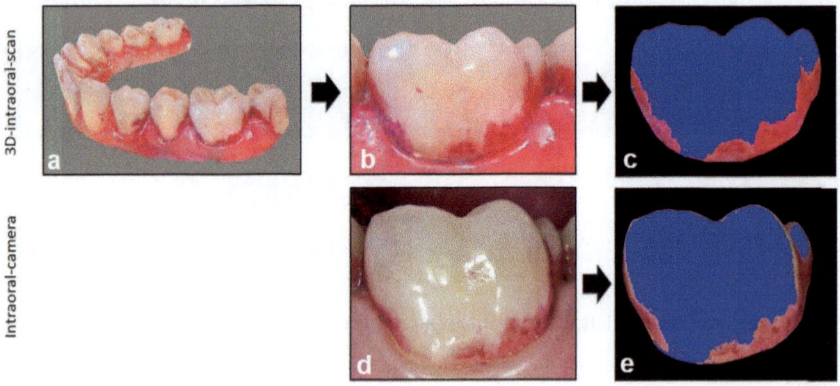

Fig. 17 **a** Original 3D intraoral scan image. **b** Selected view focusing on the tooth of interest from the 3D scan. **c** The program visualizes plaque by isolating pixels with red values below a specific threshold on the extracted tooth, displaying the result on a black background. **d** Raw image from the intraoral camera. **e** Plaque visualization generated by the software, showing pixels under the red threshold on the cropped tooth against a black background. (Image courtesy: Lim et al. (2018))

Table 14 Comparison of IOS and intraoral camera plaque detection

Plaque assessment method	Baseline plaque (P%)	Plaque after 72 h without brushing (P%)	Plaque after brushing (P%)
Intraoral scanner (IOS)	6.9%	16.0% (+47%)	5.2% (−43%)
Intraoral camera (reference)	6.1%	15.2% (+44%)	4.8% (−40%)

9 Future Directions in IOS Technology

The next generation of intraoral scanners is expected to integrate:

- AI-driven automated scanning paths: AI assisting in real-time navigation for optimised scanning

- 5G connectivity: instant cloud storage and real-time data sharing for remote consultations
- Augmented reality (AR) integration: live treatment simulations for enhanced patient education
- Self-cleaning optics: anti-fogging and moisture-resistant lenses to improve scanning quality

1. Extraoral Scanners

In digital dentistry, particularly in prosthodontics, restorative dentistry and orthodontics extraoral scanners (EOSs) are indispensable. Unlike intraoral scanners (IOSs), EOS scans indirect imprints or physical models external to the patient's mouth, therefore offering more accuracy and precision for full-arch reconstructions. EOSs are digital technologies that use imprints, stone models, or prosthetic frameworks rather than directly scanning the patient's oral cavity. These scanners use structured light, laser, or photogrammetry technology to generate digital replicas of dental models for CAD/CAM processes. Popular extraoral scanner brands include: 3Shape D700/D1000, Straumann CARES 3Series and 7Series, Medit T710, and Zirkonzahn S600 ARTI.

EOS allows full-facial 3D capture, which is critical for Digital Smile Design (DSD), facial aesthetics assessment, orthognathic surgery planning, and integration with intraoral scanning for comprehensive digital rehabilitation. The use of AI in digital scanning improves facial recognition accuracy and predicts intermaxillary correlations, thereby improving occlusion-based restorations. The integration of intraoral and extraoral images allows for more accurate aesthetic and prosthetic planning. Future research should look on AI-driven automation for scan alignment and occlusion prediction (Brunetto et al. 2024).

A study by Sason et al. (2018) was conducted to evaluate and compare the accuracy of IOS and EOS in obtaining digital dental impressions (Table 15). IOSs are more precise and truer to the actual tooth dimensions since they capture data directly without relying on impression materials or cast models. EOSs are dependent on the quality of the impression and cast and may introduce additional distortions, although they are still within the clinically acceptable range.

Similarly, Shah et al. (2023) conducted a comprehensive assessment of the accuracy, precision, and clinical utility of EOS versus IOS in the fields of prosthodontics, orthodontics, and maxillofacial rehabilitation. EOS exhibits enhanced precision in full-arch and extensive-span restorations. EOS demonstrates greater precision than IOS in the scanning of stone models, impressions, and occlusal surfaces. Hybrid scanning, which integrates EOS and IOS, provides an optimal balance of accuracy and usability (Fig. 18). However, EOS needs extra processes (impression/model scanning), making it unsuitable for chairside use. AI-based alignment solutions enhance EOS procedures, although user intervention is still necessary.

2. Photogrammetry

Dentistry needs precise 3D representations of the teeth, dental arches, and facial features to enhance treatment planning, occlusion assessment, and prosthesis repair.

Table 15 Comparison between IOS and EOS

Feature	Intraoral scanner (IOS)	Extraoral scanner (EOS)
Definition	A scanner that captures direct digital impressions inside the patient's mouth	A scanner that captures digital impressions from a dental cast made from conventional impressions
Scanning process	Directly scans the teeth inside the oral cavity	Requires making an impression first, pouring a dental cast, and then scanning the cast
Equipment used	CS 3500 (Carestream Dental)	LAVA™ Scan ST Design system (3 M™ ESPE)
Data format	Standard Tessellation Language (STL)	Standard Tessellation Language (STL)
Precision (μm)	20.7–33.35 μm (higher precision)	19.5–37 μm (slightly lower precision)
Trueness (μm)	Mean trueness: 413 μm (closer to actual tooth measurement of 459 μm)	Mean trueness: 396 μm
Mean deviations	Mesiodistally (MD): 19.6 μm Buccolingually (BL): 16.4 μm	Mesiodistally (MD): 24.0 μm Buccolingually (BL): 22.5 μm
Scanning efficiency	Faster process as it eliminates conventional impressions	Takes longer due to impression-making and casting steps
Error possibilities	Possible minor stitching errors due to intraoral scanning limitations	Potential errors from material distortions during impression-making and model pouring
Clinical accuracy	Higher accuracy as it captures data directly from the oral cavity	Accuracy depends on the impression material and model stability
Material influence	No need for impression material; direct scanning reduces material-related errors	Uses addition silicone impression material, which may introduce slight distortions
Best for	Chairside restorations, same-day dentistry, digital workflows	Laboratory-based workflows, traditional impression workflows
Disadvantages	Requires a learning curve for scanning techniques; may not work well in deep or hard-to-reach areas	More steps involved; potential for material shrinkage/distortion

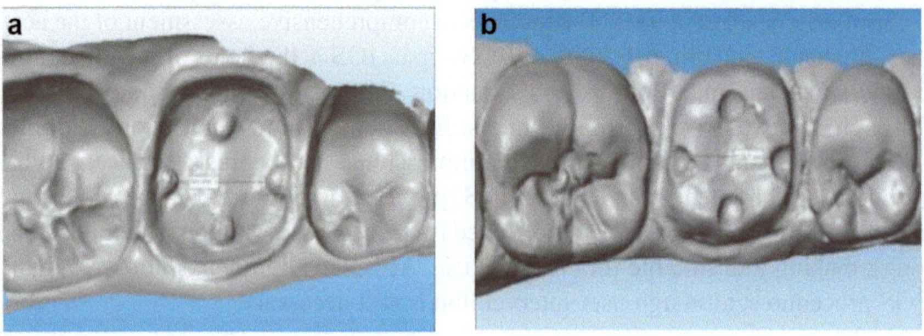

Fig. 18 STL file obtained from **a** IOS and **b** EOS to make measurements (Image courtesy: Sason et al. (2018))

Conventional techniques, including plaster models, mechanical articulators, and 2D photographs, are prevalent yet exhibit considerable deficiencies in accuracy, reproducibility, and visualisation efficacy. To solve these issues, photogrammetry-based digital approaches are recommended as a replacement for human impression-taking, physical model creation, and classical occlusion analysis (Fig. 19).

Photogrammetry is a sophisticated imaging technology that uses many images taken from various angles to create a very accurate 3D model (Fig. 20). In dentistry, photogrammetry is transforming digital workflows by producing precise, non-invasive, and reproducible digital imprints that increase the precision of prosthodontic, orthodontic, and maxillofacial reconstructions.

Principles of Photogrammetry in Dentistry

Photogrammetry is the study of extracting precise measurements and spatial data from images. It is frequently employed in a variety of industries, including architecture, engineering, medicine, and especially dentistry. The core concepts of

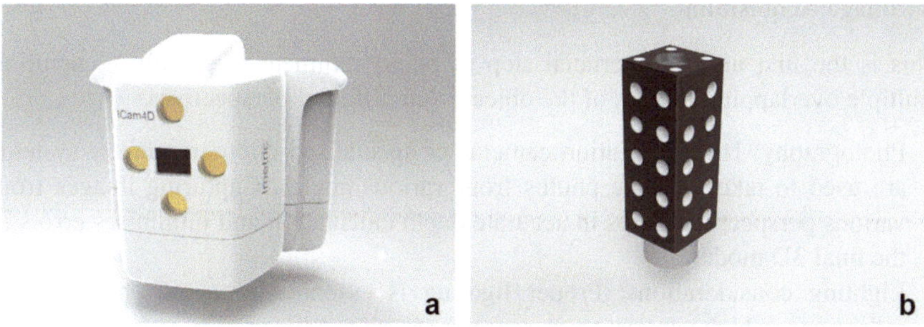

Fig. 19 **a** Schematic representation of the iCam4D® system with four cameras and a projector **b** iCamBody marker, fixed to the implant fixture

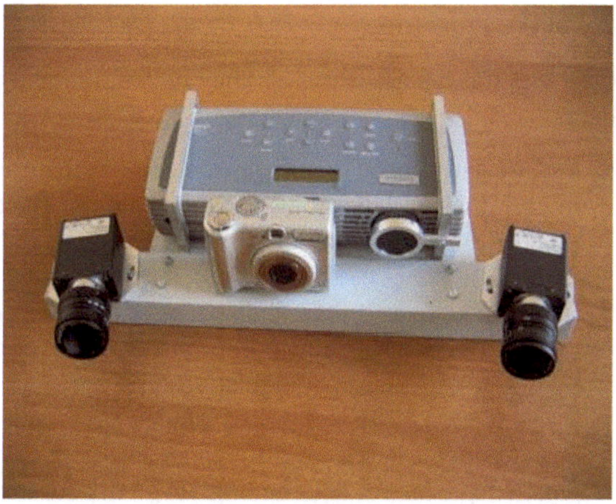

Fig. 20 Photogrammetric system (Image courtesy: Gaboutchian et al. (2019))

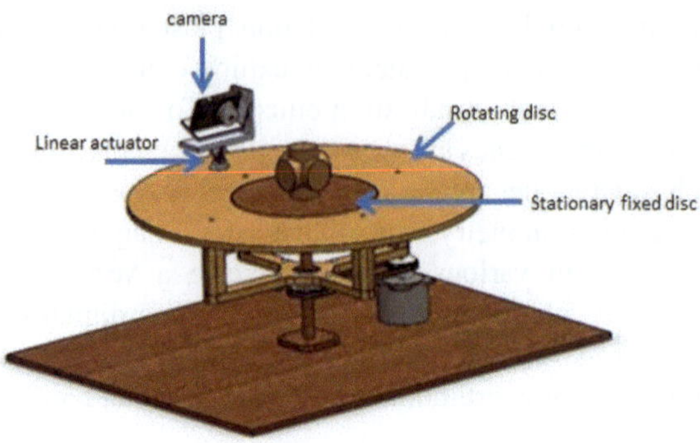

Fig. 21 Hardware design (Image courtesy: Alyaman et al. (2019))

photogrammetry are taking several photographs of an item from various perspectives and utilising software to recreate its 3D representation (Fig. 21) (Alyaman et al. 2019; Stuani et al. 2019; Ma et al. 2021).

1. Image Acquisition

This is the first and most crucial step in photogrammetry. It involves capturing multiple overlapping images of the object from different perspectives.

- Photography: High-resolution cameras or specialised photogrammetry systems are used to take multiple photos from various angles. Capturing images from various perspectives helps in accurate depth calculation and minimises errors in the final 3D model.
- Lighting considerations: Proper lighting is essential to avoid shadows and reflections, which can distort measurements.
- Camera calibration: Proper calibration of cameras is essential to correct distortions and ensure accuracy in the final 3D reconstruction. Camera settings, including lens distortion and focal length, are calibrated to ensure accuracy.

2. Image Processing

Once the images are captured, they undergo digital processing to extract essential data.

- Feature detection: The software detects key features (edges, textures, and corners) in each image. Algorithms such as scale-invariant feature transform (SIFT) and speeded-up robust features (SURF) are commonly used to detect key points in images.
- Image matching: It then finds common features across multiple images to align them correctly. Matching algorithms compare common features across multiple images to establish spatial relationships.
- Triangulation: The system calculates the depth and 3D coordinates of each detected point based on differences in perspective between images. The mathematical process of determining 3D point coordinates is based on the differences in camera angles.

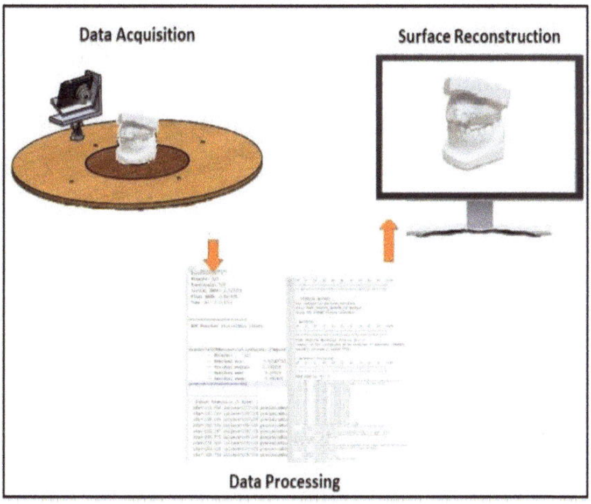

Fig. 22 Phases involved in 3D reconstruction process (Alyaman et al. 2019)

3. 3D Reconstruction

The triangulated points are used to construct a digital 3D model (Fig. 22).

- Point cloud generation: A collection of data points in a 3D coordinate system that represents the object's surface.
- Mesh creation: The point cloud is converted into a solid surface or mesh, forming the final digital model.
- Texture mapping: The original image colours and textures are overlaid on the model for realism.

4. Accuracy and Precision

For photogrammetry to be reliable, it must be both accurate and precise.

- Calibration: Photogrammetric systems require calibration to ensure consistent results.
- Error minimisation: Techniques like bundle adjustment refine the model by optimising alignment and reducing distortions.
- Trueness versus precision:
  - *Trueness* refers to how close the digital model is to the real object.
  - *Precision* refers to the consistency of results when repeated multiple times.

Limitations

- Lighting issues: Poor lighting can cause errors in reconstruction.
- Movement sensitivity: Objects or patients must remain still for accurate results.
- Data processing requirements: High-quality photogrammetry requires powerful computers and advanced software.
- Surface limitations: Transparent or highly reflective surfaces can cause distortion.

Despite some limitations, advancements in AI-based image processing and hardware improvements continue to enhance its accuracy and usability. As photogrammetry technology evolves, it is expected to further integrate with augmented reality (AR) and artificial intelligence (AI) for improved real-time applications (Zotti et al. 2022).

10 3D Printing in Dentistry

Introduction to 3D Printing in Dentistry

3D printing, also known as additive manufacturing (AM), has revolutionised several sectors, including engineering, medicine, and dentistry. This technique enables the layer-by-layer creation of complicated structures, making it ideal for creating unique dental prostheses and models. Charles Hull introduced stereolithography (SLA) in the 1980s, which sparked the technology's development. Over time, advances resulted in the creation of numerous printing processes, making the technology more accessible and accurate. Dentistry introduced 3D printing in the early 2000s, which greatly improved efficiency and customisation in dental applications. Innovations in digital dentistry, especially CAD/CAM (computer-aided design/computer-aided manufacturing) systems, which help to smoothly combine digital impressions and additive manufacturing techniques, drive the integration of 3D printing in dentistry (Table 16). High-quality dental goods distinguished by outstanding accuracy and biocompatibility have been produced using diverse printing technologies like stereolithography (SLA), digital light processing (DLP), selective laser sintering (SLS), and fused deposition modelling (FDM).

In dentistry, 3D printing offers benefits beyond only increased production efficiency. Excellent fitting restorations and improved treatment planning have come from the ability to design highly customised dental treatments based on particular patient anatomy. Moreover, the declining labour-intensive operations and material waste makes this technology financially feasible over time. Three-dimensional (3D) printing in dentistry still presents difficulties like material restrictions, legal limitations, and costly initial investment prices, notwithstanding its numerous benefits. Constant research and technology developments help to solve these difficulties,

Table 16 Comparing 3D printing with traditional methods

Factor	3D printing	Conventional milling and casting
Speed	Faster	Slower
Customisation	Highly customisable	Limited
Material waste	Minimal	High
Precision	High	Dependent on manual skill
Cost efficiency	More cost-effective	Expensive materials and labour

thereby extending the uses of 3D printing to encompass bioprinting and the creation of new dental materials.

The fundamentals of 3D printing technology are presented in Table 17.

Table 17 Role of 3D printing in modern dentistry: types of 3D printing technologies in dentistry

Technology	Description	Applications	Advantages	Disadvantages and limitations
Stereolithography (SLA)	Uses light-sensitive resin cured layer by layer with UV light; high resolution and fine details	Surgical guides, dental models, temporary restorations, clear aligners	High accuracy, smooth surface finish, excellent detail reproduction	Expensive equipment, limited material choices, post-processing required
Fused deposition modelling (FDM)	Heats and extrudes plastic filament through a nozzle; affordable and accessible, but lower resolution	Orthodontic devices, temporary prostheses, occlusal splints, study models	Low cost, easy to use, widely available materials	Lower resolution, visible layer lines, weaker mechanical properties
Selective laser sintering (SLS)	Uses a laser to sinter powder-based materials into solid layers, providing strong and durable results	Metal dental frameworks, permanent restorations, dentures, partial denture frameworks	Strong and durable materials, complex geometries possible	High cost, time-consuming, requires post-processing
Direct metal laser sintering (DMLS)	Similar to SLS but works specifically with metals for high-strength applications; high accuracy with complex geometries	Dental implants, crowns, bridges, custom abutments, metal prosthetics	High precision, biocompatible materials, durable structures	Expensive, requires specialised equipment, potential for porosity
Inkjet bioprinting	Deposits droplets of bioinks containing ceramic or resin materials, allowing for multi-material and multi-layered printing	Temporary and permanent restorations, biocompatible dental scaffolds, custom dental prosthetics	Multi-material capability, fine resolution, potential for tissue engineering	Limited material options, high cost, requires biocompatible inks

Materials Used in 3D Printing for Dentistry

(1) Resin-Based Materials

Resin-based materials play a significant role in modern digital dentistry due to their adaptability, affordability, and high precision. They encompass materials such as light-curable resins (SLA/DLP), photopolymer resins (PolyJet), and composite resins. These materials are widely used in applications like dental models, surgical guides, temporary crowns and bridges, as well as occlusal splints and clear aligners.

Advantages

1. High precision and detail: Resin-based materials enable the creation of highly detailed and accurate dental models, as demonstrated in a study by Kwaśny et al. (2022), which found that photopolymer resin-based interim crowns fabricated via 3D printing showed superior accuracy compared to traditional methods.
2. Rapid production: Three-dimensional (3D) printing with resin-based materials allows for faster production times, reducing turnaround for dental restorations.
3. Cost-effectiveness: Digital fabrication with resin-based materials is generally more affordable compared to traditional dental methods.
4. Good aesthetics: Composite resin restorations are preferred for their ability to mimic natural tooth colour and translucency (Randolph et al. 2018).

Disadvantages

1. Not suitable for permanent restorations: Despite their advantages, resin-based materials are primarily used for temporary solutions due to their lower durability and wear resistance.
2. Prone to shrinkage: Polymerisation shrinkage remains a challenge in resin-based dental materials, leading to marginal gaps and possible failure of restorations (Wu et al. 2017).
3. Requires post-curing for mechanical stability: Proper photopolymerisation is crucial for achieving optimal mechanical properties. Studies have shown that curing duration and method significantly impact the mechanical properties of resin composites (Szalewski et al. 2022).

(2) Thermoplastics and Polymers in Dental Prosthetics

Thermoplastics and polymers, particularly polylactic acid (PLA), acrylonitrile butadiene styrene (ABS), and polyether ether ketone (PEEK), are increasingly utilised in prosthetic frameworks, custom trays, removable partial dentures (RPDs), and implant-supported prostheses due to their unique mechanical and biocompatibility properties.

Applications

1. Prosthetic Frameworks

- PEEK has been evaluated as a material for fixed prostheses supported by implants. A study comparing metal-ceramic and PEEK-based maxillary fixed

prostheses supported by four implants found that PEEK provided favourable clinical and prosthetic outcomes, with lower peri-implant marginal bone loss compared to metal but a higher rate of veneer fractures (Kortam et al. 2022).
- PEEK is also a viable alternative framework material for removable dental prostheses, particularly for patients allergic to metals or those seeking improved aesthetics (Zoidis et al. 2016).

2. Custom Trays and RPDs

- The accuracy and suitability of PEEK frameworks in RPDs have been validated using CAD/CAM technology. Studies show that PEEK frameworks have clinical accuracy and trueness comparable to traditional Co–Cr frameworks (Zhao et al. 2024).
- PEEK frameworks have been found to generate less strain on supporting structures compared to metallic frameworks, making them suitable for patients with Kennedy Class III edentulous mandibles (Chen et al. 2019).

3. Implant-Supported Prostheses

- PEEK components in implant-supported removable prostheses show durability and resistance to wear, with thermocycling tests indicating that their surface roughness and hardness remain unchanged over time.
- Additionally, clinical trials suggest that PEEK-based RPD frameworks provide similar improvements in oral health-related quality of life (OHRQoL) compared to traditional Co–Cr frameworks (Ali et al. 2020).

Advantages

High flexibility: PEEK is particularly noted for its ability to distribute stress more favourably than metal alloys.

Lightweight: PEEK is significantly lighter than metal-based prosthetic frameworks, enhancing patient comfort.

Good durability: Studies show that PEEK prostheses maintain their mechanical properties over long-term use, with no significant wear-related degradation (Gomes et al. 2024).

Biocompatibility and wear resistance: PEEK has been widely used in orthopaedic applications due to its biocompatibility. In dental prostheses, it shows resistance to plaque build-up and bacterial retention, reducing the risk of peri-implant disease (Liu et al. 2022).

Disadvantages

Limited colour choices: Unlike traditional resins and ceramics, thermoplastic prosthetics (such as those made of ABS or PLA) may not provide the most aesthetically pleasing colour options.

Biocompatibility concerns (ABS): While PEEK is highly biocompatible, some plastics like ABS may contain toxic components, making them less suitable for direct oral use.

High-temperature printing required: PEEK requires high temperatures for processing, making it challenging to fabricate using conventional 3D printing techniques (Negm et al. 2019).

(3) Metals and alloys

Titanium (Ti6Al4V), cobalt–chrome (Co–Cr), and stainless steel are commonly used in dental applications, including dental implants, crown and bridge frameworks, partial denture frameworks, and orthodontic brackets and wires due to their excellent strength, durability, high biocompatibility, and corrosion resistance. However, they come with drawbacks such as high costs, the need for advanced manufacturing techniques like direct metal laser sintering (DMLS) or selective laser melting (SLM), and surface roughness that requires polishing.

Titanium (Ti6Al4V).

- Strength and biocompatibility: Titanium and its alloys are among the most commonly used metals for dental implants due to their superior mechanical properties and biocompatibility (Blackwood 2003).
- Corrosion resistance: Ti6Al4V is known for its high corrosion resistance, making it ideal for long-term dental use.
- Concerns with ion release: The release of vanadium and aluminium ions from Ti6Al4V has raised concerns over potential cytotoxicity, which is why newer materials like Ti6Al7Nb are being explored as alternatives (Abreu-García et al. 2023).
- Success rate: Three-dimensional (3D)-printed titanium implants have demonstrated a 94.5% survival rate over a period of 3 years.
- Challenges: Surface modifications are required to reduce roughness and improve osseointegration, often through coatings like hydroxyapatite (Nahum and Lugovskoy 2018).

Cobalt–Chrome (Co–Cr)

- Precision and durability: Co–Cr alloys are widely used for crown and bridge frameworks due to their high wear resistance and strength.
- Fabrication methods: A comparison between conventional and 3D-printed Co–Cr copings found that 3D-printed versions were more precise.
- Corrosion resistance: Co–Cr alloys demonstrate high corrosion resistance in dental environments, though alloying with titanium can further enhance their properties.
- Challenges: Some studies report allergic responses to elements within Co–Cr alloys, necessitating proper surface treatments and coatings (Ghiban et al. 2012).

Stainless Steel (SS316L)

- Applications: Stainless steel is commonly used for orthodontic brackets, wires, and temporary prosthetic frameworks due to its good mechanical strength and corrosion resistance.

- Limitations: SS316L's corrosion resistance is highly dependent on pH, with increased ion release in acidic conditions (Goharian and Abdullah 2017).

4. Biocompatible and Hybrid Materials

Biocompatible and hybrid materials such as zirconia ceramics, glass ceramics (lithium disilicate, leucite), and bioactive composites have been widely studied for various dental applications, including permanent restorations (crowns, bridges), custom dental implants, and bone graft substitutes. These materials exhibit high strength and aesthetics, excellent biocompatibility, and the ability to integrate with surrounding tissues, making them ideal for dental use. However, challenges such as shrinkage during printing, the need for post-sintering, and high costs remain significant drawbacks.

Zirconia ceramics: Zirconia ceramics have demonstrated superior mechanical properties and biocompatibility, making them a reliable choice for dental implants. Research has shown that zirconia-based materials provide excellent long-term stability and favourable osseointegration, especially when modified with bioactive coatings. Osman et al. successfully 3D-printed zirconia dental implants using digital light processing (DLP), achieving high accuracy, while Cheng et al. developed custom zirconia implants using 3D slurry printing, showing promising mechanical properties. Additionally, modifications with bioactive coatings such as bioactive glass have been shown to enhance osseointegration and soft tissue sealing (Wei and Wei 2022). Akermanite-modified zirconia ceramics have further demonstrated improved bioactivity and osseointegration potential (Zhang et al. 2023).

Glass ceramics (lithium disilicate, leucite): Glass ceramics, particularly lithium disilicate and leucite-based ceramics, are valued for their excellent aesthetics, translucency, and biocompatibility. Studies indicate that lithium disilicate provides high strength and bioactivity, making it a viable option for dental restorations (Daguano et al. 2019). However, challenges remain regarding their long-term mechanical properties and susceptibility to wear against opposing materials. Advances in lithium disilicate and zirconia-reinforced glass–ceramic composites are being explored to improve durability and clinical performance (Zarone et al. 2019).

Bioactive composites: Bioactive composites, particularly those incorporating bioactive glass, have gained attention for their ability to promote bone regeneration and enhance implant integration. Research on bioactive glass coatings on zirconia has shown that they accelerate the formation of a bond between bone and the implant surface. Similarly, bioactive glass–ceramic composites have been developed with enhanced biocompatibility and osteo-inductive properties for bone grafting applications (Pant et al. 2024).

Despite their advantages, these materials present certain manufacturing and clinical challenges. The printing of zirconia ceramics remains difficult due to shrinkage, requiring precise sintering to maintain dimensional accuracy. The high cost of both zirconia and lithium disilicate materials also limits their widespread adoption in clinical practice. Research is ongoing to optimise processing techniques, including the development of novel hybrid materials that balance mechanical strength, aesthetics, and cost-effectiveness (Upadhyay et al. 2024).

Workflow in Dental 3D Printing

- Digital scanning and CAD/CAM technology
- 3D modelling and design software:
  - PreForm (by Formlabs)—Slicer software for preparing STL files for printing
  - CHITUBOX—used for resin-based 3D printers in dental applications
- Slicing and printing preparation
- Post-processing and finishing

Applications of 3D Printing in Dentistry

(1) Restorative dentistry: Three-dimensional (3D) printing has revolutionised restorative dentistry by enabling high-precision fabrication of diagnostic models, prostheses, wax patterns, and surgical guides. The technology allows for improved accuracy, reproducibility, and efficiency in dental restorations compared to traditional methods (Anadioti et al. 2018).

(1.1) Diagnostic models and casting patterns: Digital dental models provide superior accuracy and reproducibility compared to conventional plaster models. A comparative study using digital light processing (DLP), photopolymer jetting, and stereolithography (SLA) found that 3D-printed models had high reproducibility (ICC = 0.935) and were clinically equivalent to traditional plaster models. These digital models also facilitate efficient diagnostic workflows and treatment planning in prosthetic and orthodontic dentistry (Fig. 23) (Anadioti et al. 2018).

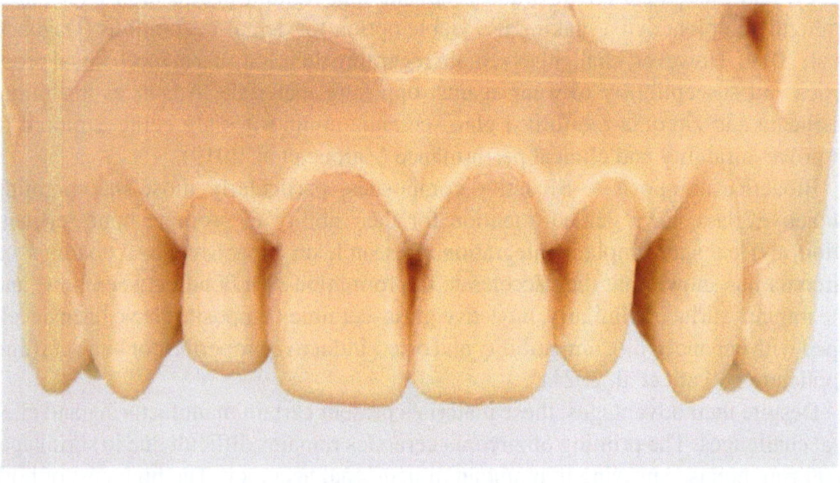

Fig. 23 Diagnostic model made using resin-based 3D printing (Image courtesy: Anadioti et al. (2018))

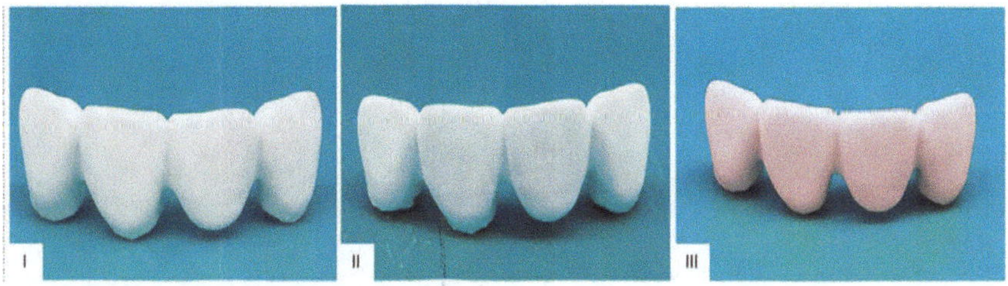

Fig. 24 Zirconia bridge prepared using 3D printing (Khorsandi et al. 2021)

(1.2) 3D-printed crowns, bridges, and veneers: Crowns and bridges are among the most common dental restorations fabricated using 3D printing technology. Traditionally, they are manufactured through CAD/CAM milling or conventional casting, which often results in material wastage and extended production time. Three-dimensional (3D) printing allows for precise, rapid, and cost-effective production of both temporary and permanent crowns and bridges (Fig. 24).

Advantages

- Improved fit and accuracy: A study comparing 3D-printed wax patterns versus conventional milling and casting found that 3D-printed restorations demonstrated superior marginal accuracy (36 ± 5 μm versus 141 ± 31 μm), enhancing the precision of crowns and bridges (Schönhoff et al. 2021).
- Interim restorations: Photopolymer-jetting 3D printing has been shown to outperform traditional milling and compression moulding techniques in the fabrication of temporary crowns by improving fit, durability, and efficiency.
- Customisation and patient-specific designs: Unlike prefabricated or milled restorations, each crown or bridge is uniquely designed for the patient.

2. Surgical guides for dental implant: Three-dimensional (3D) printing has improved implant placement accuracy, efficiency, and predictability in dental implantology. Its main use is making surgical guides to place implants precisely and reduce procedural mistakes. Rouzé l'Alzit et al. (2022) found that computer-guided surgery with 3D-printed guides improves implant placement and prosthesis results over freehand techniques. SLA, DLP, FDM, SLS, and inkjet printing have been tested for implant surgical guide production. Research shows that SLA and DLP technologies are best for clinical applications due to their accuracy and precision. Smaller guides are more precise than full-arch guides. The benefits of 3D-printed surgical guides go beyond precision. They offer minimally invasive operations, save chairside time, and improve patient comfort. Integrating CBCT and IOS data to digitally design and produce guides speeds up the procedure (Fig. 25) (Rouzé l'Alzit et al. 2022).

Three-dimensional (3D)-printed surgical guides facilitate minimally invasive operations, diminishing surgical mistakes and enhancing success rates. The research

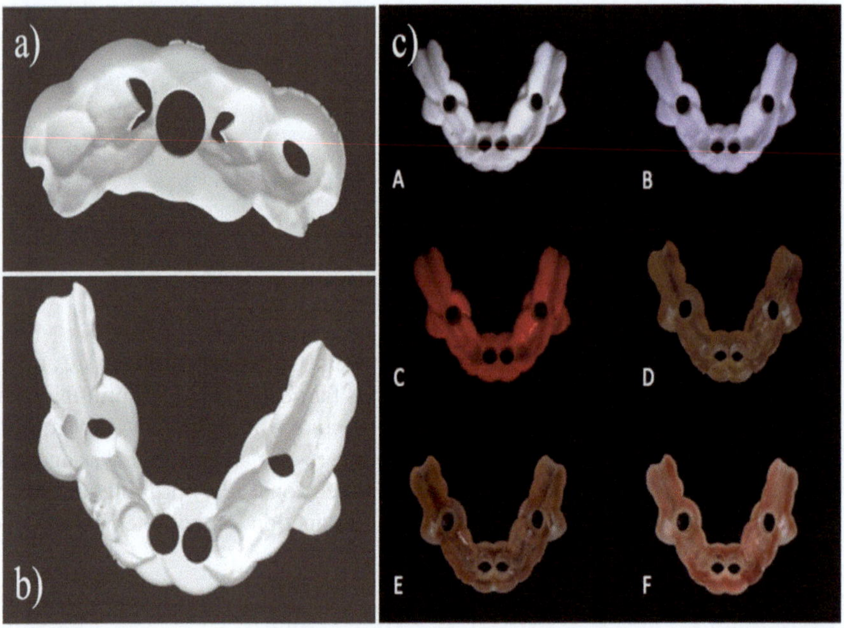

Fig. 25 **a** STL files of limited surgical guides and **b** extensive surgical guides. **c** Extensive surgical guides produced by **A.** Stratasys J750, **B.** Prodways P1000, **C.** Raise 3D Pro2, **D.** Form 2, **E.** Rapid Shape D40, and **F.** cara Print 4.0 (Image courtesy: Rouzel'Alzit et al. (2022))

by Mistry et al. (2021) utilised CBCT and intraoral scanning to strategise implant placements on 3D-printed mandibular models, employing both freehand (FH) and fully guided (FG) procedures. The findings indicated that FG surgery markedly decreased angular deviation (0.78° versus 6.43° in FH) and offered superior control over implant placement, with FG attaining a mean apical deviation of 0.43 mm against 1.88 mm in FH. The study determined that FG surgery provides enhanced precision and safety, minimising the risk of iatrogenic injury to essential anatomical structures and increasing implant success rates. Although 3D-guided surgery provides improved precision and predictability, the study recognised certain constraints, such as the possibility of manufacturing flaws in 3D-printed guides and reliance on operator proficiency during execution (Fig. 26). Notwithstanding these limitations, FG surgery showed superior consistency in implant placement and reduced hazards to surrounding anatomical structures, making it a preferred technique for implant placement in vital areas.

Advantages

Studies indicate that in-office 3D-printed implant surgical guides are as accurate as laboratory-fabricated ones, showing no significant deviation in implant placement.

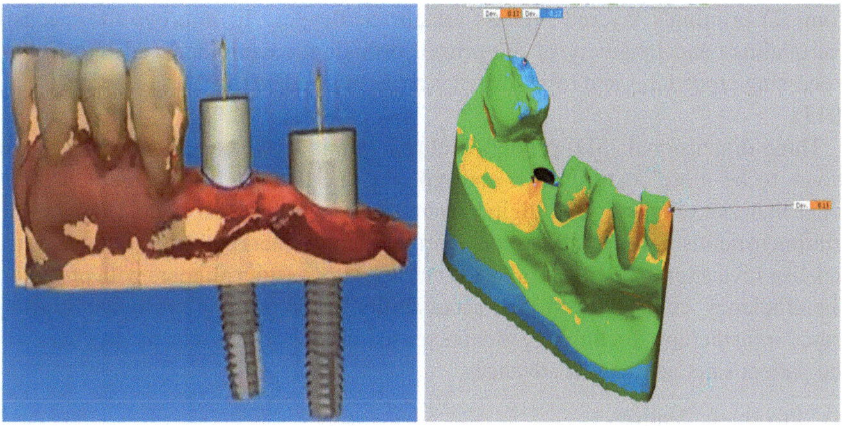

Fig. 26 3D-printed STL demonstrating a model accuracy deviation of less than 0.13 mm from the intended position in the FH surgical method (Image courtesy: Mistry et al. (2021))

Limitations

Despite its benefits, material restrictions, post-processing needs, and prices prevent broad implementation. Continued improvements in printer resolution, material biocompatibility, and software optimisation should make implantology 3D-printed solutions more reliable and accessible.

(3) Orthodontic treatment: Three-dimensional (3D) printing has improved orthodontics by making transparent aligners, retainers, and customised devices. Stereolithography, fused deposition modelling, and digital light processing provide accurate and economical orthodontic device fabrication, improving fit and accuracy. A comparison of rapid prototyping (RP) and computer numerical control (CNC) clear removable orthodontic appliances showed that 3D-printed aligners were adaptable but needed post-processing to reduce the staircase effect, a surface imperfection caused by layer-by-layer printing. However, 3D printing reduced manufacturing time and allowed mass customisation, making it a viable alternative for milling. Three-dimensional (3D)-printed aligners took longer to treat than CNC-milled aligners (3 weeks versus 2 weeks per aligner), but they were cheaper and more scalable.

Digital processes in 3D-printed orthodontic equipment allow orthodontists to create treatment plans based on 3D scans, virtual simulations, and digital models. By reducing chairside visits, this improves patient experience and treatment result predictability. Patients choose 3D-printed transparent aligners for their comfort and appearance. Transparent, removable aligners cause less irritation than metal braces. High-resolution printer requirements, material restrictions, and surface roughness from 3D printing's layered process remain challenges. To improve the mechanical qualities and longevity of 3D-printed orthodontic equipment, advanced post-processing procedures and resin formulas are being studied (Revilla-León and Özcan 2017).

Three-dimensional (3D)-printed occlusal splints and clear aligners have been shown to be more cost-effective and reproducible than traditional methods, with better material efficiency and digital accuracy. One of the most popular uses of 3D printing in dentistry is the fabrication of orthodontic aligners and appliances. Companies like Invisalign® use 3D printing to manufacture custom aligners with precision. The efficiency, customisation, and accessibility of 3D printing are revolutionising orthodontic therapy. Technology is expected to improve orthodontic treatment results and patient satisfaction as it advances.

(4) Prosthetic dentistry:

- Complete dentures: Three-dimensional (3D)-printed complete removable dental prostheses (CRDPs) offer higher precision and trueness compared to conventionally fabricated dentures (Fig. 27). However, some patients prefer the aesthetics of conventionally processed dentures due to minor differences in surface texture (Jawahar and Maragathavalli 2019).
- Removable partial dentures (RDPs): Early research and case reports suggest that 3D-printed cobalt–chromium partial removable dental prosthesis (PRDP) frameworks show promising results in terms of structural integrity and biocompatibility, although long-term studies are still needed.
- Maxillofacial prosthetics: Three-dimensional (3D) printing is widely used in craniofacial reconstruction by printing negative moulds for prostheses fabrication. Definitive obturator prostheses for patients with maxillofacial defects have been successfully fabricated using 3D-printing-based approaches, offering highly personalised and functional results (Khorsandi et al. 2021).

(5) Maxillofacial surgery:

- Training of surgeons: Three-dimensional (3D) printing has revolutionised preoperative planning, surgical training, and personalised treatment in maxillofacial surgery. Additive manufacturing enables the creation of tailored anatomical models, allowing surgeons to visualise complex cases prior to surgical procedures. The application of 3D printing in creating personalised implants, providing surgical guidance, and facilitating prosthetic reconstructions extends well beyond traditional training methods (Fig. 28). Enhancements in post-surgical recovery can be achieved through the use of tailored implants and established protocols for bone cutting and implant positioning. Studies indicate that mock operations utilising 3D-printed models assist surgeons in enhancing their skills and reducing intraoperative errors. Utilising realistic 3D-printed models for pre-surgical simulations significantly reduces surgery time, minimises complications, and lowers patient risk. The primary advantage of utilising 3D printing is the

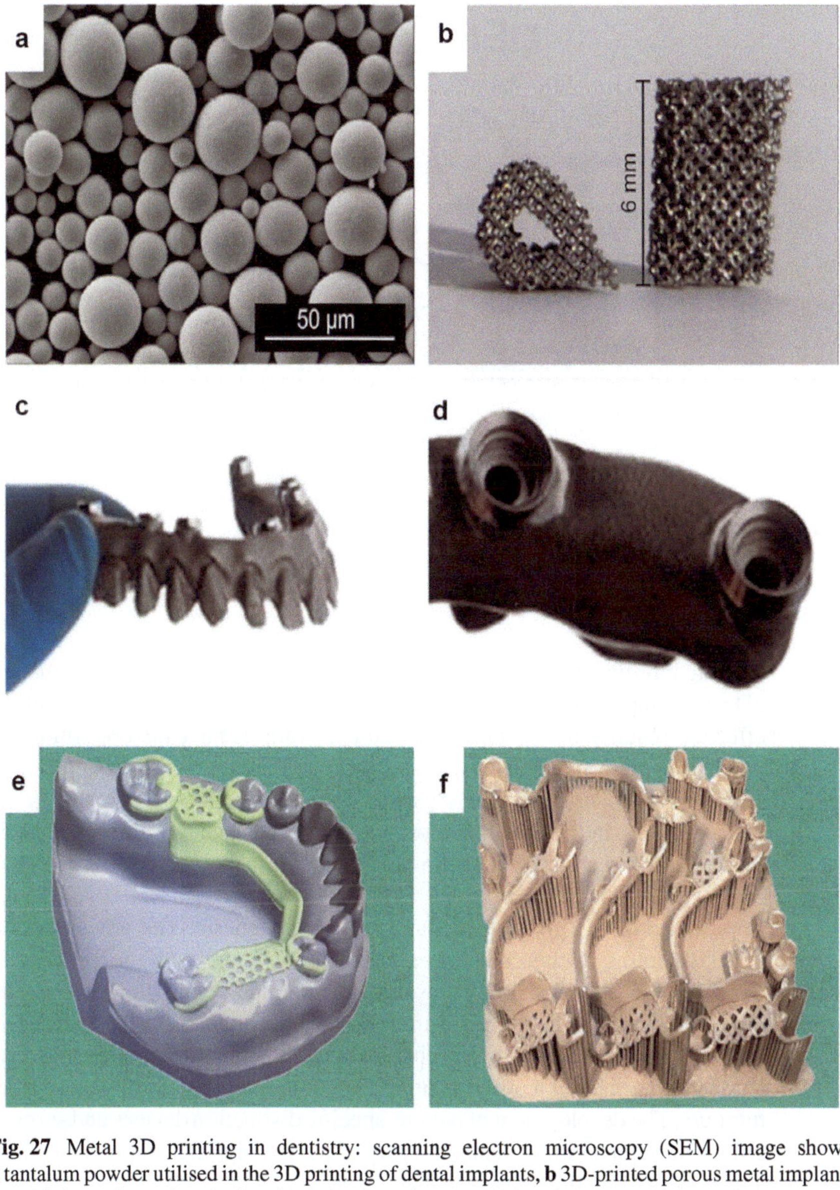

Fig. 27 Metal 3D printing in dentistry: scanning electron microscopy (SEM) image shows **a** tantalum powder utilised in the 3D printing of dental implants, **b** 3D-printed porous metal implant, **c** and **d** three-dimensional printed cobalt–chromium-based denture implant framework, **e** design of a detachable partial denture structure before 3D printing, and **f** a detachable partial denture framework composed of Co–Cr powder, fabricated using 3D printing, together with support elements that must be eliminated post-printing (Revilla-León and Özcan 2017)

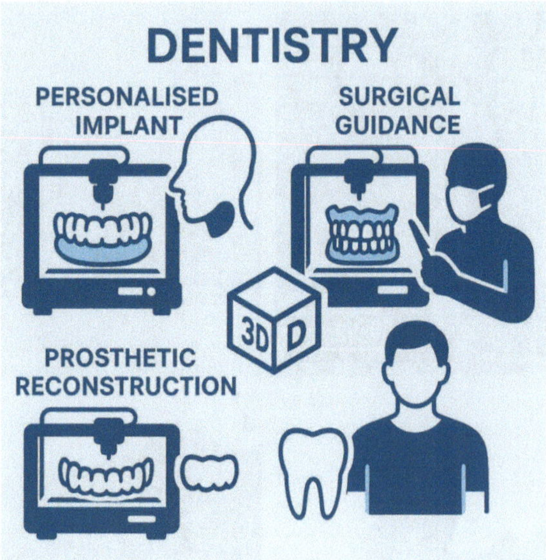

Fig. 28 Applications of 3D printing in dentistry

training it provides to emerging maxillofacial surgeons. Cadaver models and 2D photography failed to provide the necessary depth and tactile feedback for effective practice in conventional training. Trainees have the opportunity to practise on 3D-printed medical models prior to conducting orthognathic operations (Fig. 29), tumour resections, and TMJ reconstructions in real patients. Investigations indicate that 3D-printed models enhance trainee precision, skilfulness, and assurance, leading to better surgical outcomes (Reddy et al. 2018).

- Importance of 3D printing in distraction osteogenesis: The advancements in 3D printing technology have significantly enhanced the process of distraction osteogenesis (DO), a surgical technique in maxillofacial surgery aimed at lengthening and reconstructing bone irregularities. This advanced, methodical technique for bone separation and regeneration is well-suited for repairing the mandible after trauma, congenital defects, or the excision of tumours. The development of patient-specific distraction devices and surgical guides through additive manufacturing (AM) has significantly enhanced the accuracy of DO procedures (Mohan Alwala et al. 2018).

The ability to customise is a significant advantage of 3D printing. Three-dimensional (3D) printing of patient-specific mandibular models can be achieved through the utilisation of CT scan data, enabling the design of osteotomy incisions, the identification of distraction vectors, and the simulation of bone movement. This enhances the placement of distraction devices, reducing surgical errors and improving outcomes. Studies indicate that 3D-printed models can decrease surgical time by

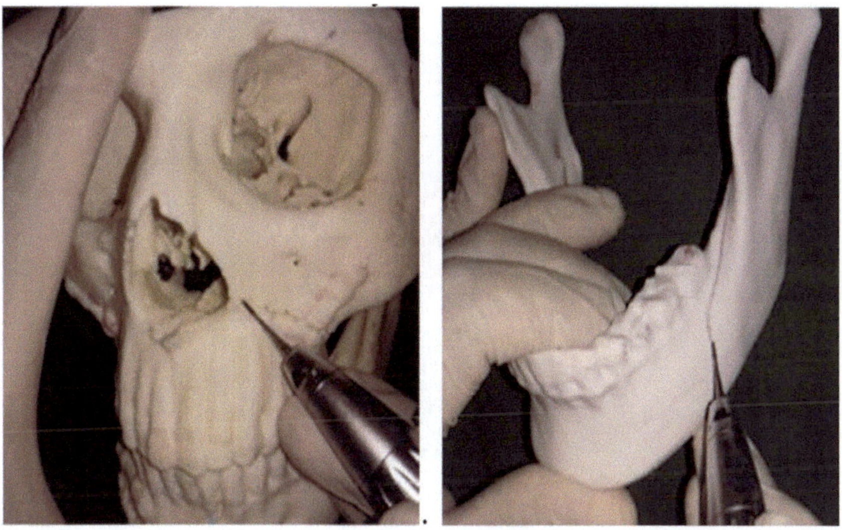

Fig. 29 Medical model used for training in orthognathic surgery (Reddy et al. 2018)

40–50 min, enhance the accuracy of distractor placement, and minimise significant structural damage (Fig. 30). Surgeons can utilise 3D printing not only for surgical planning but also to visually demonstrate procedures and obtain informed consent. Utilising pre-bent plates and crafting distractors from 3D-printed models enhance surgical efficiency and promote better bone healing outcomes.

- Reconstructive surgery: The development of patient-specific anatomical models, implants, and surgical guidance through 3D printing has significantly advanced the field of reconstructive surgery. The utilisation of this technology in preoperative planning enables surgeons to gain insights into complex anatomical structures, rehearse surgical procedures, and accurately address trauma, tumours, and congenital deformities.

A meticulous reconstruction of the orbital floor using 3D printing is crucial for preserving functionality and ensuring facial symmetry. Studies indicate that 3D-printed medical models can facilitate the pre-adaptation of titanium plates prior to surgery, thereby removing the need for intraoperative adjustments. The process of pre-bending and customising implants using 3D-printed models led to a significant reduction in surgery time by 40 min, as well as decreased patient morbidity and improved implant fit in a case study utilising fused deposition modelling (FDM).

In addition to its applications in orbital surgery, 3D printing is utilised in craniofacial reconstruction, mandibular reconstruction, and the treatment of maxillofacial defects. Surgeons have the capability to create accurate implants and grafts through the replication of patient anatomy, thereby enhancing both functional and aesthetic results. Simulated procedures utilising 3D-printed models enhance surgical techniques and reduce errors (Fig. 31).

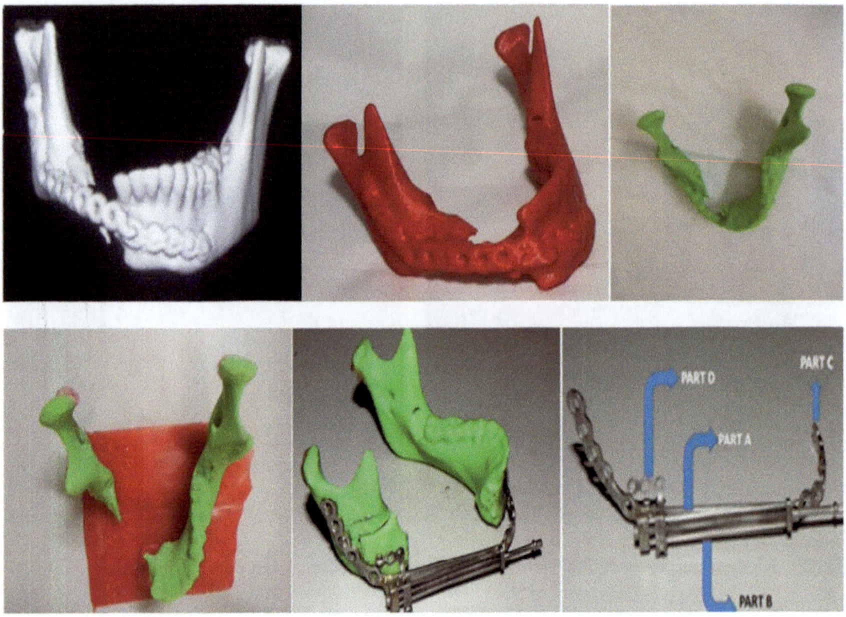

Fig. 30 3D model of mandible with planned distractor (Mohan Alwala et al. 2018)

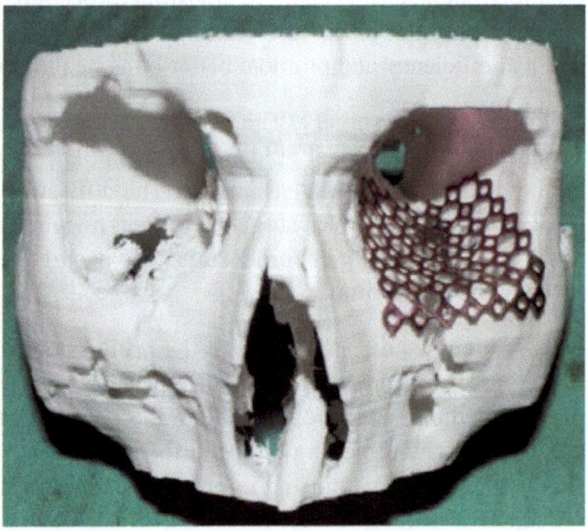

Fig. 31 Mock surgery and plate adaptation on model (Image courtesy: Kumar Malyala et al. (2017))

Despite these advancements, challenges such as elevated manufacturing costs, material limitations, and the necessity for specialised equipment persist. With the progression of technology, the application of 3D printing in maxillofacial surgery is set to enhance safety, precision, and personalisation in treatment solutions.

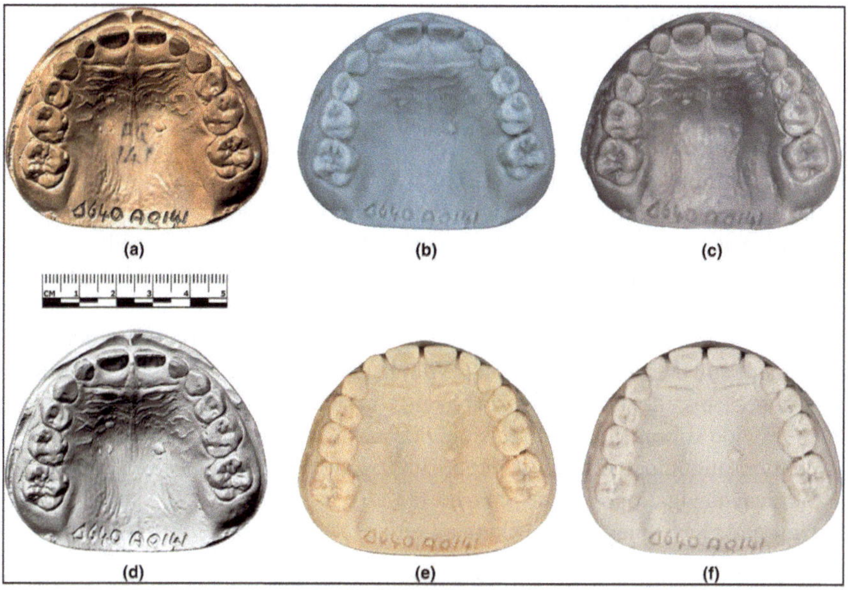

Fig. 32 **a** Textured polygonal model, **b** FDM print, **c** SLA print, **d** monochromatic polygonal model, **e** material-jetting print, and **f** binder-jetting print

(6) 3D printing in dental anthropology collections: Three-dimensional (3D) printing provides dental anthropology collections with high-resolution digital and physical copies that accurately recreate dental specimen morphology. The method allows stereolithography (SLA), fused deposition modelling (FDM), binder jetting, and material jetting to scan and duplicate dental casts without damage. Precision and resolution vary, with SLA and material-jetting processes reproducing detail better. A study of the Yuendumu Australian Aboriginal tooth collection found that 3D-printed reproductions accurately retained macro- and micro-morphological traits of the original specimens, with slight metric deviations (Fig. 32).

Besides preservation, 3D printing allows institutions to digitally exchange and reproduce dental collections, improving research accessibility. This reduces the need to handle fragile anthropological materials, reducing wear and injury. Computerised 3D models enable advanced morphometric analysis, comparative study, and dental anthropology training. Despite its benefits, 3D printing in dental anthropology has challenges such high costs, long printing times, and printing technology limits. As the technology becomes more cost-effective and efficient, dental anthropology will use it more, ensuring the preservation and accessibility of important anthropological collections (Fiorenza et al. 2018).

11 Navigation in Dentistry

1. Introduction to Navigation in Dentistry

Navigation technology in dentistry has changed several dental operations by boosting precision, efficiency, and predictability. Computer-assisted navigation (CAN) devices provide real-time guidance for implantology, endodontics, orthodontics, and maxillofacial surgery, minimising mistakes and enhancing clinical results. Initially, dental operations relied on 2D radiographic imaging and freehand approaches, resulting in unpredictable outcomes. The development of CBCT, intraoral scanning, and artificial intelligence (AI)-assisted planning has greatly improved preoperative assessment and execution. Precision is vital in dental operations to provide minimal invasiveness, excellent aesthetics, and long-term success. Navigation-assisted procedures provide sub-millimetre precision, decreasing issues such as nerve injury and implant misalignment (Birkfellner et al. 2000; Landaeta-Quinones et al. 2018).

Surgical navigation systems can be broadly categorised into optical tracking systems and electromagnetic tracking systems:

1. Optical tracking systems utilise infrared cameras to detect reflective markers attached to surgical instruments. These systems offer high accuracy but require an unobstructed line of sight.
2. Electromagnetic tracking systems employ low-frequency magnetic fields to determine the position of surgical instruments. They allow greater flexibility but are susceptible to interference from metallic objects.

2. Principles of Dental Navigation Systems

Dental navigation systems have revolutionised modern dentistry by integrating real-time tracking, 3D imaging, and computerised guidance to enhance surgical precision (Fig. 33). These systems, broadly classified into static and dynamic navigation, provide a significant improvement in treatment accuracy, safety, and efficiency. Dynamic navigation systems (DNS), in particular, have become an essential component of digital dentistry, offering real-time guidance during complex procedures such as dental implant placement, oral and maxillofacial surgeries, and endodontic treatments (Tang et al. 2024).

Fundamental Principles of Dental Navigation Systems

A dental navigation system operates on three primary principles: imaging and virtual planning, registration and calibration, and real-time tracking.

1. Imaging and virtual planning: DNS relies on preoperative imaging data obtained through CBCT scans to reconstruct a 3D model of the patient's oral structures. This imaging enables the practitioner to pre-plan the surgical procedure, selecting the optimal implant position or surgical path while ensuring the avoidance of critical anatomical structures.

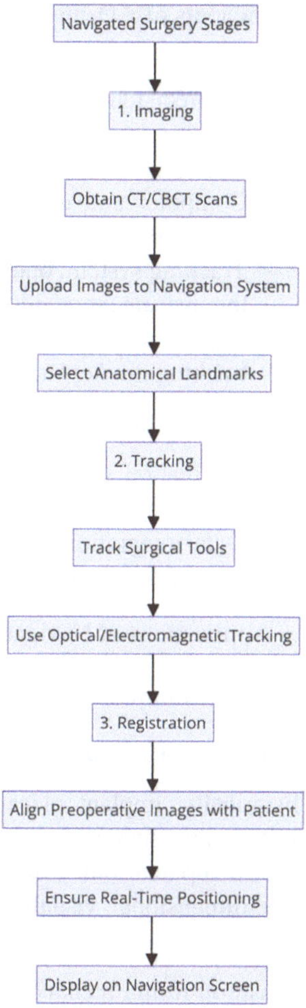

Fig. 33 Workflow of navigation

2. Registration and calibration: To synchronise the virtual 3D model with the physical patient anatomy, the system undergoes a registration process. Registration techniques are divided into marker-based and marker-free methods. Marker-based registration utilises fiducial markers placed around the surgical site, while marker-free approaches rely on anatomical landmarks. Calibration ensures that the tracking instruments and software accurately correspond to real-time surgical movements.
3. Real-time tracking and navigation: The core functionality of DNS is its ability to track surgical instruments dynamically in real time. This tracking is achieved using optical or electromagnetic sensors, which continuously relay data to the navigation software. Optical tracking, based on stereoscopic triangulation, is the most commonly employed technique in dental procedures, utilising infrared cameras and reflective markers to guide surgical movements with high precision.

Components of a Dental Navigation System

A DNS comprises both hardware and software elements that work together to facilitate precision in dental procedures.

- Hardware Components
  - Computer and display screen: provides real-time visualisation of surgical instruments and patient anatomy
  - Tracking system: optical or electromagnetic sensors that continuously monitor the instrument position
  - Tracer instruments: Specialised handpieces and positioners equipped with tracking markers to facilitate navigation.
- Software Components
  - Navigation software: supports preoperative planning, 3D visualisation, and real-time intraoperative guidance
  - Data integration system: processes CBCT scans and converts them into a navigable 3D model for precision planning.

3. Applications of Navigation systems

(i) Guided Implantology and Surgical Navigation

Evolution of Computer-Assisted Navigation in Dental Implantology.

Historically, implant placement was performed freehand, relying solely on 2D radiographic imaging and the clinician's experience. The introduction of cone beam computed tomography (CBCT) revolutionised implant planning by allowing three-dimensional visualisation of anatomical structures (Sukegawa and Kanno 2021).

Transition from Freehand to Navigation Systems

- Freehand surgery: high variability in accuracy and increased risk of complications such as nerve damage and improper angulation
- Static guided surgery: uses prefabricated surgical guides for implant placement but lacks intraoperative flexibility
- Dynamic navigation systems (DNS): provides real-time guidance, allowing intraoperative adjustments for improved precision (Pinter et al. 2022).

Static versus Dynamic Navigation in Implant Surgery

Static Navigation (Guided Surgery)

- Process: uses CBCT and CAD/CAM-designed surgical guides
- Advantages: high accuracy (<1.0 mm deviation), shorter surgery time, and predictable outcomes
- Limitations: no intraoperative flexibility and challenges in limited interocclusal space case.

Dynamic Navigation (Real-Time Guidance)

- Process: uses optical tracking for real-time implant guidance
- Advantages: allows real-time modifications, reduces surgical invasiveness, and provides accuracy similar to static guides (~1.2-mm deviation)
- Limitations: requires a learning curve and is susceptible to errors due to patient movement.

Workflow of Navigation-Assisted Implant Surgery

1. Preoperative Planning
   - CBCT imaging for anatomical assessment
   - Digital implant planning using intraoral scan data
2. Calibration and Registration

   Static navigation: Fabrication of surgical guides
   - Dynamic navigation: Calibration of tracking markers
3. Intraoperative Navigation
   - Real-time tracking of drill position and implant placement
4. Post-Operative Evaluation
   - CBCT verification and assessment of implant accuracy.

Accuracy and Clinical Outcomes

- Dynamic Navigation achieves ~0.4 mm coronal deviation and 4° angular deviation.
- A comparison of techniques is shown in Table 18.
- Clinical studies confirm superior precision and reduced complications compared to freehand techniques.
- Meta-analyses show dynamic navigation is comparable to static but offers greater intraoperative flexibility.

Clinical Applications and Case Studies

- Single implant placement: Dynamic navigation enhances precision in aesthetically critical areas.
- Full-arch rehabilitation: Static guides are preferred for multiple implants, but dynamic navigation is advantageous in complex cases.

Table 18 Comparison of techniques

Technique	Deviation (mm)
Freehand placement	1.5–2.0
Static navigation	1.0
Dynamic navigation	<0.9

Future Perspectives in Computer-Assisted Navigation

- Integration of AI and augmented reality: AI-driven navigation may further improve precision and efficiency.
- Technological advancements: Improved tracking systems and machine learning algorithms could optimise workflow and reduce errors.

Computer-assisted navigation (CAN) has significantly improved dental implant placement by enhancing accuracy and minimising errors. Static guides ensure high pre-planned precision, while dynamic navigation provides intraoperative flexibility. As technology continues to evolve, the integration of AI and augmented reality is expected to further refine navigation-assisted implant surgery (Bhochhibhoya and Guragain 2022).

(ii) Endodontic Navigation

Endodontics has experienced notable technology breakthroughs, particularly through navigation systems—both static and dynamic—that have significantly enhanced precision, accuracy, and therapeutic outcomes. Endodontic navigation largely emphasises guided access, canal identification, and minimally invasive techniques. The advent of dynamic navigation systems (DNS) has transformed endodontic practice by offering real-time tracking and enhancing results in complex patients. This scholarly analysis examines the concepts, applications, benefits, and constraints of navigation in endodontics, drawing on recent research and systematic reviews. The notion of navigation in dentistry emerged from implantology, where guided surgery was created to improve the precision of implant placement. This idea was subsequently used for endodontics to enhance access cavity preparation and the treatment of intricate root canal systems (Martinho et al. 2023).

Endodontic navigation is classified into static and dynamic systems.

- Static navigation involves preoperative planning with CBCT-based guides, which dictate the exact trajectory of access cavity preparation. The limitation is that once fabricated, the guide does not allow intraoperative modifications (Langaliya et al. 2024).
- Dynamic navigation, on the other hand, offers real-time tracking using optical markers and motion sensors, allowing adjustments during treatment (Vasudevan 2022).

The shift towards dynamic navigation is largely due to its higher precision, reduced iatrogenic errors, and conservation of dentine compared to conventional freehand techniques (Jonaityte et al. 2022).

Principles of Dynamic Navigation in Endodontics

Dynamic navigation is based on computer-aided navigation technology, which integrates CBCT data with real-time motion tracking. The key components of DNS include:

1. Preoperative CBCT imaging: Digital volumetric imaging is used to assess root canal morphology.

2. Tracking system: Optical cameras and motion sensors track the bur position in real time.
3. Software integration: The system overlays the planned drill path onto the CBCT data for intraoperative guidance.
4. Real-time feedback: The clinician receives instant visual guidance, ensuring precise drilling and minimal deviation from the pre-planned path (Huth et al. 2024).

Studies comparing freehand, static guided, and dynamic navigation techniques reveal that DNS significantly reduces angular and positional deviations, leading to better preservation of dentine and fewer procedural errors.

Applications of Navigation in Endodontics

- Guided Endodontic Access

The principal use of DNS in endodontics is in the preparation of access cavities, especially in calcified canals, atypical root anatomies, and minimally invasive endodontic procedures (Fig. 34). Vasudevan et al. (2022) discovered that dynamic navigation diminishes iatrogenic mistakes by facilitating accurate access preparation with minimum dentine loss. A systematic review by Langaliya et al. (2024) demonstrated that DNS is superior to freehand techniques in accuracy and preservation of dentine, making it highly effective in guided endodontics. DNS has shown promising results in conservative access cavity designs, which are crucial for maintaining tooth strength and long-term prognosis (Mujumdar et al. 2022).

- Locating Calcified and Obliterated Canals

A significant challenge in endodontics is the detection and navigation of calcified root canals. DNS enables doctors to traverse pulp canal obliterations (PCOs) with exceptional accuracy. Studies indicate that freehand approaches have a high rate of missed canals and perforations, whereas DNS significantly improves success rates (Jonaityte et al. 2022). Research by Liu et al. (2024) highlighted the learning curve of DNS in locating obliterated canals, showing that clinicians master navigation within seven attempts, thereby improving confidence and efficiency in clinical practice.

- Endodontic Microsurgery

DNS has also been utilised in apical microsurgery, where precision is critical for apicoectomies and retrograde fillings (Fig. 35). A study by Liu et al. (2024) confirmed that real-time navigation enhances accuracy in apical surgery, reducing the risk of root perforations and ensuring optimal resection angles. Dynamic guidance allows for smaller osteotomies and reduced trauma, making it an excellent tool for endodontic retreatment cases (Martinho et al. 2023).

Comparative Evaluation: Freehand versus Static versus Dynamic Navigation.

Multiple in vitro and systematic review studies have compared freehand, static, and dynamic navigation approaches as summarized in Table 19:

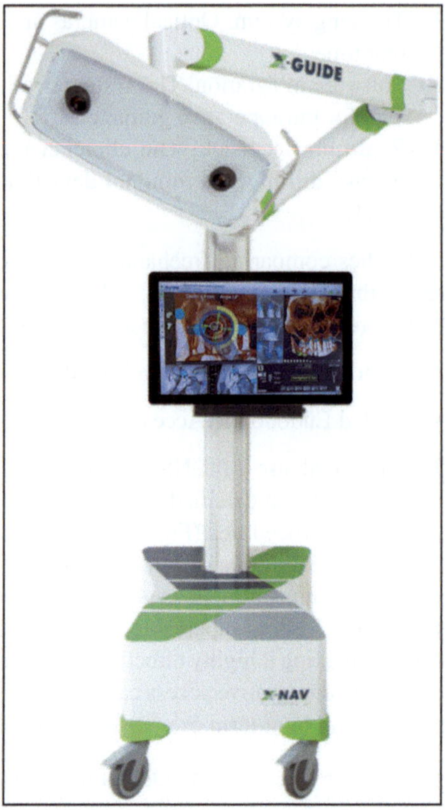

Fig. 34 Dynamic navigation system (Image courtesy: X-Mark® system)

- DNS provides the highest accuracy among the three techniques, with minimal deviations in bur placement (Huth et al. 2024).
- While static navigation also improves accuracy, its rigidity limits intraoperative flexibility (Langaliya et al. 2024).
- DNS allows real-time modifications, making it the most adaptable approach in complex endodontic cases (Mujumdar et al. 2022).

Limitations of Dynamic Navigation in Endodontics

Despite its advantages, DNS has certain challenges that need to be addressed:

1. High cost and accessibility: The technology requires expensive hardware and software integration, limiting its widespread adoption.
2. Learning curve: Clinicians require training to efficiently use DNS, though studies indicate rapid skill acquisition within a few cases.
3. Set-up complexity: DNS requires CBCT imaging, software planning, and calibration, which may increase clinical chair time.
4. Given the advancements in artificial intelligence and augmented reality, the future of endodontic navigation may include AI-powered guidance, haptic feedback

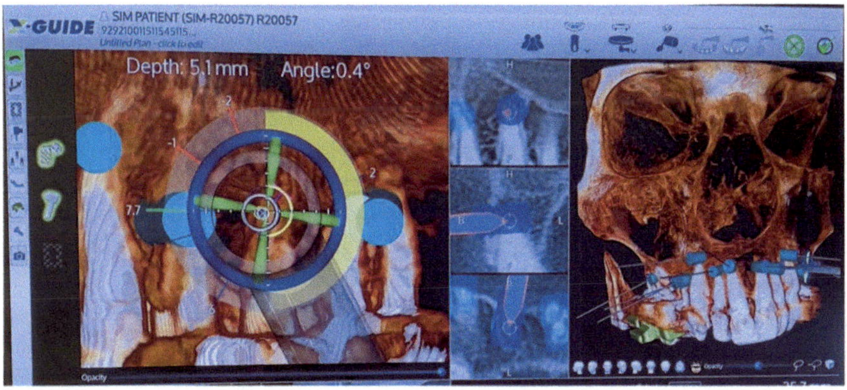

Fig. 35 DNS system while performing endodontic microsurgery (Image courtesy: X-Guide® system)

Table 19 Comparative evaluation of navigation techniques

Technique	Accuracy	Dentine preservation	Time efficiency	Clinical adjustability
Freehand	Low	High dentine loss	Fast	No adjustability
Static navigation	High	Moderate	Moderate	No adjustability
Dynamic navigation	Highest	Maximal preservation	Moderate	Real-time adjustability

technology, and fully automated endodontic workflows, leading to predictable and highly successful root canal treatments.

(iii) Orthodontics and Digital Navigation

Significant advances in orthodontics have been made possible by technologically advanced techniques that increase treatment results' accuracy, effectiveness, and predictability. Orthodontic procedures have been revolutionised by navigation technologies including three-dimensional (3D) surgical guidance, computer-aided design/computer-aided manufacturing (CAD/CAM), and augmented reality (AR). These tools allow surgeons to increase surgical accuracy, help with mini-implant insertion, and improve bracket placement.

- Augmented Reality in Orthodontic Navigation

Orthodontists can properly visualise bracket position, mini-implant implantation, and cephalometric parameters using augmented reality (AR), a new technique. Ströbele et al. (2023) found that AR navigation systems provide real-time feedback, reducing positioning errors without physical guides or 3D radiographic imaging in orthodontic bracket placement. AR technology superimposes digital bracket templates onto a patient's teeth to enhance bracket position and reduce human installation errors. A comparative study by Lo et al. (2021) found that AR-assisted bracket navigation reduced vertical positioning variations, improving treatment efficiency and outcomes. Dua et al. (2021) showed that AR-based learning models improved bracket positioning comprehension in orthodontic students.

Despite its benefits, augmented reality in orthodontics is limited by cost, software complexity, and training. Smartphone-based augmented reality apps may become more accessible and integrated into orthodontic procedures.

- 3D Surgical Guides in Orthodontic Mini-Implant Placement

Three-dimensional (3D)-printed surgical guides are crucial for mini-implant insertion, facilitating accurate positioning and minimising the likelihood of procedural mistakes (Fig. 36). Pop et al. (2025) examined the progression of surgical guides in orthodontics, emphasising their customisability, mechanical characteristics, and biocompatibility. Contemporary surgical guides use CBCT imaging and CAD/CAM technology, enabling physicians to meticulously pre-plan mini-implant placement with millimetre precision.

Research conducted by Liang (2023) indicated that CAD/CAM surgical guides enhance mini-screw stability, lower failure rates, and mitigate root injury in comparison to freehand methods. Hou et al. (2019) presented a 3D-printed computer-assisted piezocision guide (CAPG) to expedite orthodontic procedures. This guide aims to enhance irrigation, increase visibility, and minimise surgical problems, resulting in notable advancements in treatment efficacy.

Comparative Evaluation: Freehand versus Surgical Guides.

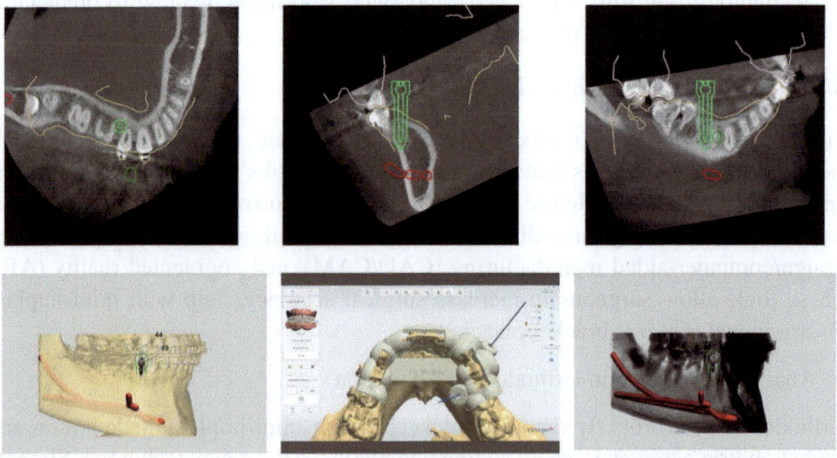

Fig. 36 Surgical guide for pre-drilling—digitally designed and manufactured (Image courtesy: Wenyong Liang (2023))

Table 20 Comparative evaluation of different techniques

Technique	Accuracy	Root damage risk	Clinical adjustability
Freehand	Low	High	No
AR navigation	High	Low	Real time
3D surgical guides	Very high	Minimal	Fixed path

A comparative study by Deglow et al. (2023) analysed freehand mini-implant placement versus AR-assisted and CAD/CAM-guided techniques. The study found that (Table 20):

The study concluded that navigation techniques significantly improve accuracy and reduce root perforation risks compared to conventional freehand methods.

- Digital Workflows and AI Integration in Orthodontic Navigation

The incorporation of digital processes, including intraoral scanning, AI-enhanced treatment planning, and automated navigation systems, is influencing the future of orthodontic navigation. Chen et al. (2020) emphasised the significance of CBCT-integrated CAD software in orthodontic surgery planning, allowing real-time modifications and personalised mini-implant positioning. Advanced AI-driven systems are being created to autonomously determine ideal bracket placements using cephalometric analysis and tooth morphology, hence minimising human error and treatment variability.

Lee et al. (2023) examined AI-driven adaptive learning algorithms that forecast optimal force distribution for orthodontic motions, hence improving treatment efficacy and minimising relapse probabilities. Notwithstanding these gains, issues like elevated computational expenses, software integration impediments, and the necessity for regulatory permissions persist as hurdles to extensive clinical implementation.

- Computer-Guided Piezocision in Accelerated Orthodontics

Orthodontic treatments sometimes necessitate surgical procedures to expedite tooth mobility. Piezocision, a minimally invasive corticotomy method, has been enhanced by computer-assisted navigation devices. Hou et al. (2019) developed a 3D-printed piezocision guide (CAPG) to improve surgical precision, cooling efficacy, and visibility. The research indicated that CAPG-assisted piezocision decreased surgical complications and enhanced healing rates.

Dibart et al. (1995) examined minimally invasive piezocision procedures, highlighting the significance of navigation-guided incisions to avert injury to soft tissue and alveolar bone (Fig. 37).

(iv) Navigation in Oral and Maxillofacial Surgery

The complexity of maxillofacial anatomy, which includes essential structures like nerves, blood vessels, and the cranial base, necessitates the use of navigational technologies that offer real-time intraoperative guidance. This approach reduces complications and enhances surgical outcomes. Surgical navigation has progressed from

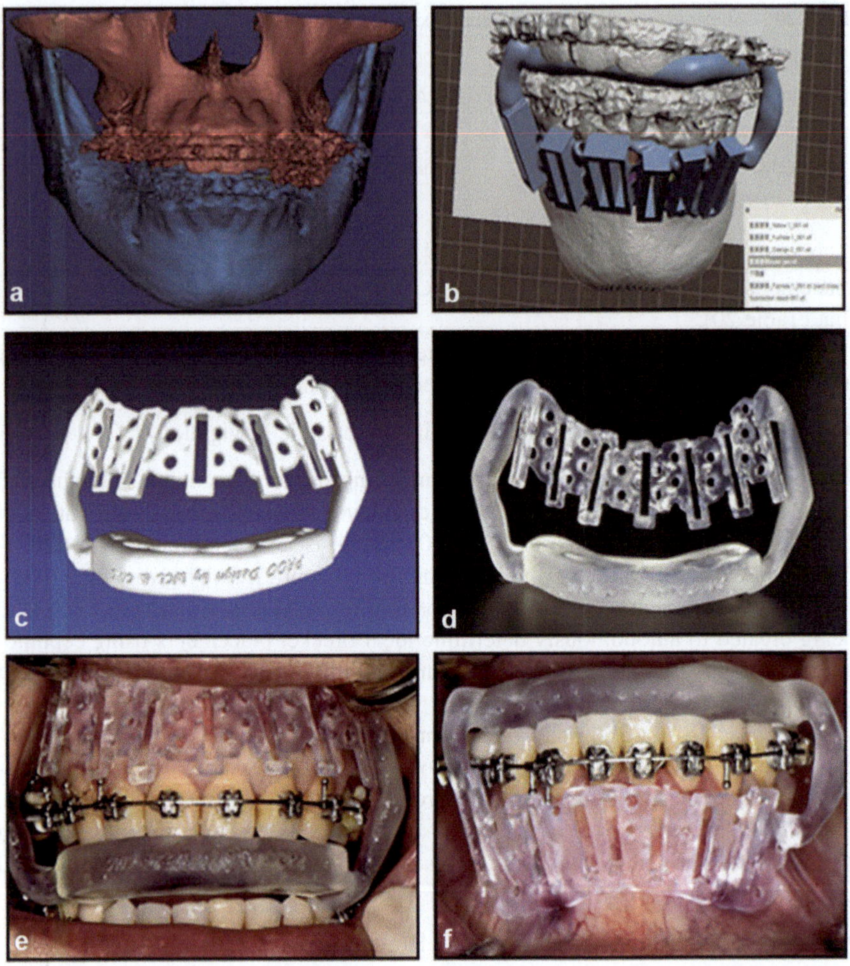

Fig. 37 Three-dimensional printed CAPG for pre-surgical planning and production. **a** Medical imaging software generated 3D models from maxilla and mandible DICOM data, with 3D CBCT images of maxillary and mandibular stone models superimposed. **b** Piezocision cutting incision slots were constructed using 3D CAD. **c** The irrigated cooling system reduces thermal damage with many drainage openings and holes. **d** Stereolithography was used to create CAPG files on solid material for fast prototyping. 3D-printed transparent CAPGs **e** and **f** were tested for operational placement and stability (Image courtesy: Hou et al. (2024))

the use of stereotactic techniques in neurosurgery to the implementation of advanced frameless optical and electromagnetic tracking systems in maxillofacial procedures (Novelli et al. 2023). Initial methods utilised fixed headframes, constraining intraoperative adaptability and necessitating mathematical computations for target localisation (Bukhsh et al. 2023).

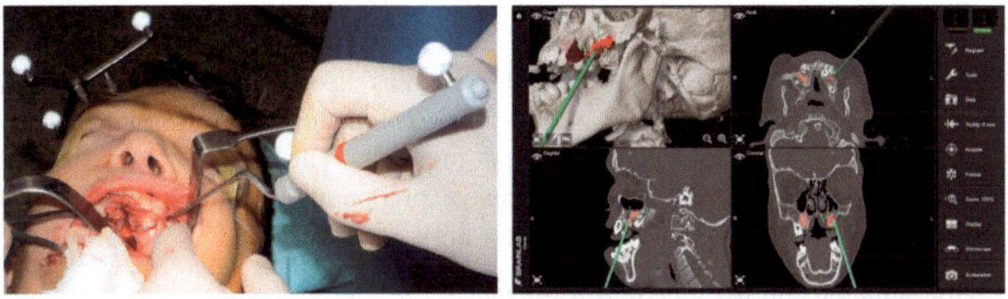

Fig. 38 Intraoperative image during tooth removal (Image courtesy: Novelli et al. (2023))

The introduction of computed tomography (CT) and magnetic resonance imaging (MRI) has facilitated real-time tracking and digital overlays, thereby enhancing surgical precision. Modern navigation systems incorporate computer-aided design and manufacturing (CAD/CAM), augmented reality (AR), and virtual surgical planning (VSP), enabling surgeons to accurately visualise intricate anatomical structures and meticulously plan procedures (Landaeta-Quinones et al. 2018).

- Removal of Impacted Teeth

The extraction of impacted teeth, especially third molars and supernumerary teeth, stands out as a significant application of surgical navigation in the field of oral surgery. Conventional methods depend on radiographic imaging and the skill of the surgeon, while navigation-assisted procedures improve safety by accurately pinpointing anatomical structures like the inferior alveolar nerve and maxillary sinus. Surgical navigation systems provide real-time guidance during surgical procedures to determine the exact location of impacted teeth within the osseous structure, identify the optimal extraction trajectory to minimise the risk of damage to essential anatomical structures, such as the inferior alveolar nerve and maxillary sinus, and enhance accessibility to deeply embedded or displaced teeth, minimising iatrogenic injury.

The research carried out by Novelli et al. (2023) explored the application of computer-assisted surgery for the extraction of impacted teeth in individuals with craniofacial syndromes, showcasing an impressive accuracy of $\leq$1 mm in target registration error (Fig. 38). This degree of accuracy notably diminishes the likelihood of unintended complications and enhances the results following surgery.

- Removal of Foreign Objects

Cases that involve foreign bodies, particularly those related to orthodontic arch fragments, present significant surgical challenges owing to their restricted visibility on standard imaging techniques. Surgical navigation enhances the accuracy of localisation and supports minimally invasive removal, thereby minimising the potential for collateral tissue damage.

- Management of Craniofacial Syndromes

Individuals with craniofacial abnormalities, such as Apert and Pfeiffer syndromes, often exhibit impacted teeth, dental crowding, and anatomical variations that may pose challenges to conventional surgical methods. The incorporation of navigation technology facilitates comprehensive preoperative planning and precise intraoperative execution, thereby reducing surgical morbidity.

- Orthognathic and Reconstructive Surgery

The use of navigation-assisted surgery has become increasingly prominent in orthognathic and reconstructive procedures, especially in intricate cases that involve facial asymmetry or significant bone grafting. The integration of virtual planning with intraoperative anatomy significantly improves the accuracy of osteotomies, implant placements, and facial contour reconstructions during surgical navigation. Precision osteotomies and maxillomandibular repositioning are essential components of orthognathic surgeries, highlighting the significance of navigation-assisted techniques.

Applications encompass:

- Virtual planning is performed for osteotomies prior to surgery in instances of malocclusion, facial asymmetry, and maxillomandibular deformities.
- Monitoring of bony segment movement during surgery is essential to ensure the accurate execution of planned corrections.
- Integration with CAD/CAM splints facilitates precise guidance of bone cuts to the millimetre.

Alkhayatt et al. (2024) demonstrated that navigation in bimaxillary surgery facilitates accurate bone segmentation and alignment, thereby improving aesthetic and functional outcomes. Bukhsh et al. (2023) demonstrated that the integration of virtual surgical planning (VSP) with navigation leads to decreased operative times and enhanced accuracy in complex skeletal corrections (Fig. 39).

- Maxillofacial Trauma Reconstruction

Surgical navigation has markedly improved the accuracy of treating intricate facial trauma cases, especially concerning zygomatic, orbital, and midfacial fractures. High-impact trauma may result in orbital fractures, zygomatic fractures, and mandibular disruptions that necessitate accurate realignment.

Surgical navigation assists in:

- Realigning bone fragments with sub-millimetre accuracy
- Restoration of orbital volume in cases of blowout fractures
- Virtual mirroring techniques that utilise the unaffected side as a surgical guide for reconstruction.

The integration of real-time 3D imaging, augmented reality (AR), and artificial intelligence (AI)-driven analytics enhances the accuracy of navigation systems and

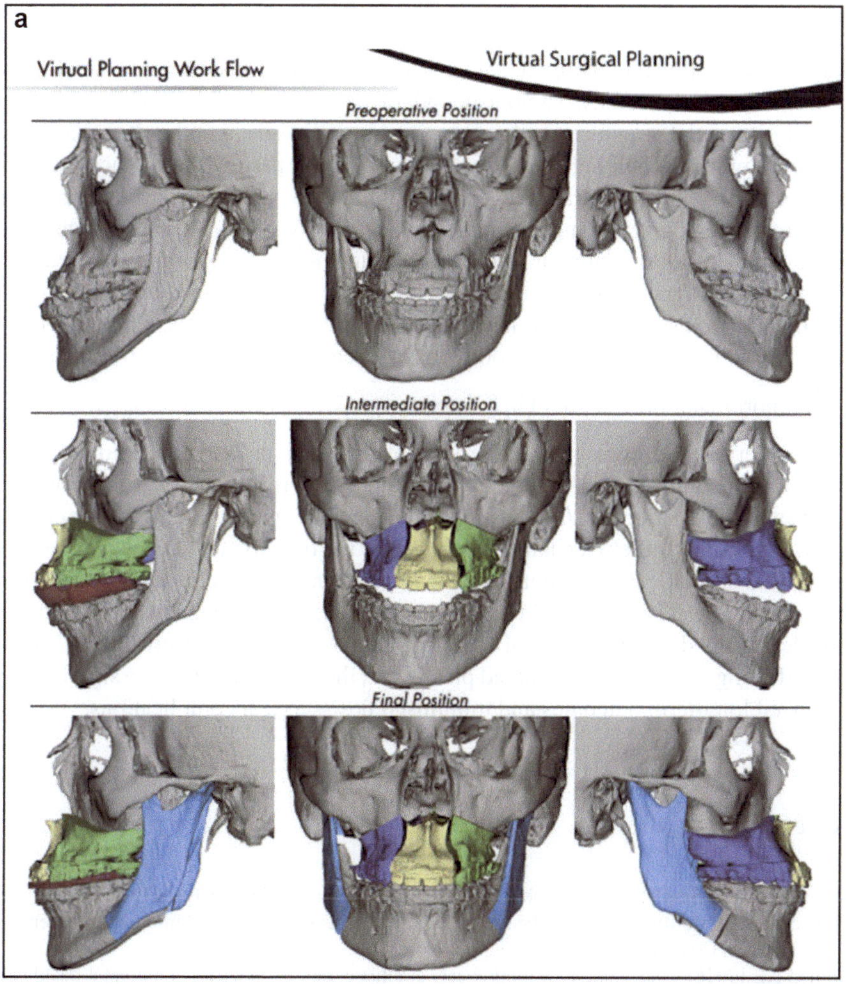

Fig. 39 Virtual surgery planning utilising DICOM software to treat facial asymmetry and occlusion by segmented LeFort I and BSSO (Image courtesy: Edward Ellis, DDS, MS, San Antonio, TX)

improves surgical outcomes. Yu et al. (2013) conducted an analysis of 104 cases of maxillofacial trauma, demonstrating that real-time navigation decreased post-operative deviations to 1.46 ± 0.24 mm, thereby significantly enhancing accuracy compared to conventional method. Sukegawa et al. (2021) demonstrated improved reduction accuracy in comminuted unilateral fractures, resulting in better post-operative facial symmetry. Demian et al. (2019) highlighted that navigation reduces the necessity for revision surgeries, thereby decreasing patient morbidity and overall healthcare expenses.

- Tumour Resection and Skull Base Surgery

Surgical navigation has altered oncologic excision in skull base tumours, ameloblastomas, and osteosarcomas. Tumour boundaries are delineated with great accuracy, avoiding essential structures such as nerves, blood vessels, and the dura mater and aiding in tumour debulking while maintaining healthy tissue. Maxillofacial tumour resection necessitates accurate excision to maintain the integrity of surrounding vital structures, thereby rendering navigation essential. Yu et al. (2013) demonstrated that navigation-assisted tumour resections resulted in a mean error margin of merely 1 mm, thereby significantly enhancing oncological outcomes. Sukegawa et al. (2021) highlighted the essential role of navigation in skull base surgeries, where the close proximity to cranial nerves and blood vessels necessitates millimetre precision.

- Temporomandibular Joint (TMJ) Surgery

TMJ surgeries encompass intricate procedures in which precise navigation is essential for achieving optimal prosthetic placement and restoring joint functionality. Landaeta-Quinones et al. (2018) observed that navigation effectively minimises joint space deviations, thereby enhancing post-operative function and decreasing relapse rates. Bukhsh et al. (2023) indicated that navigation notably decreases operative time and improves precision in TMJ reconstruction. Recent advancements in technology have led to the development of 3D-printed, patient-specific TMJ prostheses. When utilised alongside navigation-guided placement, these innovations have significantly enhanced long-term outcomes and minimised post-surgical complications.

References

Abreu-García A, Souto RM, Izquierdo J (2023) Corrosion performance of Ti6Al7Nb alloy in simulated body fluid for implant application characterized using macro- and microelectrochemical techniques. Coatings 13(6):1121

Ahmed KE (2016) Management of tooth wear: a holistic, dental, medical, and mental healthcare approach. Prim Dent J 5(3):35–37

Akl MA, Mansour DE, Zheng F (2023) The role of intraoral scanners in the shade matching process: a systematic review. J Prosthodont 32(3):196–203

Ali Z, Baker S, Sereno N, Martin N (2020) A pilot randomized controlled crossover trial comparing early OHRQoL outcomes of cobalt-chromium versus PEEK removable partial denture frameworks. Int J Prosthodont 33(4):386–392

Alkhayatt NM, Alzahrani HH, Ahmed S, Alotaibi BM, Alsaggaf RM, ALAlmuaysh AM et al (2024) Computer-assisted navigation in oral and maxillofacial surgery: a systematic review. Saudi Dent J 36(3):387–94

Alyaman M, Abd-Raheem A, AlDeiri F (2019) Design of an automated extraoral photogrammetry 3D scanner 16(3)

Anadioti E, Kane B, Soulas E (2018) Current and emerging applications of 3D printing in restorative dentistry. Curr Oral Health Rep 5(2):133–139

Ayoub A, Khan A, Aldhanhani A, Alnaser H, Naudi K, Ju X et al (2021) The validation of an innovative method for 3D capture and analysis of the nasolabial region in cleft cases. Cleft Palate Craniofacial J 58(1):98–104

Benitez BK, Brudnicki A, Surowiec Z, Wieprzowski Ł, Rasadurai A, Nalabothu P et al (2022) Digital impressions from newborns to preschoolers with cleft lip and palate: a two-centers experience. J Plast Reconstr Aesthet Surg 75(11):4233–4242

Beuer F, Schweiger J, Edelhoff D (2008) Digital dentistry: an overview of recent developments for CAD/CAM generated restorations. Br Dent J 204(9):505–511

Bhochhibhoya A, Guragain M (2022) Dynamic navigation: a novel tool for dental implant surgery. J Nepal Prosthodont Soc [Internet] [cited 2025 Feb 27] 5(1). https://www.nepjol.info/index.php/jnprossoc/article/view/53388

Birkfellner W, Wanschitz F, Watzinger F, Huber K, Figl M, Schopper C et al (2000) Accuracy of a navigation system for computer-aided oral implantology. In: Delp SL, DiGoia AM, Jaramaz B (eds) Medical image computing and computer-assisted intervention—MICCAI 2000 [Internet]. Berlin, Heidelberg: Springer Berlin Heidelberg; 2000 [cited 2025 Feb 26], pp 1061–7 (Goos G, Hartmanis J, Van Leeuwen J, editors. Lecture Notes in Computer Science; vol. 1935). http://link.springer.com/10.1007/978-3-540-40899-4_110

Blackwood DJ (2003) Biomaterials: past successes and future problems. Corros Rev 21(2–3):97–124

Bronkhorst H, Bronkhorst E, Kalaykova S, Pereira-Cenci T, Huysmans MC, Loomans B (2023) Inter- and intra-variability in tooth wear progression at surface-, tooth- and patient-level over a period of three years: a cohort study. J Dent 138:104693

Brunetto JL, Adriazola Ique MM, Melo Neto CLDM, Sachi VP, Dos Santos DM, Goiato MC (2024) Intraoral and extraoral scanning technologies in the digital workflow era: an integrative review with artificial intelligence. Odovtos—Int J Dent Sci 26:166–174

Bukhsh A, Alanazi M, Alnaim M, Hamdi N, Al-ghamdi H, Alsanamah F et al (2023) Benefits and limitations of computer-assisted surgery in maxillofacial surgery. J Healthc Sci 03(09):289–295

Burhardt L, Livas C, Kerdijk W, Van Der Meer WJ, Ren Y (2016) Treatment comfort, time perception, and preference for conventional and digital impression techniques: a comparative study in young patients. Am J Orthod Dentofacial Orthop 150(2):261–267

Chen X, Mao B, Zhu Z, Yu J, Lu Y, Zhang Q et al (2019) A three-dimensional finite element analysis of mechanical function for 4 removable partial denture designs with 3 framework materials: CoCr, Ti-6Al-4V alloy and PEEK. Sci Rep 9(1):13975

Chen L, Liang X, Shen C, Jiang S, Wang J (2020) Synthetic CT generation from CBCT images via deep learning. Med Phys 47(3):1115–1125

Christopoulou I, Kaklamanos EG, Makrygiannakis MA, Bitsanis I, Perlea P, Tsolakis AI (2022) Intraoral scanners in orthodontics: a critical review. Int J Environ Res Public Health 19(3):1407

Connert T, Weiger R, Krastl G (2022) Present status and future directions—guided endodontics. Int Endod J 55(S4):995–1002

Daguano JKMB, Milesi MTB, Rodas ACD, Weber AF, Sarkis JES, Hortellani MA et al (2019) In vitro biocompatibility of new bioactive lithia-silica glass-ceramics. Mater Sci Eng C 94:117–125

Demian N, Pearl C, Woernley TC, Wilson J, Seaman J (2019) Surgical navigation for oral and maxillofacial surgery. Oral Maxillofac Surg Clin N Am. 31(4):531–538

Dibart S, Sebaoun JD, Surmenian J (2009) Piezocision: a minimally invasive, periodontally accelerated orthodontic tooth movement procedure. Compend Contin Educ Dent Jamesburg NJ 1995 30(6):342–4, 346, 348–50

Diniz MB, Boldieri T, Rodrigues JA, Santos-Pinto L, Lussi A, Cordeiro RCL (2012) The performance of conventional and fluorescence-based methods for occlusal caries detection. J Am Dent Assoc 143(4):339–350

Doi K, Yoshiga C, Kobatake R, Kawagoe M, Wakamatsu K, Tsuga K (2021) Use of an intraoral scanner to evaluate oral health. J Oral Sci 63(3):292–294

Dua VS, Sikri A, Kaur A, Sachdeva M (2021) Augmented reality in orthodontics: the way ahead. Int J Oral Health Dent. 7(3):195–198

Eggmann F, Blatz MB (2024) Recent advances in intraoral scanners. J Dent Res 103(13):1349–1357
Estai M, Bunt S, Kanagasingam Y, Kruger E, Tennant M (2016) Diagnostic accuracy of teledentistry in the detection of dental caries: a systematic review. J Evid Based Dent Pract 16(3):161–172
Fiorenza L, Yong R, Ranjitkar S, Hughes T, Quayle M, McMenamin PG et al (2018) Technical note: the use of 3D printing in dental anthropology collections. Am J Phys Anthropol 167(2):400–406
Fried D (2020) Optical methods for monitoring demineralization and caries. In: Wilder-Smith P, Ajdaharian J (eds) Oral diagnosis [Internet]. Cham: Springer International Publishing [cited 2025 Feb 8], pp 1–27. http://link.springer.com/10.1007/978-3-030-19250-1_1
Friedland B, Miles DA (2014) Liabilities and risks of using cone beam computed tomography. Dent Clin North Am 58(3):671–685
Gaboutchian AV, Knyaz VA, Leybova NA, Petrosyan G, Simonyan H, Vasilyev SV (2019) Application of photogrammetric techniques in palaeoodontological studies trough automated digital shape analysis of human teeth. Int Arch Photogramm Remote Sens Spat Inf Sci XLII-2/W12:75–80
Ghiban A, Ghiban B, Borţun CM, Ghiban N, Antoniac I (2012) Heat treatments influence on corrosion resistance of some new dental cobalt alloys. Solid State Phenom 14(188):93–97
Goharian A, Abdullah MR (2017) Bioinert metals (Stainless Steel, Titanium, Cobalt Chromium). In: Trauma plating systems [Internet]. Elsevier [cited 2025 Feb 26], pp 115–42. https://linkinghub.elsevier.com/retrieve/pii/B9780128046340000070
Goracci C, Franchi L, Vichi A, Ferrari M (2016) Accuracy, reliability, and efficiency of intraoral scanners for full-arch impressions: a systematic review of the clinical evidence. Eur J Orthod 38(4):422–428
Gupta J, Ali S (2013) Cone beam computed tomography in oral implants. Natl J Maxillofac Surg 4(1):2
Hou HY, Li CH, Chen MC, Lin PY, Liu WC, Cathy Tsai YW et al (2019) A novel 3D-printed computer-assisted piezocision guide for surgically facilitated orthodontics. Am J Orthod Dentofacial Orthop. 155(4):584–591
Huth KC, Borkowski L, Liebermann A, Berlinghoff F, Hickel R, Schwendicke F et al (2024) Comparing accuracy in guided endodontics: dynamic real-time navigation, static guides, and manual approaches for access cavity preparation—an in vitro study using 3D printed teeth. Clin Oral Investig 28(4):212
Imburgia M, Logozzo S, Hauschild U, Veronesi G, Mangano C, Mangano FG (2017) Accuracy of four intraoral scanners in oral implantology: a comparative in vitro study. BMC Oral Health 17(1):92
Jacobs R, Salmon B, Codari M, Hassan B, Bornstein MM (2018) Cone beam computed tomography in implant dentistry: recommendations for clinical use. BMC Oral Health 18(1):88
Jonaityte EM, Bilvinaite G, Drukteinis S, Torres A (2022) Accuracy of dynamic navigation for non-surgical endodontic treatment: a systematic review. J Clin Med 11(12):3441
De Josselin De Jong E, Sundström F, Westerling H, Tranaeus S, Ten Bosch JJ, Angmar-Månsson B (1995) A new method for in vivo quantification of changes in initial enamel caries with laser fluorescence. Caries Res 29(1):2–7
Khorsandi D, Fahimipour A, Abasian P, Saber SS, Seyedi M, Ghanavati S et al (2021) 3D and 4D printing in dentistry and maxillofacial surgery: printing techniques, materials, and applications. Acta Biomater 122:26–49
Kiarudi AH, Eghbal MJ, Safi Y, Aghdasi MM, Fazlyab M (2015) The applications of cone-beam computed tomography in endodontics: a review of literature. Iran Endod J. 10(1):16–25
Kim S hyang, Lee SM, Park JH, Yang S, Kim JW. Effectiveness of individualized 3D titanium-printed Orthognathic osteotomy guides and custom plates. BMC Oral Health 3;23(1):255
Kochar SP, Reche A, Paul P (2022) The etiology and management of dental implant failure: a review. Cureus 14(10):e30455
Kortam S, ELsyad M, Awad S, ElHelbawy N (2022) Metal-ceramic and polyether ether ketone–composite maxillary fixed prosthesis supported by four implants and opposed by removable

distal extension partial dentures: a comparative study of clinical and prosthetic outcomes. Int J Oral Maxillofac Implants 37(1):181–9
Kugel G (2014) Impression-taking: conventional methods remain steadfast as digital technology progresses. Compend Contin Educ Dent Jamesburg NJ 1995 35(3):202–3
Kumar Malyala S, Kumar YR, Mohan Alwala A, Vasamsetty P (2017) Benefits of additive manufacturing medical model in orbital floor reconstruction surgery: a case study. Jurnalul Chir [Internet] [cited 2025 Feb 26] 13(2). https://www.omicsonline.org/open-access/benefits-of-additive-manufacturing-medical-model-in-orbital-floor-reconstruction-surgery-a-case-study-1584-9341-13-2-6.php?aid=92012
Landaeta-Quinones CG, Hernandez N, Zarroug NK (2018) Computer-assisted surgery. Dent Clin North Am 62(3):403–420
Langaliya A, Kritika S, Shah A, Shah J, Mahalaxmi S (2024) Does dynamic navigation system preserve more dentine?—a systematic review. BMC Oral Health 24(1):678
Lawson NC, Burgess JO (2015) Clinicians reaping benefits of new concepts in impressioning. Compend Contin Educ Dent Jamesburg NJ 1995 36(2):152–3
Lee SJ, MacArthur RX, Gallucci GO (2013) An evaluation of student and clinician perception of digital and conventional implant impressions. J Prosthet Dent 110(5):420–423
Lee JH, Lee HL, Park IY, On SW, Byun SH, Yang BE (2023) Effectiveness of creating digital twins with different digital dentition models and cone-beam computed tomography. Sci Rep 13(1):10603
Liang W (2023) Application of surgical guide for pre-drilling for the successful placement of orthodontic mini-screws using CAD/CAM technology in two cases. J Orthod 50(2):243–251
Lim JH, Park JM, Kim M, Heo SJ, Myung JY (2018) Comparison of digital intraoral scanner reproducibility and image trueness considering repetitive experience. J Prosthet Dent 119(2):225–232
Liu Y, Fang M, Zhao R, Liu H, Li K, Tian M et al (2022) Clinical applications of polyetheretherketone in removable dental prostheses: accuracy, characteristics, and performance. Polymers 14(21):4615
Liu SM, Peng L, Zhao YJ, Han B, Wang XY, Wang ZH (2024) The learning curve of a dynamic navigation system used in endodontic apical surgery. J Dent Sci 19(4):2247–2255
Ma B, Yue X, Sun Y, Peng L, Geng W (2021) Accuracy of photogrammetry, intraoral scanning, and conventional impression techniques for complete-arch implant rehabilitation: an in vitro comparative study. BMC Oral Health 21(1):636
Mangano F, Bazzoli M, Tettamanti L, Farronato D, Maineri M, Macchi A et al (2013) Custom-made, selective laser sintering (SLS) blade implants as a non-conventional solution for the prosthetic rehabilitation of extremely atrophied posterior mandible. Lasers Med Sci 28(5):1241–1247
Manjunatha VA, Parisarla H, Parasher S (2024) A systematic review on recent advancements in 3D surface imaging and artificial intelligence for enhanced dental research and clinical practice. IP Int J Maxillofac Imaging 10(4):132–139
Marti AM, Harris BT, Metz MJ, Morton D, Scarfe WC, Metz CJ et al (2017) Comparison of digital scanning and polyvinyl siloxane impression techniques by dental students: instructional efficiency and attitudes towards technology. Eur J Dent Educ 21(3):200–205
Martinho FC, Griffin IL, Corazza BJM (2023) Current applications of dynamic navigation system in endodontics: a scoping review. Eur J Dent 17(03):569–586
Michou S, Vannahme C, Ekstrand KR, Benetti AR (2020) Detecting early erosive tooth wear using an intraoral scanner system. J Dent 100:103445
Michou S, Lambach MS, Ntovas P, Benetti AR, Bakhshandeh A, Rahiotis C et al (2021) Automated caries detection in vivo using a 3D intraoral scanner. Sci Rep 11(1):21276
Mikolicz A, Simon B, Gáspár O, Shahbazi A, Vag J (2023) Reproducibility of the digital palate in forensic investigations: a two-year retrospective cohort study on twins. J Dent 135:104562
Mirosław K, Polkowski J, Bombalska A (2022) A study on the photopolymerization kinetics of selected dental resins using Fourier infrared spectroscopy (FTIR). Mater Basel Switz. 15(17):5850

Mistry A, Ucer C, Thompson J, Khan R, Karahmet E, Sher F (2021) 3D guided dental implant placement: impact on surgical accuracy and collateral damage to the inferior alveolar nerve. Dent J 9(9):99

Mohan Alwala A, Arvind U, Kumar Malyala S, Vasamsetty P (2018) Customization of patient specific distraction device using additive manufacture technology. Mater Today Proc 5(2):4134–4137

Muir JD, Calvert EJ (1988) Vomiting during the taking of dental impressions. Two case reports of the use of psychological techniques. Br Dent J 165(4):139–41

Mujumdar S, Borkar A, Maral S, Nighot N, Aras S (2022) Use of dynamic navigation system in endodontics: a literature review. J Int Clin Dent Res Organ 14(1):17

Nahum E, Lugovskoy S (2018) A comparative study of hydroxyapatite coating produced with plasma electrolytic oxidation and hydrothermal treatment on titanium alloys: Ti6Al4V and Ti6Al7Nb for dental implants [Internet] [cited 2025 Feb 26]. http://www.preprints.org/manuscript/201810.0694/v2

Negm EE, Aboutaleb FA, Alam-Eldein AM (2019) Virtual evaluation of the accuracy of fit and trueness in maxillary poly(etheretherketone) removable partial denture frameworks fabricated by direct and indirect CAD/CAM techniques. J Prosthodont 28(7):804–810

Novelli G, Moretti M, Meazzini MC, Cassé CMA, Mazzoleni F, Sozzi D (2023) Introduction to surgical navigation in oral surgery: a case-series. Oral 3(2):146–154

Obaid AS (2020) Three dimensional digitally designed surgical guides in periodontal and implant surgeries: a review. Int J Dent Sci Res 8(6):150–154

Pant G, Krishna BV, Abed NK, Nagpal A, VA, Meheta A (2024) Advances in dental materials: bioactive glass and ceramic composites: a review. In: Msomi V, Ngonda T (eds) E3S Web conferences 505:01026

Patil S, Kulkarni V, Bhise A (2019) Algorithmic analysis for dental caries detection using an adaptive neural network architecture. Heliyon 5(5):e01579

Pinter GT, Decker R, Szenasi G, Barabas P, Huszar T (2022) Dynamic navigation for dental implant placement. J vis Exp 187:63400

Pop SI, Bud E, Jánosi KM, Bud A, Kerekes-Máthé B (2025) Three-dimensional surgical guides in orthodontics: the present and the future. Dent J 13(2):74

Pretty IA, Ellwood RP (2013) The caries continuum: opportunities to detect, treat and monitor the re-mineralization of early caries lesions. J Dent 41:S12-21

Randolph LD, Palin WM, Leprince JG (2018) Composition of dental resin-based composites for direct restorations. In: Miletic V (ed) Dental composite materials for direct restorations [Internet]. Cham: Springer International Publishing [cited 2025 Feb 25], pp 11–24. http://link.springer.com/10.1007/978-3-319-60961-4_2

Reddy GV, Vasamsetty P, Kumar Malyala S, Alwala A (2018) Training young maxillofacial surgeons or trainees using additive manufacturing. Mater Today Proc 5(2):4046–4049

Revilla-León M, Özcan M (2017) Additive manufacturing technologies used for 3D metal printing in dentistry. Curr Oral Health Rep. 4(3):201–208

Riad Deglow E, Zubizarreta-Macho Á, González Menéndez H, Lorrio Castro J, Galparsoro Catalán A, Tzironi G et al (2023) Comparative analysis of two navigation techniques based on augmented reality technology for the orthodontic mini-implants placement. BMC Oral Health 23(1):542

Rouzé l'Alzit F, Cade R, Naveau A, Babilotte J, Meglioli M, Catros S (2022) Accuracy of commercial 3D printers for the fabrication of surgical guides in dental implantology. J Dent 117:103909

Saini M, Singh Y, Arora P, Arora V, Jain K (2015) Implant biomaterials: a comprehensive review. World J Clin Cases WJCC 3(1):52–57

Sakornwimon N, Leevailoj C (2017) Clinical marginal fit of zirconia crowns and patients' preferences for impression techniques using intraoral digital scanner versus polyvinyl siloxane material. J Prosthet Dent 118(3):386–391

Salimov F, Tatli U, Kürkçü M, Akoğlan M, Öztunç H, Kurtoğlu C (2014) Evaluation of relationship between preoperative bone density values derived from cone beam computed tomography and implant stability parameters: a clinical study. Clin Oral Implants Res 25(9):1016–1021

Sarment D (ed) Cone beam computed tomography: oral and maxillofacial diagnosis and applications [Internet], 1st ed. Wiley [cited 2025 Feb 2]. https://onlinelibrary.wiley.com/doi/book/10.1002/9781118769027

Sason G, Mistry G, Tabassum R, Shetty O (2018) A comparative evaluation of intraoral and extraoral digital impressions: an in vivo study. J Indian Prosthodont Soc. 18(2):108

Schlenz MA, Schupp B, Schmidt A, Wöstmann B, Baresel I, Krämer N et al (2022) New caries diagnostic tools in intraoral scanners: a comparative in vitro study to established methods in permanent and primary teeth. Sensors 22(6):2156

Schönhoff LM, Mayinger F, Eichberger M, Reznikova E, Stawarczyk B (2021) 3D printing of dental restorations: mechanical properties of thermoplastic polymer materials. J Mech Behav Biomed Mater 119:104544

Schwendicke F, Samek W, Krois J (2020) Artificial intelligence in dentistry: chances and challenges. J Dent Res 99(7):769–774

Shah N, Thakur M, Gill S, Shetty O, Alqahtani NM, Al-Qarni MA et al (2023) Validation of digital impressions' accuracy obtained using intraoral and Extraoral scanners: a systematic review. J Clin Med 12(18):5833

Shanbhag G, Pandey S, Mehta N, Kini Y, Kini A (2020) A virtual noninvasive way of constructing a nasoalveolar molding plate for cleft babies, using intraoral scanners, CAD, and prosthetic milling. Cleft Palate Craniofacial J 57(2):263–266

Da Silva RLB, Kim JH, Markarian RA, Falacho R, Cortes DN, Costa AJM et al (2022) Introduction to digital dentistry. In: Cortes ARG (ed) Digital dentistry [Internet], 1st ed. Wiley [cited 2025 Feb 2], pp 1–17. https://onlinelibrary.wiley.com/doi/10.1002/9781119852025.ch1

Steinmeier S, Wiedemeier D, Hämmerle CHF, Mühlemann S (2020) Accuracy of remote diagnoses using intraoral scans captured in approximate true color: a pilot and validation study in teledentistry. BMC Oral Health 20(1):266

Stimmelmayr M, Güth JF, Erdelt K, Edelhoff D, Beuer F (2012) Digital evaluation of the reproducibility of implant scanbody fit—an in vitro study. Clin Oral Investig 16(3):851–856

Ströbele DA, Othman A, Meier MA, Aboulazm K, Von See C (2023) Augmented reality in orthodontics for bracket placement using conventional mobile devices: technical note. J World Fed Orthod. 12(6):280–283

Stuani VT, Ferreira R, Manfredi GGP, Cardoso MV, Sant'Ana ACP (2019) Photogrammetry as an alternative for acquiring digital dental models: a proof of concept. Med Hypotheses 128:43–9

Sukegawa S, Kanno T (2021) Computer-assisted navigation surgery in oral and maxillofacial surgery. In: Bonanthaya K, Panneerselvam E, Manuel S, Kumar VV, Rai A (eds) Oral and maxillofacial surgery for the clinician [Internet]. Singapore: Springer Nature Singapore [cited 2025 Feb 27], pp 841–62. https://link.springer.com/10.1007/978-981-15-1346-6_41

Szalewski L, Wójcik D, Sofińska-Chmiel W, Kuśmierz M, Różyło-Kalinowska I (2022) How the duration and mode of photopolymerization affect the mechanical properties of a dental composite resin. Materials 16(1):113

Tabatabaian F, Namdari M, Mahshid M, Vora SR, Mirabbasi S (2024) Accuracy and precision of intraoral scanners for shade matching: a systematic review. J Prosthet Dent 132(4):714–725

Tang WL, Chao XY, Ye Z, Liu MW, Jiang H (2024) The use of dynamic navigation systems as a component of digital dentistry. J Dent Res 103(2):119–128

Upadhyay A, Pradhan L, Yenurkar D, Kumar K, Mukherjee S (2024) Advancement in ceramic biomaterials for dental implants. Int J Appl Ceram Technol 21(4):2796–2817

Vasudevan A (2022) Dynamic navigation in guided endodontics—a systematic review. Eur Endod J [Internet] [cited 2025 Feb 27]. https://eurendodj.com/jvi.aspx?un=EEJ-96168&volume

Vitai V, Németh A, Sólyom E, Czumbel LM, Szabó B, Fazekas R et al (2023) Evaluation of the accuracy of intraoral scanners for complete-arch scanning: a systematic review and network meta-analysis. J Dent 137:104636

Wei Z, Wei L (2022) Application of zirconia ceramic biomaterial implants in the restoration of tooth loss caused by periodontal disease. Sci Adv Mater 14(1):1–10

Wismeijer D, Mans R, Van Genuchten M, Reijers HA (2014) Patients' preferences when comparing analogue implant impressions using a polyether impression material versus digital impressions (Intraoral Scan) of dental implants. Clin Oral Implants Res 25(10):1113–1118

Witecy C, Ganss C, Wöstmann B, Schlenz MB, Schlenz MA (2021) Monitoring of erosive tooth wear with intraoral scanners in vitro. Caries Res 55(3):215–224

Wu X, Liu Y, Xie W (2017) Development and characterization of novel light-curable composite resins with calcium phosphate silicate cement. In: Goulbourne NC (ed) Portland, Oregon, United States [cited 2025 Feb 25], pp 101651I. http://proceedings.spiedigitallibrary.org/proceeding.aspx?doi=10.1117/12.2263167

Yu H, Shen SG, Wang X, Zhang L, Zhang S (2013) The indication and application of computer-assisted navigation in oral and maxillofacial surgery—Shanghai's experience based on 104 cases. J Cranio-Maxillofac Surg. 41(8):770–774

Zarone F, Di Mauro MI, Ausiello P, Ruggiero G, Sorrentino R (2019) Current status on lithium disilicate and zirconia: a narrative review. BMC Oral Health 19(1):134

Zhang W, Fu W, Wang X, Ye J (2023) Improving the osseointegration and soft tissue sealing of zirconia ceramics by the incorporation of akermanite *via* sol infiltration for dental implants. J Mater Chem B 11(19):4237–4259

Zhao K, Wu S, Qian C, Sun J (2024) Suitability and trueness of the removable partial denture framework fabricating by polyether ether ketone with CAD-CAM technology. Polymers 16(8):1119

Zimmermann M, Mehl A, Mörmann WH, Reich S (2015) Intraoral scanning systems—a current overview. Int J Comput Dent 18(2):101–129

Zoidis P, Papathanasiou I, Polyzois G (2016) The use of a modified poly-ether-ether-ketone (PEEK) as an alternative framework material for removable dental prostheses: a clinical report. J Prosthodont 25(7):580–584

Zotti F, Rosolin L, Bersani M, Poscolere A, Pappalardo D, Zerman N (2022) Digital dental models: is photogrammetry an alternative to dental Extraoral and intraoral scanners? Dent J 10(2):24

Application of AI in Orthodontics

Karan Maheshwari, Alisha, and Sharnjeet Kaur

In the rapidly evolving field of orthodontics, artificial intelligence (AI) is increasingly playing a pivotal role in enhancing diagnostic accuracy, streamlining treatment planning, and improving overall patient care (Fig. 1). Integrating AI technology in orthodontics is reshaping traditional methodologies, providing orthodontists with powerful tools to deliver more precise, personalized, and efficient care. AI systems can analyze complex datasets, recognize patterns, and make predictions that may be difficult or time-consuming for human practitioners to identify (Kiełczykowski et al. 2023). AI has several impactful applications in orthodontics, significantly improving patient care, treatment efficiency, and practice management. In this chapter, we will discuss some key applications.

1 Diagnosis and Treatment Planning

Traditional Diagnostic Approaches

Orthodontists typically begin the diagnostic process by gathering detailed patient history, conducting physical examinations, and reviewing imaging such as panoramic radiographs (X-rays), cephalometric analysis, and photographs. Traditional diagnosis and treatment planning methods rely heavily on the orthodontist's expertise and experience. The process involves the following:

- **Manual Assessment**: Orthodontists manually analyze X-rays and photographs to identify malocclusions (misalignments), impacted teeth, and other irregularities.

K. Maheshwari (✉) · Alisha · S. Kaur
Department of Orthodontics and Dentofacial Orthopaedics, Adesh Institute of Dental Sciences and Research, Bathinda, Punjab, India
e-mail: karan245m@gmail.com

A. Gupta et al. (eds.), *Application of Robotics in Dentistry*, Lecture Notes in Bioengineering, https://doi.org/10.1007/978-981-95-1470-0_8

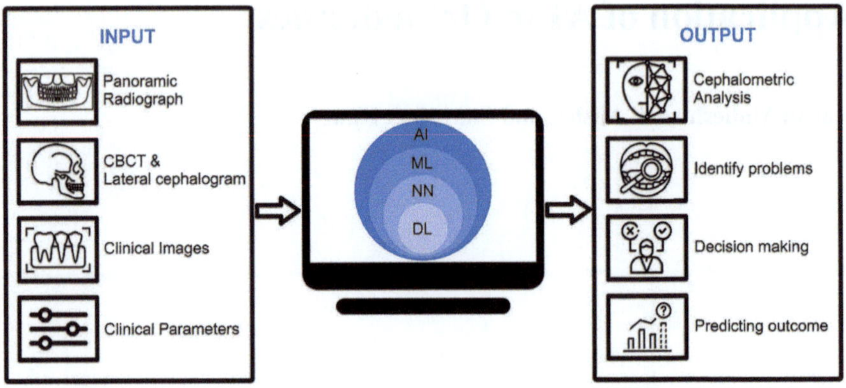

Fig. 1 Input and output of AI applications in orthodontics AI: artificial intelligence; ML: machine learning; NN: neural networks; DL: deep learning (Gracea January 2025)

- **Cephalometric Analysis**: Cephalometric X-rays, which capture lateral and frontal views of the head, are analyzed to measure skeletal relationships and determine optimal bite positions.
- **Manual Modeling**: Orthodontists create physical models of a patient's dental impressions to study tooth position and plan treatment.

While these traditional diagnostic techniques have been effective, they are time-consuming, subjective, and prone to human error (Wong et al. 2019). As a result, there is increasing interest in adopting artificial intelligence (AI)-powered systems to enhance diagnostic accuracy and streamline treatment planning.

Role of AI in Automated Diagnostics

AI-Driven Image Analysis

One of AI's most significant applications in orthodontics is image analysis. Machine learning (ML) and deep learning algorithms have revolutionized the interpretation of diagnostic images such as X-rays, cone-beam computed tomography (CBCT) scans, and intraoral photographs (Obermeyer and Emanuel 2016). AI can detect patterns and anomalies in dental images that may be difficult to spot through manual examination.

- **Radiographic Interpretation**: AI models can identify signs of malocclusion, caries, bone loss, impacted teeth, and even early-stage periodontal disease. These systems use convolutional neural networks (CNNs) to analyze radiographs and generate detailed diagnostic reports.
- **Three-Dimensional (3D) CBCT and Computed Tomography (CT) Scans**: AI-powered software can process 3D imaging from cone-beam computed tomography (CBCT) scans to accurately identify jawbone abnormalities, tooth eruptions, and root positions. The AI analyzes volumetric data, which are more complex than traditional 2D X-rays, providing a more accurate diagnosis.

- **Intraoral Scans**: Intraoral scanners capture detailed 3D images of the teeth and gums. AI algorithms can detect irregular tooth position, alignments, and bite relationships, offering a more accurate representation of the patient's dental anatomy than traditional impressions.

Precision in Diagnosis

AI systems can process vast amounts of data from a variety of sources, including clinical records, imaging, and genetic data. By analyzing these large datasets, AI can make predictions regarding the development of malocclusions or other dental conditions based on patterns observed in similar cases (Subramanian et al. 2022). This allows orthodontists to do the following:

- **Detect Hidden Issues**: AI can flag potential issues that may not be immediately visible to the human eye, allowing for early intervention and more timely treatment.
- **Accuracy and Speed**: The use of AI tools significantly reduces diagnostic time. AI can analyze images and make diagnoses almost instantly, which can streamline clinical workflows and enhance the overall patient experience.

AI-Powered Decision Support Systems

AI can act as a decision-support tool by providing orthodontists with evidence-based recommendations. These systems analyze patient data and suggest potential treatment options based on prior outcomes from similar cases. AI tools help orthodontists make informed decisions by highlighting possible treatment alternatives and offering insights into the likely success of each approach.

- **Predictive Analysis**: AI can predict treatment outcomes based on historical data, helping orthodontists assess the most likely scenarios for tooth movement, treatment duration, and potential risks.

AI-Optimized Treatment Plans

Once a diagnosis has been made, treatment planning is the next critical step in orthodontic care. AI assists orthodontists in developing more personalized and optimized treatment plans by analyzing patient data and predicting how teeth will move over time (Amann et al. 2020). To develop an individualized treatment plan, AI systems can consider numerous factors, such as the patient's skeletal structure, age, tooth morphology, and bite relationships.

- **Personalized Treatment Approaches**: AI analyzes historical treatment data to understand the most effective methods for patients with similar characteristics. By applying these insights, AI can recommend specific treatment modalities such as clear aligners, braces, or retainers.
- **Predicting Treatment Outcomes**: AI algorithms can simulate how a patient's teeth will move under different treatment methods. This simulation allows the

orthodontist to visualize the progression of the treatment, adjust the plan as needed, and set realistic expectations for the patient.

- **Optimized Tooth Movement**: AI-powered systems can determine the most efficient sequence for moving teeth, ensuring that the movement occurs in the least invasive and most comfortable manner for the patient. AI can adjust wire thickness, bracket placement, and appliance configurations in real time based on the patient's progress.

Simulation of Treatment Progress

AI-driven software enables orthodontists to simulate the entire treatment journey, showing how teeth will shift over time and the final result. This simulation not only aids in treatment planning but also serves as a valuable communication tool with patients.

- **Patient Communication**: Simulations visually represent their treatment outcome, helping them understand the projected changes to their smile. This can lead to higher patient satisfaction, improved compliance, and a better overall experience.
- **Treatment Time Prediction**: AI can predict the estimated duration of the treatment based on the patient's specific condition, helping the orthodontist manage patient expectations and optimize scheduling.

Virtual Braces and Aligners Design

For patients undergoing treatment with clear aligners, AI is essential in customizing each aligner to the individual's teeth. AI-powered systems generate a series of custom aligners based on the patient's current dental anatomy and predicted tooth movements (Khanagar et al. 2021a).

- **Aligner Design Optimization**: AI can design each aligner in a series to move teeth progressively, ensuring that they fit well and function effectively for the patient. This reduces the need for adjustments and enhances treatment efficiency.
- **Minimizing Treatment Time**: By optimizing the aligner design, AI can reduce the overall duration of treatment. Aligners are precisely calibrated to move teeth most efficiently, decreasing the need for frequent visits or appliance modifications.

Advantages of AI in Diagnosis and Treatment Planning

- **Increased Accuracy**

AI offers a higher degree of precision in diagnosis and treatment planning by analyzing large datasets and identifying patterns that may be difficult for human practitioners to spot. This reduces the likelihood of errors and improves the quality of care.

- **Personalization**

AI enables more personalized treatment plans by taking into account individual patient characteristics. This results in customized treatment approaches that address specific needs, leading to faster and more successful outcomes.

- **Efficiency and Time-Saving**

The use of AI reduces the time spent on manual diagnostics, image analysis, and treatment planning. This not only improves workflow efficiency in the clinic but also allows orthodontists to manage more cases in a shorter amount of time.

- **Predictability and Risk Mitigation**

AI's predictive capabilities allow orthodontists to foresee potential treatment challenges, such as delayed tooth movement or complications. This information can help mitigate risks and ensure that the treatment progresses smoothly.

Challenges and Considerations in AI Adoption

- **Data Privacy and Security**

The use of AI in orthodontics requires the collection and analysis of large volumes of patient data, raising concerns about data privacy and security—ensuring that patient information is protected and compliant with regulations such as Health Insurance Portability and Accountability Act (HIPAA) is essential for maintaining patient trust and meeting legal standards (Thrall et al. 2018).

- **Ethical Considerations**

AI-based systems must be transparent and unbiased, ensuring that treatment recommendations are based on clinical evidence and not influenced by external factors. Ethical concerns regarding the use of AI, particularly in terms of decision-making in patient care, must be addressed.

- **Integration into Existing Practices**

Integrating AI tools into established orthodontic practices requires time, training, and financial investment. The cost of implementing AI systems and the need for continuous updates can be barriers for some practitioners. Ensuring that orthodontists are adequately trained to use AI systems effectively is also essential for their success (Talaat et al. 2020).

2 Three-Dimensional Imaging and Modeling

3D imaging and modeling in orthodontics have revolutionized the way dental professionals diagnose, plan, and treat orthodontic issues. Here is how it is impacting the field:

3D Imaging Technology

- **Cone-Beam Computed Tomography (CBCT)**: This is one of the most commonly used 3D imaging techniques. It allows orthodontists to get detailed, high-resolution images of the teeth, jawbones, and surrounding tissues. Unlike traditional X-rays, CBCT provides a 360-degree view of the patient's anatomy, offering insights into bone structure, tooth positioning, and even airways, which can be important for treatment planning (Kunz et al. 2020).
- **Intraoral Scanners**: These devices capture high-definition 3D images of the inside of the mouth without the need for physical impressions. It allows for more accurate measurements and quicker, more comfortable procedures for the patient.
- **Facial Scanning**: Some systems now include facial 3D scanning to analyze the relationship between the teeth, jaw, and overall facial structure.

3D Modeling

- **Customized Treatment Plans**: With 3D imaging, orthodontists can create digital models of a patient's teeth and jaws. These models are used to design treatment plans with greater accuracy. For example, the exact movements of the teeth can be simulated using software, showing how braces or aligners will affect the smile over time.
- **Clear Aligners**: Companies like Invisalign use 3D imaging and modeling to create precise, custom-fit patient aligners. The digital models ensure that each aligner is tailored to the patient's specific needs and progress (Amasya et al. 2020).
- **Surgical Planning**: In more complex cases, such as jaw surgery (orthognathic surgery), 3D imaging and modeling can help plan the surgery with high precision, making the process more predictable and reducing the risk of errors.

Advantages of 3D Imaging and Modeling in Orthodontics

- **Precision**: These technologies provide highly accurate visualizations of the patient's anatomy, leading to more precise treatment planning.
- **Visualization and Communication**: Patients can see a digital model of their teeth and how they will look after treatment. This helps in setting clear expectations and improving patient satisfaction. It also allows orthodontists to explain the treatment process better.
- **Treatment Speed and Comfort**: Digital impressions are more comfortable for patients and faster for orthodontists. 3D modeling also speeds up the overall workflow, reducing the time needed for custom appliances.
- **Predictability**: Treatment outcomes can be more accurately predicted, as 3D models simulate tooth movements over time. This reduces the likelihood of trial and error.

Examples of 3D Technologies in Use

- **3D-printed Braces**: Some orthodontists are using 3D printing technology to create customized braces that fit each patient's teeth more precisely.

- **Virtual Treatment Simulation**: With software like ClinCheck (used by Invisalign), orthodontists can simulate how the teeth will move over time, ensuring that the patient receives the most efficient treatment possible (Real et al. 2022).

Future of 3D Imaging and Modeling in Orthodontics

- **AI and Machine Learning**: These technologies are being integrated into the planning and analysis process to predict the best treatment options based on historical data and outcomes.
- **Augmented Reality (AR)**: Some emerging systems use AR to visualize treatment in real time, providing even more dynamic interaction with patients and treatment simulations (Alowais et al. 2023).

Overall, 3D imaging and modeling are changing orthodontics by improving accuracy, patient comfort, and the overall treatment experience.

3 AI in Orthodontic Education

AI is transforming orthodontic education by enhancing learning, training, and practical skills acquisition. Here are several ways AI is being applied in orthodontic education:

Virtual and Augmented Reality Simulations

- **Immersive Training**: AI-driven virtual reality (VR) and augmented reality (AR) systems allow dental students to practice complex orthodontic procedures in a risk-free, simulated environment. Students can perform tasks such as bracket placements, wire adjustments, and diagnosis of malocclusions on virtual patients (Maleki Varnosfaderani and Forouzanfar 2024).
- **3D Simulation of Orthodontic Treatments**: AI-powered 3D modeling tools enable students to visualize and manipulate dental structures, helping them understand how tooth movement occurs over time during treatment (Fig. 2). This enhances their understanding of treatment mechanics and biomechanics.

Personalized Learning and Adaptive Systems

- **Customized Learning Pathways**: AI can assess students' individual learning progress and offer personalized content based on their performance. This includes providing targeted tutorials, quizzes, and case studies to help students focus on areas where they need improvement.
- **Real-Time Feedback**: AI systems can analyze students' performance during practical exercises (e.g., digital simulations or manual tasks) and provide instant feedback on areas requiring attention. This allows students to learn through trial and error while refining their skills.

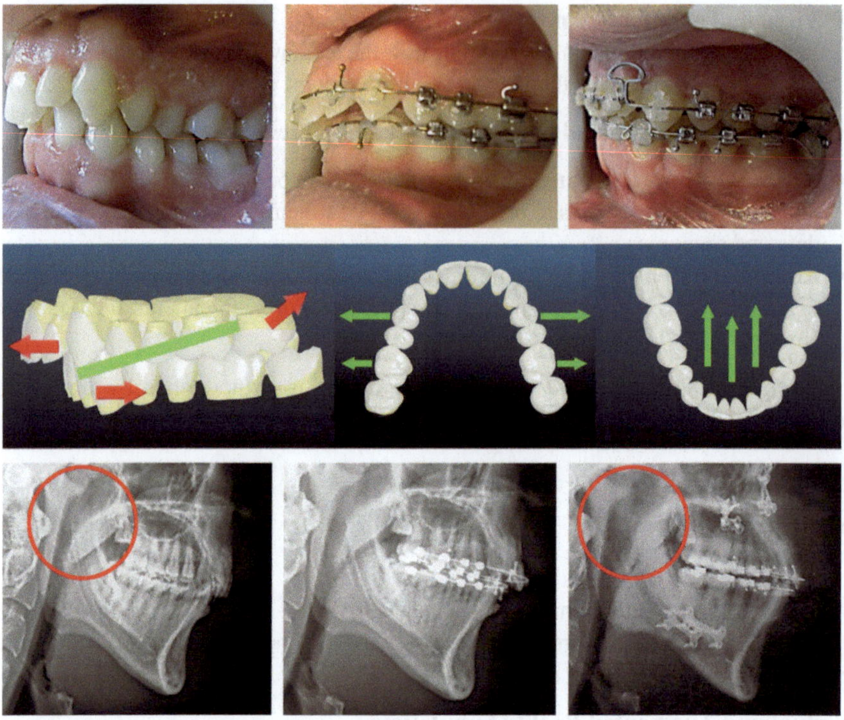

Fig. 2 AI-powered 3D modeling tools for patient and student education

- **Progress Tracking**: AI can track student progress over time, identifying strengths and weaknesses. It can then recommend further study materials or interventions to help students progress independently.

AI-Enhanced Case Studies and Problem-Solving

- **AI-Powered Case Simulations**: Dental students can be exposed to a variety of orthodontic cases, with AI offering realistic case studies for students to diagnose and develop treatment plans. AI-generated simulations can model how different treatment approaches might affect the patient's dental alignment, improving the critical thinking skills of students (Fachada and David 2024).
- **Treatment Planning Assistance**: AI systems can help students develop treatment plans based on real patient data, offering suggestions for appliance design, estimated treatment duration, and possible outcomes. This enables students to experience the decision-making process in a structured environment, supported by AI.

Automated Grading and Assessment

- **Objective Grading Systems**: AI tools can grade student assignments and practical exams more efficiently and consistently, ensuring fair assessments. For example,

AI can evaluate a student's diagnostic skills or their ability to design treatment plans and provide detailed feedback.

- **Assessment of Clinical Skills**: AI-powered systems can assess students' clinical skills in real time during simulated exercises. By analyzing student performance, AI can identify areas where students need additional practice or guidance, ensuring continuous improvement (Bouletreau et al. 2019).

AI for Anatomy and Physiology Learning

- **3D Anatomy Models**: AI-driven 3D anatomy software allows students to explore and understand the structures of the oral cavity, jaw, and facial bones. By interacting with detailed anatomical models, students can learn how orthodontic treatments affect different structures and how to tailor interventions to individual patients.
- **Simulating Tooth Movement**: AI can simulate tooth movement in response to forces applied through braces or clear aligners. This helps students understand the biological mechanisms behind orthodontic treatment and the impacts of various appliances.

AI-Powered Chatbots and Virtual Tutors

- **24/7 Assistance**: AI chatbots can answer students' questions about orthodontic theory, procedures, or case management, making educational support more accessible at any time (Ganzer et al. 2018). Virtual tutors can provide personalized explanations and guide students through complex topics or case studies.
- **Clinical Decision Support**: AI-powered virtual tutors can assist in clinical decision-making by suggesting treatment options or alerting students to possible errors during case assessment, thus improving clinical reasoning and decision-making.

Research and Evidence-Based Learning

- **AI-Driven Literature Review**: AI tools can help students and educators find relevant research articles, summarize key findings, and analyze large volumes of research data. This allows students to stay up-to-date with the latest advancements in orthodontics and base their learning on evidence-based practices (Makaremi 2016).
- **Data-Driven Insights for Education**: By analyzing trends in orthodontic research and treatment outcomes, AI can guide the curriculum development process, ensuring that students are taught the most current and relevant techniques.

AI-Assisted Collaborative Learning

- **Group Learning Platforms**: AI can create collaborative learning experiences by matching students with complementary skill sets. These platforms use AI to assess individual abilities and create study groups where students can share knowledge, discuss cases, and work together on simulated treatments.

- **Peer Feedback Systems**: AI-powered tools can facilitate peer review processes in educational settings, helping students assess each other's treatment plans or clinical skills and provide constructive feedback.

Facilitating Clinical Exposure

- **Simulated Clinical Experiences**: AI can create virtual or simulated clinical scenarios where students must interact with virtual patients to make diagnoses, create treatment plans, and perform treatments. This provides students with extensive practice before they treat real patients.
- **Remote Learning for Clinical Cases**: AI can allow remote learning in clinical orthodontics, enabling students to interact with AI-powered systems or virtual patients to practice diagnosis and treatment planning from anywhere in the world (Gracea 2025).

Early Detection of Learning Gaps

- **AI for Identifying Struggling Students**: AI can analyze performance trends across multiple students and identify those who are struggling. This allows educators to intervene early and provide additional support before these gaps hinder students' overall progress.

Benefits of AI in Orthodontic Education

- **Increased Access to Learning**: AI tools make it easier for students to access educational content at their own pace, anytime and anywhere.
- **Efficiency**: Automating administrative tasks (grading, assessment) and providing real-time feedback allows educators to focus on mentoring and one-on-one student interactions.
- **Hands-on Experience**: AI-powered simulations and VR/AR tools give students more hands-on experience, which is crucial for mastering orthodontic techniques.

4 AI in Aligners and Braces

AI plays a critical role in designing, customizing, and optimizing **clear aligners** (Fig. 3) and **braces**, enhancing the precision, efficiency, and effectiveness of orthodontic treatments (Krishnan n.d.). Here are the key ways AI is transforming the design process of these orthodontic devices:

Personalized Treatment Plans

- **Data-Driven Design**: AI analyzes the patient's dental scans (3D images, X-rays, or intraoral photographs) to create highly personalized treatment plans. It helps orthodontists understand the patient's unique oral anatomy, bite issues, and other factors, allowing for the design of customized aligners or braces that fit the individual's needs.

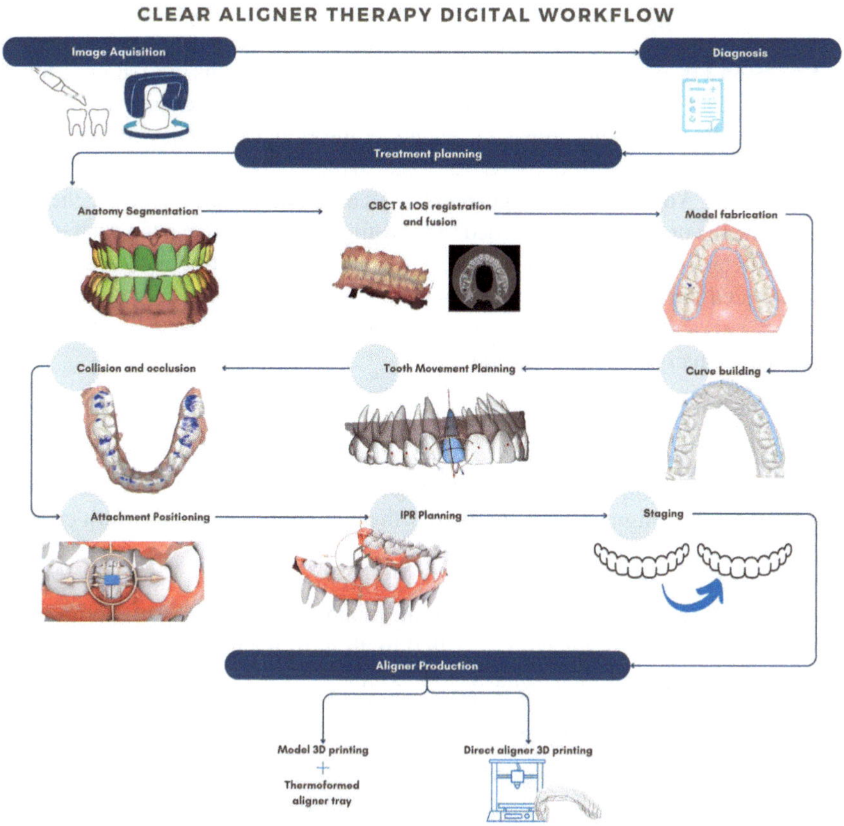

Fig. 3 Clear aligner therapy digital workflow (Ruiz March 2025)

- **Optimizing Tooth Movement**: AI can simulate tooth movement over time and suggest the best sequence for gradually shifting teeth. It can predict how the teeth will move, the forces needed, and the timeline for each phase of the treatment. (Takeshita et al. 2024)

3D Simulation and Modeling

- **Virtual 3D Models**: AI algorithms can generate 3D digital models of a patient's teeth, which can be adjusted to plan and visualize the orthodontic treatment. These models are used to design clear aligners or braces with precise details, such as specific contours and adjustments, ensuring that they fit correctly.
- **Predicting Outcomes**: With the help of AI, orthodontists can simulate different treatment options to see how each will affect the patient's teeth over time. The ability to visualize these outcomes before actual treatment starts helps in fine-tuning the design of aligners or braces.

Custom Clear Aligners Design

- **Precision Fit**: AI algorithms take digital impressions or scans of a patient's mouth and generate a series of custom clear aligners tailored to the exact dimensions of the patient's teeth. This allows for greater comfort and efficiency throughout the treatment.
- **Automatic Adjustment Suggestions**: AI can automatically propose the ideal adjustments or refinements needed in each aligner set to achieve the desired tooth movement, ensuring a smoother and more predictable treatment course.
- **Enhanced Patient Comfort**: AI's precision in designing clear aligners also minimizes gaps and ensures that aligners are comfortable, with less pressure on teeth and gums than traditional methods.

Braces Design Optimization

- **Brackets and Wire Design**: AI assists in the precise placement of brackets and wires for traditional braces. By analyzing 3D scans and treatment goals, AI helps orthodontists design wire configurations that will move teeth in the most effective manner.
- **Customized Arch wires**: AI can design custom arch wires that are specifically tailored to the patient's dental anatomy and treatment objectives. This optimization results in more accurate and controlled tooth movement, improving the overall treatment experience (KhanagarS et al. 2021).

Efficient Production Process

- **Automated Manufacturing**: AI-integrated systems streamline the production of clear aligners and braces. Once the design is finalized, AI systems can help with the automated production process, including 3D printing or molding of aligners and precise fabrication of brackets and wires for braces.
- **Rapid Iteration**: AI allows orthodontists to generate quickly and test design modifications, speeding up the process of making adjustments or designing new aligners or braces without the need for time-consuming manual processes (Chung et al. 2020).

Continuous Monitoring and Adaptation

- **Tracking Tooth Movement**: AI software can track the progress of tooth movement using digital images, scans, or sensors. As the treatment progresses, the system can compare the actual results with the planned treatment, providing insights into whether adjustments to the design of aligners or braces are needed.
- **Real-Time Feedback**: Some AI systems can offer real-time feedback on the effectiveness of aligners or braces. For example, if a patient is not adhering to their treatment plan (e.g., wearing their aligners as instructed), AI can alert the orthodontist to take corrective action (Lo et al. 2021).

Enhancing Predictability of Treatment

- **Outcome Prediction**: AI uses large datasets and historical treatment results to predict the success of a specific aligner or braces design. It can identify patterns and outcomes from similar cases, allowing orthodontists to make more informed decisions about the best approach for each patient.
- **Treatment Duration**: AI algorithms can more accurately estimate how long the treatment will take by analyzing similar cases and individual factors, helping patients set realistic expectations.

Posttreatment Design and Retention

- **Retention Device Design**: After orthodontic treatment, AI can assist in designing custom retainers to maintain the teeth in their new positions. AI helps ensure that the retainer fits perfectly and provides adequate support to avoid relapse (Ruiz et al. 2025).
- **Relapse Prevention**: In cases where relapse is likely (based on the patient's dental condition or compliance history), AI can suggest specific changes to the retention plan, improving long-term results.

Optimizing Treatment for Specific Conditions

- **Addressing Complex Malocclusions**: AI can be especially useful in treating complex malocclusions (misaligned bites) or severe crowding, where clear aligners or traditional braces need to be adjusted in unique ways. AI helps develop custom solutions that would be more challenging to create manually.
- **Targeting Specific Teeth Movements**: Whether it is extrusion, intrusion, or rotation, AI allows for targeted movements of specific teeth. For example, if one tooth needs to be rotated while others remain in place, AI can design aligners or braces that apply the necessary forces only to the right teeth (Ruiz 2025).

Patient Engagement and Monitoring

- **AI-Powered Apps for Patients**: Some orthodontic companies use AI-powered apps that help patients monitor their treatment. These apps can provide reminders, track progress, and even offer virtual consultations or checkups using AI to detect potential issues (e.g., missed aligner wear).
- **Compliance Monitoring**: AI systems can analyze data from wearable devices or smartphone apps to track if a patient is following the prescribed treatment plan (e.g., wearing their aligners for the correct amount of time). This helps ensure optimal results and adjust treatment plans as needed (Thurzo and Kurilová 2021).

5 Role of Robotics and AI Integration

Robotics and AI-assisted procedures in orthodontics are transforming the way orthodontic treatments are delivered, improving both the precision of the procedures and overall efficiency. By integrating AI with robotics, orthodontists can enhance treatment outcomes, minimize human error, and automate routine tasks. Here are some of the key roles robotics and AI play in orthodontics:

Precise Placement of Brackets and Appliances

- **Robotic Bracket Placement**: One of the most promising applications of robotics in orthodontics is using robotic systems to place braces and brackets. AI-powered robots can precisely place orthodontic brackets on each tooth according to the 3D treatment plan. This precision reduces human error and ensures the brackets are placed at the correct angle and position for optimal tooth movement (Khanagar et al. 2021b).
- **Customization for Each Patient**: Robotics can adapt to the specific dental anatomy of each patient, ensuring that every bracket is aligned perfectly. This level of precision helps to reduce the need for adjustments during the treatment, speeding up the process and improving the effectiveness of the treatment.

Automated Wire Bending

- **Customized Arch Wires**: Robotics and AI can assist in bending arch wires to the specifications needed for each patient's treatment plan. The robotic system can create customized wires based on the tooth movements required, ensuring a more effective and comfortable treatment process.
- **Consistency and Precision**: Robots ensure that the wire bending is consistent across all patients, resulting in fewer adjustments and a more predictable treatment outcome. This also ensures that the forces applied to the teeth are uniform, improving the overall efficiency of the treatment (Maspero and Tartaglia 2020).

Robotic-Assisted Orthodontic Procedures

- **Robotic Assistance in Surgery**: In more complex orthodontic cases, such as jaw surgery or surgical orthodontics (e.g., for patients with severe malocclusion or skeletal problems), AI-assisted robotic systems can assist in the planning and executing surgical procedures. For example, AI can assist in the virtual planning of jaw repositioning and guide the surgeon during surgery to achieve more accurate outcomes.
- **Minimally Invasive Surgery**: Robots can assist with minimally invasive techniques for orthodontic procedures, reducing the amount of trauma to surrounding tissues. This results in quicker recovery times and less discomfort for the patient (Li and Wang 2016).

AI-Powered Diagnostic and Treatment Planning

- **Predictive Modeling**: AI can analyze a patient's 3D dental scans, X-rays, and other diagnostic data to create highly personalized treatment plans. By using machine learning algorithms, AI can predict how a patient's teeth will move over time and optimize the forces and movements required for treatment.
- **Automated Treatment Adjustments**: AI can continuously monitor the progress of the treatment and suggest adjustments to the treatment plan in real time. For example, if a particular tooth is not responding as expected to the applied forces,

AI can recommend changes to the appliance design or treatment sequence to address the issue (Lee et al. 2022).

- **Virtual Assistants for Case Analysis**: AI-powered virtual assistants can analyze patient data and offer insights, which can assist orthodontists in making quicker, more informed decisions. AI can analyze large datasets from similar cases to predict the most effective treatment strategy.

Remote Monitoring and Virtual Checkups

- **AI-Based Monitoring Tools**: AI tools can help monitor the progress of treatment remotely by analyzing images or scans sent by the patient or taken using intraoral scanners. The AI system can track how teeth are moving and compare them to the planned progress, alerting orthodontists to any issues or delays that may require intervention.
- **Robotic Assistance in Virtual Follow-Ups**: Robotics combined with AI can enable orthodontists to conduct virtual follow-up consultations. This may include robotic assistants that help examine a patient's dental structures remotely, using AI to analyze the patient's progress and suggest follow-up actions (Kuziemsky et al. 2019).
- **Monitoring Treatment Compliance**: Robots equipped with AI can also track how well patients are following their prescribed treatment regimen (e.g., wearing aligners or attending regular checkups) and provide feedback to both the patient and the orthodontist.

AI and Robotics in Patient Education

- **Interactive Learning Tools**: AI-powered robots can be used as interactive educational tools to help patients better understand their treatment process. For example, virtual assistants can explain the purpose of braces or aligners, demonstrate how appliances work, and show how treatment will progress using animations or simulations.
- **Virtual Treatment Simulations**: AI-driven systems can simulate the progression of orthodontic treatment, allowing patients to visualize how their teeth will move and how different appliances or treatment strategies will impact their smile. This can help set patient expectations and improve compliance (Friedman et al. 2015).

Enhanced Precision in Complex Cases

- **Handling Complex Malocclusions**: In cases where patients have complex malocclusions (misalignments), AI and robotics can assist in designing more accurate treatment plans and appliances. The robotic systems can take into account the finer details of tooth movement, such as the angle, rotation, and forces required to correct the bite, leading to more effective treatment for patients with challenging conditions.
- **Multidisciplinary Treatment Coordination**: For patients undergoing both orthodontic and surgical treatment, AI can help coordinate between different

specialists. It can assist in planning and visualizing how orthodontic appliances and surgical interventions can work together to achieve optimal results (Kuziemsky et al. 2019).

Improved Workflow and Efficiency in Orthodontic Practices

- **Robotic Workflow Optimization**: In orthodontic offices, robotics can assist with routine tasks such as sterilizing instruments, preparing treatment materials, or organizing patient records, allowing orthodontists to focus on more complex aspects of patient care.
- **Automated 3D Printing**: AI and robotics can also optimize the 3D printing process for creating custom aligners or orthodontic appliances, automating the design and production steps, improving precision, and speeding up the time required to create these devices (Loh 2018).

Patient Comfort and Experience

- **Less Painful Treatment**: By improving the precision of bracket placement, wire bending, and overall treatment planning, AI and robotics reduce the risk of discomfort or injury during orthodontic procedures. This contributes to an overall more comfortable patient experience.
- **Faster Treatment**: Robotic systems enable orthodontists to deliver more efficient and accurate treatments, reducing the amount of time patients spend in the orthodontist's chair and improving treatment timelines.

6 AI in Growth Prediction

Growth Prediction and Modeling

- **Simulating Facial Growth**: AI uses large datasets of facial development patterns to simulate how a patient's face will grow in the future. These simulations incorporate factors such as age, gender, genetics, and current facial morphology, enabling AI to predict how the jaw, teeth, and overall facial structure will evolve (Fig. 4).
- **Long-Term Growth Predictions**: With the help of AI, orthodontists can predict how skeletal structures, like the maxilla and mandible, will grow during different stages of development (childhood, adolescence, and early adulthood). By comparing individual growth patterns with those of similar patients, AI models can forecast changes in the facial profile, bite, and other key aspects of facial symmetry (Larkin et al. 2024).
- **Data-Driven Predictions**: AI can combine data from different diagnostic tools—such as X-rays, CT scans, and growth charts—to provide more accurate growth predictions than traditional methods. This allows orthodontists to identify potential concerns earlier and plan treatments accordingly.

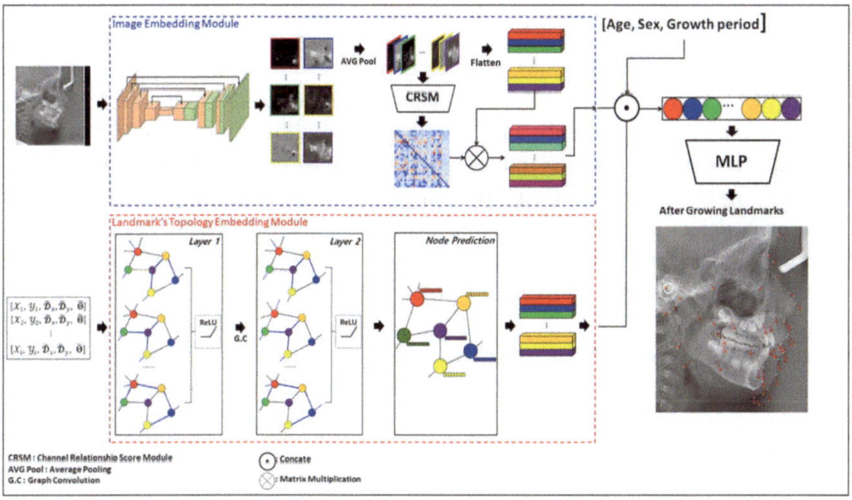

Fig. 4 Model description of the growth-prediction graph convolution neural network (GP-GCNN) (Larkin et al. 2024)

Assessing Soft Tissue Growth

- **Analyzing Soft Tissue Changes**: Facial growth is related to not only bone development but also soft tissues such as the lips, cheeks, and skin. AI systems can analyze soft tissue growth by studying how these tissues adapt in response to changes in underlying bone structures. This can help predict how a patient's facial appearance will change with treatment or natural growth (Larkin et al. 2024).
- **Facial Aesthetics Evaluation**: AI can evaluate changes in facial aesthetics by comparing pretreatment and posttreatment facial images. This can help orthodontists assess how the balance between hard (bone) and soft (tissue) tissues will affect the overall appearance of the face and ensure that treatments are aligned with the patient's aesthetic goals.

Predicting the Impact of Orthodontic Treatment

- **Modeling Treatment Effects**: AI can simulate the effects of different orthodontic treatments (e.g., braces, clear aligners, or jaw surgery) on facial growth. By creating 3D models of the patient's face, AI can predict how certain treatments will influence the development of the facial skeleton and soft tissues over time. This helps orthodontists choose the most effective treatment plan based on the patient's individual growth potential.
- **Customized Treatment Plans**: Using AI to predict facial growth allows orthodontists to develop highly customized treatment plans. For instance, in cases where jaw growth is necessary (e.g., for patients with a severe overbite or underbite), AI can help plan interventions like functional appliances, growth modification, or surgery at the right stage of facial development (Loh 2018).

Tracking Growth Progress

- **Continuous Monitoring**: AI enables continuous, real-time tracking of facial growth by comparing periodic 3D scans or photographs. With each scan, AI can assess how the patient's face is changing, highlighting areas of concern or unexpected growth patterns that may require adjustments in treatment.
- **Detecting Growth Deviations**: By using AI to monitor facial growth, orthodontists can detect any deviations from expected growth patterns. For example, if a child's jaw growth is not progressing as expected, AI can alert the orthodontist to potential issues, allowing for timely intervention to guide the development process.
- **Automated Growth Measurements**: AI tools can automatically measure key parameters of facial growth, such as changes in the distance between facial landmarks or the angle of the jaw. These objective measurements help orthodontists assess facial development more accurately, leading to more informed decisions about the treatment approach.

Predicting Facial Aesthetics and Symmetry

- **Facial Symmetry Analysis**: AI algorithms can assess facial symmetry by analyzing the relationship between the left and right sides of the face. This is particularly important in orthodontics, as treatment often aims to improve the balance of facial features, such as the alignment of the jaw, nose, and chin. AI helps identify areas where imbalances may exist and guides orthodontists in achieving better facial harmony.
- **Aesthetic Outcomes**: AI can also help predict the aesthetic impact of orthodontic treatments, helping orthodontists design plans that meet both functional and aesthetic goals. By simulating the posttreatment face, AI provides insights into how changes in the teeth, jaws, and bone structure will affect the overall facial appearance.

Integrating Growth and Treatment Planning with AI

- **Growth and Treatment Synchronization**: AI allows orthodontists to synchronize facial growth and treatment plans by combining growth predictions with treatment objectives. For example, AI can help determine when to start certain interventions to align with a patient's natural growth patterns (e.g., initiating jaw expansion treatments at the right stage of craniofacial development).
- **Multidisciplinary Collaboration**: In complex cases, such as those requiring both orthodontic and surgical intervention, AI can assist in integrating the growth assessment with input from oral surgeons, pediatricians, and other specialists. This collaborative approach ensures that treatments are tailored to the patient's growth potential, maximizing both functional and aesthetic outcomes.

Enhancing Patient Communication

- **Visualizing Growth and Treatment Effects**: AI can generate detailed visualizations of how a patient's face will look at various stages of treatment, helping patients and their families understand the expected outcomes. This can be especially useful in motivating patients, particularly young ones, as they can see how their treatment will impact both their appearance and function.
- **Interactive Treatment Simulations**: AI-driven software can allow patients to interact with 3D models of their face, showing how different treatments may alter their appearance. This provides a clearer understanding of potential results, fostering greater patient engagement and satisfaction.

7 AI in Patient Monitoring

AI plays a pivotal role in patient monitoring and remote follow-up in orthodontics, enhancing the effectiveness of care while improving convenience for both patients and orthodontists. Integrating AI with digital tools and telehealth platforms allows for real-time monitoring of treatment progress, reduces the need for frequent office visits, and ensures that any issues are addressed promptly (Friedman et al. 2015). Here is how AI contributes to patient monitoring and remote follow-ups in orthodontics:

Real-Time Monitoring of Treatment Progress

- **Automated Image Analysis**: AI tools, such as intraoral cameras, smartphone apps, and scanners, can capture images or scans of a patient's teeth and gums. AI analyzes these images in real time to assess the alignment of teeth, the fit of aligners, or the position of braces. This allows orthodontists to monitor progress remotely, without requiring the patient to come into the office for every checkup.
- **Detecting Misalignments and Treatment Deviations**: AI can automatically identify discrepancies in the patient's treatment plan. For example, if an aligner is not fitting properly, or if teeth are not moving as expected, AI can flag these issues and alert the orthodontist. This helps orthodontists address potential problems before they become significant, ensuring the treatment stays on track.

Remote Monitoring Through Wearables and Sensors

- **Smart Braces and Aligners**: Modern orthodontic appliances, such as **smart braces** or **clear aligners with embedded sensors**, are often equipped with AI-driven capabilities. These sensors can monitor the force applied to the teeth and the amount of time an aligner is worn and even track whether a patient is adhering to the prescribed treatment plan. AI algorithms can then analyze these data and send feedback to both the patient and the orthodontist.
- **Real-Time Feedback**: For example, clear aligner systems like **Invisalign** can track the wear time of aligners and alert patients if they have not been worn for the recommended number of hours per day. The AI system also gives orthodontists

a detailed report of a patient's compliance, which can be reviewed during a remote consultation.

Telehealth and Virtual Consultations

- **Remote Video Consultations**: AI-powered telehealth platforms allow orthodontists to conduct virtual consultations with patients. Through these consultations, patients can share updates on their treatment progress by sending photographs or scans. AI can assist in analyzing these images and automatically assessing changes in the patient's dental structure.
- **AI-Based Case Assessment**: AI systems can assist orthodontists during virtual consultations by providing objective assessments of a patient's condition based on their images or data. This enables orthodontists to make data-backed decisions on whether the treatment needs any adjustments, without needing an in-person visit.
- **Follow-Up Appointments via AI**: AI chatbots or virtual assistants can guide patients through follow-up procedures. For example, patients can be asked to submit pictures of their braces, bite, or smile, and AI can assess whether the treatment is progressing as expected. In case there are issues or deviations, the system can alert the orthodontist for further review (Chapter 2023; El-Sherif et al. 2022).

Tracking Treatment Adherence and Compliance

- **AI-Driven Reminder Systems**: AI can be integrated into patient apps that send automatic reminders about when to wear aligners, adjust appliances, or schedule checkups. This ensures that patients are adhering to their treatment plan, improving the overall effectiveness of their care.
- **Monitoring Wear Compliance**: AI can track how consistently patients wear their aligners or braces. For example, AI can use data from aligner tracking devices or wearables to determine whether the patient is following the recommended wear time. If wear time is insufficient, the system can send notifications to both the patient and the orthodontist, who can then intervene if needed.

Predicting and Preventing Complications

- **Early Detection of Issues**: AI can predict potential complications before they become serious problems. By continuously analyzing patient data (e.g., tooth movement, pressure on the teeth, and oral health conditions), AI can alert the orthodontist about potential risks such as gum irritation, bracket failure, or misalignment. This early detection can prevent delays in treatment and reduce the need for emergency visits.
- **Continuous Adjustment Recommendations**: If a patient's progress deviates from the expected treatment plan, AI can suggest small adjustments, such as modifications to the aligner design, changes in force application, or alternative treatment strategies. This helps keep the treatment plan on track even with limited in-person visits.

Long-Term Treatment Tracking and Posttreatment Monitoring

- **Posttreatment Retention**: AI can continue to monitor a patient's teeth after they have completed their primary orthodontic treatment. For instance, AI systems can track the patient's adherence to retainer wear, ensuring that teeth do not return to their original positions. The system can provide reminders and follow-up assessments to prevent relapse.
- **Post-Correction Progress**: After treatment, AI can continue to track any minor movements in the teeth and recommend corrective actions if needed. This ensures long-term stability and prevents the need for re-treatment.

Patient Engagement and Education

- **Interactive AI Assistants**: AI-powered virtual assistants or chatbots can engage patients throughout their treatment journey, answering their questions and providing guidance on how to care for their appliances, adjust their oral hygiene habits, and follow through with treatment requirements (Nordblom et al. 2024). This helps keep patients informed and actively engaged in their care.
- **Treatment Progress Visualization**: AI can generate dynamic, visual representations of a patient's progress, showing how their teeth are shifting over time. This motivates patients to remain committed to their treatment and provides them with a tangible sense of progress.
- **Feedback and Support**: AI chatbots or virtual assistants can provide real-time answers to patients' concerns, whether it is about adjusting braces, managing discomfort, or understanding the next steps in treatment. This accessibility enhances the patient experience and increases treatment satisfaction.

Data-Driven Insights for Treatment Optimization

- **Big Data Analytics**: AI can process and analyze large datasets of patient information, including treatment histories, outcomes, and compliance rates. These data can provide valuable insights for orthodontists to improve treatment strategies for individual patients and across a broader patient base.
- **Optimizing Follow-Up Frequency**: AI can suggest the optimal frequency for follow-up visits based on the patient's progress and treatment type. For instance, if a patient's treatment is progressing well and no issues are detected, AI can recommend longer intervals between checkups, which helps reduce the number of in-office visits, saving time for both the patient and the orthodontist.

Increased Efficiency for Orthodontic Practices

- **Automated Record-Keeping**: AI can automate the management of patient records, including treatment progress, compliance data, and follow-up schedules. This improves the efficiency of the orthodontic practice by reducing administrative work and allowing orthodontists to focus more on direct patient care (Dalessandri et al. 2021).
- **Reducing the Need for In-Office Appointments**: By using AI for remote monitoring, orthodontists can reduce the need for frequent in-person visits, making

their practices more efficient. This is especially beneficial for patients who live far away or have busy schedules, as they can receive quality care without needing to come into the office frequently.

8 Conclusion

AI and robotics in orthodontics are improving the quality, precision, and efficiency of treatments, while also providing more personalized and effective care for patients. From the automated design and placement of braces to the use of AI for treatment planning and monitoring, these technologies are reshaping the orthodontic field. The combination of robotics and AI reduces human error, enhances patient outcomes, and optimizes the entire orthodontic treatment process, offering a more streamlined and high-quality experience for both patients and orthodontists.

References

Alowais SA, Alghamdi SS, Alsuhebany N et al (2023) Revolutionizing healthcare: the role of artificial intelligence in clinical practice. BMC Med Educ 23:689. https://doi.org/10.1186/s12909-023-04698-z

Amann J, Blasimme A, Vayena E, Frey D, Madai VI (2020) Explainability for artificial intelligence in healthcare: a multidisciplinary perspective. BMC Med Inform Decis Mak 20:310. https://doi.org/10.1186/s12911-020-01332-6

Amasya H, Yildirim D, Aydogan T, Kemaloglu N, Orhan K (2020) Cervical vertebral maturation assessment on lateral cephalometric radiographs using artificial intelligence: comparison of machine learning classifier models. Dentomaxillofac Radiol 49:20190441. https://doi.org/10.1259/dmfr.20190441

Andrikopoulou E (2023) Chapter 13 - The rise of AI in telehealth. Emerging practices in telehealth. Best practices in a rapidly changing field, 183–207

Bouletreau P, Makaremi M, Ibrahim B, Louvrier A, Sigaux N (2019) Artificial Intelligence: applications in orthognathic surgery. J Stomatol Oral Maxillofacial Surg 120(4):347–354

Chung M, Lee J, Song W, Song Y, Yang IH, Lee J, Shin YG (2020) Automatic registration between dental cone-beam CT and scanned surface via deep pose regression neural networks and clustered similarities. IEEE Trans Med Imaging 39:3900–3909

Dalessandri D, Sangalli L, Tonni I, Laffranchi L, Bonetti S, Visconti L, Signoroni A, Paganelli C (2021) Attitude towards telemonitoring in orthodontists and orthodontic patients. Dent J (Basel). 9(5):47

El-Sherif DM, Abouzid M, Elzarif MT, Ahmed AA, Albakri A, Alshehri MM (2022) Telehealth and Artificial Intelligence Insights into Healthcare during the COVID-19 Pandemic. Healthcare (Basel) 10(2):385. https://doi.org/10.3390/healthcare10020385

Fachada N, David N (2024) Artificial intelligence in modeling and simulation. Algorithms 17(6):265. https://doi.org/10.3390/a17060265

Friedman C, Rubin J, Brown J, Buntin M, Corn M, Etheredge L et al (2015) Toward a science of learning systems: a research agenda for the high-functioning learning health system. J Am Med Inform Assoc 22:43–50. https://doi.org/10.1136/amiajnl-2014-002977

Ganzer N, Feldmann I, Liv P, Bondemark L (2018) A novel method for superimposition and measurements on maxillary digital 3D models-studies on validity and reliability. Eur J Orthod 40(1):45–51. https://doi.org/10.1093/ejo/cjx029

Gracea RS (2025) Artificial intelligence for orthodontic diagnosis and treatment planning: a scoping review. J Dent 152:105442

Krishnan V, Integrating artificial intelligence: A step forward in orthodontic education. World Federation Orthodontists 13(4):153–154

Khanagar SB, Al-Ehaideb A, Vishwanathaiah S, Maganur PC, Patil S, Naik S, Baeshen HA, Sarode SS (2021a) Scope and performance of artificial intelligence technology in orthodontic diagnosis, treatment planning, and clinical decision-making—a systematic review. J Dent Sci 16:482–492. https://doi.org/10.1016/j.jds.2020.05.022

Khanagar SB, Al-Ehaideb A, Maganur PC, Vishwanathaiah S, Patil S, Baeshen HS et al (2021b) Developments, application, and performance of artificial intelligence in dentistry - a systematic review. J Dent Sci 16:508–522. https://doi.org/10.1016/j.jds.2020.06.019

Khanagar SB, AlEhaideb A, Vishwanathaiah S, Maganur PC, Patil S, Naik, Baeshen HA, Sarode SS (2021) Scope and performance of artificial intelligence technology in orthodontic diagnosis, treatment planning, and clinical decision-making—a systematic review. J Dent Sci 16:482–492

Kiełczykowski M, Kamiński K, Perkowski K, Zadurska M, Czochrowska E (2023) Application of artificial intelligence (AI) in a cephalometric analysis: a narrative review. Diagnostics (Basel) 13(16):2640. https://doi.org/10.3390/diagnostics13162640

Kunz F, Stellzig-Eisenhauer A, Zeman F, Boldt J (2020) Artificial intelligence in orthodontics: Evaluation of a fully automated cephalometric analysis using a customized convolutional neural network. J Orofac Orthop 81:52–68. https://doi.org/10.1007/s00056-019-00203-8

Kuziemsky C, Maeder AJ, John O, Gogia SB, Basu A, Meher S, Ito M (2019) Role of artificial intelligence within the telehealth domain. Yearb Med Inform 28(1):35–40. https://doi.org/10.1055/s-0039-1677897

Larkin A, Kim J-S, Kim N et al (2024) Accuracy of artificial intelligence-assisted growth prediction in skeletal Class I preadolescent patients using serial lateral cephalograms for a 2-year growth interval. Orthod Craniofac Res 27:535–543. https://doi.org/10.1111/ocr.12764

Lee S-C, Hwang H-S, Lee KC (2022) Accuracy of deep learning-based integrated tooth models by merging intraoral scans and CBCT scans for 3D evaluation of root position during orthodontic treatment. Prog Orthod 23:15. https://doi.org/10.1186/s40510-022-00410-x

Li Z, Wang H (2016) Interactive tooth separation from dental model using segmentation field PLoS. One 11:Article e0161159. https://doi.org/10.1371/journal.pone.0161159

Lo LJ, Yang CT, Ho CT, Liao CH, Lin HH (2021) Automatic assessment of 3-dimensional facial soft tissue symmetry before and after orthognathic surgery using a machine learning model: a preliminary experience. Ann Plast Surg 1:86

Loh E (2018) Medicine and the rise of the robots: a qualitative review of recent advances of artificial intelligence in health. BMJ Leader 2:59–63

Makaremi M (2016) The role of cognitive sciences in orthodontic treatments: optimizing the interface between practitioners and new technologies. J Dentofac Anomalies Orthod 19(4):410. https://doi.org/10.1051/odfen/2018116

Maleki Varnosfaderani S, Forouzanfar M (2024) The role of AI in hospitals and clinics: transforming healthcare in the 21st century. Bioengineering (Basel) 11(4):337. https://doi.org/10.3390/bioengineering11040337

Maspero C, Tartaglia GM (2020) 3D printing of clear orthodontic aligners: where we are and where we are going. Materials (Basel) 13:5204. https://doi.org/10.3390/ma13225204

Nordblom NF, Büttner M, Schwendicke F (2024) Artificial Intelligence in orthodontics: critical review. J Dent Res 103(6):577–584. https://doi.org/10.1177/00220345241235606

Obermeyer Z, Emanuel EJ (2016) Predicting the future—big data, machine learning, and clinical medicine. N Engl J Med 375:1216–1219. https://doi.org/10.1056/NEJMp1606181

Real AD, Real OD, Sardina S, Oyonarte R (2022) Use of automated artificial intelligence to predict the need for orthodontic extractions. Korean J Orthod 52:102–111. https://doi.org/10.4041/kjod.2022.52.2.102

Ruiz DC (2025) Unveiling the role of artificial intelligence applied to clear aligner therapy: a scoping review. J Dent 154:105564

Ruiz DC, Mureşanu S, Du X, Elgarba BM, Fontenele RC, Jacobs R (2025) Unveiling the role of artificial intelligence applied to clear aligner therapy: a scoping review. J Dentistry 154:105564

Subramanian AK, Chen Y, Almalki A, Sivamurthy G, Kafle D (2022) Cephalometric analysis in orthodontics using artificial intelligence-a comprehensive review. Biomed Res Int 2022:1880113. https://doi.org/10.1155/2022/1880113

Takeshita WM, Silva TP, Trindade de Souza LL, Tenorio JM (2024) State of the art and prospects for artificial intelligence in orthognathic surgery: a systematic review with meta-analysis. J Stomatol Oral Maxillofacial Surg 125(6):101787

Talaat S, Kaboudan A, Talaat W, Kusnoto B, Sanchez F, Elnagar MH, Ghoneima A, Bourauel C (2020) Improving the accuracy of publicly available search engines in recognizing and classifying dental visual assets using convolutional neural networks. Int J Comput Dent 23:211–218

Thrall JH, Li X, Li Q, Cruz C, Do S, Dreyer K, Brink J (2018) Artificial intelligence and machine learning in radiology: opportunities, challenges, pitfalls, and criteria for success. J Am Coll Radiol 3:504–508

Thurzo, Kurilová V, Varga I (2021) Artificial intelligence in orthodontic smart application for treatment coaching and its impact on clinical performance of patients monitored with AI-telehealth system. Healthcare (Basel) 9:1695. https://doi.org/10.3390/healthcare9121695

Wong SH, Al-Hasani H, Alam Z, Alam A (2019) Artificial intelligence in radiology: how will we be affected? Eur Radiol 29:141–143. https://doi.org/10.1007/s00330-018-5644-3

Artificial Intelligence in Conservative Dentistry and Endodontics

Ashish J. Johnson, Tarun Kumar Singh, and Aakash Gupta

1 Current AI Models and Techniques in Endodontics

Adoption of artificial intelligence (AI) in dentistry brought a suite of computational models that work on decision enhancements and improving clinical workflows. Among many, one of the foremost roles of machine learning (ML) and deep learning (DL) is the analysis of patient data and images.

1.1 Machine Learning in Diagnostics

Machine learning algorithms excel in pattern recognition, hence finding abnormalities on radiographs, cone-beam computed tomography (CBCT) scans, and other diagnostic tools. For example, supervised ML models trained on vast dental datasets may highlight the early signs of caries, fractures, or periapical lesions that might have been missed upon manual interpretation. Such systems assist clinicians in diagnosing dental pathologies more efficiently and accurately. A study demonstrated that ML-based algorithms achieved diagnostic accuracies comparable to experienced clinicians in identifying caries and apical periodontitis on periapical radiographs, particularly when used as an adjunct to clinical expertise (Shamaun and Scoping 2023).

A. J. Johnson · T. K. Singh (✉) · A. Gupta
Division of Conservative Dentistry and Endodontics, Department of Dentistry, All India Institute of Medical Sciences, Bathinda, India
e-mail: drtarunkumarsingh@gmail.com

A. Gupta et al. (eds.), *Application of Robotics in Dentistry*, Lecture Notes in Bioengineering, https://doi.org/10.1007/978-981-95-1470-0_9

1.2 Deep Learning for Image Analysis

Deep learning, a more advanced subset of ML, uses artificial neural networks to process complex imaging data. DL-based algorithms can analyze three-dimensional (3D) CBCT scans, segment anatomical structures, and detect abnormalities with remarkable precision. For example, convolutional neural networks (CNNs) have been developed to identify root fractures, calcifications, and apical lesions. A study by Ylisiurua et al. (2024) found that DL algorithms reduced noise in CBCT analysis compared to traditional methods, emphasizing their potential in enhancing diagnostic accuracy.

1.3 Natural Language Processing (NLP)

Natural language processing (NLP) systems process unstructured textual data, such as patient records, clinical notes, and research articles. Such systems subsequently extract meaningful insights through summarization of patient history or pointing out recent evidence-based findings relevant to a particular case; NLP tools can assist in synthesizing complex medical histories to identify risk factors for treatment failure or provide clinicians with the latest guidelines for managing specific dental conditions.

1.4 Case-Based Reasoning (CBR)

Case-based reasoning is an AI methodology for solving new problems by using solutions applied in similar past cases. It holds, of course, that analogous situations will usually have analogous solutions—a notion surely of great relevance for dentistry, whose clinical decisions rest so frequently upon past experience and a base of evidence-based practice (Fig. 1). CBR involves four steps:

a. **Retrieving** relevant past cases from a database.
b. **Reusing** the information and solutions from those cases.
c. **Revising** the proposed solution based on the specific context of the current case.

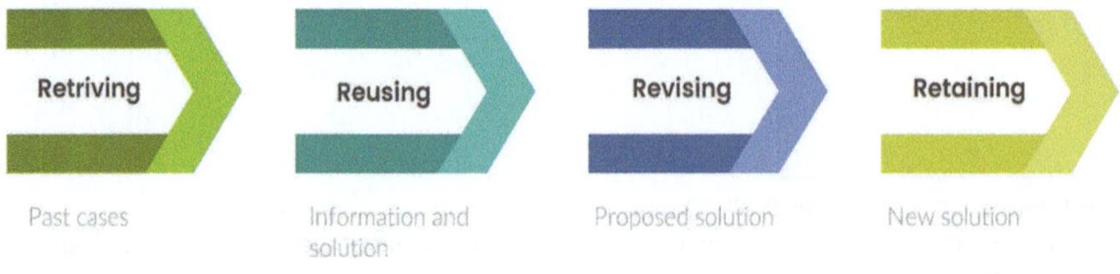

Fig. 1 Case based reasoning data flow

d. **Retaining** the new solution for future use in similar scenarios.

In dental retreatment and restorative material selection, CBR can streamline decision-making and improve outcomes.

1.5 Neuro-Fuzzy Inferencing

Neuro-fuzzy inferencing combines neural networks' adaptability with fuzzy logic's human-like reasoning, making it valuable for regenerative dental procedures and cavity management. In regeneration, it helps assess case suitability, predict outcomes, and optimize protocols like scaffold and biomaterial selection. For cavities, it aids in early detection, lesion classification, material selection, and prognosis, ensuring minimally invasive and durable solutions. By analyzing patient-specific data, neuro-fuzzy systems personalize treatment plans, enhance decision-making, and predict risks, improving clinical outcomes while minimizing errors. Its potential lies in real-time learning and integration with diagnostic tools, offering a promising future for precision dentistry.

2 Applications of AI in Conservative Dentistry and Endodontics

The utility of AI in dentistry is gaining momentum, from improving diagnostic precision to optimizing treatment planning and enhancing procedural outcomes (Fig. 2).

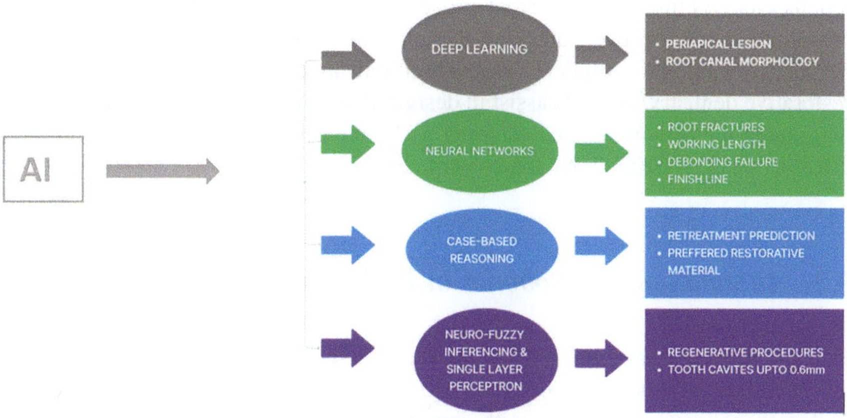

Fig. 2 AI models used in conservative dentistry and endodontics

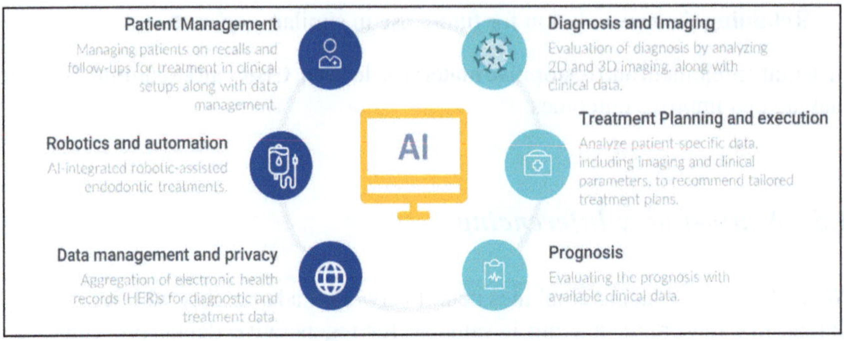

Fig. 3 Application of AI in conservative dentistry and endodontics

2.1 *Diagnosis and Imaging*

AI is changing the face of dental imaging by offering tools that can analyze and detect pathologies with greater precision. For instance, ML algorithms can point out changes in bone density indicative of early osteoporosis on panoramic radiographs or highlight periapical lesions of endodontic importance on CBCT scans that are barely discernible to the human eye. AI also helps mitigate errors caused by clinician fatigue or inexperience, thus standardizing diagnostic accuracy across practitioners (Fig. 3).

2.2 *Treatment Planning and Virtual Simulation*

AI systems analyze patient-specific data, including imaging and clinical parameters, to recommend tailored treatment plans. The AI-powered virtual treatment simulations enable clinicians to predict procedural challenges, such as complex canal anatomies or calcifications, and plan accordingly. These simulations provide a visual roadmap of potential complications and highlight areas requiring special attention. In restorative dentistry, AI tools assist in designing custom prosthetics and restorations that match the patient's dental anatomy with unmatched precision (Alshadidi et al. 2023; Chen et al. 2024; Tabatabaian et al. 2023).

2.3 *Automation and Robotics in Endodontics*

Robotic systems integrated with AI are pushing the boundaries of what is possible in endodontics (Ivashchenko et al. 2020). These systems perform delicate tasks, such as canal instrumentation, with consistency and precision that surpass manual techniques. AI algorithms guide robotic arms during canal cleaning and shaping, ensuring uniformity while adapting dynamically to the canal's anatomy. Moreover, robotic systems equipped with real-time feedback mechanisms can adjust torque, pressure, and speed, minimizing the risk of procedural errors like perforations or file separation (Cheng et al. 2023).

2.4 Predictive Analytics for Prognosis

AI systems apply predictive analytics models to determine probable outcomes of different treatments, using patients' history and characteristics (Shruti 2023). They can predict complications such as reinfection or failure in a restoration, hence giving actionable insight that could reduce the risks involved. For example, artificial intelligence-driven prognostic models make predictions on the size of the lesion, the patient's compliance, and morphology of the canal before predicting the healing possibility from the root canal treatment results. Such insight would greatly facilitate clinicians in informed decision-making about treatment options and follow-up care.

2.5 Data Management and Integration

Artificial intelligence enhances the aggregation of electronic health records (HERs) for diagnostic and treatment data so that full visualization of a patient's oral status becomes possible and a better decision might become obtainable. Predictive analytics streamline patterns, like the frequency of cancellations, which in many aspects depict either very minimal to nil risks during treatment or even behaviors likely to change treatment outcomes. However, data security and privacy remain significant concerns, requiring robust encryption and adherence to regulatory standards like Health Insurance Portability and Accountability Act (HIPAA) and General Data Protection Regulation (GDPR) to protect patient information (Herzog et al. 2024; Ghassemi et al. 2019).

3 Key Challenges in Conservative Dentistry and Endodontics

Conservative dentistry and endodontics aim to restore and preserve natural tooth structures with minimal intervention while ensuring optimal functionality. These fields face significant challenges that stem from the complexity of dental anatomy, diagnostic limitations, and procedural precision (Huang et al. 2024; Johnsen et al. 2023).

One major challenge lies in the anatomical complexity of the root canal system. The variability in root canal morphology, particularly in posterior teeth, includes intricate features such as accessory canals, lateral canals, apical deltas, and isthmuses. These anatomical variations complicate canal preparation and cleaning during endodontic treatment, leading to potential treatment failures. For example, studies highlight that traditional instrumentation techniques fail to contact 35–50% of canal walls, leaving residual infected tissue that could compromise the long-term prognosis of treatment (Siqueira Junior et al. 2018; Siqueira et al. 2019). Advanced technologies like cone-beam computed tomography (CBCT) have enhanced the visualization of these anatomical intricacies, but the interpretation of CBCT images demands expertise and remains time-intensive.

Diagnostic limitations present another significant hurdle. The two-dimensional nature of periapical radiographs, one of the most common imaging techniques in endodontics, usually misses the detection of early periapical changes or subtle fractures. Overlapping of anatomical structures obscures fine details, hence increasing the possibility of undiagnosed cases. While CBCT provides three-dimensional imaging, the increased radiation exposure, cost, and operator variability limit its routine application. Clinical studies demonstrate that small apical radiolucencies may go undetected on conventional radiographs, leading to delayed interventions (McGuigan et al. 2018).

Treatment precision remains a cornerstone of success in both conservative and endodontic procedures. Minor errors in cleaning, shaping, or obturation of the root canal system can compromise outcomes. For instance, over-instrumentation during canal preparation risks apical perforation, while under-filling leaves untreated spaces that could harbor residual pathogens. Additionally, restorative procedures often fail due to marginal discrepancies or improper material selection, resulting in secondary caries or structural failure.

Finally, patient-specific factors, such as dental anxiety, systemic health conditions, and inconsistent compliance with posttreatment care, exacerbate these challenges. Addressing these multifactorial issues requires a combination of advanced diagnostic tools, precise treatment modalities, and patient-centered care strategies.

4 AI in Diagnosis

4.1 Radiographic Image Analysis

Radiographic imaging, such as periapical and panoramic radiographs, is the cornerstone of diagnosis in conservative dentistry and endodontics. Conventional radiographic interpretation relies highly on the skill and experience of the clinician; hence, variability and diagnostic errors are common. Recently, AI has emerged as a transformative tool in enhancing the accuracy and consistency of radiographic analysis through the use of ML algorithms (Yu 2016; Roosanty et al. 2022).

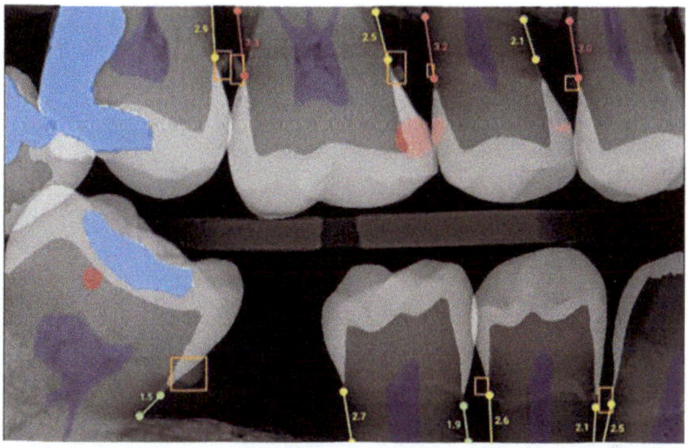

Fig. 4 AI used to evaluate the bone loss, calculus, and caries present in radiographic image analysis. *Courtesy* Overjet AI

CNNs, a subset of ML, have proven to be very effective in the analysis of radiographs. These models detect abnormalities, such as carious lesions, root fractures (Abdelazim and Fouad 2024), and periapical pathologies, by identifying subtle variations in pixel intensity that may not be visible to the naked human eye. Clinical studies have demonstrated that AI-based systems are able to detect dental caries with 93.93% accuracy, outperforming traditional diagnostic methods (Forouzeshfar et al. 2023).

Apart from the detection of visible pathologies, AI algorithms predict the progression of diseases. For example, they analyze early-stage carious lesions (Surdilovic et al. 2023) for their estimated risk of advancement to dentin or pulp involvement (Fig. 4). Such predictions allow clinicians to adopt preventive measures, such as fluoride application or remineralization therapies (Singh and Asthana 2024), rather than invasive procedure.

4.2 AI in CBCT Analysis

CBCT provides three-dimensional imaging of dental and maxillofacial structures; therefore, the possibilities for identifying complex anatomical variations are great. However, manual interpretation of CBCT images is a time-consuming procedure burdened with a certain amount of variability. AI-driven automation provides consistent and precise analysis in this respect.

Deep learning models trained on CBCT datasets can map complex root canal anatomies, identify calcified canals, and detect periapical radiolucencies indicative of infections or cysts (Alshomrani 2024). One study by Pauwels et al. in 2021 demonstrated that AI-assisted CBCT analysis improved the detection of periapical lesions compared to manual interpretation (Pauwels et al. 2021). These tools are especially helpful in diagnosing challenging cases, such as vertical root fractures or resorptive defects, which are often missed on conventional radiographs.

It also assists in performing volumetric analysis in CBCT by segmenting the structures like alveolar bone, periodontal ligaments, and pulp chamber (Fig. 5). Further,

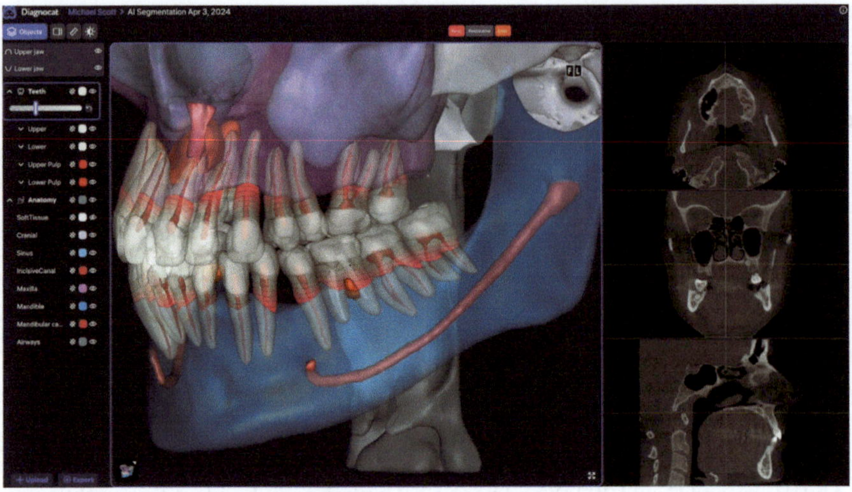

Fig. 5 CBCT segmentation using AI integration. *Courtesy* Diagnocat

this segmentation allows for studies of bone density and periodontal health for proper treatment planning.

4.3 Natural Language Processing for Diagnostic Data

Natural language processing (NLP) algorithms enhance diagnostic workflows by processing unstructured clinical data from electronic health records (EHRs). NLP systems extract meaningful patterns from patient histories, treatment notes, and imaging reports, enabling clinicians to make data-driven decisions.

NLP algorithms can identify trends in repeated restorations or persistent caries in specific quadrants, flagging areas requiring preventive or corrective intervention. Moreover, these systems integrate evidence-based recommendations by cross-referencing patient data with the latest scientific literature (Mollaei et al. 2022).

5 AI in Treatment Planning and Execution

AI has significantly improved both the planning and execution in conservative dentistry and endodontics. Using individualized information, like imaging, medical history, and clinical outcomes, AI can optimize treatment workflows to more accurate, efficient, and personalized experiences. These systems can foresee not only which procedures may have complications but also guide in real time (Yin et al. 2016) to improve outcomes and reduce complications.

5.1 *Personalized Treatment Simulations*

AI-powered treatment simulations will help the clinician foresee any issues that might arise and sharpen treatment strategies in advance of the procedures. In the case of endodontics, this involves simulations integrating highly detailed imaging data, such as CBCT scans, used in modeling the complex anatomy of the root canal system. This is how practitioners are able to identify anatomical variations, such as accessory canals, bifurcations, and apical deltas, which usually cannot be found during conventional planning.

AI systems can predict the likelihood of complications such as canal blockages, perforations, or incomplete cleaning, allowing clinicians to adjust their instrumentation techniques and select appropriate files. The expert consensus on digital AI-guided treatment planning recommended the reduced procedural errors in cases involving complex canal systems, significantly improving long-term outcomes (Wei et al. 2023).

In restorative dentistry, AI-based simulations analyze factors such as occlusal forces, material properties, and esthetic requirements to optimize restoration design. These simulations predict stress distribution across restorative materials, enabling clinicians to choose materials that balance durability and esthetics. The new predictive models simulate the wear patterns of crowns and veneers under dynamic forces, ensuring that the restorations withstand long-term functional demands.

5.2 *AI-Optimized Restorative Designs*

Computer-aided design and manufacturing (CAD/CAM) systems have deeply integrated AI algorithms that greatly enhance the capability for highly accurate, patient-specific restorations. These systems analyze intraoral scans to design restorations with perfect marginal fit, thus ensuring that restorations integrate seamlessly with the natural dentition (Fig. 6). Marginal integrity is critical in preventing secondary caries and maintaining the longevity of restorations (Revilla-León et al. 2023).

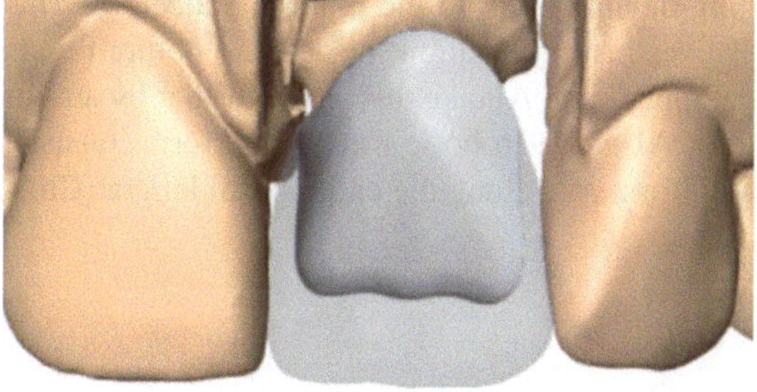

Fig. 6 AI-automated crown design. *Courtesy* 3Shape

AI also optimizes occlusal adjustments by analyzing bite dynamics and occlusal forces. Algorithms simulate the functional interaction of restorations with opposing and adjacent teeth, ensuring balanced occlusion and minimizing the risk of post-treatment discomfort or TMJ disorders (Farook and Dudley 2024). Clinical studies revealed that there is reduction in postoperative occlusal adjustments when AI-optimized CAD/CAM systems were employed, highlighting their precision and clinical utility (Yeslam et al. 2024).

5.3 Integration with Endodontic Instrumentation

AI systems integrated into endodontic instruments have transformed the way root canal therapies are performed. These systems use real-time data to guide clinicians during canal preparation, ensuring that instruments follow the natural curvature of the canal while avoiding critical structures. AI algorithms analyze tactile feedback from rotary systems to adjust torque and speed dynamically, reducing the risk of file separation or canal transportation and also analyze the longevity of instruments (Thakur et al. 2023).

AI-driven navigation systems, such as guided endodontic templates, leverage CBCT data to create precise access guides for complex canal anatomies (Lin et al. 2021). These templates reduce the risk of procedural errors, particularly in calcified or obstructed canals, where traditional approaches may fail. Research has shown that guided templates improve access cavity precision by 30% compared to freehand methods, leading to better procedural outcomes (Chen et al. 2022).

5.4 Real-Time Feedback During Procedures

Real-time feedback systems powered by AI provide invaluable support during treatment execution. These systems analyze procedural data continuously, offering visual and auditory cues to clinicians. For example, in root canal therapy, AI systems monitor canal length measurements, apical preparation, and obturation quality, flagging deviations from the planned trajectory. This feedback minimizes errors such as over-instrumentation, inadequate obturation, or missed canals. Robotic systems equipped with AI take this a step further by automating certain aspects of the procedure. AI-guided robotic arms can perform consistent and precise obturation, ensuring a uniform seal along the entire canal length (Cheng et al. 2023).

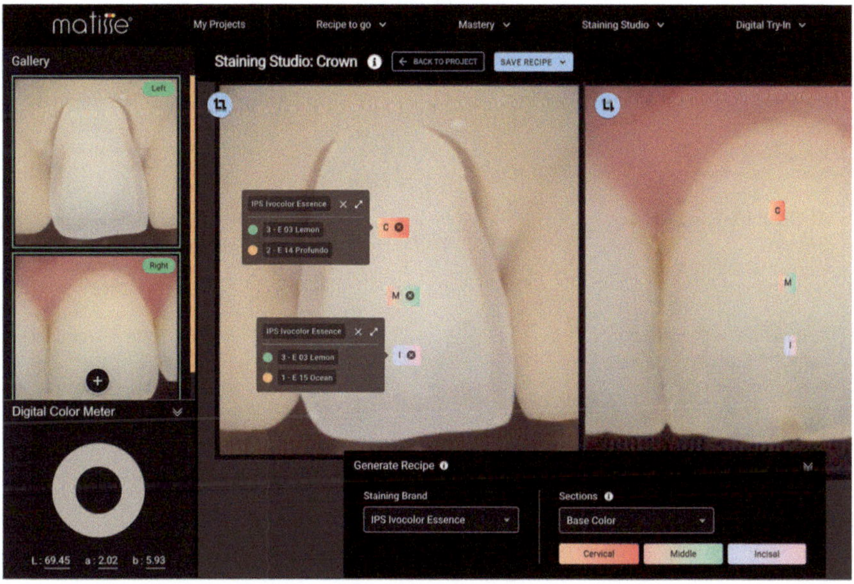

Fig. 7 AI-guided shade selection. *Courtesy* Matisse.ai

5.5 Enhanced Decision Support for Material Selection

AI systems analyze patient-specific factors, such as bite force, dietary habits, and oral hygiene, to recommend the most suitable restorative materials. For example, in patients with high occlusal forces or bruxism, AI models may suggest zirconia-based restorations for their superior strength, while prioritizing composite materials for aesthetically demanding anterior restorations (Fig. 7). These systems also factor in cost, durability, and patient preferences, ensuring a comprehensive and personalized approach to material selection (Rivera et al. 2024).

5.6 Automation in Restorative Execution

AI-powered automation extends beyond treatment planning to the physical execution of restorative procedures (Li et al. 2022). Robotic systems guided by AI algorithms handle intricate tasks such as milling and placement of restorations with extreme precision. These systems eliminate inconsistencies in manual execution, ensuring superior fit and finish (Dobrzański and Dobrzański 2020).

Robotic systems can place veneers with micrometer precision, greatly reducing marginal discrepancies. The augmented reality platforms, combined with AI, further enable the clinician to enhance visualization of the operative field through overlaying, in real time, anatomical guides and occlusal maps (Fig. 8) (Xia et al. 2024).

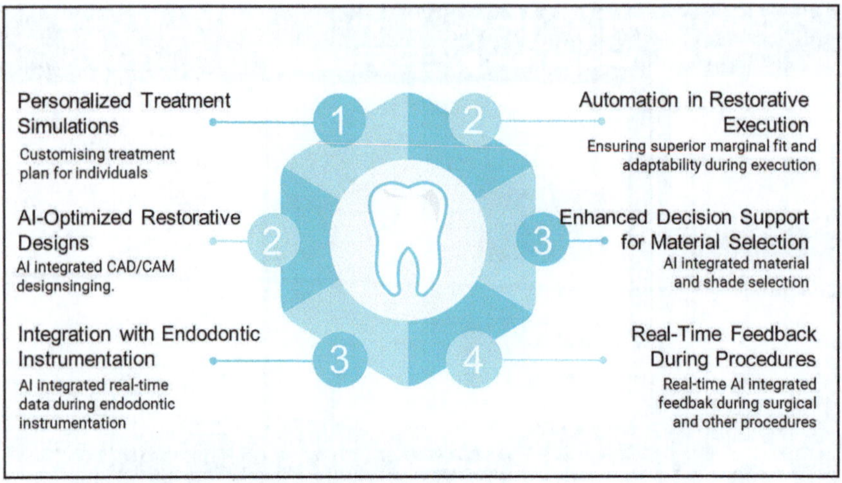

Fig. 8 AI in treatment planning and execution

6 AI in Prognosis

Prognosis in conservative dentistry and endodontics is a key area, allowing the clinician to forecast the outcome and the success rate of a dental treatment. Artificial intelligence has upgraded the prognostic model, bringing with it huge datasets and powerful computational algorithms in analyzing variables that could influence treatment results. AI enables clinicians to assess potential complications, determine the need for follow-up appointments, and adjust treatment plans according to the results predicted by this powerful technology.

6.1 Predictive Modeling in Endodontic Success

Predictive models in endodontics are designed to evaluate the likelihood of successful root canal therapy (RCT) based on patient-specific and procedural factors. These models use machine learning (ML) algorithms to analyze data such as the complexity of the canal system, preoperative conditions (e.g., presence of periapical lesions or calcified canals), and intraoperative variables like instrumentation quality and obturation technique (Chugal et al. 2001).

Studies have demonstrated that AI-driven models can predict the success of RCT with acceptable accuracy. Deep learning models trained on thousands of clinical cases were able to assess the healing potential of periapical lesions based on the size of the lesion, canal preparation quality, and postoperative radiographic outcomes. These models also incorporate data on patient compliance (Kayaoglu et al. 2016), such as adherence to follow-up visits, which is critical for long-term success.

AI systems also evaluate the likelihood of posttreatment complications, such as persistent infection or apical periodontitis, by identifying subtle patterns in imaging and clinical data (Jang et al. 2024). By providing a quantified risk assessment, these tools empower clinicians to preemptively address potential issues through additional interventions or modifications to the treatment plan (Signor et al. 2021).

6.2 *Prognosis of Restorative Procedures*

The longevity and performance of such treatments as crowns, inlays, and veneers depend on several factors in restorative dentistry, including material properties and occlusal forces, along with the oral hygiene practices of the patient. AI algorithms analyze these variables to predict restoration durability and identify factors that may compromise success (Hashem et al. 2019).

AI models assess the marginal fit of crowns and the quality of adhesive bonds, which are critical determinants of restoration longevity. AI-driven systems can accurately predict the survival rates of ceramic crowns based on occlusal stress simulations and patient-specific bite dynamics (Cho et al. 2024). These predictions enable dentists to recommend appropriate materials and design restorations tailored to individual patient needs.

AI tools provide even more insight into how environmental factors such as acidic diets or bruxism may impact restorative outcomes. Simulate the effects of bruxism on dental restorations and recommend preventive measures, including night guards. This level of personalization enhances treatment outcomes and decreases the chances of restoration failure.

6.3 *Long-Term Outcomes in Complex Cases*

In more challenging cases, such as those involving teeth with extensive decay, fractures, or failed previous treatment, AI tools may help make informed decisions about the prediction of most likely courses of long-term outcomes associated with various treatment modalities (Bennasar et al. 2023). Thus, AI compares the likelihood of retreatment success to that of extraction and implant placement and provides evidence-based suggestions that conform to the patient's clinical and personal preferences (Karobari et al. 2023).

More recently, advanced AI models now incorporate patient demographics, systemic health, and biomechanical analyses in predicting the functional and aesthetic outcomes of different treatment option.

6.4 Posttreatment Monitoring and Follow-Up

AI has a very important role in posttreatment follow-up, analyzing patient-reported results and clinical follow-up. Using AI-driven mobile applications, patients can send photographs or report symptoms, and data are analyzed by the system to identify marks of complications such as swelling, discoloration, or sensitivity. This allows early intervention by the clinician before the small issues turn into big problems. AI-powered tools also automate reminders for follow-up appointments and maintenance care, ensuring that patients stay on course with their treatment plans (Santos et al. 2024).

7 AI in Patient Management

Patient management in conservative dentistry and endodontics ranges from pretreatment planning to intra-treatment guidance and posttreatment follow-up. AI has emerged as one important tool that can enhance patient care by offering tailor-made solutions, smoothing administrative tasks, and improving communication between clinicians and patients. The insights gained through AI come after analyzing a large amount of data from various aspects of patients' information. These insights allow the clinician to address the needs of individual patients more accurately, enhance compliance, and better overall results.

During the pretreatment stage, AI applications focus on patient education (Johnson et al. 2024) and engagement. Dental anxiety is one of the common barriers to treatment acceptance. AI-driven applications, such as virtual assistants and chatbots, help alleviate this anxiety, for these systems are programmed to answer patient questions about the procedures, possible outcomes, and risks associated with them, so that patients can make informed decisions. Moreover, AI platforms can run through the history, risk factors, and past dental treatment of a patient in order to provide them with the right information and suggestions.

During treatment, AI elevates the management of the patient by improving communication and workflow efficiency. For instance, AI systems in dental management software automate appointment scheduling, patient reminders, and consent documentation. This not only saves time but also ensures that treatment timelines are adhered to.

Follow-up after treatment is an integral part of the management of patients, as this ensures the durability of the treatment outcomes and prevents complications. Using AI-powered mobile applications, patients can report symptoms, upload images, and receive feedback from clinicians without necessarily visiting in person. They become particularly useful in the monitoring of postoperative healing in endodontic procedures or after the success of restorative treatments. For example, an AI application could analyze images of the wound and patient reports on pain levels for signs of infection or delayed healing and thereby provide timely interventions.

AI also plays a critical role in personalized care plans. By analyzing data on a patient's oral hygiene habits, dietary patterns, and systemic health conditions, AI systems generate customized maintenance protocols that include recommendations for brushing techniques, fluoride treatments, or professional cleanings.

8 AI in Automation and Robotics in Endodontics

Automation and robotics, guided by AI, are revolutionizing the endodontics landscape with enhanced precision, efficiency, and predictability of dental procedures. Such technologies overcome certain limitations of traditional root canal therapy and the challenges of complex canal anatomy, operator variability, and procedural fatigue. Allowing for better decision-making and execution through a combination of data-driven insight and mechanical precision, AI-integrated robotic systems stand to change the face of endodontics and other related modalities (Sankar et al. 2025).

8.1 AI-Driven Robotic Systems for Root Canal Therapy

Robotic systems integrated with AI algorithms provide exceptional accuracy and consistency in performing root canal therapy. These systems utilize preoperative imaging data, such as cone-beam computed tomography (CBCT) scans, to construct a detailed 3D model of the root canal system. This model is then used to guide robotic arms during instrumentation, ensuring optimal cleaning and shaping.

A notable example of manually operated partial robotic technology in endodontics is the use of dynamic navigation systems (DNSs), such as the "X-Guide." These systems allow for real-time feedback and adaptation to the anatomical challenges of each canal, including extreme curvatures, bifurcations, and calcifications (Dianat et al. 2020). The learning curve and achieving technical proficiency were found to be significantly higher while using the DNS (Sharma et al. 2024). With the integration AI, there can be predicted enhancement of the accuracy and efficiency.

Moreover, AI-powered robotics can control torque and speed dynamically with enhanced haptic feedback, preventing file separation and enhancing the safety of rotary instrumentation. The introduction of the "Dentibot" (Cheng et al. 2023) is a significant remark in the endodontic society. These capabilities are particularly beneficial for treating teeth with challenging anatomies, such as those with C-shaped canals or calcifications, where manual techniques often fall short (Fig. 9).

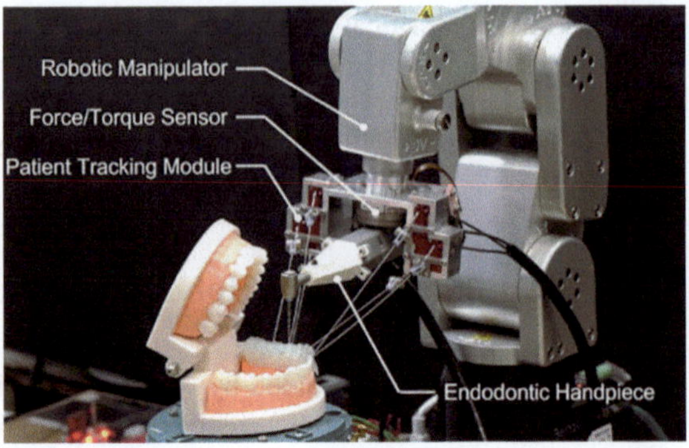

Fig. 9 Denti-bot, designed for performing robot-assisted endodontic treatment. *Courtesy* YouTube video

8.2 AI in Robotic Guidance for Access Cavity Preparation

Access cavity preparation is a critical step in endodontic therapy, requiring precise location of canal orifices without compromising tooth structure. Robotic systems equipped with AI algorithms use CBCT data to generate virtual guides that assist in creating access cavities with minimal deviation. These guides provide real-time visualization of the tooth's anatomy, reducing the risk of errors such as excessive removal of dentin or missed canals (Momen 2022).

8.3 Robotic-Assisted Irrigation and Disinfection

Thorough irrigation and disinfection are necessary to eliminate biofilm and residual debris in the root canal system. AI-augmented robotic systems automate the delivery of irrigants with precision, optimizing flow rates and pressure to achieve maximal debridement while minimizing the risk of extrusion into periapical tissues.

Recent studies of irrigant activation using Er: YAG laser where a prototype robot was used, which vaporizes water in the pulp chamber, causing micro-explosions that destroy organic and inorganic particles, reducing the need for mechanical preparation (He et al. 2023).

8.4 Augmented Reality (AR) Integration with Robotics

The combination of augmented reality (AR) and robotics represents a cutting-edge approach in endodontics (Farronato et al. 2023). AR systems overlay 3D anatomical models onto the operative field, providing clinicians with enhanced visualization and real-time guidance. When integrated with robotics, AR systems enable precise navigation of endodontic instruments within complex canal systems (Jiang et al. 2022).

8.5 Robotic Applications in Endodontic Surgery

Robotic systems, associated with AI, offer the advantage of incomparable precision—calculating optimal trajectory for surgical instruments, so minimal collateral tissue damage is sustained, and resection of infected periapical tissues is accurate, in those cases where surgical interventions such as apicoectomy or root-end resections are indicated.

Robotic surgery in endodontics is associated with better patient-related outcomes because there is less postoperative pain and swelling (Liu et al. 2024; Isufi et al. 2024).

9 Data Management and Privacy

The coordination of digital technologies and artificial intelligence in dentistry relies on efficient management of vast data. High-quality datasets such as radiographic images, CBCT scans, and clinical records form the basis for training sophisticated computational models that will be able to assist diagnostic and therapeutic decisions. Nevertheless, a number of challenges involved in acquiring, storing, and securing data inhibit their best use.

One of the main issues is the absence of standardization in data collection and annotation between dental clinics. Differences in imaging protocols and clinical reports generate inconsistencies that hinder the creation of solid datasets. As an example, CBCT images employed to assess periapical pathologies are frequently saved in incompatible formats, making it difficult to integrate them for large-scale analysis. Studies emphasize the need for standardized datasets to enhance the accuracy and generalizability of diagnostic algorithms.

Interoperability continues to be the major hurdle in using clinical data for sophisticated purposes. The majority of dental electronic health record (EHR) systems are not connected, confining the unhindered sharing of patient data among institutions. Such fragmentation hinders the integration of heterogeneous datasets needed to train universal diagnostic tools.

Patient confidentiality and data protection are of prime importance, especially in the context of legislative guidelines such as the Health Insurance Portability and Accountability Act (HIPAA) and the General Data Protection Regulation (GDPR). These legislations require strict data anonymization protocols, encryption policies, and secure access mechanisms. Data security breaches can undermine patient confidence and attract legal actions against institutions. Research indicates that strong encryption methods and automated anomaly detection systems are imperative to protect patient data.

AI-powered solutions themselves are able to improve data handling procedures. Automated systems for data validation can detect discrepancies in record-keeping, and datasets can be kept as reliable for use in a clinical context. Predictive analytics can anticipate security vulnerabilities in advance, enabling timely intervention to contain risks. Ethical issues of patient consent and data ownership need to be resolved, though, to maintain transparency and foster trust in AI-enabled systems.

10 Challenges and Limitations of AI in Endodontics and Conservative Dentistry

The promise of artificial intelligence (AI) in endodontics and conservative dentistry is transformative but also plagued by a range of challenges and limitations that need to be overcome for successful implementation to occur. The limitations include technological, ethical, cost, and clinical barriers, each one of which is a major impediment to adoption and mainstream use. Knowledge of these limitations is critical to the prospect of AI technology improving, rather than diminishing, clinical practice.

One of the largest challenges is the reliance on high-quality, standardized data for training AI models. AI systems depend on large datasets that span a variety of clinical scenarios, imaging techniques, and patient populations to make precise predictions and recommendations. Without standardization in the collection of data in dental practices at present, variations in the quality of datasets exist. For example, radiographic images can differ enormously in resolution, exposure levels, and file types, making it difficult to create consistent training datasets. In addition, missing or incorrect data contributes biases that may invalidate the AI models' credibility. This is especially true for endodontics, where the anatomy of canals and the outcome of treatments are extremely case-dependent, needing extremely high-resolution and refined datasets.

Computational complexity is another hurdle to the deployment of AI in dentistry. Sophisticated AI algorithms, particularly those using deep learning, are computationally intensive and require high-end machines. Such requirements are challenging to meet for small dental clinics and low-resource environments, where necessary human and economic resources to set up such a system are unavailable. Cloud-based alternatives have been suggested to counteract these limitations, but they raise data security and latency issues. The expense of creating and sustaining AI-based innovations is also still prohibitive, which may discourage usage, especially in thin-budget practice.

The most important issues with the integration of AI into the clinical environment are legal and ethical. Patient information is at the heart of creating and implementing AI systems, but it creates very serious issues with privacy and confidentiality. Compliance systems like the European Union's General Data Protection Regulation (GDPR) and the United States' Health Insurance Portability and Accountability Act (HIPAA) require strict protection of patient data. Yet, these rules have been breached by cyberattacks, unintended data leakage, or malicious data handling. Also, issues regarding data ownership complicate ethical usage of AI. For example, the ownership of the data on which AI technology is trained usually remains unknown whether the data concerns patients, institutions, or developers, and that creates potential issues in commercialization.

The "black box" character of much AI technology is a second important limitation. Deep learning models, on which so much of the success of AI depends, are black boxes where the logic for their predictions or decisions is not readily understandable. That lack of transparency threatens to deny clinicians and patients trust, as AI system decisions may seem arbitrary or hard to audit. For example, an AI system can recommend a certain treatment plan based on the patterns in the data, but as it cannot explain why it is recommending this, it gets difficult for evidence-based practice. To overcome this constraint, explainable AI (XAI) systems that give interpretable, understandable outputs to clinicians must be developed (O' Shaughnessy et al. 2020).

Another challenge lies in the overreliance on AI systems, which may inadvertently reduce the clinical expertise and decision-making skills of practitioners. While AI is intended to augment human capabilities, there is a risk that clinicians may become overly dependent on AI tools, leading to diminished critical thinking and diagnostic acumen. This risk is particularly relevant in endodontics, where complex cases often require nuanced judgment and a deep understanding of anatomy, pathology, and treatment principles. Balancing the use of AI with the retention of essential clinical skills is crucial to maintaining high standards of care.

Another practical constraint of AI in conservative dentistry and endodontics is integration with current workflows. Most dental clinics utilize more than one electronic health record (EHR) system and imaging software, some of which are not compatible with AI platforms. This prevents the potential of AI to be easily integrated into standard clinical workflows. In addition, proper use and interpretation of AI results necessitate extensive training of clinicians, dental assistants, and administrative personnel. Skeptical mindsets and the high learning curve for new technology are obstacles that can discourage adoption by some.

Economic accessibility is one of the challenges, especially where there are few healthcare budgets available in the region or for small-sized practices with no means of affording the upfront cost of installing AI technology. The price of AI robotics systems, medical diagnostic equipment, and software subscription will probably be extremely expensive, making it available only to well-funded organizations or private practitioners. Steps toward subsidizing such technologies or creating low-cost alternatives are also crucial toward democalization of access to AI in dentistry.

Lastly, validation and regulation of AI systems are still issues (Karobari et al. 2023; Johnson et al. 2024). The fast pace of AI development has a propensity to outpace the capacity of regulatory agencies to create guidelines and standards for their safe and effective application. AI models need to be tested by rigorous clinical validation to ascertain their accuracy, reliability, and applicability across various populations. Yet, the heterogeneity of dental treatments and patient populations can make it challenging to generalize AI models with the need for ongoing monitoring and updating to keep them up to date.

The limitations and challenges AI poses to endodontics and conservative dentistry require a concerted effort to its implementation. Clinicians, researchers, technology innovators, and policymakers must join hands in addressing such barriers and utilizing AI as a useful tool toward dental care development.

11 Conclusion and Future Directions

AI has come as a revolutionizing element in conservative dentistry and endodontics, bringing new remedies to age-old challenges. From increasing the accuracy and precision of diagnosis and treatment planning to improving patient management and robotic systems, AI has reformed the dental care landscape. Even though the promise of applications of AI has been vast, their implementation is in its developmental stages, and much needs to be done to leverage their true potential.

Integration of AI with diagnostics has bridged key shortcomings of conventional methods, especially radiographic interpretation and analysis of CBCT. AI tools provide improved sensitivity and specificity to allow clinicians to detect pathologies and anatomical complexities at earlier stages more effectively. AI, in turn, has facilitated improvements in treatment planning and its performance through its ability to mimic patient-specific cases and offer feedback on a real-time basis during intervention. Such technological advancements have refined procedural results, minimized complications, and generally heightened patient satisfaction levels. The introduction of AI in other departments has already on its future path (Sankar et al. 2024, 2025), so innovative movements has to be introduced in conservative dentistry and endodontics also.

Even as these results are being achieved, some challenges to the widespread utilization of AI technology include data dependency, ethics, and budgetary restrictions. All of these are going to need solving by all stakeholders from a unified effort between the research community, policymakers, clinicians, and technologists. There are regulatory mechanisms that need to be implemented in order to avoid dangerous and unethical applications of AI, especially where data privacy is involved and patient consent. In addition, coordination across institutions to synchronize data collection and labeling will be essential for creating strong and generalizable AI models.

The future of AI in conservative dentistry and endodontics is promising and complex. The most exciting area of development is the design of explainable AI (XAI) systems. These systems try to do away with the "black box" issue by giving intelligible outputs that can be seen and confirmed by practitioners. By having more openness, XAI will enable trust between patients and practitioners, rendering AI a good tool and never the cause of confusion.

Another area of future research includes creating low-cost AI technologies. Present systems are costly, which restricts their use to well-funded practices or organizations. In order to democratize AI, developers and researchers need to ensure that low-cost solutions are created without sacrificing functionality. For example, open-source AI platforms can allow small practices to take advantage of AI features without forking out tremendous sums.

The integration of AI with other cutting-edge technologies, including augmented reality (AR) and virtual reality (VR), is another potential area. AR and VR platforms have already demonstrated the ability to increase surgical accuracy and patient education. Their fusion with AI could deliver immersive data-driven visualizations that improve diagnostic and procedural results. For instance, clinicians can utilize AI-enhanced AR to visualize real-time internal tooth anatomy, informing endodontic instrumentation with previously unknown precision.

Personalized dental care will become the bedrock of AI implementation over the next two years. Through the study of each patient's genetic susceptibility, microbiome signature, and lifestyle indicators, AI software might provide treatment protocols of unheralded personalization. This would not only improve the quality of care but also preventive treatment by detecting risk factors at an early stage in their evolution so that interventions can be targeted appropriately. AI will also transform dentistry education and training. AI-based virtual simulators would give students and professionals real simulation environments to hone complex procedures and receive immediate feedback. These systems would be especially beneficial in endodontics, where the complexity of canal morphology demands skill development at a high level. On a larger scale, AI can redefine dental public health by spotting trends and areas of care needs. Predictive analysis can help distribute resources more efficiently, formulate prevention programs for specific groups, and solve access disparities in the dental sector. For instance, AI systems could scrutinize population-level data in a bid to determine high ratios of untreated caries or periodontal illness so that policymakers can target intervention to underserved communities.

As AI advancements evolve, interdisciplinary cooperation will be most critical to enable its effective implementation into clinical practice. Interdisciplinary cooperation between dental clinicians, computer scientists, and regulatory agencies will promote the creation of user-friendly and ethically appropriate AI systems. Continuous clinical trials and longitudinal studies will also be essential to guarantee the safety, efficacy, and long-term implications of AI technologies in dentistry. AI has already progressed extensively in conservative dentistry and endodontics and provides new cutting-edge solutions to enhance clinical effectiveness, precision, and patient results. Issues do still exist, but the on-going development efforts of AI technologies, together with solutions to remove the impediments to its integration, hold the potential for gigantic advancements in dental care in the future. By embracing such innovation in a sustainable and collaborative fashion, the dental community is enabled to move toward an oral care treatment future where AI serves to enhance human potential without sacrificing it.

References

Abdelazim R, Fouad EM (2024) Artificial intelligent-driven decision-making for automating root fracture detection in periapical radiographs. BDJ Open 10(1):76

Alshadidi AAF, Alshahrani AA, Aldosari LIN, Chaturvedi S, Saini RS, Hassan SAB et al (2023) Investigation on the application of artificial intelligence in prosthodontics. Appl Sci 13(8):5004

Alshomrani F (2024) Cone-beam computed tomography (CBCT)-based diagnosis of dental bone defects. Diagnostics 14(13):1404

Bennasar C, García I, Gonzalez-Cid Y, Pérez F, Jiménez J (2023) Second opinion for non-surgical root canal treatment prognosis using machine learning models. Diagnostics 13(17):2742

Boreak N (2020) Effectiveness of artificial intelligence applications designed for endodontic diagnosis, decision-making, and prediction of prognosis: a systematic review. J Contemp Dent Pract 21(8):926–934

Chen C, Wang FS, Zhang R, Bian Z, Meng LY (2022) An in vitro model study of computer-guided endodontic microsurgery. Zhonghua Kou Qiang Yi Xue Za Zhi Zhonghua Kouqiang Yixue Zazhi Chin J Stomatol 57(1):44–51

Chen D, Yu MQ, Li QJ, He X, Liu F, Shen JF (2024) Precise tooth design using deep learning-based templates. J Dent 144:104971

Cheng HF, Ho YC, Chen CW (2023) DentiBot: system design and 6-dof hybrid position/force control for robot-assisted endodontic treatment. https://arxiv.org/abs/2310.09691

Cho JH, Çakmak G, Yi Y, Yoon HI, Yilmaz B, Schimmel M (2024) Tooth morphology, internal fit, occlusion and proximal contacts of dental crowns designed by deep learning-based dental software: a comparative study. J Dent 141:104830

Chugal NM, Clive JM, Spångberg LSW (2001) A prognostic model for assessment of the outcome of endodontic treatment: effect of biologic and diagnostic variables. Oral Surg Oral Med Oral Pathol Oral Radiol Endod 91(3):342–352

Dianat O, Nosrat A, Tordik PA, Aldahmash SA, Romberg E, Price JB et al (2020) Accuracy and efficiency of a dynamic navigation system for locating calcified canals. J Endod 46(11):1719–1725

Dobrzański LA, Dobrzański LB (2020) Dentistry 4.0 concept in the design and manufacturing of prosthetic dental restorations. Processes 8(5):525

Farook TH, Dudley J (2024) Understanding occlusion and temporomandibular joint function using deep learning and predictive modeling. Clin Exp Dent Res 10(6):e70028

Farronato M, Torres A, Pedano MS, Jacobs R (2023) Novel method for augmented reality guided endodontics: an in vitro study. J Dent 132:104476

Forouzeshfar P, Safaei AA, Ghaderi F, Hashemikamangar S, Kaviani H, Haghi S (2023) Dental caries diagnosis from bitewing images using convolutional neural networks. https://www.researchsquare.com/article/rs-3044180/v1

Ghassemi M, Naumann T, Schulam P, Beam AL, Chen IY, Ranganath R (2019) Practical guidance on artificial intelligence for health-care data. Lancet Digit Health 1(4):e157–e159

Hashem M, Al-Kheraif AA, Wahba AA (2019) Examining the longevity of dental restoration using Hebbian adversarial networks clustering with gradient boosting recurrent neural network. Measurement 141:313–323

He X, Li Y, Nie M, Yu Y, Chen H, Pan C et al (2023) Transient apical peak pressure measurement of Er: YAG laser–activated irrigation in different in vitro tooth models using a high-frequency sensor system. Lasers Med Sci 38(1):123

Herzog NJ, Celik D, Sulaiman RB (2024) Artificial intelligence in healthcare and medical records security. In: Jahankhani H, Bowen G, Sharif MS, Hussien O (eds) Cybersecurity and artificial intelligence. Springer, Cham, pp 35–57. https://doi.org/10.1007/978-3-031-52272-7_2

Huang D, Wang X, Liang J, Ling J, Bian Z, Yu Q et al (2024) Expert consensus on difficulty assessment of endodontic therapy. Int J Oral Sci 16(1):22

Isufi A, Hsu TY, Chogle S (2024) Robot-assisted and haptic-guided endodontic surgery: a case report. J Endod 50(4):533-539.e1

Ivashchenko AV, Fedyaev IM, Yablokov AE, Kondrashin DV, Tselkovich LS, Sadykov MI (2020) Robot-assisted and robotic systems used in dentistry. Biomed Eng 53(5):322–326
Jang YE, Kim Y, Kim SY, Kim BS (2024) Predicting early endodontic treatment failure following primary root canal treatment. BMC Oral Health 24(1):327
Jiang J, Guo Y, Huang Z, Zhang Y, Wu D, Liu Y (2022) Adjacent surface trajectory planning of robot-assisted tooth preparation based on augmented reality. Eng Sci Technol Int J 27:101001
Johnsen I, Bårdsen A, Haug SR (2023) Impact of case difficulty, endodontic mishaps, and instrumentation method on endodontic treatment outcome and quality of life: a four-year follow-up study. J Endod 49(4):382–389
Johnson AJ, Singh TK, Gupta A, Sankar H, Gill I, Shalini M et al (2024) Evaluation of validity and reliability of AI Chatbots as public sources of information on dental trauma. Dent Traumatol 13000
Karobari MI, Adil AH, Basheer SN, Murugesan S, Savadamoorthi KS, Mustafa M et al (2023) Evaluation of the diagnostic and prognostic accuracy of artificial intelligence in endodontic dentistry: a comprehensive review of literature. Comput Math Meth Med 2023(1):7049360
Kayaoglu G, Gürel M, Saricam E, Ilhan MN, Ilk O (2016) Predictive model of intraoperative pain during endodontic treatment: prospective observational clinical study. J Endod 42(1):36–41
Li H, Sakai T, Tanaka A, Ogura M, Lee C, Yamaguchi S et al (2022) Interpretable AI explores effective components of CAD/CAM resin composites. J Dent Res 101(11):1363–1371
Lin X, Fu Y, Ren G, Yang X, Duan W, Chen Y et al (2021) Micro-computed tomography–guided artificial intelligence for pulp cavity and tooth segmentation on cone-beam computed tomography. J Endod 47(12):1933–1941
Liu C, Liu X, Wang X, Liu Y, Bai Y, Bai S et al (2024) Endodontic microsurgery with an autonomous robotic system: a clinical report. J Endod
McGuigan MB, Duncan HF, Horner K (2018) An analysis of effective dose optimization and its impact on image quality and diagnostic efficacy relating to dental cone beam computed tomography (CBCT). SWISS Dent J SSO Sci Clin Top128(4):297–316
Mollaei N, Cepeda C, Rodrigues J, Gamboa H (2022) Biomedical text mining: applicability of machine learning-based natural language processing in medical database. In: Proceedings of the 15th international joint conference on biomedical engineering systems and technologies. SCITEPRESS—Science and Technology Publications. https://doi.org/10.5220/0010819500003123
Momen R (2022) Comparison of accuracy and efficiency of robotic-assisted haptic guidance versus freehand access preparation in calcified teeth
O' Shaughnessy M, Canal G, Connor M, Rozell C, Davenport M (2020) Generative causal explanations of black-box classifiers. In: Larochelle H, Ranzato M, Hadsell R, Balcan MF, Lin H (eds), Advances in neural information processing systems. Curran Associates, Inc, pp 5453–5467. https://proceedings.neurips.cc/paper_files/paper/2020/file/3a93a609b97ec0ab0ff5539eb79ef33a-Paper.pdf
Pauwels R, Brasil DM, Yamasaki MC, Jacobs R, Bosmans H, Freitas DQ et al (2021) Artificial intelligence for detection of periapical lesions on intraoral radiographs: comparison between convolutional neural networks and human observers. Oral Surg Oral Med Oral Pathol Oral Radiol 131(5):610–616
Revilla-León M, Gómez-Polo M, Vyas S, Barmak AB, Gallucci GO, Att W et al (2023) Artificial intelligence models for tooth-supported fixed and removable prosthodontics: a systematic review. J Prosthet Dent 129(2):276–292
Rivera KP, Whang K, Joshi K, Son H, Kim YS, Flores M (2024) Dental composite performance prediction using artificial intelligence. https://doi.org/10.1101/2024.10.08.24314998
Roosanty A, Widyaningrum R, Diba SF (2022) Artificial intelligence based on convolutional neural network for detecting dental caries on bitewing and periapical radiographs. J Radiol Dentomaksilofasial Indones JRDI 6(2):89

Sankar H, Alagarsamy R, Lal B, Rana SS, Roychoudhury A, Agrawal A et al (2025) Role of artificial intelligence in treatment planning and outcome prediction of jaw corrective surgeries by using 3-D imaging: a systematic review. Oral Surg Oral Med Oral Pathol Oral Radiol 139(3):299–310

Sankar H, Alagarsamy R, Lal B, Rana SS, Roychoudhury A, Barathi A et al (2024) Role of artificial intelligence in magnetic resonance imaging-based detection of temporomandibular joint disorder—a systematic review. Br J Oral Maxillofac Surg S0266435624005497

Santos M, Peyroteo M, Lapão L (2024) AI-powered post-discharge monitoring to prevent patients readmissions and reduce workforce burden. Eur J Public Health 34(suppl 3):ckae144.1209

Shamaun M, Field J (2023) A scoping review of machine learning in dental radiography: its current applications and relevance in dentistry. https://www.researchsquare.com/article/rs-2865258/v1

Sharma S, Haldar P, Kumar V, Chawla A, Logani A (2024) Learning curve for dynamic navigation procedure during endodontic management of permanent maxillary anterior teeth with pulp canal calcification: a risk-adjusted cumulative summation analysis of a single operator's experience. J Endod S0099239924006824

Shruti TNK (2023) Predictive analytics in healthcare using machine learning. In: 2023 14th international conference on computing communication and networking technologies (ICCCNT). IEEE, Delhi, India, pp 1–5. https://ieeexplore.ieee.org/document/10306782/

Signor B, Blomberg LC, Kopper PMP, Augustin PAN, Rauber MV, Rodrigues GS et al (2021) Root canal retreatment: a retrospective investigation using regression and data mining methods for the prediction of technical quality and periapical healing. J Appl Oral Sci 29:e20200799

Singh S, Asthana G (2024) Artificial intelligence: a futuristic tool for advanced endodontics. J Conserv Dent Endod 27(5):447–448

Siqueira JF, Rôças IN, Ricucci D (2019) Internal tooth anatomy and root canal instrumentation. In: Versiani MA, Basrani B, Sousa-Neto MD (eds) The root canal anatomy in permanent dentition. Springer, Cham, pp 277–302. https://doi.org/10.1007/978-3-319-73444-6_10

Siqueira Junior JF, Rôças IDN, Marceliano-Alves MF, Pérez AR, Ricucci D (2018) Unprepared root canal surface areas: causes, clinical implications, and therapeutic strategies. Braz Oral Res 32(suppl 1). http://www.scielo.br/scielo.php?script=sci_arttext&pid=S1806-83242018000500600&lng=en&tlng=en

Surdilovic D, Abdelaal H, D'Souza J (2023) Using artificial intelligence in preventive dentistry: a narrative review. J Datta Meghe Inst Med Sci Univ 18(1):146

Tabatabaian F, Vora SR, Mirabbasi S (2023) Applications, functions, and accuracy of artificial intelligence in restorative dentistry: a literature review. J Esthet Restor Dent 35(6):842–859

Thakur VS, Kankar PK, Parey A, Jain A, Jain PK (2023) Health prediction of reciprocating endodontic instrument based on the machine learning and exponential degradation models. Proc Inst Mech Eng 237(10):1202–1214

Wei X, Du Y, Zhou X, Yue L, Yu Q, Hou B et al (2023) Expert consensus on digital guided therapy for endodontic diseases. Int J Oral Sci 15(1):54

Xia Z, Ahmad F, Deng H, Jiang L, Qin W, Zhao Q et al (2024) Robotics application in dentistry: a review. IEEE Trans Med Robot Bionics 6(3):851–867

Yeslam HE, Freifrau Von Maltzahn N, Nassar HM (2024) Revolutionizing CAD/CAM-based restorative dental processes and materials with artificial intelligence: a concise narrative review. PeerJ 12:e17793

Yin MS, Haddawy P, Suebnukarn S, Rhienmora P (2016) Toward intelligent tutorial feedback in surgical simulation: Robust outcome scoring for endodontic surgery. In: International conference on intelligent user interfaces, proceedings IUI. Association for computing machinery, vol 07–10-March-2016, pp 402–406. https://www.scopus.com/inward/record.uri?eid=2-s2.0-84963749730&doi=10.1145%2f2856767.2856810&partnerID=40&md5=9ffc7e8b73857d0e6c669fd83a301196

Ylisiurua S, Sipola A, Nieminen MT, Brix MAK (2024) Deep learning enables time-efficient soft tissue enhancement in CBCT: proof-of-concept study for dentomaxillofacial applications. Phys Med 117:103184

Yu Y (2016) Machine learning for dental image analysis

Application of Artificial Intelligence and Robotics in Prosthodontics

Chetan Mukund Modgi, Tarun Kumar Singh, and Aakash Gupta

1 Robotics in Prosthodontics

Showa Hanako, the first artificially intelligent (AI) robot ever made, was able to imitate human movements and responses. Boesecke et al. introduced the first robot-guided dental implant insertion in 2002 (Karnik et al. 2024a). The robot system's operating area was 70 cm, and it was capable of placing 48 dental implants within 1–2 mm of the apical boundary and executing an implant osteotomy drilling guide. Furthermore, a stereo camera-equipped three-degrees-of-freedom (DOF) robotic system was created. By identifying and managing the dental handpiece, this method could guarantee that implants were positioned in compliance with the preoperative guidelines. Introduced in 2017, YOMITM (Neocis, Miami, FL, USA) is the first FDA-approved computerized navigation robotic system to increase the clinical accuracy of dental implant surgery. In order to solve the lack of qualified dentists and prevent surgical errors, Beijing University and Fourth Military Medical University Hospital (Xi'an, China) also created an autonomous dental implant robot in 2017. CRS Robots, a Canadian company, created a single manipulator robotic system that uses six degrees of freedom (DOF) to fabricate entire denture prostheses (Ali et al. 2024).

Robotic articulators can mimic jaw movements with or without the aid of jaw movement tracking sensors. In one experiment, a robotic articulator was used to build a full veneer crown on a single patient's working cast. A commercially accessible robot known as the "Bionic Jaw Motion" (Bionic Technology, Vercelli, Italy) is the most recent advancement. To mimic mandibular kinematics, the robot combines a

C. M. Modgi (✉)
Department of Prosthodontics, Government Dental College, Silchar, India
e-mail: dr.chetanmodgi@gmail.com

T. K. Singh · A. Gupta
Division of Conservative Dentistry and Endodontics, Department of Dentistry, All India Institute of Medical Sciences, Bathinda, India

A. Gupta et al. (eds.), *Application of Robotics in Dentistry*, Lecture Notes in Bioengineering, https://doi.org/10.1007/978-981-95-1470-0_10

robot articulator with a movement analyzer, which is a high-speed camera (Putra et al. 2022; Singi et al. 2022a).

2 Applications in Prosthodontics

Due to its substantial influence and innovation in the field of intelligence, artificial intelligence is becoming a growing popularity globally. Since it facilitates the creation of functional maxillofacial appliances and the design of prostheses, it is vital in dentistry, particularly throughout the field of prosthodontics (Marinello and Brugger 2021). By analyzing patient data, including digital impressions, radiographs, and facial scans, AI can help in prosthodontic treatment planning by producing virtual 3D models of the patient's oral anatomy. By optimizing the shape, fit, and aesthetics of prosthodontic restorations—such as dental crowns, bridges, and dentures—based on patient-specific factors and preferences, artificial intelligence (AI) algorithms can help with their design and production. Digital imprints and intraoral scans can be analyzed by AI-powered software to precisely identify and define the edges of tooth preparations. By enabling perfect fit and minimizing the need for manual corrections, automated margin detection can increase the accuracy of prosthetic restorations. Artificial intelligence (AI) systems are able to analyze digital dental models and simulate virtual articulation in order to evaluate functional dynamics, find interferences, and assess occlusal relationships. Planning a prosthetic treatment can be aided by virtual articulation and occlusal analysis, which guarantee appropriate occlusal alignment and harmony for the best possible functional and cosmetic results (Lo Russo and Salamini 2018). Artificial intelligence (AI) technologies may scan digital photos of patients' natural teeth to predict how prosthetic restorations will look in different lighting scenarios and offer shade-matching recommendations. Prosthodontists can benefit from guided implant surgery using AI-powered augmented reality (AR) platforms, which offer real-time navigation and visibility of the implant insertion procedure (Doshi et al. 2024; Koralakunte and Aljanakh 2014).

2.1 Limitations

The application of AI in prosthodontics is theoretically limitless. Unfortunately, financial considerations frequently drive the creation and widespread adoption of new AI technologies in the most lucrative fields. They also sometimes stifle innovative dental applications because a market seems too tiny for the dentistry sector. However, we may look forward to more AI research and advancements in the future. Future studies on AI technology in (reconstructive) dentistry must also rigorously analyze the cost–benefit ratio and the moral implications of using patient-specific data, in addition to the technical potential (Sreelekshmi et al. 2017).

Biases may be ingrained in AI programming, leading to unfair or discriminatory outcomes. The possibility of dental technicians losing their jobs when AI replaces them is another issue brought up. When applying AI to address problems, a comprehensive algorithm with several uses is needed to respond to a specific query. Artificial intelligence is unable to interpret directly; instead, misinterpretations may result from algorithmic flaws. Because of their complexity, robotic systems require certain knowledge and skills to operate at their best. The dentist might not have the skills and knowledge necessary to program and manage the robotic equipment. Additionally, the dentists' cooperation and acceptance of the unidentified patient could be another important consideration (Thomas et al. 2022).

3 Role of AI in Complete Denture Fabrication: From Planning to Delivery

The production of digitally engineered complete dentures has gained prominence with the rise of advanced digital tools and evolving clinical protocols. These innovations not only simplify the overall treatment process by reducing clinical appointments but also lead to better-fitting prostheses with improved retention and comfort. This translates to increased satisfaction for both patients and practitioners. The *Glossary of Digital Terms* describes a digital denture as a complete prosthesis designed and produced using automated systems such as computer-aided design (CAD), computer-aided manufacturing (CAM), and computer-aided engineering (CAE), as a replacement for traditional manual methods (Polizzi A et al. 2024).

3.1 Digital Impression Acquisition

Intraoral scanners have made it possible to transition to fully digital workflows for complete denture creation. These digital impressions offer several benefits, such as avoiding discomfort from traditional materials, eliminating risks of allergic reactions, and preventing distortions caused by material shrinkage or expansion during setting. This approach is especially advantageous for mucostatic impression techniques, which are ideal for patients with mobile or flat ridges. The mucostatic technique utilizes surface tension between the denture base and soft tissues, often requiring less flange extension while maintaining good retention. However, overly short borders may affect stability and lip support.

Though conventional impressions still demonstrate slightly higher accuracy for full-arch scans, clinical studies have shown that the variance in trueness (38.2 μm) and precision (19.9 μm) between digital and conventional methods is not clinically significant (Kong and Kim 2024).

3.2 *Recording Jaw Relations with Virtual Articulators*

Virtual articulators (VAs) allow for the simulation of mandibular dynamics in both static and functional scenarios, offering a three-dimensional view for occlusion evaluation and patient communication. These systems are categorized into mathematically simulated (MS) and completely adjustable (CA) articulators. The foundation for virtual articulator technology was laid by Szentpetery in the 1990s, with operational models developed by Bisler et al. by 2002 (Silva et al. 2020).

Kordass and Gartner (2001) introduced a system integrating 3D laser scans with a jaw motion analyzer (JMA) to replicate patient-specific temporomandibular joint (TMJ) movements (Fig. 1). Essential components of this system include the following:

- Digital impressions via scanning
- Real-time TMJ motion capture with ultrasonic sensors and a facebow
- Digitally mapped occlusion
- Functional mandibular simulations

If a JMA is not accessible, the articulator can be preset using average values for movements such as condylar guidance and lateral shifts.

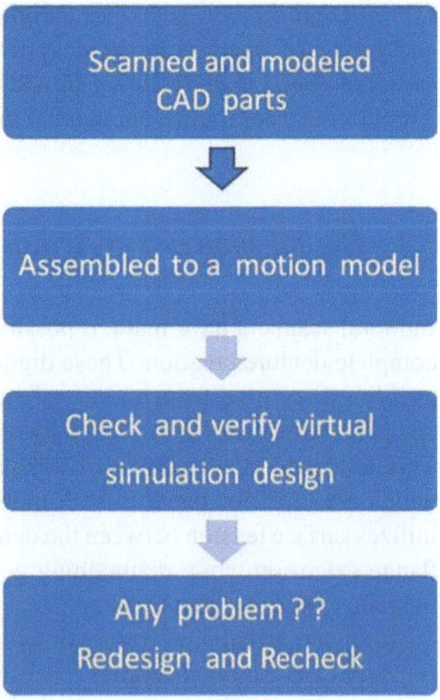

Fig. 1 Virtual articulator mimics jaw relation

3.3 Robotic Systems for Tooth Placement

Manual placement of denture teeth has been replaced in some systems with robotic manipulators. One of the first innovations in this space was a six-DOF robotic arm developed by CRS Robotics (Fig. 2). This eventually led to the creation of a more complex system featuring 84 degrees of freedom, enabling highly accurate multi-axis control for tooth arrangement (Fig. 3).

Despite offering remarkable precision (±0.05 mm), the complexity and bulk of the 84-DOF system limited its practicality. To address this, a more efficient 50-DOF robotic assembly was designed, incorporating a dental arch model and slipway track mechanism (Fig. 4). Fourteen manipulators, each with three movement axes and vertical adjustability, facilitated smoother operation and reduced mechanical complexity (Fig. 5). The updated design cut down on motor use, improved system

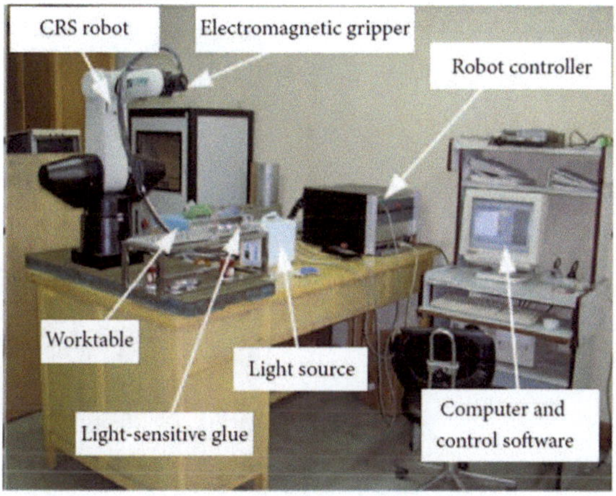

Fig. 2 Single manipulator tooth arrangement robot system for complete denture

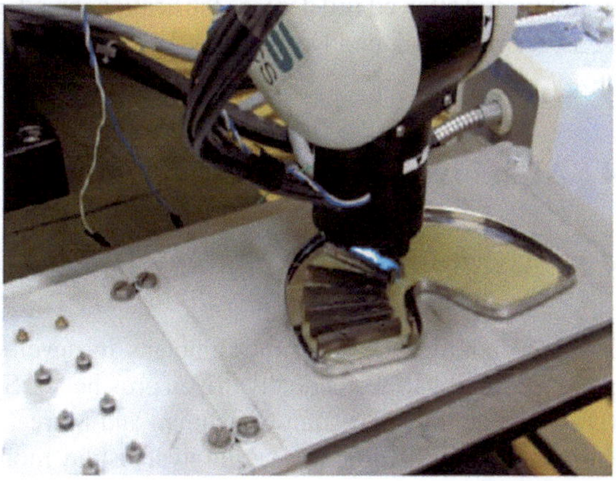

Fig. 3 Working process of the single manipulator robot tooth arrangement robot system for complete denture

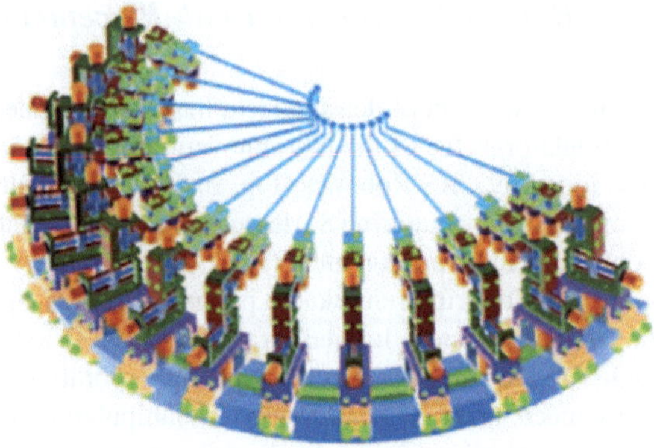

Fig. 4 Structure of the 84-DOF multimanipulator tooth arrangement robot

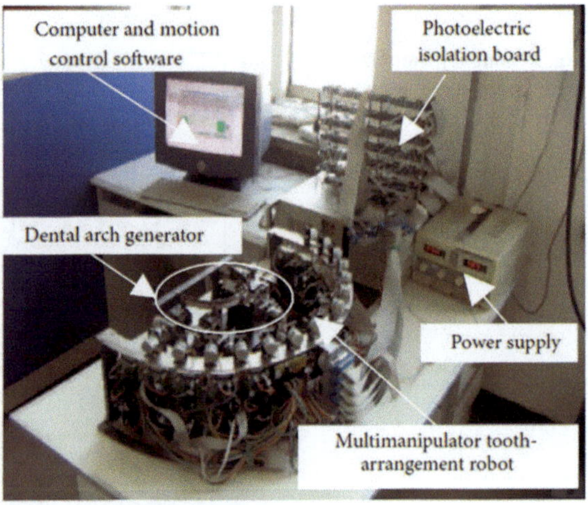

Fig. 5 50-DOF multimanipulator tooth arrangement robot system

usability, and allowed full denture fabrication in under 30 min, achieving an accuracy of ±0.1 mm (Cevik and Kocacikli 2019; Shah et al. 2014).

4 AI in Fixed Dental Prosthodontics

4.1 Assessment and Planning

Artificial intelligence supports clinicians in developing comprehensive treatment plans, especially in aesthetically driven prosthetics. Systems like digital smile design (DSD), created by Christian Coachman and Marcelo Calamita, help analyze facial harmony, tooth positioning, and gingival display more precisely than the human eye.

These tools assess parameters such as dental midline, tooth width-to-height ratio, and smile dynamics.

The digital planning protocol generally includes the following:

1. Capturing intraoral scans
2. Importing facial photographs
3. Aligning digital facial guidelines
4. Overlaying tooth templates and assessing symmetry
5. Digitally marking areas for esthetic correction
6. Transferring the plan to physical models via analog or digital calipers.

AI tools also assist in evaluating abutment teeth by analyzing crown–root ratios and predicting periodontal risks, supporting more informed decision-making (Park and Han 2018).

4.2 Tooth Preparation Using Robotics and AR

Conventional tooth preparation techniques emphasize minimal invasiveness and anatomical fidelity. Inadequate reduction can compromise esthetics or endanger pulp vitality. CAD/CAM systems guided by AI and robotics ensure more accurate finish lines, while augmented reality (AR) solutions offer enhanced precision in managing preparation depth (Park et al. 2021; Murdoch 2021; Jiang et al. 2017; Karnik et al. 2024b).

4.3 Digital Impression Techniques and Scanner Technologies

Digital impressions with intraoral scanners (IOS) provide a real-time, accurate, and more comfortable alternative to traditional methods. These systems minimize material deformation and provide enhanced visualization during scanning. Different scanning principles include triangulation, confocal microscopy, structured light, and stereophotogrammetry.

- **Triangulation** determines spatial depth using geometric angles from multiple beams (Fig. 6a).
- **Confocal imaging** captures images at various depths for 3D reconstruction (Fig. 6b).
- **Wavefront sampling** uses off-center apertures to map oral topography.
- **Stereophotogrammetry** passively captures spatial data through multiple camera angles, offering a low-cost and user-friendly option.

Together, these imaging technologies lay the groundwork for AI-powered restorative workflows, improving diagnostic accuracy and the precision of prosthetic outcomes (Sonkar et al. 2023).

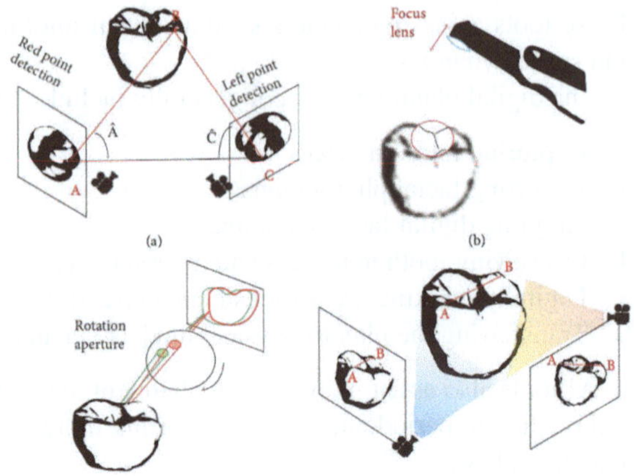

Fig. 6 Confocal imaging calculating positions of points (**a**), measuring distances and reconstructing the object (**b**)

5 Computer-Aided Designing and Manufacturing

Dental CAD/CAM systems rely on three key components: The first as discussed is the scanner, the second is a digital design program, and the last is the manufacturing device.

There are three main types of CAD/CAM production systems for dental restorations:

1. Chair-side Systems: These, such as the CEREC System (Dentsply Sirona, Charlotte, NC, USA), enable same-visit restoration creation and placement.
2. Laboratory Systems: Systems like the CEREC in Lab MC XL (Dentsply Sirona) produce restorations or copings from scanned impressions, stone casts, or dies, with technicians applying esthetic veneers.
3. Central Machining Networks: These outsource laboratory work online for producing high-strength ceramic frameworks with specialized requirements.

Fabrication can be either subtractive (milling) or additive (3D printing). Subtractive techniques, often favored for ceramic restorations, minimize material waste and lower costs. Additive manufacturing, increasingly used for resin-based restorations, is still evolving for ceramics like zirconia. Milling machines, classified by their number of axes (three, four, or five), enhance production efficiency. Five axis machines, though more expensive, complete tasks faster and with greater precision, reducing errors and enhancing restoration durability.

Artificial intelligence plays a transformative role in modern dental CAD/CAM systems, revolutionizing the design, fabrication, and implementation of dental restorations (Fig. 7). In restorative workflows, AI enhances chair-side CAD systems by enabling real-time analysis and design. And its application extends to chair-side digital scanners, which use intelligent algorithms to refine digital impressions and improve design consistency, minimizing errors caused by soft tissue interference (Fig. 8). Virtual reality (VR) and augmented reality (AR) have further amplified the potential of AI in CAD/CAM. These technologies allow for precise simulations of

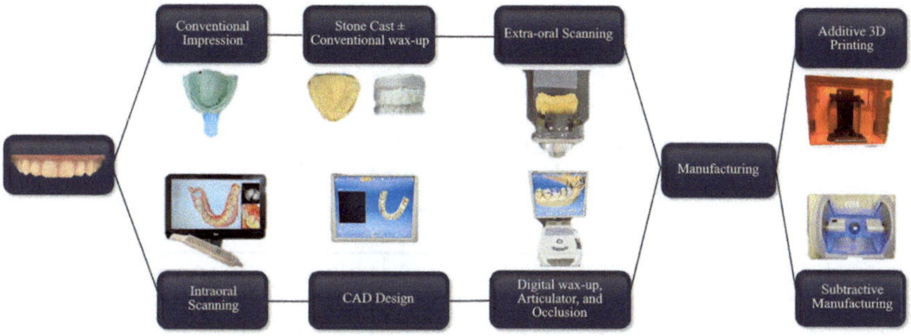

Fig. 7 CAD/CAM-based restorative dental processes and materials with artificial intelligence (Li et al. 2020)

occlusion, jaw movements, and facial features, providing clinicians with an unparalleled level of accuracy in treatment planning and restoration design. Virtual articulators equipped with AI offer dynamic occlusion analysis and facilitate adjustments to optimize masticatory efficiency and occlusal pressure distribution.

AI automates repetitive tasks such as preparation margin detection and undercut designation, streamlining manufacturing workflows. This enhances the efficiency of dental laboratories and ensures consistent quality across restorations. Intelligent systems in CAM also incorporate advanced machining flexibility, accommodating the nuances of different dental materials and restoration designs. Artificial intelligence (AI) plays an emerging role in enhancing the design, fabrication, and application of maxillofacial prostheses by streamlining and optimizing various processes (Yeslam et al. 2024a).

5.1 *Digital Planning and Design*

AI assists in analyzing imaging data obtained from magnetic resonance imaging (MRI) or computed tomography (CT) scans to create detailed 3D models of the patient's soft and hard tissues. These models are integral to the precise planning and customization of prostheses.

5.2 *Integration with CAD/CAM Technology*

AI-powered tools embedded in CAD/CAM systems enable the automated design of prostheses by interpreting anatomical data. AI can also facilitate the use of digital libraries to select or adapt preexisting forms for immediate prosthesis creation, reducing design time.

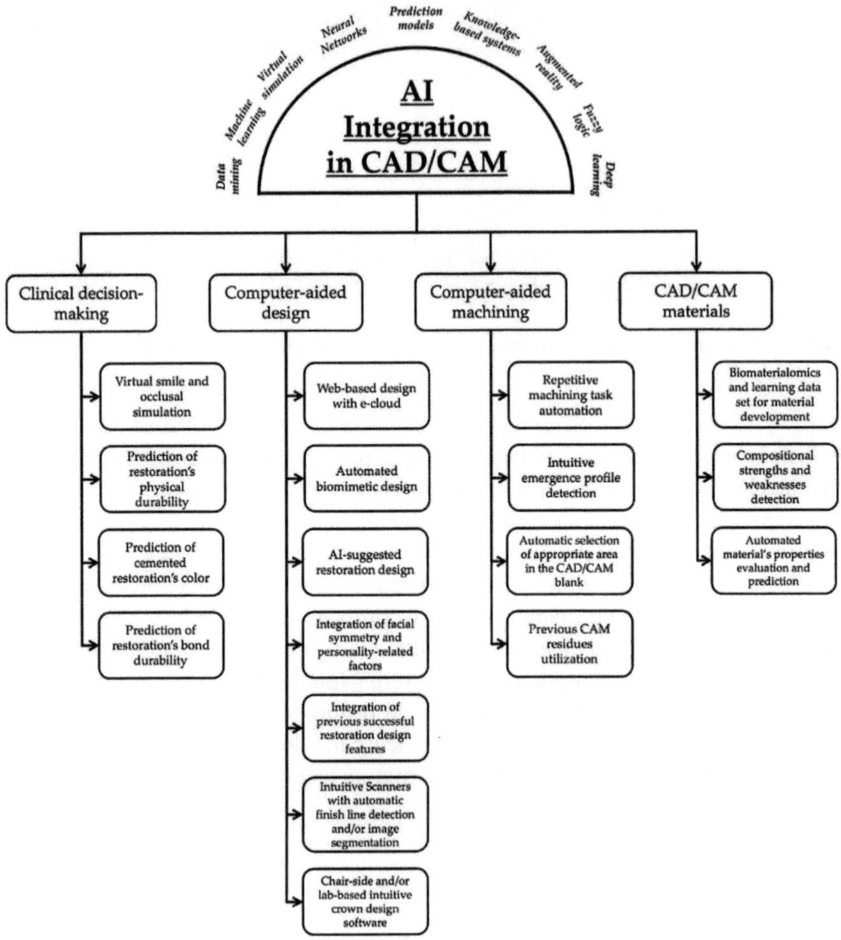

Fig. 8 AI integration in CAD/CAM

5.3 Rapid Prototyping and Refinement

AI enhances rapid prototyping (RP) techniques by improving the accuracy of 3D-printed models. These models serve as the basis for prosthetic fabrication, ensuring high precision in fit and function.

5.4 Automation in Aesthetic Adjustments

AI algorithms can predict and simulate skin curvature, which aids in the customization of prostheses. While final manual adjustments are still required, AI reduces the extent of hand carving by providing a more accurate starting point.

5.5 Efficiency and Time-Saving

AI significantly reduces the overall time required for prosthesis design and production by automating repetitive tasks and leveraging predictive modeling. By integrating AI with imaging, design, and manufacturing technologies, the field of maxillofacial prosthetics achieves greater precision, efficiency, and customization, ultimately improving patient outcomes.

Steps in Fabrication Using an Optical Facial Scanner and 3D Printer (Park et al. 2021; Gerhardt et al. 2022).

1. **Scanning**: A noncontact optical 3D scanner is used to scan the healthy side of the patient's ear. A mirror image of the scanned ear is created in the software.
2. **Mold Fabrication**: Negative and positive molds are designed using the mirror image. Parallel lines are transferred to the casts, ensuring the accurate placement of the missing ear by referencing the healthy side.
3. **Silicone Mixture**: The platinum room temperature vulcanizing (RTV) silicone elastomer is mixed according to manufacturer's instructions, and the color is matched using an intrinsic coloring system.
4. **Prosthesis Formation**: The silicone mixture was poured into the 3D-printed mold, and a cast was placed onto the mold, aligning the parallel lines. The silicone was left to polymerize at room temperature (Fig. 9).
5. **Mold Separation**: After polymerization, the prosthesis was separated from the mold, with any residual silicone trimmed. An extrinsic coloring kit was used for final color matching.

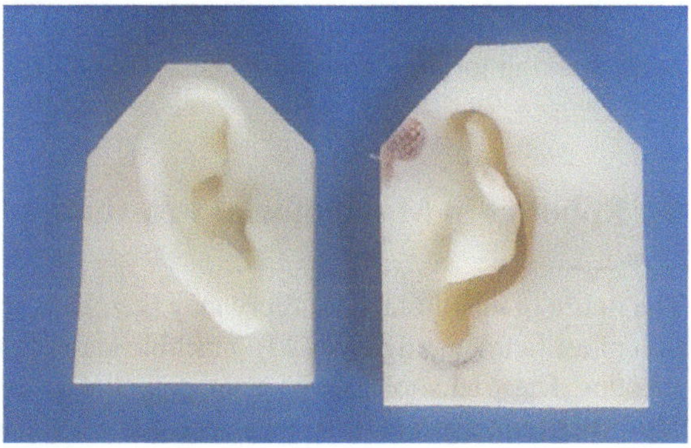

Fig. 9 Silicone mixture poured into 3D model

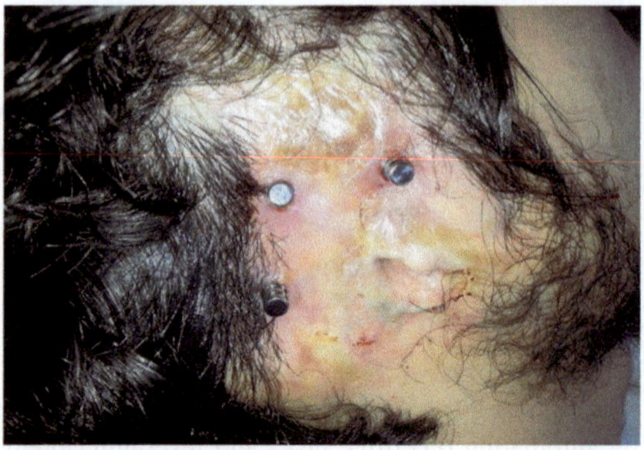

Fig. 10 Implants were placed, and a magnet-retained auricular prosthesis was planned

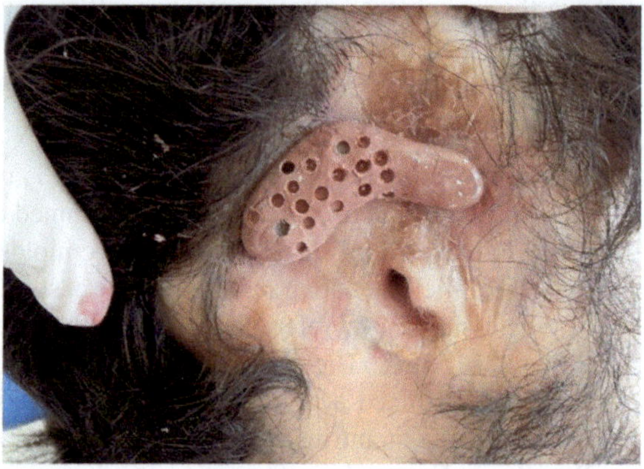

Fig. 11 Retention holes were created for mechanical retention

6. **Magnet Placement**: Implant impression copings are placed, and an impression is made with polyvinyl siloxane (PVS). A stone cast was obtained, and a polymethyl methacrylate framework was fabricated to hold the magnets (Fig. 10).

Acrylic Fabrication: An acrylic mixture (translucent acrylic powder with pigments) was poured over the magnets, excess material was removed, and retention holes were created for mechanical retention (Fig. 11). This acrylic framework served as the backing for the silicone prosthesis (Fig. 12).

6 Robotics in Maxillofacial Prosthetics

The future of maxillofacial surgery may be significantly transformed by the integration of artificial intelligence (AI), machine learning (ML), deep learning (DL), and robotics. These technologies have the potential to revolutionize both the educational and procedural aspects of surgical practice by enhancing accuracy and improving

Fig. 12 Silicone prosthesis placement

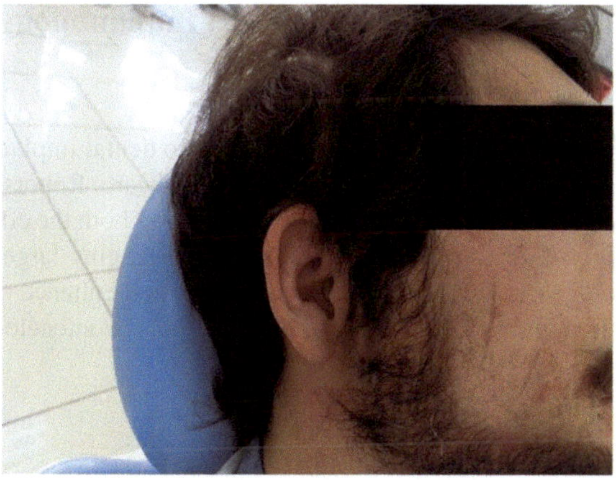

outcomes (Sikri et al. 2023; Hadj Saïd et al. 2020). Robotic-assisted surgery employs systems with robotic arms equipped with surgical instruments, which are controlled via a console operated by the surgeon. This setup translates the surgeon's hand movements into refined robotic actions, allowing greater precision and stability, especially in delicate head and neck operations (Johnson et al. 2023; Lyakhov et al. 2022).

While AI has not surpassed human expertise in surgery, it has shown comparable performance to skilled surgeons in evaluating technical proficiency through computer vision. This indicates a growing potential for AI to contribute to standardized assessments of surgical skills (Bernauer et al. 2021a). AI technologies also support various facets of surgery—ranging from preoperative planning and navigation to real-time decision-making and training. Continued innovation is expected to pave the way for widespread adoption of AI-enhanced robotic systems in maxillofacial procedures. However, as this technology advances, robust frameworks for data protection—including secure storage and disposal—will be necessary to maintain patient confidentiality. Establishing clear guidelines for managing AI-derived data will be key to fostering trust among both clinicians and patients.

Moreover, effective collaboration between healthcare professionals and AI systems will be essential for fully realizing the benefits of these tools. Such synergy could improve diagnostic accuracy, enable personalized treatments, and streamline patient care. If coupled with strict data governance and well-structured cooperation, AI holds immense promise for transforming healthcare delivery and elevating the patient experience (Lee and Jeong 2020; Moufti et al. 2023).

7 AI and Robotics in Oral Implantology and Prosthodontics

The integration of AI and robotics into dental implantology represents a significant advancement in personalized oral healthcare. Robots, guided by precise algorithms, can optimize implant placement, boosting both the effectiveness and longevity of the prosthesis. AI complements this by leveraging large-scale data analysis to support diagnosis, customize treatment plans, and enhance surgical accuracy through real-time feedback and decision-making tools (Fontenele et al. 2023).

7.1 AI-Powered Diagnostics

AI algorithms can interpret the substantial volume of data from CBCT scans, identifying patterns and anomalies in tooth structures that aid in accurate diagnoses (Kwak et al. 2020; Oliveira-Santos et al. 2023; Morgan et al. 2022; Mangano et al. 2023).

7.2 AI in Treatment Planning

General practitioners may lack the expertise needed for detailed implant planning using CBCT data. AI can bridge this gap by autonomously merging CBCT and intraoral scan data to create 3D jaw models. It then plans the restoration and selects the ideal implant for accurate placement, streamlining the design and surgical guide fabrication process (Sakai et al. 2023; Oh et al. 2023). Traditional CAD/CAM methods can introduce errors in cementation and positioning. AI systems help minimize such issues by accurately identifying abutment margins and ensuring proper alignment of zirconia crowns, which has resulted in high survival (91%) and success (93%) rates in clinical studies (Fontenele et al. 2023; Zhang et al. 2023).

7.3 Bone Assessment and Segmentation

AI tools can precisely evaluate bone density and detect potential bone loss using CBCT imagery (Bonny et al. 2023; Altalhi et al. 2023). Comparisons between AI and human-led segmentation show promising accuracy, with AI models performing segmentation tasks much faster. These tools also support anatomical landmark detection, like identifying the mandibular canal with deep learning models (Johnson et al. 2023; Singi et al. 2022b; Ahmad et al. 2021; Leung et al. 2021). Automated sinus segmentation and 3D modeling further enhance surgical planning (Yakin and Linden 2021).

7.4 Augmented Reality and Predictive Modeling

The combination of AI and AR in guided implant surgeries has shown efficiency in simpler cases. Predictive AI models have also demonstrated strong accuracy in estimating primary implant stability and potential treatment outcomes, particularly when supported by preoperative drilling protocols (https://www.coursera.org; Thurzo et al. 2023). Although the body of literature is still limited, early neural network models have shown encouraging results in predicting implant survival with high accuracy, although they are not yet standalone tools (Karnik et al. 2024c; Wolgin et al. 2018). AI has also been explored for detecting peri-implant bone loss and predicting implant failure over five years through clinical and radiographic data integration (Yeslam et al. 2024b; Alshadidi et al. 2023).

7.5 Implant Identification Systems

Identifying implant brands and specifications post-placement remains a challenge, particularly when prior records are unavailable. While online databases and questionnaires exist for manual identification, they are prone to human error. AI-based radiograph analysis—primarily using two-dimensional (2D) images like panoramic or periapical radiographs—has shown high accuracy but requires broader datasets and validation across diverse conditions for consistent results (Morgan et al. 2022; Mangano et al. 2023; Sakai et al. 2023; Oh et al. 2023; Cha et al. 2021; Huang et al. 2022; Leung et al. 2021; Yakin and Linden 2021).

7.6 Design Optimization

AI is being used to enhance implant designs through finite element analysis (FEA), which evaluates mechanical stress at the bone–implant interface. Neural network models have helped reduce interface stress and improve design parameters like implant length and thread geometry. Combining AI with genetic algorithms shows potential in optimizing micro-strain for improved osseointegration (Huang et al. 2022; Zhang et al. 2023; Bonny et al. 2023).

7.7 Robotics in Dental Implantology

Robot-assisted implant surgery relies on precise intraoperative navigation. The first such system was introduced in 2002, followed by advancements like the YOMITM system—approved by the FDA in 2017—which provides physical guidance for implant depth and angle, reducing the need for custom guides. In 2017, fully automated systems capable of performing procedures without human intervention were introduced. However, more research is needed to validate the decision-making capabilities and consistency of robotic systems in real clinical scenarios (Moufti et al. 2023; https://www.coursera.org; Thurzo et al. 2023).

AI-driven planning is reshaping implantology, allowing data-driven decisions and predictive modeling for improved precision. As this field evolves, combining clinical insight with AI tools will continue to enhance treatment outcomes and procedural accuracy (Karnik et al. 2024c).

8 Artificial Intelligence in Prosthodontic Education: A Preview of Educator

The integration of artificial intelligence (AI) in prosthodontic education is an emerging trend that promises to revolutionize how students are taught and trained in this specialized field of dentistry. As AI technologies advance, they offer new possibilities to enhance both theoretical learning and practical skills acquisition for dental students, providing personalized learning experiences, real-time feedback, and simulations of clinical scenarios.

8.1 Applications of AI in Prosthodontic Education

A. Simulation and Virtual Reality (VR)

AI-driven simulation platforms allow students to practice prosthodontic procedures in a virtual environment. These simulations can replicate complex clinical scenarios, such as crown preparation, implant placement, and occlusal analysis. Educators see the advantage of VR and AI in offering a safe, risk-free setting for students to refine their skills, making it an essential tool for skill development and assessment.

Example Tool: DentSim by Simodont (Fig. 13) uses haptic feedback and AI to simulate tactile experiences, helping students refine their manual dexterity.

A study showed 30% improvement in students' crown preparation accuracy after using Simodont compared to traditional methods (Wolgin et al. 2018).

B. Adaptive Learning Platforms and Personalized Learning

AI-powered platforms customize content delivery based on individual student performance. These systems identify gaps in knowledge and adapt teaching methods accordingly. AI can track a student's progress over time, identifying strengths and areas for improvement. Based on these data, AI systems can recommend personalized learning paths and adapt course content to the student's pace and needs. Prosthodontic

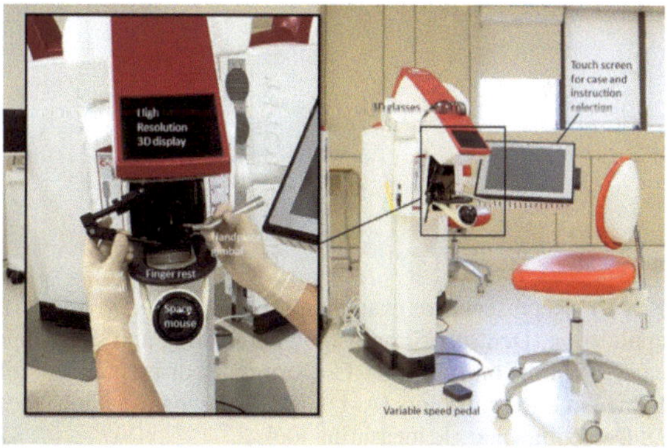

Fig. 13 Components of Simodont

educators are increasingly incorporating AI-driven educational platforms to create a more personalized and dynamic learning experience (Yeslam et al. 2024b). Example Application: Coursera's AI-based algorithms used in dental courses adjust lecture depth and quizzes based on student progress (Alshadidi et al. 2023).

C. AI-Assisted Diagnosis and Treatment Planning

AI can assist students in learning how to diagnose and plan treatment for prosthodontic cases. For example, AI algorithms can analyze radiographic images, such as CT scans or intraoral scans, and suggest treatment options based on patterns observed in large datasets. Educators value this as a tool for teaching students how to interpret complex diagnostic information and make informed clinical decisions (Bernauer et al. 2021b).

AI-based software like *Dentsply Sirona's Primescan* is used in training for real-world applications of digital impressions.

8.2 3Shape Trios Intraoral Scanner with AI

3Shape Trios intraoral scanner with AI captures highly detailed digital impressions using AI for image stitching and defect detection. It teaches students to assess impression quality. It allows exploration of AI-driven occlusal analysis and treatment planning. It reduces material wastage and patient discomfort.

D. Automated Feedback and Assessment

AI systems can provide immediate feedback on students' performance during hands-on exercises or virtual simulations. Educators find that AI-driven assessment tools can objectively evaluate a student's proficiency in various prosthodontic tasks, providing valuable insights into areas of strength and weakness. This feedback can be used to tailor individualized learning plans for students.

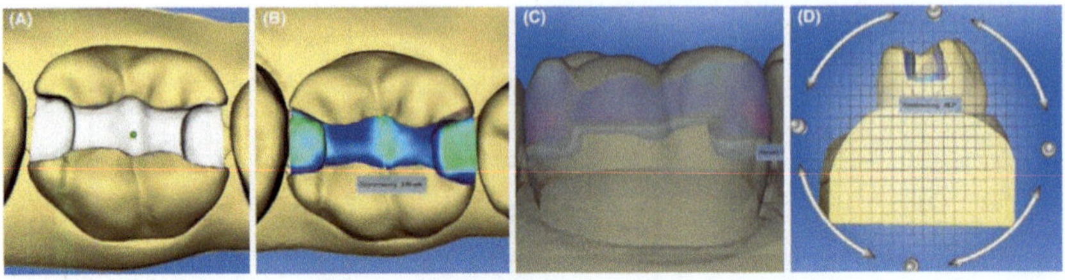

Fig. 14 Representative example of a sample cavity from different perspectives. The PrepCheck application (Dentsply Sirona) allows a layering and superimposition of the sample and the master cavity (sample on approval). Conformity or discrepancy of different values is automatically highlighted in different colors (A–D). B, Displaying a distance measuring tool of the CEREC software. D, Depicting an angle measuring tool

Tools like PrepCheck by Dentsply Sirona (Fig. 14) evaluate preparation dimensions, taper, undercut, and finish lines. It provides numerical scores and visual feedback (Li et al. 2020).

E. Automation in Laboratory Work

CAD/CAM systems, supported by AI, allow students to design and fabricate prostheses with high precision. Automated generation of digital wax-ups and guided adjustments to optimize occlusal forces. AI enhances the learning curve for manual skills by providing guided instructions during the design process.

Case Example: AI in CAD/CAM software, such as Exocad, guides students in designing complex implant-supported prostheses.

Exocad Dental CAD: Exocad dental CAD is AI-powered design tools for creating crowns, bridges, implants, and removable dentures. It enhances student understanding of digital prosthetic design workflows and enables exploration of patient-specific anatomical considerations. It reduces fabrication errors by providing real-time design validation. It bridges the gap between theory and clinical practice in digital prosthodontics (Puleio et al. 2024).

F. Research and Data-Driven Insights

AI tools like machine learning algorithms process large datasets from clinical studies, enabling students to analyze trends in prosthodontic failures or successes and predict patient-specific outcomes based on treatment variables (Iosif et al. 2024).

Example: AI tools like Waikato Environment for Knowledge Analysis (Weka) are used for research-driven learning in prosthodontics.

8.3 Simulated Implant Planning

Tool Used: Nobel Clinician by Nobel BioCare (AI-enhanced implant planning software).

Forty dental students practiced implant placement in edentulous and partially edentulous cases. AI guided students through bone density analysis, nerve mapping, and implant angulation.

For example, the use of AI-driven systems for dental implant placement has been shown to improve precision in both virtual planning and real-time procedures. Research on AI applications, such as in radiographic analysis or CAD software for designing prosthetics, has demonstrated significant advantages in accuracy and reduced errors (Puleio et al. 2024). One study found that AI could be used for precise 3D implant planning, which likely contributes to better patient outcomes by optimizing implant positioning (Iosif et al. 2024).

8.4 *VR and AI in Complete Denture Fabrication*

The integration of HoloLens AR with AI overlay for denture design represents a significant advancement in dental education and clinical practice. In this approach, students and practitioners use augmented reality (AR) to visualize holographic models of dentures, guided by AI to assist with design adjustments. Specifically, during maxillary denture try-ins, this system overlays real-time error visualization such as overextensions, undercuts, or other potential fitting issues directly onto the model, giving immediate feedback to the user. This technology has shown promising results in enhancing learning and reducing errors in denture fabrication.

Improved Confidence and Learning: A study revealed that 90% of students reported a significant increase in confidence when fabricating dentures using this AR and AI-driven system. The interactive feedback mechanism helps students better understand their mistakes and make adjustments quickly.

Reduced Clinical Errors: Objective metrics from first-year clinical denture cases showed a 40% reduction in errors during denture try-ins, demonstrating the system's effectiveness in improving the accuracy of initial designs. By providing visual feedback during the try-in process, the system helps identify and correct potential issues before proceeding with final fabrication.

This combination of AR and AI offers a powerful tool for teaching, as well as for clinical applications, by reducing error rates and improving the speed and accuracy of the denture creation process, thus optimizing patient outcomes. It provides both immersive learning environments and real-time clinical support, contributing to more confident practitioners and better-quality prosthodontics (Li et al. 2020).

8.5 *Benefits of AI in Prosthodontic Education*

A. Enhanced Learning Efficiency

AI can help streamline the learning process by providing instant feedback and personalized content. This allows students to spend more time on areas that need improvement, making their learning experience more efficient and targeted. Educators believe that AI can shorten the learning curve, allowing students to progress more quickly (Bernauer et al. 2021b).

B. Increased Accessibility

AI-driven platforms can make prosthodontic education more accessible to students, especially in underserved regions. Virtual simulations, online learning modules, and AI-assisted teaching tools can be accessed remotely, allowing students to learn at their convenience. This can be particularly beneficial for students in geographically remote areas or those who have scheduling constraints.

C. Improved Accuracy and Objectivity

AI systems offer a high level of accuracy and consistency in assessments, which can reduce human bias in evaluating students' performance. By automating repetitive tasks such as grading, AI ensures that assessments are standardized, leading to fairer evaluations (Karnik et al. 2024c).

D. Bridging the Gap Between Theory and Practice

AI's ability to integrate theoretical knowledge with practical applications helps bridge the gap between classroom learning and clinical practice. Educators appreciate how AI can present real-world clinical situations for students to solve, thus preparing them for actual patient care in a way that traditional methods cannot (Yakin and Linden 2021).

8.6 Challenges and Concerns

Despite the many benefits, the integration of AI in prosthodontic education also comes with several challenges and concerns:

A. Lack of Human Touch

Prosthodontics, like other dental fields, requires hands-on, patient-centered care. While AI can simulate clinical scenarios, educators worry that it cannot replace the experience and empathy needed when treating real patients. Clinical experience remains crucial for developing communication skills and learning the subtleties of patient management.

B. Resistance to Change

Some educators may resist adopting AI in the curriculum due to concerns about its complexity, the need for training, or skepticism about its ability to replicate the human experience of teaching and mentoring. Resistance to technological changes can slow down the integration of AI into educational settings.

C. Ethical and Privacy Concerns

The use of AI in education raises ethical issues such as data privacy, especially when dealing with sensitive patient data for training purposes. The potential for data breaches or misuse of personal information requires careful consideration and adherence to privacy regulations.

D. Costs and Accessibility

The implementation of AI in prosthodontic education may involve significant financial investment in software, hardware, and faculty training. While the technology promises long-term benefits, its high initial cost can be a barrier for some institutions, especially in developing countries (Thurzo et al. 2023).

8.7 Future Directions

As AI technology continues to evolve, its role in prosthodontic education will likely expand. Future trends may include the development of more advanced AI tools for diagnosing and planning complex prosthodontic cases, further integration with augmented reality (AR) for hands-on training, and the use of machine learning to predict student success and personalize learning even further.

8.8 Future Directions in AI for Prosthodontic Education

Hybrid AI Models: Combining AI with Internet of Things (IoT) (e.g., smart dental chairs) for real-time training and monitoring.

AI-Assisted Patient Interaction Training: Simulations incorporating conversational AI to train students in patient communication during prosthodontic procedures.

AI-Driven Interoperability: Seamless integration of AI tools across educational and clinical platforms for continuity in training and practice (Zhang et al. 2023).

9 Conclusion

The integration of AI in prosthodontic education holds great promise, with many educators recognizing its potential to enhance learning, improve clinical skills, and create more personalized educational experiences. However, it is important to address the challenges related to ethical considerations, the cost of implementation, and the balance between AI and human interaction in the learning process. The future of prosthodontic education is likely to see an increasing role for AI, provided that its application is thoughtfully integrated into curricula, with ongoing support for both educators and students. Gao et al. (2020, Logozzo et al. (2014), Otani et al. (2015), Richert et al. (2017), Yang et al. (2022).

References

Ahmad P, Alam MK, Aldajani A, Alahmari A, Alanazi A, Stoddart M et al (2021) Dental robotics: a disruptive technology. Sensors 21(10):3308. https://doi.org/10.3390/s21103308

Ali IE, Tanikawa C, Chikai M, Ino S, Sumita Y, Wakabayashi N (2024) Applications and performance of artificial intelligence models in removable prosthodontics: a literature review. J Prosthodont Res 68(3):358–367

Alshadidi AAF, Alshahrani AA, Aldosari LIN, Chaturvedi S, Saini RS, Hassan SAB, Cicciù M, Minervini G (2023) Investigation on the application of artificial intelligence in prosthodontics. Appl Sci 13:5004. https://doi.org/10.3390/app13085004

Altalhi AM, Alharbi FS, Alhodaithy MA et al (2023) The impact of artificial intelligence on dental implantology: a narrative review. Cureus 15(10):e47941. https://doi.org/10.7759/cureus.47941

Bernauer SA, Zitzmann NU, Joda T (2021a) The use and performance of artificial intelligence in prosthodontics: a systematic review. Sensors 21(19):6628. https://doi.org/10.3390/s21196628

Bernauer SA, Zitzmann NU, Joda T (2021b) The use and performance of artificial intelligence in prosthodontics: a systematic review. Sensors 21:6628. https://doi.org/10.3390/s21196628

Bonny T, Al Nassan W, Obaideen K, Al Mallahi MN, Mohammad Y, El-Damanhoury HM (2023) Contemporary role and applications of artificial intelligence in dentistry. F1000Research 12:1179

Cevik A, Kocacikli G (2019) Three-dimensional printing technologies in the fabrication of maxillofacial prosthesis: a case report. Int J Artif Organs 42(9):527–532

Cha JY, Yoon HI, Yeo IS, Huh KH, Han JS (2021) Peri-implant bone loss measurement using a region-based convolutional neural network on dental periapical radiographs. J Clin Med 10:1009. https://doi.org/10.3390/jcm10051009

Doshi KN, Sathe S, Dubey SA, Bhoyar A, Dhamande M, Jaiswal T (2024) A comprehensive review on virtual articulators. Cureus

Fontenele RC, Gerhardt MD, Picoli FF et al (2023) Convolutional neural network-based automated maxillary alveolar bone segmentation on cone-beam computed tomography images. Clin Oral Implants Res 34:565–574. https://doi.org/10.1111/clr.14063

Gao J, Li C, Liu C, Lin F, Yu J, Yu H (2020) A stereolithographic template for computer-assisted teeth preparation in dental esthetic ceramic veneer treatment. J Esthet Restor Dent 32(6):1–7

Gerhardt MDN, Fontenele RC, Leite AF, Lahoud P, Van Gerven A, Willems H et al (2022) Automated detection and labelling of teeth and small edentulous regions on cone-beam computed tomography using convolutional neural networks. J Dent 122(7):104139. https://doi.org/10.1016/j.jdent.2022.104139

Hadj Saïd M, Le Roux MK, Catherine JH, Lan R (2020) Development of an artificial intelligence model to identify a dental implant from a radiograph. Int J Oral Maxillofac Implants 36(6):1077–1082. https://doi.org/10.0.11607/jomi.8060

https://www.coursera.org/learn/ai-and-machine-learning-algorithms-andtechniques?msockid=17a114fc3fe167123c2606cf3e7a66e7

Huang N, Liu P, Yan Y et al (2022) Predicting the risk of dental implant loss using deep learning. J Clin Periodontol 49:872–883. https://doi.org/10.1111/jcpe.13689

Iosif L, Tâncu, AMC, Amza OE, Gheorghe GF, Dimitriu B, Imre M (2024) AI in prosthodontics: a narrative review bridging established knowledge and innovation gaps across regions and emerging frontiers. Prosthesis 6:1281–1299. https://doi.org/10.3390/prosthesis6060092

Jiang F, Jiang Y, Zhi H, Dong Y, Li H, Ma S, Wang Y, Dong Q, Shen H, Wang Y (2017) Artificial intelligence in healthcare: past, present and future. Stroke Vasc Neurol 2:230–243

Johnson L, Upadhyay P, Mishra S (2023) Dentronics, robotics, artificial intelligence and its application in dentistry. Eur Chem Bull 12:2630–2645. https://doi.org/10.48047/ecb/2023.12.7.204 2023.19/06/2023

Karnik AP, Chhajer H, Venkatesh SB (2024) Transforming prosthodontics and oral implantology using robotics and artificial intelligence. Front Oral Health 5

Karnik AP, Chhajer H, Venkatesh SB (2024b) Transforming prosthodontics and oral implantology using robotics and artificial intelligence. Front Oral Health 5:1442100. https://doi.org/10.3389/froh.2024.1442100

Karnik AP, Chhajer H, Venkatesh SB (2024c) Transforming Prosthodontics and oral implantology using robotics and artificial intelligence. Front Oral Health 5:1442100. https://doi.org/10.3389/froh.2024.1442100

Kong HJ, Kim (2024) Application of artificial intelligence in dental crown prosthesis: a scoping review. BMC Oral Health

Koralakunte PR, Aljanakh M (2014) The role of virtual articulator in prosthetic and restorative dentistry. J Clin Diagn Res 8(7)

Kordass B and Gartner Ch. The virtual articulator—concept and development of VR-tools to analyse the dysfunction of dental occlusion. International Congress Series Volume 1230, June 2001, Pages 689-694

Kwak GH, Kwak EJ, Song JM et al (2020) Automatic mandibular canal detection using a deep convolutional neural network. Sci Rep 10:5711. https://doi.org/10.1038/s41598-020-62586-8

Lee JH, Jeong SN (2020) Efficacy of deep convolutional neural network algorithm for the identification and classification of dental implant systems, using panoramic and periapical radiographs: a pilot study. Medicine (Baltimore) 99(26):e20787. https://doi.org/10.1097/MD.0000000000020787

Leung AL-S, Yeung C, Chu S, Wong AW-Y, Yu OY, Chu C-H (2021) Use of computer simulation in dental training with special reference to simodont. Dent J 9:125. https://doi.org/10.3390/dj9110125

Li J, Chen Z, Dong B et al (2020) Registering maxillomandibular relation to create a virtual patient integrated with a virtual articulator for complex implant rehabilitation: a clinical report. J Prosthodont

Lo Russo L, Salamini A (2018) Single-arch digital removable complete denture: a workflow that starts from the intraoral scan. J Prosthet Dent 120(1):20–24

Logozzo S, Zanetti EM, Franceschini G, Kilpelä A, Mäkynen A (2014) Recent advances in dental optics—part I: 3D intraoral scanners for restorative dentistry. Opt Lasers Eng 54:203–221

Lyakhov PA, Dolgalev AA, Lyakhova UA, Muraev AA, Zolotayev KE, Semerikov DY (2022) Neural network system for analyzing statistical factors of patients for predicting the survival of dental implants. Front Neuroinform 16:1067040. https://doi.org/10.3389/fninf.2022.1067040

Mangano FG, Admakin O, Lerner H, Mangano C (2023) Artificial intelligence and augmented reality for guided implant surgery planning: a proof of concept. J Dent 133:104485

Marinello CP, Brugger R (2021) Digital removable complete denture—an overview. Current oral health reports, vol 8. Springer Science and Business Media, pp 117–31

Morgan N, Van Gerven A, Smolders A, de Faria VK, Willems H, Jacobs R (2022) Convolutional neural network for automatic maxillary sinus segmentation on cone-beam computed tomographic images. Sci Rep 12:7523. https://doi.org/10.1038/s41598-022-11483-3

Moufti MA, Trabulsi N, Ghousheh M, Fattal T, Ashira A, Danishvar S (2023) Developing an artificial intelligence solution to autosegment the edentulous mandibular bone for implant planning. Eur J Dent. https://doi.org/10.1055/s0043-1764425

Murdoch B (2021) Privacy and artificial intelligence: challenges for protecting health information in a new era. BMC Med Ethics 22:122

Oh S, Kim YJ, Kim J, Jung JH, Lim HJ, Kim BC, Kim KG (2023) Deep learning-based prediction of osseointegration for dental implant using plain radiography. BMC Oral Health 23:208. https://doi.org/10.1186/s12903-023-02921-3

Oliveira-Santos N, Jacobs R, Picoli FF, Lahoud P, Niclaes L, Groppo FC (2023) Automated segmentation of the mandibular canal and its anterior loop by deep learning. Sci Rep 13:10819. https://doi.org/10.1038/s41598-023-37798-3

Otani T, Raigrodski AJ, Mancl L, Kanuma I, Rosen J (2015) In vitro evaluation of accuracy and precision of automated robotic tooth preparation system for porcelain laminate veneers. J Prosthet Dent 114(2):229–235

Park SH, Han K (2018) Methodologic guide for evaluating clinical performance and effect of artificial intelligence technology for medical diagnosis and prediction. Radiology 286:800–809

Park SH, Choi J, Byeon J-S (2021) Key principles of clinical validation, device approval, and insurance coverage decisions of artificial intelligence. Korean J Radiol 22:442–453

Polizzi A, Quinzi V, Lo Giudice A, Marzo G, Leonardi R, Isola G (2024) Accuracy of artificial intelligence models in the prediction of periodontitis: a systematic review. JDR Clin Transl Res

Puleio F, Tosco V, Pirri R, Simeone M, Monterubbianesi R, Lo Giudice G, Lo Giudice R (2024) Augmented reality in dentistry: enhancing precision in clinical procedures—a systematic review. Clin Pract 14:2267–2283. https://doi.org/10.3390/clinpract14060178

Putra RH, Doi C, Yoda N, Astuti ER, Sasaki K (2022) Current applications and development of artificial intelligence for digital dental radiography. Dentomaxillofacial Radiol 51

Richert R, Goujat A, Venet L, Viguie G, Viennot S, Robinson P, Farges JC, Fages M, Ducret M (2017) Intraoral scanner technologies: a review to make a successful impression. J Healthc Eng 2017:8427595. https://doi.org/10.1155/2017/8427595

Sakai T, Li H, Shimada T et al (2023) Development of artificial intelligence model for supporting implant drilling protocol decision making. J Prosthodont Res 67:360–365. https://doi.org/10.2186/jpr.JPR_D_22_00053

Shah J, Vyas A, Vyas D (2014) The history of robotics in surgical specialties. Am J Robot Surg 1:12–20

Sikri A, Sikri J, Gupta R (2023) Artificial intelligence in prosthodontics and oral implantology—a narrative review. Glob Acad J Dent Oral Health 5(2):13–19. https://doi.org/10.36348/gajdoh.2023.v05i02.001

Silva P, Stanley K, Gardee J (2020) Laminate veneers: preplanning and treatment using digital guided tooth preparation. J Esthet Restor Dent 32(7):1–11

Singi SR, Sathe S, Reche AR, Sibal A, Mantri N (2022a) Extended arm of precision in prosthodontics: artificial intelligence. Cureus

Singi SR, Sathe S, Reche AR, Sibal A, Mantri N (2022b) Extended arm of precision in prosthodontics: artificial intelligence. Cureus 14(11):e30962. https://doi.org/10.7759/cureus.30962

Sonkar A, Jaiswal RK, Dagli N, Patel M, Patel S, Kumar S et al (2023) Advancements and challenges of artificial intelligence in prosthodontics: from diagnosis to treatment planning and future directions. Eur Chem Bull 12(8):4136–4142

Sreelekshmi S, Varghese K, Abraham JP, Jaysa JJ (2017) Applications of robotics in prosthodontics—a review. https://www.ijiras.com

Thomas PA, Krishnamoorthi D, Mohan J, Raju R, Rajajayam S, Venkatesan S (2022) Digital smile design. J Pharm Bioallied Sci

Thurzo A, Strunga M, Urban R, Surovková J, Afrashtehfar KI (2023) Impact of artificial intelligence on dental education: a review and guide for curriculum update. Educ Sci 13:150. https://doi.org/10.3390/educsci13020150

Wolgin M, Grabowski S, Elhadad S, Frank W, Kielbassa AM (2018) Comparison of a prepCheck-supported self-assessment concept with conventional faculty supervision in a pre-clinical simulation environment. Eur J Dent Educ 22(3):e522–e529. https://doi.org/10.1111/eje.12337

Yakin M, Linden K (2021) Adaptive e-learning platforms can improve student performance and engagement in dental education. https://doi.org/10.1002/jdd.12609

Yang JH, Goodman ED, Dawes AJ, Gahagan JV, Esquivel MM, Liebert CA, Kin C, Yeung S, Gurland BH (2022) Using AI and computer vision to analyze technical proficiency in robotic surgery. Surg Endosc 37:3010–3017

Yeslam HE, Freifrau von Maltzahn N, Nassar HM (2024a) Revolutionizing CAD/CAM-based restorative dental processes and materials with artificial intelligence: a concise narrative review. PeerJ 12:e17793. https://doi.org/10.7717/peerj.17793

Yeslam HE, Freifrau von Maltzahn N, Nassar HM (2024) Revolutionizing CAD/CAM-based restorative dental processes and materials with artificial intelligence: a concise narrative review. PeerJ 12:e17793 https://doi.org/10.7717/peerj.17793

Zhang C, Fan L, Zhang S, Zhao J, Gu Y (2023) Deep learning based dental implant failure prediction from periapical and panoramic films. Quant Imaging Med Surg 13:935–45. https://doi.org/10.21037/qims-22-457

[illegible]

Application of Artificial Intelligence in Implantology

Ragavi Alagarsamy, Babu Lal, Jitendra Chawla, and Hariram Sankar

1 Introduction

Dental implants provide a permanent, biomechanically integrated replacement that mimics natural dentition in both form and function (Duong et al. 2000; Boven et al. 2015). The field of prosthetic rehabilitation with dental implants has witnessed exponential advancement through the integration of digital dentistry, profoundly impacting patient care and clinical outcomes. Dental implant placement is an intricate procedure that demands meticulous planning. The treatment plan serves as a blueprint and roadmap that determines the prognosis and overall success of the dental implants. Recent advances in digital technology and artificial intelligence (AI) have demonstrated a significant escalation in procedure success, as evidenced by emerging literature, through strategic pretreatment planning and increased surgical precision (Schwendicke et al. 2025).

Effective treatment planning is more than mere placement of an implant. Multiple domains of clinical assessment are required for successful implant placement. The clinician evaluation must encompass a detailed history, examination, advanced

R. Alagarsamy (✉)
Department of Oral and Maxillofacial Surgery, Maulana Azad Institute of Dental Sciences, New Delhi, India
e-mail: drragavialagar@gmail.com

B. Lal
Department of Trauma and Emergency Medicine, All India Institute of Medical Sciences, Bhopal, India
e-mail: blsoni.tem@aiimsbhopal.edu.in

J. Chawla
Department of Dentistry, All India Institute of Medical Sciences, Mangalagiri, Andhra Pradesh, India

H. Sankar
Department of Dentistry, All India Institute of Medical Sciences, Bathinda, India

A. Gupta et al. (eds.), *Application of Robotics in Dentistry*, Lecture Notes in Bioengineering, https://doi.org/10.1007/978-981-95-1470-0_11

imaging, strategic planning, and prosthetic considerations. Each implant represents a calculated intervention demanding meticulous presurgical planning and exceptional technical execution. A tailored approach to each patient helps achieve anatomic, aesthetic, and functional requirements, ultimately enhancing the quality of life.

Traditional implant planning consists of clinical evaluation of both edentulous area assessment and patient's systemic health for potential case selection, followed by manual analysis of two-dimensional radiographs, navigating complex anatomy, considering bone density, volume, and quality, and identifying anatomical limitations (Juodzbalys and Kubilius 2013). This method has inherent limitations in spatial understanding and predictive accuracy. Freehand placement, while offering flexibility for experienced surgeons, remains highly skill-dependent and carries risks of positional deviations and complications.

With the paralleling advent of imaging techniques and CAD/CAM technologies, computer-assisted implant surgery (CAIS) was introduced comprising static (s-CAIS) and dynamic (d-CAIS) navigation techniques (Sankar et al. 2025). Static templates emerged as sophisticated tools enabling preplanning, which were initially fabricated by clinicians and later advanced through three-dimensional (3D)-printed guides. These guides, created through computer-aided design and manufacturing, allowed precise transferring of preoperative digital plans into surgical execution. They significantly reduced intraoperative time and uncertainties by providing predetermined drilling trajectories and depth measurements. However, the depth of drilling was not controlled.

Dynamic surgical navigation systems subsequently emerged, introducing real-time tracking capabilities (Panchal et al. 2019). Unlike static guides, these systems offered intraoperative feedback, allowing surgeons to visualize their positioning relative to preplanned trajectories (Yao et al. 2025). Optical or electromagnetic technologies enabled continuous monitoring, enhanced surgical precision, and reduced potential human error.

Artificial intelligence represents the most recent revolutionary paradigm in implant planning and execution (Altalhi et al. 2023). The intersection of artificial intelligence and dental implant planning emerges as a transformative frontier and has negated the continued complexity in this field. This assists in augmentation of clinician's decision, identification of risk factors, and reduction of failures due to biological and mechanical reasons. Virtual and augmented reality technologies complement the use of AI in research, implant training, and patient education.

Robotics and artificial intelligence are revolutionizing dental implantology by enhancing precision, predictability, and patient outcomes (Sankar et al. 2025). The introduction of AI-driven robotic-assisted implant surgery (r-CAIS) enables computer-guided surgical interventions with millimeter-level accuracy, allowing for minimally invasive procedures and optimal implant placement (Fortin et al. 2002). While challenges such as cost and training persist, AI-driven implantology is set to redefine surgical standards, bridging the gap between automation and human expertise.

This chapter explores the intricate landscape of artificial intelligence in dental implantology—analyzing current technological capabilities and projecting future innovative trajectories that promise to redefine dental surgical interventions.

2 AI in Implant Planning

Preplanning the implant placement has traditionally relied on clinical expertise and is subjective decision-making. Automation and standardization of planning aspect have been feasible with advent of AI aiding in surgical precision and efficiency. AI models have been employed in automation of critical steps such as patient selection, radiographic analysis, implant positioning, drilling protocols, and bone augmentation procedures.

2.1 Patient Selection: Clinical Evaluation and Risk Assessment

The success of implant therapy depends heavily on proper patient selection. AI models analyze large datasets to identify patients at higher risk for implant failure by evaluating systemic health conditions such as diabetes, smoking, osteoporosis, and cardiovascular diseases (Alharbi and Almutiq 2022). Machine learning (ML) algorithms process clinical and radiographic data to stratify patients based on individualized risk profiles, allowing for personalized treatment planning. These AI-driven assessments enable clinicians to preemptively modify treatment approaches, such as altering implant positioning or opting for additional procedures like bone grafting, to improve prognosis.

2.2 Radiographic Imaging and Bone Quality Assessment

AI-powered image analysis enhances radiographic interpretation by automating segmentation of anatomical structures, including the mandibular canal, maxillary sinus, and adjacent teeth. Kurt Bayrakdar et al. (2021) developed a deep learning (DL) model that successfully detected vital anatomical landmarks, such as sinuses and the inferior alveolar nerve, demonstrating its potential for improving preoperative implant assessments (Kurt Bayrakdar et al. 2021).

Deep learning models trained on cone-beam computed tomography (CBCT) and periapical radiographs provide highly accurate assessments of bone mineral density, cortical thickness, and ridge morphology, enabling precise preoperative evaluation. Fontenele et al. (2023) reported that AI-based bone segmentation tools were 116 times faster than manual segmentation, significantly reducing planning time. AI's ability to detect subtle variations in bone quality helps clinicians determine the ideal implant site and anticipate the need for bone augmentation, ridge expansion, or sinus lifting procedures (Fontenele et al. 2023).

Despite these advancements, CBCT-based bone quality assessment remains susceptible to image artifacts and variations in gray values. Further research is needed to improve AI models' ability to standardize bone density interpretation across different imaging modalities.

2.3 Implant Positioning: Length, Width, and Orientation

Optimal implant positioning is crucial for ensuring long-term stability, prosthetic compatibility, and aesthetic outcomes (Kopp et al. 2003). AI-driven virtual implant planning systems integrate CBCT, intraoral scans (IOS), and digital impressions to generate 3D models of the patient's dentition. These models assist in determining implant length, diameter, orientation, and angulation, ensuring proper load distribution and minimizing biomechanical complications. Mangano et al. (2023) demonstrated that AI-assisted planning improved the alignment of CBCT segmentation and intraoral digital scanning, optimizing implant positioning accuracy (Mangano et al. 2023).

Several studies have demonstrated AI's effectiveness in automating implant placement recommendations. Roongruangsilp et al. (2021) investigated AI's learning curve for posterior maxillary implant planning, concluding that AI-based decision support improved implant positioning while maintaining high interpretability (2021). However, while AI enhances preoperative planning, real-time intraoperative adjustments still require clinician expertise, particularly in cases involving anatomical variations or unexpected surgical challenges.

2.4 Number of Implants and Drilling Protocol Optimization

Determining the appropriate number of implants for full-arch or multi-unit restorations is another area where AI has shown promise. AI-based models analyze occlusal forces, bone density, and prosthetic requirements to recommend the optimal number and distribution of implants, reducing the risk of overload and prosthetic failures. Lyakhov et al. (2022) proposed an AI-based decision support system that could predict single implant survival rates, providing invaluable knowledge about long-term implant success (Lyakhov et al. 2022).

Additionally, AI has been integrated into drilling protocol optimization, where ML algorithms suggest drilling sequences tailored to individual patients based on bone density and implant dimensions. Takahiko et al. (2023) demonstrated that AI-based prediction models can effectively determine the correct drilling protocol before surgery, improving primary stability and reducing surgical complications (Sakai et al. 2023).

2.5 *Immediate Placement, Sinus Augmentation, and Ridge Splitting*

AI has significantly impacted immediate implant placement protocols, where implants are inserted at the time of tooth extraction. Predictive modeling helps clinicians assess socket morphology, residual bone volume, and primary stability potential, enabling real-time decision support for immediate loading cases. Chen et al. (2024) assessed AI-assisted implant planning software and found that higher bone density correlated with increased implant deviations, emphasizing the importance of AI-guided surgical precision (Chen et al. 2024).

For sinus augmentation and ridge splitting, AI can assist in preoperative assessment by analyzing bone deficiencies and predicting the success rates of grafting procedures. AI-driven planning software provides virtual simulations of sinus lift procedures, ensuring proper graft volume estimation and minimizing risks associated with sinus perforation.

3 AI in Implant Design

The design optimization of dental implants is possible by leveraging finite element analysis. They help in enhancing the mechanical behavior of implant systems by simulating stress distribution and biomechanical interactions (Chang et al. 2018). Li et al. used computational modeling to evaluate stress at the bone–implant interface. By meticulously analyzing parameters like implant length, thread length, and thread pitch, their model resulted in a 36.6% reduction in interface stress compared to conventional design (Li et al. 2018).

Furthermore, studies have integrated artificial neural networks (ANNs) and genetic algorithms to optimize the microstrain at the implant–bone junction by simultaneously modifying the design parameters, including length, porosity, and diameter (Roy et al. 2018). Neural networks have been employed for measuring the elastic modulus of the bone–implant interface, facilitating design changes (Zaw et al. 2009). All these contribute to a more precise, data-driven approach in implant designing, simulating loading forces, identifying regions of mechanical failure, and refining implant geometry iteratively. Future research should focus on continuous validation of AI-enhanced design frameworks through experimental studies and clinical trials to ensure the long-term efficacy and durability of optimized implant systems.

4 AI in Dental Implant Placement

Artificial intelligence (AI) plays a crucial role in implant placement by enhancing precision, efficiency, and patient outcomes. During surgery, robotic-assisted systems provide real-time guidance, reducing errors and improving procedural success. AI-powered predictive analytics assess patient data to anticipate complications, while advanced diagnostics evaluate bone density and tissue conditions for optimal implant selection.

The precise 3D placement of implants is the foundation of prosthetically driven implant dentistry. By seamlessly integrating treatment planning with decision-making, AI enhances precision and efficiency in implant placement. Robotics, driven by AI's ability to analyze vast datasets, further refines diagnosis, treatment planning, and surgical execution, ultimately leading to better patient outcomes (Altalhi et al. 2023).

4.1 AI in Conventional (Intra-Alveolar) Implant Placement

In implant dentistry, robotics has emerged as an advanced extension of AI, transforming treatment planning and execution. By integrating AI-driven diagnostics, predictive analytics, and real-time surgical guidance, robotics enables highly accurate implant placement with minimal human error, improving precision, which is essential to prevent any complications in both surgical and prosthetic phases. Based on CBCT scans, the implant position is planned by the dentist, and the robotic arm performs the surgery with the dentist observing the procedure in real time—which allows the dentist the flexibility to change any angulations intraoperatively.

The first Food and Drug Administration (FDA)-approved robotic system for dental implant surgery, YOMI, was introduced in 2017. This semi-active system was designed to assist with autonomous drilling and implant placement using a coordinate system mapped onto teeth autonomously. Other dental implant robot systems have been introduced following Yomi's introduction, including the Remebot and Dentibot. Over time, fully automated robotic systems emerged, incorporating presurgical treatment planning, autonomous drilling, and implant placement using advanced tracking and guidance mechanisms. These systems help minimize errors caused by human fatigue and have demonstrated greater accuracy in implant placement. However, dentists maintain oversight throughout the surgical process and can intervene if complications arise, ensuring both precision and patient safety (Jain et al. 2023; Huynh and Mangui 2024).

4.2 AI in Bone Augmentation and Simultaneous Implant Placement

Despite advancements in one-step surgery for alveolar bone augmentation and simultaneous dental implant placement, achieving predictable outcomes remains a significant challenge. Robotic-assisted implant placement has proven effective in complex cases with limited bone height and sinus complications. Using robotic guidance, procedures such as sinus augmentation, lateral window approaches, and closed sinus lifts can be performed with enhanced precision. These systems aid in accurate osteotomy preparation, membrane elevation, and graft placement, ensuring successful implant integration even in challenging anatomical conditions. Postoperative imaging confirms the effectiveness of robotic assistance in achieving stable and predictable outcomes for dental implant procedures.

Dr. Mergelmeyer (2022) documented cases where Yomi robotic guidance was used for complex implant placements, including a 67-year-old patient requiring a lateral window sinus augmentation and a 56-year-old patient undergoing a closed sinus lift with simultaneous implant placement. Both cases demonstrated successful bone augmentation and implant stability, confirming the precision and effectiveness of robotic-assisted surgery (Mergelmeyer 2022).

4.3 AI in Severely Atrophic Edentulous Jaws and Extra-Alveolar Dental Implant Placement

The challenge of rehabilitating atrophic edentulous jaws arises from limited bone quality and quantity, which complicates implant placement for oral surgeons. AI plays a transformative role in full-arch rehabilitation by enhancing the accuracy and predictability of implant placement. In complex cases, such as zygomatic implant placement, AI optimizes positioning and improves surgical safety. Compared to freehand techniques, precision in implant spacing and angulation is ensured by advanced dynamic navigation systems that continuously update instrument positioning during surgery (Lopes et al. 2020).

Armando Lopes, in his case report, detailed the workflow of a new dynamic navigation system for dental implant placement in the rehabilitation of edentulous jaws, emphasizing the critical role of artificial intelligence (AI) in enhancing precision and treatment outcomes. In the first case, a 57-year-old female patient required maxillary full-arch rehabilitation, necessitating a CBCT scan following the placement of fiducial markers. AI-driven DTX Studio Implant Software was employed to assess anatomical conditions and optimize implant positioning (Lopes et al. 2020). The X-Guide system, calibrated with fiducial markers and handpiece tracking, facilitated real-time AI-assisted navigation, ensuring accuracy during osteotomy preparation. Precision drills, guided by AI-generated depth and angulation data, were used to prevent damage to vital anatomical structures. Four NobelParallel CC implants were placed following the All-on-4 concept, achieving angulations of 30–45° and optimal prosthetic alignment. AI integration streamlined data processing, instrument tracking, and intraoperative guidance, significantly reducing human error and improving procedural efficiency.

In the second case, a 70-year-old hypertensive female patient required full-arch rehabilitation after the failure of a previously inserted tilted implant. AI-assisted planning was conducted using CBCT imaging and DTX Studio Implant Software, which facilitated the strategic insertion of a zygomatic implant via the extra-maxillary surgical technique. Unlike the conventional dynamic navigation protocol requiring TriStar screws and an X-Guide receptor, a modified clip was fabricated and fixed onto two anterior implants, simplifying the workflow. AI-enhanced real-time navigation provided continuous tracking of both patient and surgical instruments, ensuring optimal osteotomy preparation while preventing damage to critical anatomical structures. A Nobel Zygoma 0° 45-mm implant was inserted with over 50 N/cm torque, emerging at the second premolar position and anchoring exclusively in the zygomatic bone. A 45° multi-unit abutment was then connected to ensure accurate prosthetic alignment. In both cases, AI played a pivotal role in integrating CBCT data, facilitating precise real-time guidance, and enhancing surgical precision, ultimately improving the safety, efficiency, and success rate of implant placement in edentulous patients (Lopes et al. 2020).

4.4 Navigation Versus Robotics in Implantology: Key Differences

Dynamic guidance systems, including navigation and robotics, eliminate the need for a physical guide. Robotic systems offer additional benefits over navigation systems by providing real-time visual, audio, and haptic feedback to ensure precise implant placement. The robot actively resists movements that deviate from the planned position, allowing the surgeon to guide the handpiece only toward the correct location for accurate osteotomy. In contrast, navigation systems depend entirely on the surgeon's hand–eye coordination, without robotic resistance, to position the implant at the intended site.

4.5 AI and Immersive Reality

Immersive technologies, such as virtual reality (VR), augmented reality (AR), and mixed reality (MR), are revolutionizing how digital and physical environments interact. While AR and MR overlay virtual elements onto the real world, VR creates a fully immersive, computer-generated experience that engages visual, auditory, and other senses. Initially driven by the gaming industry, VR has expanded into dentistry, playing a crucial role in preoperative planning, education, and patient-specific simulations. These innovations enhance learning, improve precision, and provide a more interactive approach to dental procedures.

Precision in implant dentistry is essential, particularly regarding implant type, positioning, and angulation. To ensure accurate placement, surgical guides and navigation systems are commonly used. However, these tools have limitations, such as restricting intraoperative adjustments based on real-time conditions, limiting surgeon access, and interfering with tactile perception and coolant delivery to the target area. Ultimately, surgeons must rely on their anatomical knowledge and experience to make necessary modifications during surgery.

Dynamic navigation systems address some of the mechanical limitations of surgical guides by providing real-time feedback (Younis et al. 2024). However, they require surgeons to shift their focus between the surgical site and a monitor, disrupting hand–eye coordination, affecting precision, and increasing surgical time. Augmented reality-guided navigation offers a potential solution by superimposing 3D images, including the planned path and drill, onto the real surgical environment through head-mounted VR glasses.

Mixed reality further bridges the gap between the real and virtual worlds, creating a continuous feedback loop between the two. By superimposing the surgical field and preoperative planning, MR allows surgeons to "see through" tissues and identify vital anatomical structures during procedures. This technology enables the creation and execution of highly personalized and precise surgical treatment plans with navigation system guidance. MR navigation has the potential to significantly enhance oral implantology by integrating holographic displays with real-time navigation, which improves both accuracy and surgical outcomes (Liu et al. 2023).

5 AI in Implant Prognosis

Predicting the long-term prognosis of dental implants is an essential component of treatment planning, influencing both clinical decisions and patient outcomes (Howe et al. 2019; Wu et al. 2024). The onus is on clinicians to identify and mitigate risks to prevent early and late failures, which can otherwise result in additional costs and complex retreatment procedures. The clinician needs to assess multiple factors including patient-specific health conditions like smoking status, diabetes, vitamin D levels, and hypercholesterolemia, along with anatomical factors like bone quality, primary implant stability, and periodontal health.

Early failures occur before the functional loading, typically within the first few months, and are primarily attributed to the lack of primary stability, osseointegration issues, infection, procedural errors, and systemic factors (Ma et al. 2025; Chrcanovic et al. 2016). Timely intervention is required, as research shows they are twice as common as late failures. Late failures occur after the osseointegration and prosthetic placement and are often due to peri-implantitis, occlusal overload, prosthetic wear, or systemic health deterioration and patient noncompliance (Do et al. 2020; Sakka et al.

2012; Chen et al. 2023). AI has demonstrated potential in detecting the early signs of peri-implantitis through automated radiographic bone loss analysis and identifying patients susceptible to biomechanical overload.

Implant failures generally result from patient-related risk factors, surgical and biomechanical considerations, and postoperative compliance. The subjective nature of traditional prognosis prediction methods has led to variability in treatment outcomes, which emphasizes the need for more standardized and objective approaches. AI models, particularly those based on machine learning (ML) and deep learning (DL) techniques, can process complex patterns in patient data, thereby enhancing predictive accuracy. The ability to assess osseointegration by evaluating bone density and primary stability by AI-driven models have significantly contributed to prognosis prediction (Huang et al. 2022; Oh et al. 2023).

AI can predict the risk of peri-implantitis by integrating information from periodontal and radiographic data, providing early warning to clinicians (Bornes et al. 2023). AI models aid in the detection of peri-implant bone loss, reducing human error in marginal bone assessments (Cha et al. 2021; Liu et al. 2022; Vera et al. 2023; Mameno et al. 2021; Rekawek et al. 2023). Beyond biological factors, AI models can evaluate the mechanical failure risks by considering occlusal forces and prosthetic designs, helping clinicians make more informed decisions regarding implant placement and loading protocols (Alshadidi et al. 2023). Additionally, ML algorithms have transformed risk factor analysis, which can evaluate patient histories on a large scale to quantify the impact of systemic conditions on implant success. Decision-support systems powered by AI further assist clinicians in classifying high-risk patients and tailoring treatment plans accordingly. These advancements have minimized the limitations associated with manual data interpretation, making prognosis prediction more standardized and data-driven.

Huang et al. (2022) trained a deep learning model using CBCT images and achieved an impressive 96.13% accuracy in predicting implant stability, demonstrating the potential of AI in radiographic-based prognosis assessment. However, the study noted that the effectiveness of AI depends on the quality and diversity of training datasets, which calls for further multicenter research to enhance generalizability. Lyakhov et al. (2022) developed a neural network system incorporating clinical risk factors, that achieved a 94.48% accuracy rate in prognosis prediction. While the study successfully integrated both radiographic and patient history data, it lacked external validation, emphasizing the necessity of broader clinical trials. Similarly, Rekawek et al. (2023) compared multiple machine learning models and found that random forest classifiers exhibited the highest predictive performance, with an area under the curve (AUC) of 0.870 for implant failure prediction. This study emphasized the value of feature selection in improving AI-based prognosis models but also highlighted the challenge of dataset variability affecting model performance. Although AI excels at pattern recognition and predictive modeling, the lack of contextual understanding makes it less effective in the incorporation of patient compliance and oral hygiene maintenance, which also impacts the implant success. Hence, the clinician role is entirely not mitigated. The future of prognosis prediction lies in the synergy between AI and clinicians, combining the computational power of machine learning with the nuanced decision-making of experienced practitioners.

6 Role of AI in Dental Implant Detection

With increase in the number of dental implant manufacturers and the expanding variety of designs, identification of the particular implant type has become a significant challenge in modern clinical practice (Sukegawa et al. 2020). Proper identification is essential for appropriate prosthetic rehabilitation, the replacement of components or superstructures, managing complications during long-term follow-up, and for forensic purposes (Hadj Saïd et al. 2020; Greenstein and Cavallaro 1939; Bonfanti-Gris et al. 2025). Treatment histories that span multiple clinical settings, involve different practitioners, or lack precise documentation exacerbate this challenge (Kim et al. 2020).

Traditional implant identification methods have largely relied on manual comparison and limited technological support. Two notable approaches are utilized to address this challenge: a web-based database (www.whatimplantisthat.com) and a characteristic-matching questionnaire developed by Michelinakis et al. (2006). These both methods demand the clinician to visually compare with image, making the process time-consuming and prone to human error. The advent of AI-based detection with deep learning algorithms has brought a potential transformative solution to this diagnostic challenge. The convolutional neural networks (CNNs) do unprecedented feature extraction of the intricate implants, such as shape, texture, and edge morphology. Unlike clinician-driven systems, these computational models can systematically analyze and classify dental implant systems with remarkable precision and objectivity.

Literature evidence has documented that dental implant system identification elicited impressive accuracy rates between 93.8 and 98%. These studies rely on two-dimensional radiographs such as periapical and panoramic. Recent studies have highlighted AI's significant role in improving implant detection accuracy. Lee et al. (2020) demonstrated that deep CNN algorithms could classify implant systems with over 90% accuracy using panoramic and periapical radiographs (Lee et al. 2020). Santos et al. (2021) achieved 99.78% accuracy by analyzing implant surface textures with AI (Mata Santos et al. 2021). Sukegawa et al. (2020) developed a multi-task deep learning model that classified implant brands and treatment stages with an accuracy of 99.08% (Sukegawa et al. 2020). Kim et al. (2020) compared CNN architectures and found that ResNet-50 outperformed others with 98% accuracy (Kim et al. 2020). Hadj Saïd et al. (2020) used GoogLeNet to classify Nobel Biocare, Straumann, and Zimmer Biomet implants with an accuracy of 93.8% (Hadj Saïd et al. 2020). These studies collectively reinforce AI's potential to enhance implant identification, automate classification, and improve clinical decision-making. A systematic review by Dashti et al. further reinforced the superiority of CNN-based algorithms in dental implant brand detection using two-dimensional radiographs. The study achieved a remarkable overall accuracy of 95.63%, with sensitivity at 94.55% and specificity reaching an impressive 97.91% (Dashti et al. 2025).

Among the most promising algorithms, the CNN Multitask ResNet152 achieved the highest reported accuracy of 99.08%. Notably, the deep CNN (Neuro-T version 2.0.1) exhibited near-perfect sensitivity and specificity, particularly excelling in the analysis of the Straumann SLActive Bone Level Tapered (BLT) implant brand.

The role of cone-beam computed tomography (CBCT) remains a subject of debate regarding its use in dental implant system identification due to its limited resolution and sharpness, which may restrict effective image extraction and analysis. Although evidence has demonstrated remarkable accuracy, multicenter data are required to enumerate the full capabilities of AI. Therefore, there is a need to continuously expand datasets to address diversity and enhance accuracy.

Future models based on deep learning should accommodate variations in implant systems across different geographical contexts (Alqutaibi et al. 2023). This approach necessitates a complex understanding of global dental technology landscapes and requires meticulous attention to medical ethics in developing a global implant library and model development. The ultimate vision extends beyond mere technological innovation. By creating robust, ethically developed global dental implant classification systems, artificial intelligence promises to revolutionize patient care, enhance treatment continuity, and offer previously unknown information about implant characteristics and potential complications in clinical practice.

7 AI in Resident Training (AR-/VR-Based Learning)

Cadaveric training remains the gold standard for simulation-based medical education. However, limited accessibility, high costs, and ethical constraints make it difficult. The advent of virtual reality (VR) simulators in the 1990s revolutionized surgical training, offering an immersive, cost-effective, and ethically viable alternative, including in the field of dental implantology (Chahal et al. 2024).

Artificial intelligence (AI) has revolutionized dental implant training by facilitating high-fidelity virtual simulations that enable trainees to practice implant placement, surgical procedures, and treatment planning within a risk-free, controlled environment. These AI-driven platforms provide realistic hands-on experience, allowing trainees to refine their skills while minimizing patient risk. Additionally, AI algorithms can analyze performance metrics, identify areas for improvement, and offer personalized feedback, thereby optimizing the learning process.

VR performance metrics enable trainees to recognize their mistakes and identify areas for improvement. This allows VR learning parameters to be customized to trainees' specific needs, facilitating deliberate practice of essential skills and increasing exposure to both common and low-volume surgical cases. Compared to traditional non-VR training, VR training enhances objective performance in the operating room, reduces operation times, and lowers the number of intraoperative errors (Mao et al. 2021; Toni et al. 2024).

7.1 Applications of AI in Dental Implant Training

1. Virtual Patient Simulations
   AI makes realistic 3D models that mimic real-life clinical scenarios, including variations in bone density and complex anatomical structures. This helps trainees gain hands-on experience in managing challenging implant placements.
2. Haptic Feedback Integration
   AI-powered haptic technology provides a realistic sense of touch by simulating different bone densities and soft tissue resistance. This tactile feedback enhances precision and builds confidence in surgical techniques.
3. Real-Time Performance Analysis
   Advanced AI algorithms assess implant positioning, angulation, and depth, offering immediate feedback. This allows trainees to refine their technique on the spot.
4. Adaptive Learning Pathways
   AI personalizes the learning experience by adjusting difficulty levels based on a trainee's progress. This targeted approach ensures steady skill development at an optimal pace.
5. AI-Assisted Surgical Planning
   By analyzing CBCT scans and patient-specific data, AI generates 3D surgical guides, allowing trainees to plan implant placements virtually before performing procedures on real patients.
6. Error Detection and Corrcction
   AI identifies mistakes, such as improper implant positioning, and suggests corrections in real time. This enhances accuracy and reduces surgical errors.

The use of AR in education enables real-time implant planning and offers crucial surgical information for novice surgeons. AR may also be useful in clinical practice. It is necessary to assess the benefits provided by AR in educational implantology (Bochet et al. 2024).

Advantages of AI-driven dental implant training include improved surgical skills, a faster learning curve, enhanced patient safety, and cost-effective training.

8 AI and Large Language Models (LLMs) for Patient Education

Large language models (LLMs) are advanced computer programs designed to analyze and generate text. They learn from massive amounts of written content and use feedback from humans to recognize language patterns and context. As a result, LLMs can respond to a wide range of questions in a way that sounds natural and human-like (Naveed et al. 2023). Some well-known LLMs include GPT-4.0 by OpenAI, Claude 3.5 Sonnet by Anthropic, and Gemini by Google.

Large language models (LLMs) are transforming patient care in dental implant treatment by enhancing communication, education, and postoperative management (Taymour et al. 2025). From the initial consultation, LLMs can help patients understand their treatment options by providing clear explanations of procedures, benefits, risks, and alternatives. Through interactive simulations and tailored responses, they enable patients to make more informed decisions alongside their dental professionals. Many individuals experience anxiety or doubts about implant surgery, often concerned about pain, longevity, or complications. LLMs serve as an accessible source of information, offering evidence-based answers to common questions. Studies indicate that AI models can provide over 90% accuracy in responding to health-related queries, making them a valuable tool in patient reassurance. However, since AI-generated content may lack personalization, professional review remains essential.

Beyond preoperative education, LLMs play a crucial role in postoperative care by offering step-by-step recovery guidelines, including pain management strategies, dietary restrictions, oral hygiene instructions, and signs of potential complications. Personalized reminders for follow-up visits and medication schedules further enhance patient adherence to aftercare protocols. Long-term maintenance of dental implants is also critical, requiring consistent oral hygiene and regular checkups. LLMs can assist by providing personalized maintenance plans, educating patients on best practices for cleaning around implants, and advising on lifestyle habits that promote implant longevity. Additionally, automated reminders for professional cleanings and examinations ensure ongoing engagement in oral health.

While LLMs offer significant benefits, they also present challenges. Patients may struggle to assess the reliability of AI-generated information, which could lead to misinformation or misinterpretation. Therefore, AI should be used as a supportive tool rather than a substitute for professional guidance. Ethical considerations, including accuracy, readability, and responsible integration into dental care, must be prioritized. With ongoing research and validation, LLMs have the potential to enhance patient engagement, streamline clinical workflows, and improve long-term treatment outcomes, provided they are implemented with human oversight and ethical responsibility (Umer et al. 2024).

9 Robotics in Implantology

The National Aeronautics and Space Administration (NASA) developed a remotely controlled robotic system for performing surgery on astronauts in space and soldiers on the battlefield. The da Vinci robot functions as a master–slave system, where a surgeon's hand movements are transmitted to the robot and replicated on a smaller scale, especially in hard-to-reach areas. The da Vinci robot is primarily used in urology, gynecology, maxillofacial surgery, and transoral robotic surgery. However, da Vinci surgical robots are not suitable for performing osteotomies in dental implant surgery.

Robot-assisted dental surgery combines the physical stability of static guides with the flexibility of image-based dynamic navigation, providing comprehensive guidance to the surgeon during the procedure. The first robot-guided dental implant surgery took place in 2002, where the robot held a surgical stent while the surgeon performed the osteotomy. With advancements in robotics, modern robots now have auxiliary or autonomous drilling capabilities for precise dental implant placement.

The Yomi system features auxiliary drilling capability. Before osteotomy, the handpiece is precisely positioned through a hand-guided initiation process. Once the handpiece and drill reach their final position, the system locks the handpiece in place, allowing only vertical movement while restricting horizontal movement. In this system, both osteotomy and implant placement are performed manually using the robot's operational arm, which, because of its bulk, can limit intraoral access. When the instrument is in the correct position and angle, the robot does not resist, enabling precise and controlled implant placement as planned. Its compatibility with different implant systems and real-time guidance enhances accuracy and efficiency in dental implant surgeries. If there is any deviation from the preplanned treatment in terms of position, angulation, or depth, the robot intervenes to ensure the planned procedure is followed. The surgeon can modify the implant position at any point during the surgery. The system provides haptic guidance while maintaining a clear view of the surgical site and allowing easy access for instruments and irrigation. This balance of guidance, control, and flexibility enables the surgeon to make necessary adjustments while ensuring precise implant placement (Sarhan et al. 2024).

The dental implant robot developed by the Air Force Medical University of China is a fully automated system that can simultaneously perform osteotomy and implant placement according to the treatment plan using an optical navigation system. Compared to the auxiliary drilling capability of the Yomi robot, this system offers superior precision by reducing manual errors and increasing placement accuracy (Sankar et al. 2025).

Robot-assisted dental surgery combines the advantages of static guides' physical constraints with the flexibility of image-based dynamic navigation, ensuring optimal precision and control in implant placement.

9.1 Workflow of Robotic-Assisted Implant Placement (Fig. 1)

a. **Patient Preparation and Imaging**

    - Attach **tracking arm** with intraoral splint (tooth-borne or screw-fixated).
    - Take **CBCT scan** with splint in place.

b. **Preoperative Planning**

    - Use **YOMI software** for implant planning.
    - Verify anatomical alignment by touching a **preselected landmark** with a drill tip.

- Choose **registration method**:
  - **Fiducial-based registration** (artificial markers).
  - **Trace registration** (high-contrast structures like teeth).

Registration methods play a crucial role in determining the accuracy and success of surgical outcomes in dynamic implant procedures. **Bone anchorage fiducials** are regarded as the **gold standard** due to their **firm attachment** and **high-contrast visibility** in CT scans, allowing precise alignment between the registration template and anatomical landmarks.

Registration Techniques in Dynamic Implant Surgery (Fig. 2).

1. **Fiducial-Based Registration:**
   - This technique involves placing **radiographic markers** on a **stent worn by the patient** during CBCT imaging.

Fig. 1 Workflow of robotic-assisted implant placement

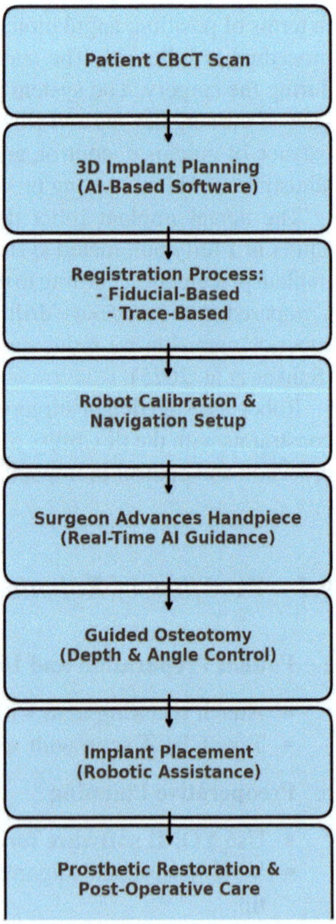

Fig. 2 Registration techniques in dynamic implant surgery

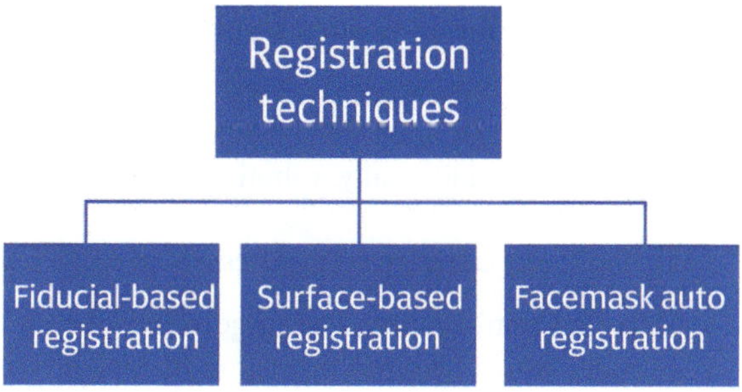

- These markers act as **reference points** for the navigation system, ensuring **alignment between the patient's anatomy and imaging data** throughout the surgery.

2. **Trace Registration:**
   - This method **utilizes high-contrast oral structures** like **teeth or radiopaque restorations** to assist in the registration process.
   - **Optical tracking devices** are attached to either the upper or lower jaw to enable accurate navigation during implant placement.

The selection of a registration method depends on the **surgical case requirements** and **capabilities of the navigation system**. However, recent research suggests that **the choice of registration technique does not significantly affect accuracy in dental implant surgery**.

c. **Navigation System Registration**
   - Sync patient anatomy with preoperative imaging.
   - Align **3D coordinate frames** (X, Y, Z axes).

d. **Surgical Execution**
   - Enter "**guided mode**"—handpiece locks implant axis.
   - Surgeon retains vertical movement control.
   - **Haptic guidance** ensures precise angulation, location, and depth.
   - If deviation occurs, **robot constrains movement**.

e. **Implant Placement and Immediate Loading**
   - Drill proceeds only in the osteotomy axis.
   - Robotic arm **stops drilling at the planned depth**.
   - **Premade prosthetic restoration** can be placed immediately.

f. **Surgeon's Flexibility**
   - Surgeon can modify the implant position **at any time**.
   - Full visualization and access to the surgical site are maintained.

Challenges in Robotic-Guided Implantology

Despite its many advantages, robotic-assisted surgery presents certain challenges. The procedure duration is often longer, and the costs are higher compared to conventional methods. Additionally, robotic surgery requires extensive training due to its steep learning curve.

Liu and Curet categorized these essential skills into two groups:

1. Console Control Skills: The surgeon must be proficient in operating the robotic console, which involves managing bimanual wrist movements, controlling the stereoscopic camera, adjusting the robotic arm, clutching, and activating energy sources simultaneously.
2. Psychomotor Skills: These include depth perception using stereoscopic vision and understanding the force applied through the robotic arm to surgical instruments.

Mastering both sets of skills is crucial for performing precise and efficient robotic-assisted dental implant procedures (Liu et al. 2018).

References

Alharbi MT, Almutiq MM (2022) Prediction of dental implants using machine learning algorithms. J Healthcare Eng 2022:7307675. https://doi.org/10.1155/2022/7307675

Alqutaibi AY, Algabri RS, Elawady D, Ibrahim WI (2023) Advancements in artificial intelligence algorithms for dental implant identification: a systematic review with meta-analysis. J Prosthet Dent. https://doi.org/10.1016/j.prosdent.2023.11.027

Alshadidi AAF, Alshahrani AA, Aldosari LIN, Chaturvedi S, Saini RS, Hassan SA Bin et al (2023) Investigation on the application of artificial intelligence in prosthodontics. Appl Sci 13. https://doi.org/10.3390/app13085004

Altalhi AM, Alharbi FS, Alhodaithy MA, Almarshedy BS, Al-Saaib MY, Al Jfshar RM et al (2023) The impact of artificial intelligence on dental implantology: a narrative review. Cureus 15:e47941. https://doi.org/10.7759/cureus.47941

Bochet Q, Raoul G, Lauwers L, Nicot R (2024) Augmented reality in implantology: virtual surgical checklist and augmented implant placement. J Stomatol Oral Maxillofacial Surgery 125:101813. https://doi.org/10.1016/j.jormas.2024.101813

Bonfanti-Gris M, Ruales E, Salido MP, Martinez-Rus F, Özcan M, Pradies G (2025) Artificial intelligence for dental implant classification and peri-implant pathology identification in 2D radiographs: a systematic review. J Dentistry 153:105533. https://doi.org/10.1016/j.jdent.2024.105533

Bornes RS, Montero J, Correia ARM, Rosa NR das N (2023) Use of bioinformatic strategies as a predictive tool in implant-supported oral rehabilitation: a scoping review. J Prosthetic Dentistry 129:322.e1–322.e8. https://doi.org/10.1016/j.prosdent.2022.12.011

Boven GC, Raghoebar GM, Vissink A, Meijer HJA (2015) Improving masticatory performance, bite force, nutritional state and patient's satisfaction with implant overdentures: a systematic review of the literature. J Oral Rehabil 42:220–233. https://doi.org/10.1111/joor.12241

Cha J-Y, Yoon H-I, Yeo I-S, Huh K-H, Han J-S (2021) Peri-implant bone loss measurement using a region-based convolutional neural network on dental periapical radiographs. J Clin Med 10. https://doi.org/10.3390/jcm10051009

Chahal B, Aydin A, Ahmed K (2024) Virtual reality versus physical models in surgical skills training. An update of the evidence. Current Opin Urolo 34:32–6. https://doi.org/10.1097/MOU.0000000000001145

Chang Y, Tambe AA, Maeda Y, Wada M, Gonda T (2018) Finite element analysis of dental implants with validation: to what extent can we expect the model to predict biological phenomena? A literature review and proposal for classification of a validation process. Int J Implant Dentistry 4:7. https://doi.org/10.1186/s40729-018-0119-5

Chen Z, Liu Y, Xie X, Deng F (2024) Influence of bone density on the accuracy of artificial intelligence-guided implant surgery: an in vitro study. J Prosthet Dent 131:254–261. https://doi.org/10.1016/j.prosdent.2021.07.019

Chen Y-C, Chen M-Y, Chen T-Y, Chan M-L, Huang Y-Y, Liu Y-L et al (2023) Improving dental implant outcomes: CNN-based system accurately measures degree of peri-implantitis damage on periapical film. Bioengineering (Basel, Switzerland) 10. https://doi.org/10.3390/bioengineering10060640

Chrcanovic BR, Kisch J, Albrektsson T, Wennerberg A (2016) Factors influencing early dental implant failures. J Dent Res 95:995–1002. https://doi.org/10.1177/0022034516646098

da Mata Santos RP, Vieira Oliveira Prado HE, Soares Aranha Neto I, Alves de Oliveira GA, Vespasiano Silva AI, Zenóbio EG et al (2021) automated identification of dental implants using artificial intelligence. Int J Oral & Maxillofacial Implants 36:918–23. https://doi.org/10.11607/jomi.8684

Dashti M, Londono J, Ghasemi S, Tabatabaei S, Hashemi S, Baghaei K et al (2025) Evaluation of accuracy of deep learning and conventional neural network algorithms in detection of dental implant type using intraoral radiographic images: a systematic review and meta-analysis. J Prosthet Dent 133:137–146. https://doi.org/10.1016/j.prosdent.2023.11.030

Do TA, Le HS, Shen Y-W, Huang H-L, Fuh L-J (2020) Risk factors related to late failure of dental implant-a systematic review of recent studies. Int J Environ Res Public Health 17. https://doi.org/10.3390/ijerph17113931

Duong H-Y, Roccuzzo A, Stähli A, Salvi GE, Lang NP, Sculean A (2000) Oral health-related quality of life of patients rehabilitated with fixed and removable implant-supported dental prostheses. Periodontol 2022(88):201–237. https://doi.org/10.1111/prd.12419

Fontenele RC, Gerhardt M do N, Picoli FF, Van Gerven A, Nomidis S, Willems H et al (2023) Convolutional neural network-based automated maxillary alveolar bone segmentation on cone-beam computed tomography images. Clin Oral Implants Res 34:565–74. https://doi.org/10.1111/clr.14063

Fortin T, Champleboux G, Bianchi S, Buatois H, Coudert J-L (2002) Precision of transfer of preoperative planning for oral implants based on cone-beam CT-scan images through a robotic drilling machine. Clin Oral Implant Res 13:651–656. https://doi.org/10.1034/j.1600-0501.2002.130612.x

Greenstein G, Cavallaro J (2014) Failed dental implants: diagnosis, removal and survival of reimplantations. J Amer Dental Assoc (1939) 145:835–42. https://doi.org/10.14219/jada.2014.28

Hadj Saïd M, Le Roux M-K, Catherine J-H, Lan R (2020) Development of an artificial intelligence model to identify a dental implant from a radiograph. Int J Oral Maxillofacial Implants 36:1077–82. https://doi.org/10.11607/jomi.8060

Howe M-S, Keys W, Richards D (2019) Long-term (10-year) dental implant survival: a systematic review and sensitivity meta-analysis. J Dent 84:9–21. https://doi.org/10.1016/j.jdent.2019.03.008

Huang N, Liu P, Yan Y, Xu L, Huang Y, Fu G et al (2022) Predicting the risk of dental implant loss using deep learning. J Clin Periodontol 49:872–883. https://doi.org/10.1111/jcpe.13689

Huynh KP, Mangui G (2024) From tradition to technology: robotic artificial intelligence in dental implantology. Cureus 16:e73340. https://doi.org/10.7759/cureus.73340

Jain S, Sayed ME, Ibraheem WI, Ageeli AA, Gandhi S, Jokhadar HF, et al (2023) Accuracy comparison between robot-assisted dental implant placement and static/dynamic computer-assisted implant surgery: a systematic review and meta-analysis of in vitro studies. Medicina (Kaunas, Lithuania) 60. https://doi.org/10.3390/medicina60010011

Juodzbalys G, Kubilius M (2013) Clinical and radiological classification of the jawbone anatomy in endosseous dental implant treatment. J Oral Maxillofacial Res 4:e2. https://doi.org/10.5037/jomr.2013.4202

Kim J-E, Nam N-E, Shim J-S, Jung Y-H, Cho B-H, Hwang JJ (2020) Transfer learning via deep neural networks for implant fixture system classification using periapical radiographs. J Clin Med 9. https://doi.org/10.3390/jcm9041117

Kopp KC, Koslow AH, Abdo OS (2003) Predictable implant placement with a diagnostic/surgical template and advanced radiographic imaging. J Prosthet Dent 89:611–615. https://doi.org/10.1016/s0022-3913(03)00198-7

Kurt Bayrakdar S, Orhan K, Bayrakdar IS, Bilgir E, Ezhov M, Gusarev M et al (2021) A deep learning approach for dental implant planning in cone-beam computed tomography images. BMC Med Imaging 21:86. https://doi.org/10.1186/s12880-021-00618-z

Lee J-H, Kim Y-T, Lee J-B, Jeong S-N (2020) A performance comparison between automated deep learning and dental professionals in classification of dental implant systems from dental imaging: a multi-center study. Diagnostics (Basel, Switzerland) 10. https://doi.org/10.3390/diagnostics10110910

Li H, Shi M, Liu X, Shi Y (2018) Uncertainty optimization of dental implant based on finite element method, global sensitivity analysis and support vector regression. Proc Inst Mech Eng [h] 233:232–243. https://doi.org/10.1177/0954411918819116

Liu M, Purohit S, Mazanetz J, Allen W, Kreaden US, Curet M (2018) Assessment of Robotic Console Skills (ARCS): construct validity of a novel global rating scale for technical skills in robotically assisted surgery. Surg Endosc 32:526–535. https://doi.org/10.1007/s00464-017-5694-7

Liu M, Wang S, Chen H, Liu Y (2022) A pilot study of a deep learning approach to detect marginal bone loss around implants. BMC Oral Health 22:11. https://doi.org/10.1186/s12903-021-02035-8

Liu L, Wang X, Guan M, Fan Y, Yang Z, Li D et al (2023) A mixed reality-based navigation method for dental implant navigation method: a pilot study. Comput Biol Med 154:106568. https://doi.org/10.1016/j.compbiomed.2023.106568

Lopes A, de Araújo Nobre M, Santos D (2020) The workflow of a new dynamic navigation system for the insertion of dental implants in the rehabilitation of edentulous jaws: report of two cases. J Clin Med 9. https://doi.org/10.3390/jcm9020421

Lyakhov PA, Dolgalev AA, Lyakhova UA, Muraev AA, Zolotayev KE, Semerikov DY (2022) Neural network system for analyzing statistical factors of patients for predicting the survival of dental implants. Front Neuroinform 16:1067040. https://doi.org/10.3389/fninf.2022.1067040

Ma B, Cruz Walma DA, Ferneini EM (2025) Long-term survival of implants placed in earlier failed implant sites. Oral Maxillofac Surg Clin North Am 37:99–108. https://doi.org/10.1016/j.coms.2024.08.008

Mameno T, Wada M, Nozaki K, Takahashi T, Tsujioka Y, Akema S et al (2021) Predictive modeling for peri-implantitis by using machine learning techniques. Sci Rep 11:11090. https://doi.org/10.1038/s41598-021-90642-4

Mangano FG, Admakin O, Lerner H, Mangano C (2023) Artificial intelligence and augmented reality for guided implant surgery planning: a proof of concept. J Dent 133:104485. https://doi.org/10.1016/j.jdent.2023.104485

Mao RQ, Lan L, Kay J, Lohre R, Ayeni OR, Goel DP et al (2021) Immersive virtual reality for surgical training: a systematic review. J Surg Res 268:40–58. https://doi.org/10.1016/j.jss.2021.06.045

Mergelmeyer BJ (2022) Dental implant surgeries with simultaneous sinus augmentation utilizing Yomi robotics, 30–3

Michelinakis G, Sharrock A, Barclay CW (2006) Identification of dental implants through the use of Implant Recognition Software (IRS). Int Dent J 56:203–208. https://doi.org/10.1111/j.1875-595x.2006.tb00095.x

Naveed H, Khan AU, Qiu S, Saqib M, Anwar S, Usman M et al (2023) A comprehensive overview of large language models. ArXiv Preprint ArXiv:230706435 2023

Oh S, Kim YJ, Kim J, Jung JH, Lim HJ, Kim BC et al (2023) Deep learning-based prediction of osseointegration for dental implant using plain radiography. BMC Oral Health 23:208. https://doi.org/10.1186/s12903-023-02921-3

Panchal N, Mahmood L, Retana A, Emery R 3rd (2019) Dynamic navigation for dental implant surgery. Oral Maxillofac Surg Clin North Am 31:539–547. https://doi.org/10.1016/j.coms.2019.08.001

Rekawek P, Herbst EA, Suri A, Ford BP, Rajapakse CS, Panchal N (2023) Machine learning and artificial intelligence: a web-based implant failure and peri-implantitis prediction model for clinicians. Int J Oral Maxillofacial Implants 38:576–582b. https://doi.org/10.11607/jomi.9852

Roongruangsilp P, Khongkhunthian P (2021) The learning curve of artificial intelligence for dental implant treatment planning: a descriptive study. Appl Sci, 11. https://doi.org/10.3390/app112110159

Roy S, Dey S, Khutia N, Roy Chowdhury A, Datta S (2018) Design of patient specific dental implant using FE analysis and computational intelligence techniques. Appl Soft Comput 65:272–9. https://doi.org/10.1016/j.asoc.2018.01.025

Sakai T, Li H, Shimada T, Kita S, Iida M, Lee C et al (2023) Development of artificial intelligence model for supporting implant drilling protocol decision making. J Prosthodont Res 67:360–365. https://doi.org/10.2186/jpr.JPR_D_22_00053

Sakka S, Baroudi K, Nassani MZ (2012) Factors associated with early and late failure of dental implants. J Investig Clin Dent 3:258–261. https://doi.org/10.1111/j.2041-1626.2012.00162.x

Sankar H, Shalini M, Rajagopalan A, Gupta S, Kumar A, Shouket R (2025) Dental implant placement accuracy with robotic surgery compared to free-hand, static and dynamic computer assisted techniques: systematic review and meta-analysis. J Oral Biolo Craniofacial Res 15:69–76. https://doi.org/10.1016/j.jobcr.2024.12.005

Sarhan MM, Ibrahim EA, Ezzelarab S, Marei MK (2024) Navigating the future of guided dental implantology: A scoping review. Int J Med Robot + Comput Assisted Surgery: MRCAS 20:e2627. https://doi.org/10.1002/rcs.2627

Schwendicke F, Mohammad Rahimi H, Tichy A (2025) Artificial Intelligence in prosthodontics. Dental clinics of north America, 69:315–26. https://doi.org/10.1016/j.cden.2024.11.009

Sukegawa S, Yoshii K, Hara T, Yamashita K, Nakano K, Yamamoto N et al (2020) Deep neural networks for dental implant system classification. Biomolecules 10. https://doi.org/10.3390/biom10070984

Taymour N, Fouda SM, Abdelrahaman HH, Hassan MG (2025) Performance of the ChatGPT-3.5, ChatGPT-4, and Google Gemini large language models in responding to dental implantology inquiries. J Prosthetic Dentistry. https://doi.org/10.1016/j.prosdent.2024.12.016

Toni E, Toni E, Fereidooni M, Ayatollahi H (2024) Acceptance and use of extended reality in surgical training: an umbrella review. Syst Rev 13:299. https://doi.org/10.1186/s13643-024-02723-w

Umer F, Batool I, Naved N (2024) Innovation and application of large language models (LLMs) in dentistry—a scoping review. BDJ Open 10:90. https://doi.org/10.1038/s41405-024-00277-6

Vera M, Gómez-Silva MJ, Vera V, López-González CI, Aliaga I, Gascó E et al (2023) Artificial intelligence techniques for automatic detection of peri-implant marginal bone remodeling in intraoral radiographs. J Digit Imaging 36:2259–2277. https://doi.org/10.1007/s10278-023-00880-3

Wu Z, Yu X, Wang F, Xu C (2024) Application of artificial intelligence in dental implant prognosis: a scoping review. J Dentistry 144:104924. https://doi.org/10.1016/j.jdent.2024.104924

Yao Y, Yang R, Lam W, Han X, Yang X (2025) A modified workflow for dynamic navigation implant surgery in fully edentulous patients utilizing a customized patient tracking module. J Stomatol Oral Maxillofacial Surgery, 102292. https://doi.org/10.1016/j.jormas.2025.102292

Younis H, Lv C, Xu B, Zhou H, Du L, Liao L et al (2024) Accuracy of dynamic navigation compared to static surgical guides and the freehand approach in implant placement: a prospective clinical study. Head Face Med 20:30. https://doi.org/10.1186/s13005-024-00433-1

Zaw K, Liu GR, Deng B, Tan KBC (2009) Rapid identification of elastic modulus of the interface tissue on dental implants surfaces using reduced-basis method and a neural network. J Biomechanics 42:634–41. https://doi.org/10.1016/j.jbiomech.2008.12.001

Application of AI in Periodontics

Anushi Mahajan and Ritesh Sood

1 Introduction

In the era of evidence-based dentistry, artificial intelligence (AI) has revolutionized the dental field by improving diagnostic accuracy, personalized treatment planning, enhancing patient engagement, streamlining clinical overflows, and providing predictive analytics for disease progression. Artificial intelligence (AI) is defined as a branch of science and engineering that involves developing a technology by training a computer/computer-controlled software/compute -controlled robot to simulate human intelligence and perform the cognitive tasks. AI involves training of algorithms and systems (Fig. 1).

The primary goals of AI are to perform automated tasks and improve efficiency. This is accomplished by enhanced decision-making. It enables machines to learn from past experiences and thereby mimic human intelligence.

2 AI Software Versus Traditional Software

The functions of traditional software are as follows:

- Input: User provides specific, well-defined data (e.g., name, date, and numbers)
- Processing: Software follows predefined rules and logic to process the input (e.g., if-else statements and loops)

A. Mahajan (✉)
Department of Periodontics, Christian Dental College, Ludhiana, Punjab, India
e-mail: anushimahajan2003@yahoo.co.in; dranushisood@gmail.com

R. Sood
Department of Conservative Dentistry and Endodontics, Rayat Bahra Dental College and Hospital, Mohali, Punjab, India
e-mail: drriteshsood@gmail.com

A. Gupta et al. (eds.), *Application of Robotics in Dentistry*, Lecture Notes in Bioengineering, https://doi.org/10.1007/978-981-95-1470-0_12

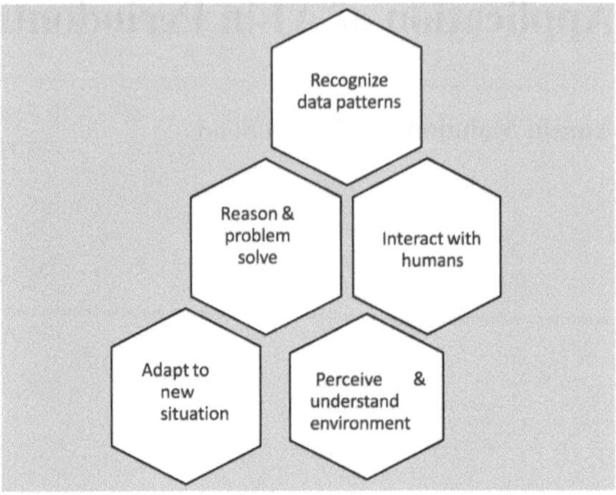

Fig. 1 Areas of training of algorithms and systems in AI

- Output: Software generates a predictable, deterministic output based on the input and rules (e.g., calculated results and printed document).

The functions of an artificial intelligence-based software include the following (Fig. 2):

- Input: User provides data, which may be unstructured, uncertain, or incomplete (e.g., images, text, and sensor readings)
- Processing: AI algorithms analyze the input using statistical models, neural networks, or machine learning techniques to identify patterns and relationships.
- Output: AI generates probabilistic, informed output based on the input and learned patterns (e.g., prediction, classification, and recommendation).

In periodontics, the input data can be in the form of

(a) Photographs, radiographs, and ultrasound images for diagnosis of periodontal diseases

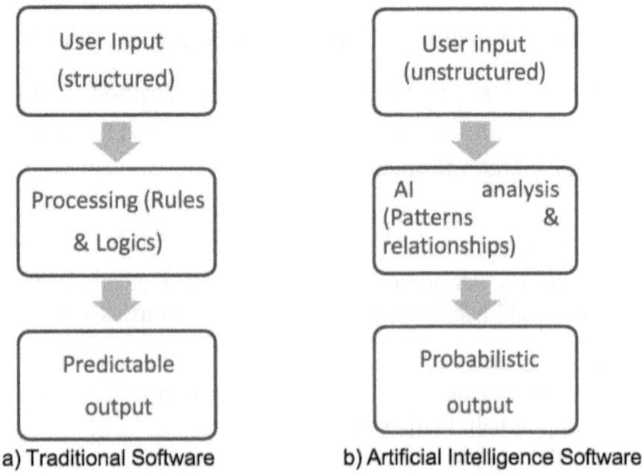

Fig. 2 Flowchart depicting difference between **a** traditional software and **b** artificial intelligence software

(b) Patient data (electronic health record) to predict dental/periodontal outcomes
(c) Metabolites and salivary markers to classify, diagnose, and predict dental/periodontal outcomes

3 Artificial Intelligence Applications in Periodontics

Diagnostic Applications: Artificial intelligence helps in timely diagnosis and quick intervention of periodontal diseases. Artificial intelligence carries out image analysis for periodontal disease detection. It involves using computer vision and machine learning algorithms to analyze dental images (Fig. 3). The images could be in the form of radiographs, intraoral scans, cone-beam computed tomography (CBCT), optical coherence tomography, and intraoral photographs. Image analysis techniques that can be incorporated are edge detection (Fig. 4a–d), segmentation, feature extraction, pattern recognition, and deep learning (Fig. 5).

Machine learning is an auxiliary domain of AI that identifies patterns by manually (by humans) extracting data from pooled data (raw, structured data from databases,

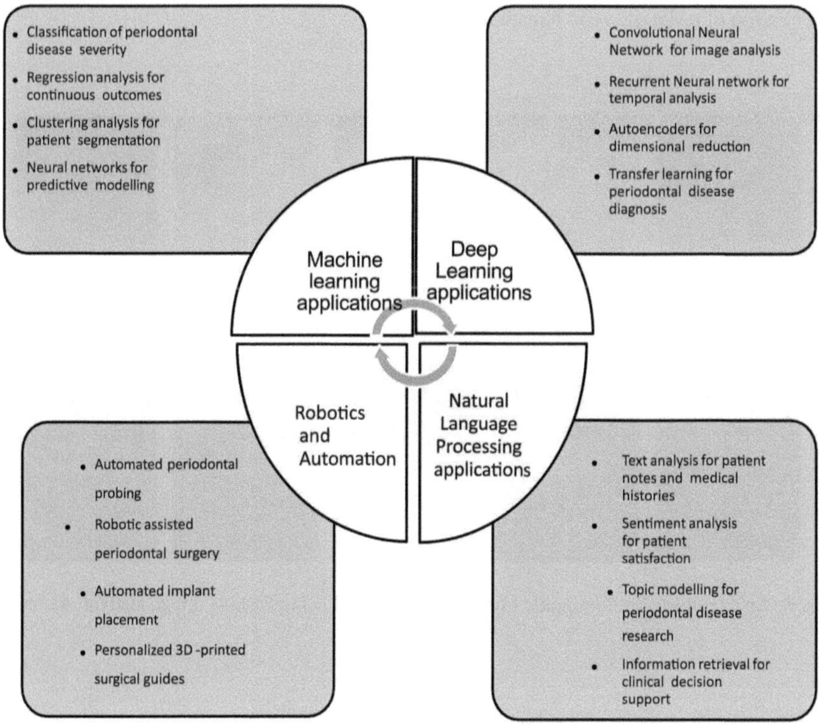

Fig. 3 Key areas of application of AI algorithms in periodontics

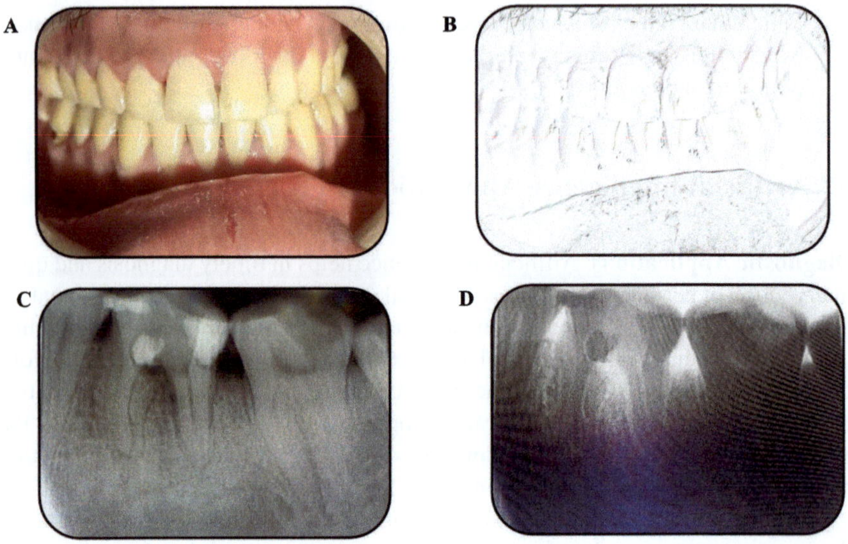

Fig. 4 **a** Original intra-oral picture, **b** Intra-oral image analysis using AI (edge detection feature), **c** Original periapical radiograph (edge detection), **d** Radiographic image analysis using AI. *Note* The contrast of restoration and furcation bone loss

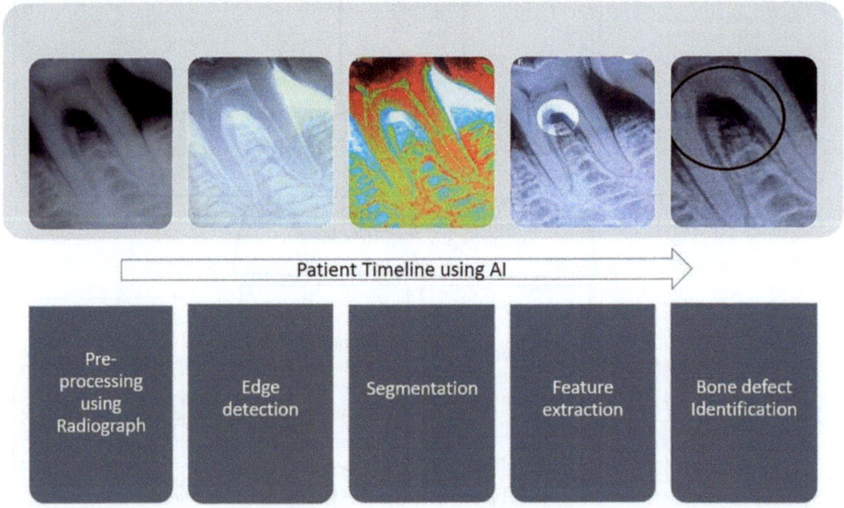

Fig. 5 An example of radiographic image analysis by AI using various image analysis techniques

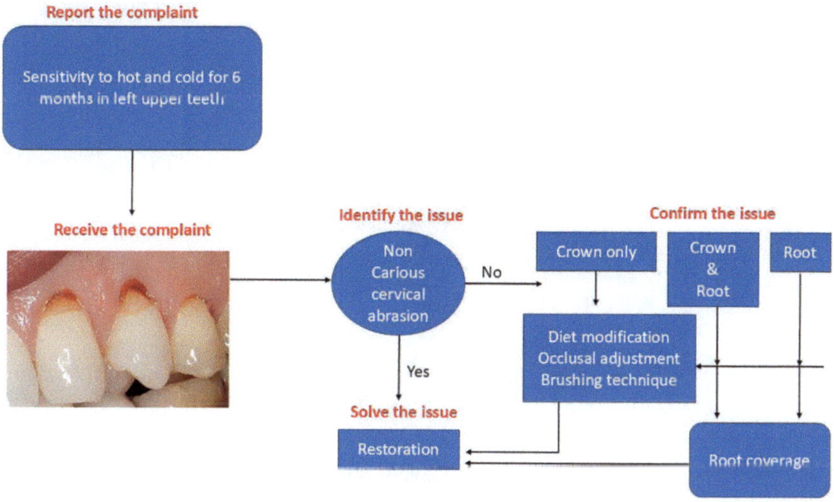

Fig. 6 Example of decision tree in machine learning

tables, etc.), selecting relevant data, and transforming and formatting data (data preprocessing) before feeding to algorithms for analysis (Fig. 6).

Deep learning, a subtype of ML, is inspired by human brain's neural networks, which handles unstructured data (e.g., images, text, and audio) by using computed neural networks to extract data, termed as feature extraction (Fig. 7).

AI assists in detecting gingival recession. It can detect furcation defects and gives an assessment of bone loss.

AI models used on intraoral photographs of patients taken before and after applying plaque disclosing agents showed high sensitivity and specificity in plaque detection (Yuksel et al. 2024).

AI models trained using intraoral photographs with marked gingival sites as healthy, diseased or questionable, accurately identify sites with and without inflammation (Chau et al. 2023). Machine learning classifier used color augmented intraoral photographs to differentiate between healthy and inflamed sites of gingiva (Rana et al. 2017).

Diagnocat is an AI-powered virtual assistant software, designed to screen and analyze data from CBCT and panoramic images and to assist healthcare providers in identifying and diagnosing periodontal disease and detecting intra-bony defects (Ezhov et al. 2021).

Ultrasonographic probe: The fifth generation periodontal probes were first reported in literature by Companion et al. in 1998 (Ramani et al. 2023). In 2009, Rudd et al. used three-dimensional (3D) parallel acoustic finite integration technique (3DPAFITT) software to create two-dimensional (2D) and three-dimensional geometry of tip and periodontal structures to simulate ultrasound echoes corresponding to depth of periodontal pocket (Rudd et al. 2009). AI-assisted features would be automated periodontal pocket detection, real-time pocket depth measurement, bone

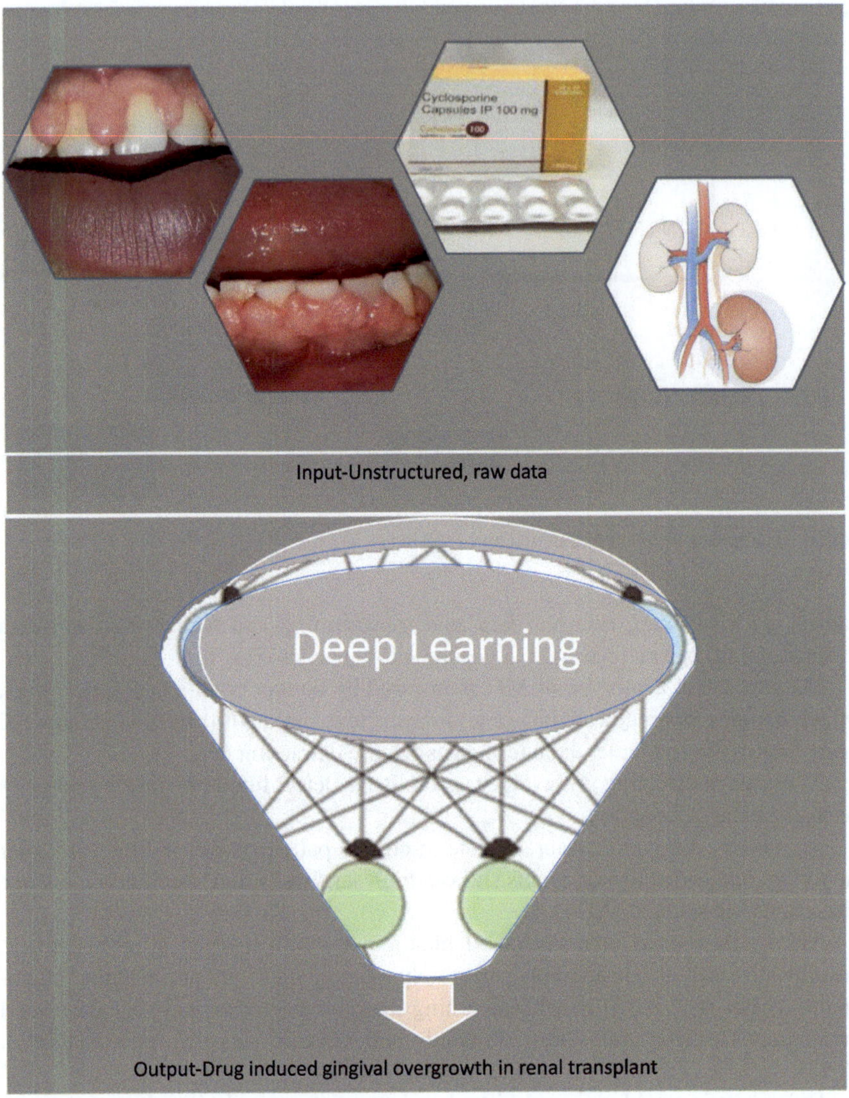

Fig. 7 An example of deep learning through AI

level evaluation, and gingival recession assessment that would be useful in providing personalized treatment plan, once completely developed.

Artificial intelligent olfaction (electric nose) essentially involves an array of AI-powered sensors (based on nanomaterials) and algorithms that detect and analyze the presence of volatile sulfur compounds. Then, pattern recognition is applied to database of breath patterns. A decision tree classifier distinguishes between oral/

extra-oral etiology and correlates it with systemic disease by assessing exhaled breaths (Ramani et al. 2023; Nakhleh et al. 2017).

Predictive modeling: AI can be used to predict periodontal disease susceptibility, treatment outcome, and periodontal disease progression and can also stratify patient's risk to periodontal disease.

Patient stratification: Subgingival biofilm samples are collected from healthy patients and patients with periodontitis. Bacterial species are isolated using DNA-DNA hybridization. Machine learning algorithm (Support vector classifier) on the basis of prevalent bacterial species differentiates between aggressive periodontitis and chronic periodontitis (Feres et al. 2018). Classification of periodontal disease can also be done using artificial neural network and support vector machine and decision tree. Patients are categorized according to risk factors, periodontal status, and radiographic bone loss (Ozden et al. 2015).

Risk assessment: Risk to periodontal disease can be correlated with patient's demographic details and disease-specific factors using machine learning model (random forest regressor) (Moosa et al. 2023). The risk assessment for periodontal disease carried out by using machine learning PRSS AI tool found 70% precision in risk assessment of periodontal disease (Patel et al. 2022).

4 Treatment Planning

Periodontal disease is a multifactorial disease. Periodontal probing, commonly used to diagnose periodontal pockets and degree of clinical attachment loss, is a technique-sensitive procedure, with the drawback of inter-examiner variability. Also, by the time the presence of periodontal pockets is established with the help of probing, the disease has already progressed. Hence, the diagnosis in periodontics is usually dependent on clinical examination and/or risk assessment of the patient, and then, all patients are usually assigned similar treatment strategies under the strata "one-size-fits-all" approach (Schwendicke and Krois 2022). A shortcoming of this kind of randomization is that patient's characteristics and physiologic variations are ignored. This brings the advent **of personalized medicine**.

Personalized medicine in periodontics involves tailoring treatment strategies to individual patients based on their unique genetic, environment, and clinical profiles.

The key components of personalized medicine are as follows:

- Genetic testing—identifying the genetic markers
- Epigenetic analysis—studying gene expression changes influenced by environmental factors
- Microbiome analysis—characterizing oral microbiota composition and function
- Clinical data integration—wherein individual's medical history, lifestyle and environmental factors are incorporated
- Advance diagnostic testing—using biomarkers, imaging, and other diagnostic tools

Personalized medicine holds relevance in assessing individual's risk to periodontal disease, personalized treatment planning, ensuing a targeted therapy, and determining the prognosis. It aids in grouping of patients on the basis of disease severity and their response to treatment, thereby leading to patient stratification (Ginsburg and McCarthy 2001; Giannobile et al. 2013; Wang et al. 2021; Abusleme et al. 2000).

AI's role in personalized medicine is in identifying high-risk patients using machine learning algorithms; stratification of patients, optimizing treatment plan for patients and providing personalized education and monitoring to patients (Pitchika et al. 2000). AI holds a promising role in early detection of periodontal diseases by focusing on biomarkers from the oral microbiome of patients.

Another term that sometimes overlaps with personalized medicine is **precision medicine**. The latter in periodontics focuses on identifying specific biologic markers or mechanisms for periodontal disease susceptibility and emphasizes on targeted therapies using advance diagnostic tools (e.g., genomics and proteomics) (Jameson and Longo 2015).

AI's role in precision medicine is to identify genetic markers for periodontal disease susceptibility, detect specific biologic markers for targeted therapy, and recommend personalized treatment plan based on genetic and biomarker profiles (Pitchika et al. 2000).

AI models have been used to calculate the radiographic bone loss thereby removing the subjective bias of the clinician. Various methods are streamlined to accurately identify the areas of bone loss and its severity; in periapical radiographs, using computer-assisted detection system based on deep convolutional neural network (CNN) algorithm (Alotaibi et al. 2022); on panoramic radiographs, using a combination of deep learning method (DL) and conventional computer assisted design (CAD) (Chang et al. 2020); and on panoramic radiographs, using deep learning tools (Krois et al. 2019).

AI consider patient-specific factors (e.g., bone density and tooth mobility) to optimize treatment strategies. The AI automated simulations predict outcomes for different treatment approaches, thereby helping the clinicians and patients in choosing the appropriate treatment strategy.

5 Clinical Decision-Support Systems

AI plays a promising role in real-time patient monitoring and alerts systems for disease progression. It can recommend various treatment options and help in patient education and engagement.

Machine learning algorithms can be incorporated to salivary metabolites sets to distinguish between different forms of oral diseases. They can distinguish oral cancer from periodontal disease with accuracy (Romm et al. 2020). Deep learning autoencoder used on salivary biomarkers can identify immune subtypes of periodontitis and pivotal immunosuppression genes that discriminate periodontitis from healthy samples (Ning et al. 2021).

AI equips the patients with tailored educational materials, remote consultations (tele-periodontics), and language translational tools. AI-driven technologies (such as virtual reality and augmented reality) and AI platforms enhance patient engagement, comprehension, and satisfaction through personalized content delivery, virtual assistants, tele-dentistry, and gamification (Thorat et al. 2024).

At home, AI-assisted dental monitoring systems use smartphone cameras for intraoral scanning and assessment. Intraoral pictures taken by the patient are evaluated by AI for providing them digital reminders for plaque control and oral hygiene maintenance between the follow-ups (Shen et al. 2022).

6 Robotics in Artificial Intelligence

Integrating AI technologies into robotic systems enhances their capabilities and enables them to perform more complex tasks.

Robotic brushing, also known as automated oral cleaning, uses robotic systems to maintain dental hygiene (Table 1).

A robotic system with a cup-shaped brush head was modified to have long filaments on outer rim for interdental penetration (Braun Oral-B EB-9) by Ernst et al. Tested in vitro on artificial plaque designed on plastic teeth, it successfully removed plaque in 2 min without a dentifrice (Ernst et al. 1985).

They are particularly indicated for patients with physical disabilities and limited manual dexterity. The brushing modes and schedules set in the robotic systems have automated brushing pressure adjustments. They provide real-time feedback and monitoring to the patient in case patient has missed any area for brushing or applies too excessive pressure.

A programmed six-axis robot found to have great plaque removal efficacy than clinical toothbrushing, when performed on artificial teeth covered with plaque-stimulating substrate (Lang et al. 2014).

Robotics in Implantology-Advancements in oral implantology have revolutionized the era of replacing and restoring the function and aesthetics of missing teeth. Static computer-assisted systems prepare a surgical guide for implant placement, whereas computer-assisted implant surgery systems guide in real-time navigation using optical tracking devices and live imaging. Both aid the dentist in placing implants with accuracy compared to free-hand surgery (Pimkhaokham et al. 2000). Yet, the expertise of the dentist plays an important role in manual placement of implants by both the systems. This led to the evolution of robotics systems (Table 2).

Surgical robots improve the precision with which the implants are placed, thereby reducing the human errors with better treatment outcomes (Shi et al. 2024). A robotic system essentially substitutes the dentist's hands with robotic operating platform, eyes with a visual system, and brain with a central control system. Robotic osteotomy deviations of less than 1 mm and angle deviations of 2° or less suggest the technology holds significant promise in implant dentistry (Wu et al. 2019).

Table 1 Examples of a few AI-enabled automated toothbrushes

Automated brushes with AI	Features	Battery charge
Oral B Genius Pro 8000	Has a pressure sensor – Alerts on applying excessive force Syncs with smartphone via Bluetooth – Maintains brushing schedules Six brushing modes – Daily clean, deep clean, whitening, gum care, tongue cleaning 3D cleaning action – 40,000 pulsations/min, 8000 oscillation/min	Charging time: 12 h Brushing charge – Brushing for 2 min, 2 times per day – Battery lasts for 12 h Rechargeable battery up to 2 weeks
Philips Sonicare ProtectiveClean 4100	2-min timer (automatic shut down after 2 min) 30 s pacer for even brushing Audible pressure sensor reduces the number of bristle movements; in case pressure is more while brushing, it alerts by changing the vibration pattern in the handle Brush -sync enabled head with incorporated microchip alerts when the brush head needs to be replaced Sonic technology (31,000 brush strokes/ min)	C Charging time: 24 h Based on 2-min brushing session two times a day, battery lasts for 2 weeks with full charge
Waterpik sensonic professional	Water flossing technology (ten pressure settings); along with Sonic toothbrush technology (30,000 brush strokes/min) Three brushing modes—clean, whiten, and massage Four brush head sizes—standard, compact, plaque control, and orthodontic 2-min brushing timer with a pacer	Charging time -24 h Rechargeable battery up to 2 weeks

(continued)

Table 1 (continued)

Automated brushes with AI	Features	Battery charge
RoboDent Robotic dental cleaning device	Automated robotic arm reaches 180-degree for three cleaning modes—prophylaxis, periodontal, and whitening Advanced computer vision and sensor system Compact, ergonomic design for maneuverability cleaning speed 30,000 brush strokes/min	Charging time: 2 h for full battery Rechargeable battery Wireless charging
BrushMonkey Automated toothbrush	360-degree brushing, Sonic technology7 (30,000 strokes/min)	Charging time: 1.5 h Rechargeable battery (2-week battery life)

It should be noted that the type of robot also determines the surgical operating time. Surgical operating time breakdown being:

- Planning and setup
- Robot calibration
- Implant placement
- Restoration (if applicable)
- Closure

Xu et al. (2023) noted that preoperative planning and setup were maximum in active robots. It included the transfer the drill's spatial position, conduct calibration and registration, and plan the movement of the robotic arm in and out of the mouth. This is contrary in case of dentist-guided passive implant robot which is directed to the osteotomy site by the dentist, thereby reducing the preoperative preparation time.

FDA-approved robotic surgery platform specific to dentistry—the Yomi dental robot (Neosis Inc., Miami, United States)—was cleared for dental implant procedures in 2016. In 2020, FDA cleared the system for the additional indication of full-arch implant treatment. In 2022, it received FDA clearance for bone reduction.

Robotics in Periodontal Microsurgery-Minimally invasive periodontal surgeries refer to the surgical techniques that minimize tissue destruction, promote faster healing, and reduce postoperative discomfort. This concept was first introduced by Fitzpatric and Wickham (Fitzpatrick and Wickham 1990) and later was refined by Hunter and Sackier (1993) (Tibbetts and Shanelec 1998) as "the ability to miniaturize our eyes and extend our hand to perform microscopic and macroscopic operations in places that could previously be reached only by large incisions."

Robotics in periodontal microsurgery aid in better ergonomics (Fig. 8a, b), thereby reducing fatigue and improving precision and dexterity. There is better visualization, minimized trauma, and improved healing outcomes. It increases magnification and resolution, thereby reducing eye strain. They are capable of integrating with digital workflows.

Table 2 Type of dental implant robots and their features depending upon human–robot interaction

Types of implant robots	Autonomy	Human intervention	Sensors	AI algorithms	Examples	Benefits	Limitations
Active	High	None	Advanced	Yes	Yekebot *(YekeBot Technology Co., Ltd, Beijing, China)*	Increased precision Reduced fatigue	High cost Technical complexity
Passive	Low	Required for robot's entry/exit; preparation of osteotomy; implant placement	Simple	No	Yomi *(Neosis Inc., Miami, United States)* DentRobot *(Dcarer Me dical Technology Co.,Ltd, Suzhou, China)*	Low-cost Simplicity	Limited functions Requires human control
Semi-active	Medium	Shared	Advanced	Some	Remebot (Baihui Weikang Technology Co., Ltd, Beijing, China)	Balanced precision and control Reduced fatigue	Higher cost than passive Requires training

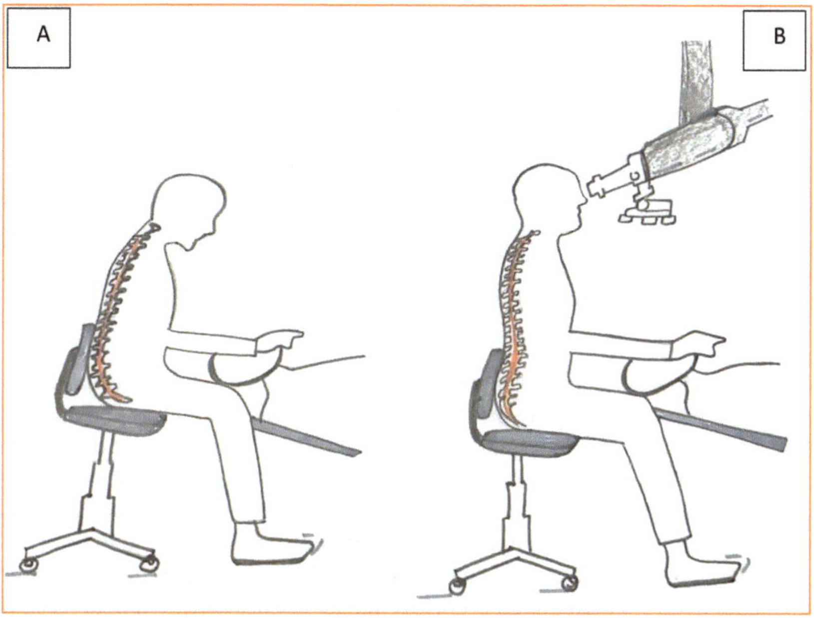

Fig. 8 **a** Ergonomics in traditional dentistry, **b** Ergonomics through robotic-aided microsurgery

Removal of plaque biofilm and calculus with resultant reduction in gingival inflammation was significant after the use of microscopy when compared with traditional SRP (Shanelec 2003; Kuang et al. 2017).

7 ChatGPT in Artificial Intelligence

Chatbot is a software application designed to simulate conversation with the human users, especially over the Internet. It uses text or voice to interact with the users and provides automated patient support and answers frequently asked questions.

ChatGPT is a generative pretrained transformer chatbot tool of artificial intelligence to create humanlike conversation. It is a natural language-processing algorithm and is available through various interfaces: web interface, mobile apps, desktop applications, virtual assistants, and other platforms.

Application of ChatGPT in Periodontics (Fig. 9).

ChatGPT can analyze and visualize patient data to identify trends and patterns. Thereby, it can aid in formulating of clinical diagnosis. Eroglu et al.(Eroglu et al. 2024) found ChatGPT to reasonably determine the stage, grade, and extent of untreated periodontitis, according to the latest 2017 World Workshop Classification of periodontal and peri-implant diseases. They used baseline digital radiographic data

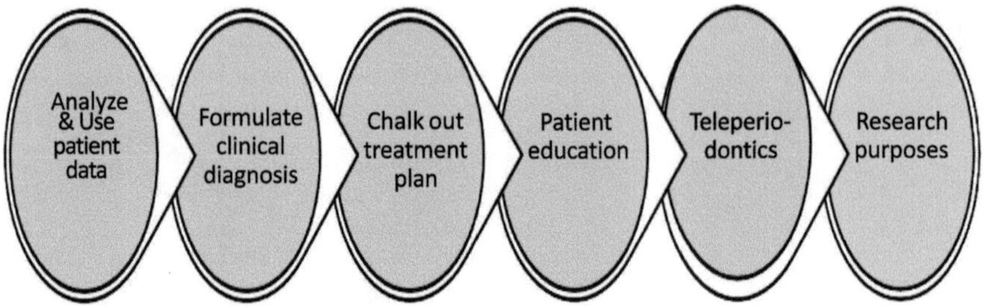

Fig. 9 Role of ChatGPT in periodontics

to compare with standardized reference diagnosis. ChatGPT does not read images, so standardized texts providing information of age, gender, clinical attachment loss in interproximal areas, radiographic bone loss, teeth lost due to periodontitis, probing depth, teeth in occlusion, tooth mobility, amount of biofilm present, and smoking and diabetic status of patient were provided. A separate chat window for each case was created, and grading and staging of periodontitis were achieved through ChatGPT.

Chalking Out the Treatment Plan-Use of ChatGPT is applicable by patients to discuss about various periodontal problems like tooth sensitivity, gingival recession, halitosis, periodontal surgery, dental implants, and peri-implant diseases and was found to give accurate responses (Babayiğit et al. 2023).

ChatGPT assists in patient education and communication by generating patient friendly content (brochures, videos, and frequently asked questions [FAQs]). Alan et al. (2023) evaluated the quality of responses generated by ChatGPT-4 on frequently googled periodontal disease related topics by the patients and found it to be good. However, close monitoring and updating of AI to provide accurate and correct information to the patient. ChatGPT aids in tele-periodontics and remote consultations.

ChatGPT summarizes research papers, identifies key findings, and provide insights. ChatGPT is used by students to complete their assignments (Lee 2023). It is also used by researchers effectively for scientific writing especially for non-native speakers (Eggmann et al. 2023). However, the issue of plagiarism also arises and has been reported during scientific writing. ChatGPT has been found useful in documentation of data and generating effective discharge summaries for the patients (Schwendicke et al. 2023).

8 AI in Dental Education

There has been a paradigm shift in teaching and learning strategies in dental training from teacher-centric, rote-based learning to student-centric, self-directed, simulation-based strategies. Schwendinke et al. (2023) has emphasized the need for change in dental curriculum to adapt to these new strategies. He has outlined four domains of learning outcomes related to artificial intelligence and suggested for these competencies to be achieved by a dental undergraduate.

Haptics and Virtual Reality Simulators-Dentistry is essentially skill-based. Simulation-based teaching has a pivotal role in training of dental graduates in giving them repeated, multiple exposures in a nonthreatening environment in realistic scenarios. "Haptics" refers to a combination of robotics and virtual reality in a simulated environment providing tactile sensitivity to the trainees. It allows for two-way exchange of information between the trainee and the virtual environment.

University of Illinois, Chicago, developed a PerioSim and a periodontal simulator (Steinberg et al. 2003; Luciano et al. 2009) that simulates a periodontal probe, scaler, and explorer. The trainees are able to learn the amount of pressure, angulation, force, etc., to correct their probing technique. Tactile sensitivity to complete removal of plaque and calculus can be mastered using haptic stylus.

Stanford Bio Robotics Laboratory has devised a visuo-haptic simulation of bone surgery that incorporates simulating bone dust, drilling sounds, even a suction, and irrigation (Konukseven et al. 2010).

BONENAVI, a computer-controlled system in Japan, has tried to simulate implant placement and surgical guide fabrication.

Augmented reality is different from virtual reality (Fig. 10). On the one hand, virtual reality (VR) creates a new environment in the form of gaming, training simulations, and virtual tours; augmented reality (AR) enhances the existing environment by blending physical with digital. It is like providing extra information of the object in line of vision, by the use of glasses, tablet, or smartphones.

Augmented reality is related to artificial intelligence, but they are distinct technologies (Fig. 11).

9 Augmented Reality Incorporation into Artificial Intelligence

The realm of dental education, concentrated mainly at tactile learning and hands-on practice, is increasing to an era of immersive and interactive learning environment by means of augmented reality. AR brings about amalgamation of real and virtual world by not only simulating dental procedures but also replicating diverse patient scenarios and giving real-time feedback. It helps in establishing patient-centric, holistic, educational modules which can be a learning opportunity for trainees for their continuous professional development as a teaching–learning and an assessment tool.

Fusion of AI and AR can bring about technological innovations in dental education (Dzyuba et al. 2022) (Fig. 12). Augmented reality (AR)-enabled smart glasses can help trainees visualize complex facial and oral anatomy, and it can help simulate real-life surgeries where interaction between trainees and holographic images is possible. In a few studies (Kivovics et al. 2022; Wang et al. 2019; Dong et al. 2023),

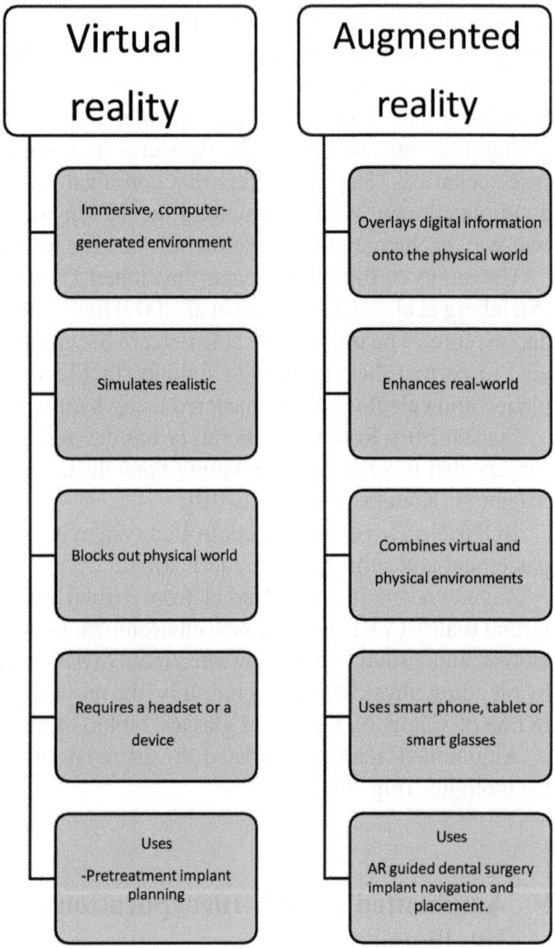

Fig. 10 Differences between virtual reality and augmented reality

AI algorithms have been used with AR-guided navigation in dental implant surgeries. The limitations involve the high investment for technological setup, technique sensitivity, limited content and customization, and enough evidence-based studies to validate its role in periodontics (Kanwal et al. 2024).

Future Trends-Artificial intelligence could be of significance in "***bioprinting***"—reconstruction of soft and hard tissues lost due to accidental or pathological conditions. It could be utilized in tissue engineering for generating 3D models of periodontal tissues, predicting tissue integration, simulating tissue growth and regeneration, and designing personalized tissue scaffolds. Bioprinting is based on inkjet printing/laser printing. It uses computed tomography (CT)/ CBCT scans to create 3D models of bone defects. Software generates design for tissue constructs (Gao et al. 2014).

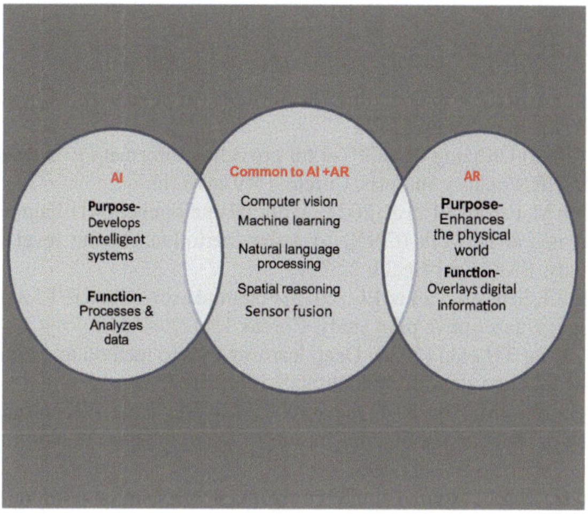

Fig. 11 Comparison of technologies of AI and AR

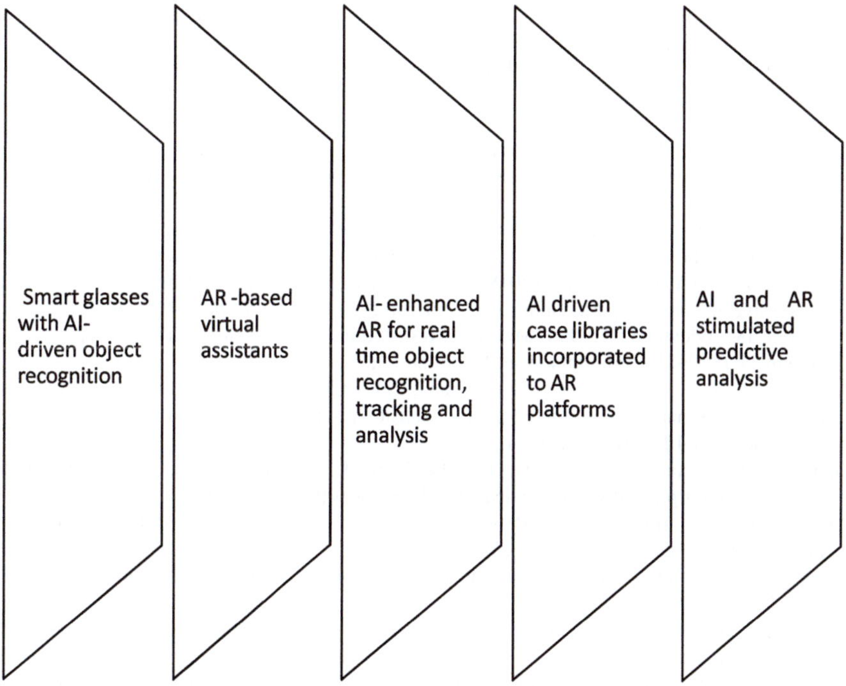

Fig. 12 Fusion of AI and AR

References

Abusleme L, Hoare A, Hong BY, Diaz PI (2021) Microbial signatures of health, gingivitis, and periodontitis. Periodontol 86(1): 57–78

Alan R, Alan BM (2023) Utilizing ChatGPT-4 for providing information on periodontal disease to patients: A DISCERN quality analysis. Cureus 15(9):e46213

Alotaibi G, Awawdeh M, Farook FF et al (2022) Artificial intelligence (AI) diagnostic tools: utilizing a convolutional neural network (CNN) to assess periodontal bone level radiographically-a retrospective study. BMC Oral Health 22:399

Babayiğit O, Eroglu ZT, Sen DO, Yarkac FU (2023) Potential use of ChatGPT for patient information in periodontology: a descriptive pilot study. Cureus 15(11):e48518

Chang HJ, Lee SJ, Yong TH et al (2020) Deep learning hybrid method to automatically diagnose periodontal bone loss and stage periodontitis. Sci Rep 10:7531

Chau RCW, Li GH, Tew IM, Thu KM, McGrath C, Lo WL, Ling WK, Hsung RT, Lam WYH (2023) Accuracy of artificial intelligence-based photographic detection of gingivitis. Int Dent J 73(5):724–730

Dong S, Du C, He B, Zhu Z, Han D, Jin W et al (2023) Application of an effective marker-less augmented reality image guidance method in dental implant surgery. Int J Med Robot 19:e2523

Dzyuba N, Jandu J, Yates J, Kushnerev E (2022) Virtual and augmented reality in dental education: The good, the bad and the better. Eur J Dent Educ Published online: Nov 6, 2022

Eggmann F, Weiger R, Zitzmann NU, Blatz MB (2023) Implications of large language models such as ChatGPT for dental medicine. J Esthet Restor Dent, 1–5

Ernst CP, Willershausen B, Driesen G, Warren PR, Hilfinger P (1997) A robot system for evaluating plaque removal efficiency of toothbrushes in vitro. Quintessence International (Berlin, Germany: 1985) 28(7):441–445

Eroglu ZT, Babayigit O, Sen DO, Yarkac FU (2024) Performance of Chat GPT in classifying periodontitis according to 2018 classification of periodontal diseases. Clin Oral Investig 28(7):407

Ezhov M, Gusarev M, Golitsyna M, Yates JM, Kushnerev E, Tamimi D et al (2021) Clinically applicable artificial intelligence system for dental diagnosis with CBCT. Sci Rep 11:15006

Feres M, Louzoun Y, Haber S et al (2018) Support vector machine-based differentiation between aggressive and chronic periodontitis using microbial profiles. Int Dent J 68:39–46

Fitzpatrick JM, Wickham JE (1990) Minimally invasive surgery. Br J Surg 77(7):721–722

Flemming TF (1999) Periodontitis. Ann Periodontol 4:32

Gao G, Schilling AF, Yonezawa T, Wang J, Dai G, Cui X (2014) Bioactive nanoparticles stimulate bone tissue formation in bioprinted three-dimensional scaffold and human mesenchymal stem cells. Biotechnol J 9(10):1304–1311

Giannobile WV, Braun TM, Caplis AK, Doucette-Stamm L, Duff GW, Kornman KS (2013) Patient stratification for preventive care in dentistry. J Dent Res 92(8):694–701

Ginsburg GS, McCarthy JJ (2001) Personalized medicine: revolutionizing drug discovery and patient care. Trends Biotechnol 19(12):491–496

Jameson JL, Longo DL (2015) Precision medicine–personalized, problematic, and promising. N Engl J Med 372(23):2229–2234

Jamison DT, Alleyne G (2006) Disease control priorities in developing countries. World Bank Publications, Herndon, VA

Kanwal L, Gulzar M, Idrees W, Ikram F, Sukhia RH, Fida M (2024) The application of virtual reality and augmented reality in dentistry—a literature review. J Pak Med Assoc 74(4 (Supple-4)): S126–S131

Kivovics M, Takács A, Pénzes D, Németh O, Mijiritsky E (2022) Accuracy of dental implant placement using augmented reality-based navigation, static computer assisted implant surgery, and the free-hand method: an in vitro study. J Dent 119:104070

Konukseven EI, Önder ME, Mumcuoglu E, Kisnisci RS (2010) Development of a visio-haptic integrated dental training simulation system. J Dent Educ 74:880–891

Krois J, Ekert T, Meinhold L et al (2019) Deep learning for the radiographic detection of periodontal bone loss. Sci Rep 9:8495

Kuang Y, Hu B, Chen J, Feng G, Song J (2017) Effects of periodontal endoscopy on the treatment of periodontitis: a systematic review and meta-analysis. J Am Dent Assoc 148:750–759

Lang T, Staufer S, Jennes B, Gaengler P (2014) Clinical validation of robot simulation of toothbrushing-comparative plaque removal efficacy. BMC Oral Health 14:82

Lee H (2023) The rise of ChatGPT: exploring its potential in medical education. Anat Sci Educ, 1–6

Luciano C, Banerjee P, De Fanti T (2009) Haptics-based virtual reality periodontal training simulator. Virtual Real 2:69–85

Moosa Y, Bacha SH, Raza SA et al (2023) Role of artificial intelligence in periodontology. Pakistan J Med Health Sci 17:363–368

Nakhleh MK, Quatredeniers M, Haick H (2017) Detection of Halitosis in breath: between past, present and future. Oral Dis 24(5):1–11

Ning W, Acharya A, Sun Z, Ogbuehi AC, Li C, Hua S et al (2021) Deep learning reveals key immunosuppression genes and distinct immunotypes in periodontitis. Front. Genet 12

Ozden FO, Özgönenel O, Özden B et al (2015) Diagnosis of periodontal diseases using different classification algorithms: a preliminary study. Niger J Clin Pract 18:416–421

Patel JS, Patel K, Vo H et al (2022) Enhancing an AI-empowered periodontal CDSS and comparing with traditional perio-risk assessment tools. AMIA Annu Symp Proc 2022:846–855

Petersen PE, Ogawa H (2000) The global burden of periodontal disease: towards integration with chronic disease prevention and control. Periodontology 60(1):15–39

Pimkhaokham A, Jiaranuchart S, Kaboosaya B, Arunjaroensuk S, Subbalekha K, Mattheos N (2022) Can computer-assisted implant surgery improve clinical outcomes and reduce the frequency and intensity of complications in implant dentistry? a critical review Periodontol 90:197–223

Pitchika V, Buttner M, Schwendicke F (2000) Artificial intelligence and personalized diagnostics in periodontology: a narrative review. Periodontol 2024(95):220–231

Ramani S, Vijayalakshmi R, Mahendra J, Burnice Nalinakumari C, Ravi N (2023) Artificial intelligence in periodontics—an overview. IP Int J Periodontol Implantol 8(2):71–74

Rana A, Yauney G, Wong LC et al (2017) Automated segmentation of gingival diseases from oral images. 2017 IEEE Healthcare innovations and point of care technologies (HI-POCT). IEEE, pp 144–7

Righolt AJ, Jevdjevic M, Marcenes W, Listl S (2018) Global-, regional-, and country-level economic impacts of dental diseases in 2015. J Dent Res 97(5):501–507

Romm E, Li J, Kouznetsova VL, Tsigelny IF (2020) Machine learning strategies to distinguish oral cancer from periodontitis using salivary metabolites. Adv Intell Syst Comput 1252:511–526

Rudd K, Bertoncini C, Hinders M (2009) Simulations of ultrasonographic periodontal probe using the finite integration technique. Open Acoust J 2:1–9

Schwendicke, F, Chaurasia A, Wiegand T, Uribe SE, Fontana M, Akota I, Tryfonos O, Krois J (2023) IADR e-oral health network and the ITU/WHO focus group AI for health. Artificial intelligence for oral and dental healthcare: core education curriculum. J Dent 128:104363

Schwendicke F, Krois J (2022) Precision dentistry-what it is, where it fails (yet), and how to get there. Clin Oral Investig 26(4):3395–3403

Shanelec DA (2003) Periodontal microsurgery, Journal of esthetic and restorative dentistry: official publication of the American Academy of Esthetic. Dentistry 15:402–407

Shen KL, Huang CL, Lin YC et al (2022) Effects of artificial intelligence-assisted dental monitoring intervention in patients with periodontitis: a randomized controlled trial. J Clin Periodontol 49(10):988–998

Shi JY, Liu BL, Wu XY, Liu M, Zhang Q, Lai HC et al (2024) Improved positional accuracy of dental implant placement using a haptic and machine-vision-controlled collaborative surgery robot: a pilot randomized controlled trial. J Clin Periodontol 5:24–32

Steinberg AD, Banerjee P, Drummond J, Zefran M (2003) Progress in the development of a haptic/virtual reality simulation program for scaling and root planning. J Dent Educ 67:161–165

Thorat V, Rao P, Joshi N, Talreja P, Shetty AR (2024) Role of artificial intelligence (AI) in patient education and communication in dentistry. Cureus. 16(5):e59799

Tibbetts LS, Shanelec DA (1998) Periodontal microsurgery. Dent Clin North Am 42(2):339–359

Wang J, Shen Y, Yang S (2019) A practical marker-less image registration method for augmented reality oral and maxillofacial surgery. Int J Comput Assist Radiol Surg 14:763–767

Wang CW, Hao Y, di Gianfilippo R et al (2021) Machine learning-assisted immune profiling stratifies peri-implantitis patients with unique microbial colonization and clinical outcomes. Theranostics. 11(14):6703–6716

Wu Y, Wang F, Fan S, Chow JKF (2019) Robotics in dental implantology. Oral Maxillofac Surg Clin 31:513–518

Xu Z, Xiao Y, Zhou L, Lin Y, Su E, Chen J, Wu D (2023) Accuracy and efficiency of robotic dental implant surgery with different human-robot interactions: an in vitro study. J Dent 137:Article 104642

Yuksel B, Ozveren N, Yesil C. Evaluation of dental plaque area with artificial intelligence model. Niger J Clin Pract 1;27(6):759–765

Application of Artificial Intelligence in Oral and Maxillofacial Surgery

Hariram Sankar, Babu Lal, Amanurrahman Zubair Ahemad, and Ragavi Alagarsamy

1 Introduction

In oral and maxillofacial surgery (OMFS), the potential of artificial intelligence (AI) becomes immediately apparent when we consider its applications in imaging and diagnosis. Imagine having an AI tool that can instantly analyse a cone-beam computed tomography (CBCT) scan or a panoramic radiograph, flagging abnormalities like impacted third molars, skeletal malocclusions, or even early signs of oral cancer (Farajollahi et al. 2023; Kazimierczak et al. 2024; Xu et al. 2023a, 2023b). These tools not only save time but can also pick up details that the human eye might miss, leading to faster and more accurate diagnosis.

Surgical planning is another area where AI is making waves. For procedures like orthognathic surgery or dental implant placement, AI can process a patient's three-dimensional (3D) scans and simulate the best possible surgical approach. This allows surgeons to visualize outcomes before making the first incision, reducing uncertainty and improving patient confidence. Moreover, AI models can predict post-surgical results, helping surgeons and patients set realistic expectations (Kato et al. 2023; Khanagar et al. 2022; Kurt Bayrakdar et al. 2021; Salazar et al. 2024; Sankar et al. 2024a).

During surgery, AI takes on an even more hands-on role. Robotic-assisted systems, guided by AI algorithms, are now being used for tasks like placing dental implants

H. Sankar · A. Z. Ahemad (✉)
Department of Dentistry, All India Institute of Medical Sciences, Bathinda, India
e-mail: amanurrahman02@gmail.com

B. Lal
Department of Trauma and Emergency Medicine, All India Institute of Medical Sciences, Bhopal, Madhya Pradesh, India

R. Alagarsamy
Department of Burns, Plastic and Maxillofacial Surgery, VMMC and Safdarjung Hospital, New Delhi, India

A. Gupta et al. (eds.), *Application of Robotics in Dentistry*, Lecture Notes in Bioengineering, https://doi.org/10.1007/978-981-95-1470-0_13

with unmatched precision or performing minimally invasive resections (Sankar et al. 2025; Wu et al. 2019; Xu et al. 2023c). These technologies reduce human error and make surgeries safer and more efficient. Augmented reality (AR), another AI-driven innovation, provides real-time overlays of a patient's anatomy during surgery, helping surgeons navigate with greater accuracy (Ayoub and Pulijala 2019; Stucki et al. 2024).

AI does not just stay in the operating room; it is also transforming how patients interact with their care. Chatbots and virtual assistants are being used to answer patient questions, provide pre- and post-operative guidance, and even help patients understand their treatment plans. While these tools are still evolving, they represent a significant step towards making healthcare more accessible and patient-focused (Azadi et al. 2024; Johnson et al. 2024).

AI becomes more integrated into OMFS, and they provide support in making decisions, handling complex data, and delivering care with greater precision. This chapter explores the many ways AI is shaping oral and maxillofacial surgery, from robotic surgery to augmented reality, while also addressing the challenges and ethical considerations that come with these advancements.

2 History and Evolution of Technology—AI, Robotics, and AR in Oral and Maxillofacial Surgery

The history of AI began in the 1950s with Alan Turing's work on computational intelligence and the Turing test, followed by the Dartmouth Conference (1956), where the term 'AI' was coined by pioneers like John McCarthy and Marvin Minsky. The 1960s saw the development of early AI programs like the Logic Theorist, but progress slowed during the AI winter of the 1970s due to funding cuts and limited advancements. In the 1980s, AI research revived with expert systems and early neural networks, leading to breakthroughs in machine learning (ML) in the 1990s, such as support vector machines and Bayesian networks. The 2000s saw the rise of big data and deep learning (DL), fuelling advancements in speech recognition and image classification. The 2010s marked an AI renaissance, with widespread adoption across industries, driven by large datasets, enhanced computing power, and improved algorithms. Today, AI is an integral part of daily life, powering virtual assistants, autonomous vehicles, and medical diagnostics, with ongoing research in reinforcement learning, explainable AI, and ethics (Bansal et al. 1990; Kaul et al. 2020).

During the late 1980s and early 1990s, the rapid growth of minimally invasive surgery (MIS) highlighted both its potential and limitations, including tremors, surgeon fatigue, reliance on two-dimensional (2D) imaging, and restricted motion. These challenges led to the evolution of robotic surgery, enhancing precision, stability, and visualization. Telerobotics, integrating telecommunications with robotic systems, enabled remote surgeries where the surgeon and patient could be in different locations. A key milestone was the introduction of the Puma 560 in the mid-1980s, the first robotic system used for brain biopsies, marking the beginning of robotics in clinical applications. These innovations laid the groundwork for modern robotic surgery, transforming MIS by addressing its limitations and enabling highly precise, remote surgical interventions (Kalan et al. 2010; Mashhadi Akbar Boojar and Ziaei 2021).

The integration of augmented reality (AR) and virtual reality (VR) in oral and maxillofacial surgery (OMFS) has evolved significantly over the past few decades, transforming surgical planning, education, intraoperative navigation, and patient communication. In the 1990s, the foundation for AR/VR in OMFS was laid with the advent of 3D imaging techniques like computed tomography (CT) and CBCT, leading to early attempts at virtual surgical planning and overlaying imaging onto patient anatomy. By the 2000s, VR-based surgical simulators emerged, allowing trainees to practice procedures like osteotomies, mandibular reconstructions, and temporomandibular joint (TMJ) surgery in a risk-free environment, while AR was introduced for real-time intraoperative navigation in craniofacial and trauma surgery. The 2010s saw the rapid adoption of AR-assisted optical tracking systems for enhanced precision in facial trauma and tumour resections, along with the integration of haptic feedback VR for realistic surgical training. By 2015, AR-based CBCT-guided surgery and holographic overlays began enhancing dental implantology and orthognathic surgery, while VR platforms for patient education allowed individuals to visualize post-surgical outcomes before undergoing procedures (Paro et al. 2022; Vertucci et al. 2023). Recent advancements in AI-driven AR and mixed reality (MR) have further improved robot-assisted surgery, dynamic 3D modelling, and precision-guided facial reconstructions. As these technologies continue to advance, AR/VR is expected to play an even greater role in improving surgical precision, training, and patient outcomes in OMFS.

3 Artificial Intelligence in Oral and Maxillofacial Surgery

In recent years, similar to other fields of medicine and dentistry, AI has begun to make significant inroads into oral and maxillofacial surgery. AI plays a pivotal role in enhancing diagnosis, treatment planning, and outcome prediction for various conditions, including impacted third molars, skeletal malocclusion, oral carcinoma, temporomandibular disorders (TMD), and dental implantology (Fig. 1) (Sankar et al. 2024a, 2025, 2024b; Johnson et al. 2024). This chapter delves into the applications of AI in these areas, highlighting its transformative potential in advancing patient care within the specialty.

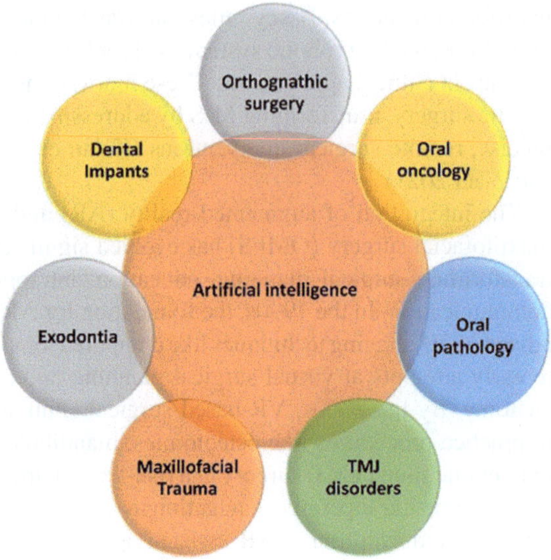

Fig. 1 Various applications of AI in OMFS

3.1 *Orthognathic Surgery*

Diagnosis

The diagnosis of orthognathic surgery involves assessing skeletal and dentofacial anomalies to determine whether surgical intervention is necessary. AI has emerged as a powerful tool in automating cephalometric landmark detection, identifying dentoskeletal discrepancies, and aiding clinical decision-making. The systematic reviews by Takeshitha et al. (Takeshita et al. 2024) Schwendicke et al. (Schwendicke et al. 2021) and Serafin et al. (Serafin et al. 2023) provide valuable insights into the role of AI in diagnosing cases requiring orthognathic surgery.

AI for Automated Cephalometric Landmark Detection

Cephalometric analysis is a crucial step in diagnosing orthognathic surgery cases. Traditionally, manual identification of cephalometric landmarks is time-consuming and subject to intra- and inter-observer variability. AI, particularly deep learning (DL) and convolutional neural networks (CNNs), has significantly improved the accuracy and efficiency of landmark detection.

Schwendicke et al. (Schwendicke et al. 2021) systematically reviewed AI-based cephalometric landmark detection in 2D and 3D radiographs. The study found that:

- AI-based landmark detection showed a mean prediction error around 2 mm, making it clinically acceptable.
- Despite promising accuracy, many studies had high risk of bias, mainly due to data selection and reference standard inconsistencies.

Serafin et al. (Serafin et al. 2023) conducted a meta-analysis on 3D cephalometric landmark detection using deep learning. The study highlighted:

- AI achieved a mean error of 2.44 mm, with some models even improving accuracy over time.
- Deep learning-based models performed better than traditional machine learning approaches, achieving greater precision in 3D landmark detection.

Takeshitha et al. (Takeshita et al. 2024) confirmed that AI can effectively identify cephalometric landmarks, reducing variability in diagnosis and providing reliable inputs for clinical decision-making.

Clinical Significance

- AI can speed up and standardize cephalometric analyses, reducing human errors.
- AI-driven cephalometric measurements are comparable to human experts, making them valuable tools for preliminary diagnostic screening.

AI for Diagnosing the Need for Orthognathic Surgery

Beyond landmark detection, AI has been applied to predict whether a patient requires orthognathic surgery based on cephalometric and clinical data. Machine learning algorithms, including CNNs and decision tree-based models (e.g. eXtreme Gradient Boosting [XGBoost]), have been trained to classify patients based on skeletal discrepancies.

Takeshitha et al. (Takeshita et al. 2024) reviewed AI models designed to assist in diagnosing whether orthognathic surgery is necessary. The study found:

- AI performed similarly to human experts in determining the need for surgery. However, heterogeneity in datasets and lack of standardization limited a comprehensive meta-analysis on this application.
- The AI models used for diagnosis typically rely on cephalometric features (e.g. SNA, SNB, ANB angles, mandibular plane angle).
- Facial photographs analysed via deep learning to assess asymmetry and skeletal discrepancies.
- Machine learning classification models trained on large datasets of diagnosed cases to make predictions.

Studies reviewed in Takeshitha et al. (Takeshita et al. 2024) and Schwendicke et al. (Schwendicke et al. 2021) confirmed that AI-assisted diagnosis can:

- Reduce subjectivity in clinical decision-making.
- Support orthodontists and maxillofacial surgeons in determining surgical necessity.
- Improve consistency in diagnosing dentoskeletal anomalies.

Clinical Significance

- AI enhances diagnostic accuracy by minimizing inter-clinician variability.
- AI-based models can serve as decision support systems, helping practitioners identify cases that may benefit from surgical intervention.
- Limitations remain, including dataset variability, lack of generalizability, and ethical concerns in AI-driven decision-making.

Treatment Planning and Outcome Prediction

Traditionally, treatment planning relied on 2D cephalometry, stone model surgery, and manual landmark identification, which were time-consuming and error-prone. AI-driven models, particularly deep learning (DL) and machine learning (ML) algorithms, now automate landmark detection, segmentation, and virtual surgical planning (VSP), reducing human dependency and increasing accuracy (Sankar et al. 2024a). AI-based models like U-Net and Skull Engine have demonstrated high Dice similarity coefficients (DSCs) of 92–96%, ensuring superior segmentation and preoperative planning. Additionally, deep learning frameworks leveraging 3D imaging can predict post-operative skeletal changes with an accuracy of 0.292 to 3.32 mm, allowing for real-time adjustments and enhanced treatment planning (Sankar et al. 2024a; Dot et al. 2022; Deng et al. 2023).

Beyond preoperative planning, AI plays a crucial role in outcome prediction and patient communication. Predicting post-operative facial soft tissue changes, a long-standing challenge, has been significantly improved using AI models like FC-Net and deep neural networks (DNNs). These models integrate preoperative bony movement vectors with facial soft tissue deformations, achieving prediction accuracies as high as 85.7% to 99.98% (Sankar et al. 2024a; Horst et al. 2021; Ma et al. 2021). AI also enhances patient education by generating 3D visualizations of expected post-surgical changes, improving informed consent and treatment acceptance. While AI has significantly improved orthognathic surgery, further prospective studies and standardization of AI models are needed to ensure widespread clinical adoption and refinement of these cutting-edge tools.

3.2 Oral Oncology

AI has shown great promise in the early diagnosis of oral cancer, improving detection accuracy and aiding clinicians in decision-making. AI has been applied in multiple areas for non-invasive oral cancer detection, including image analysis, cytology, fluorescence imaging, telemedicine, and predictive modelling (Birur et al. 2015; Uthoff et al. 2018; Welikala et al. 2020; García-Pola et al. 2021).

AI in Medical Image-Based Diagnosis of Oral Cancer

One of the most significant applications of AI in oral cancer diagnosis is image-based detection using deep learning models. AI can analyse clinical images, radiographs, and histopathological slides to identify cancerous lesions with high accuracy.

- Deep learning (DL) and convolutional neural networks (CNNs) have demonstrated high diagnostic accuracy for classifying benign, precancerous, and malignant lesions.
- CNN models trained on oral squamous cell carcinoma (OSCC) images achieved over 92% accuracy in distinguishing normal tissue from cancerous lesions (García-Pola et al. 2021).
- AI models like speeded up robust features (SURF) combined with support vector machines (SVMs) showed an 82% precision in differentiating normal and pathological mucosa (García-Pola et al. 2021).

Clinical Significance

- AI enhances early detection by identifying subtle morphological changes in lesions that may be missed by clinicians.
- AI-powered diagnostic models reduce inter-observer variability, ensuring consistent and objective analysis.

AI in Fluorescence Imaging for Oral Cancer Detection

Fluorescence imaging, combined with AI, is a promising non-invasive tool for early cancer detection.

- Confocal laser endomicroscopy (CLE) with AI showed a sensitivity of 86.6% and specificity of 90% in detecting OSCC (García-Pola et al. 2021).
- AI-assisted autofluorescence imaging (AFI) and white light imaging (WLI) enhanced accuracy in identifying high-risk lesions and cancerous transformations.
- VEL scope-based AI models predicted the most appropriate biopsy sites in dysplastic areas with 83% accuracy (García-Pola et al. 2021).

Clinical Significance

- AI-assisted fluorescence imaging enables real-time, chairside screening of suspicious lesions.
- This technology aids in early intervention, improving patient outcomes.

AI in Exfoliative Cytology for Oral Cancer Screening

Cytological analysis is another non-invasive diagnostic approach, where AI is used to assess exfoliated oral cells for malignant transformations.

- Support vector machines (SVMs) for cytological classification achieved 100% sensitivity and specificity in distinguishing oral leukoplakia from OSCC.
- AI-assisted liquid-based exfoliative cytology improved the accuracy of oral potentially malignant disorder (OPMD) detection.

- A random forest model predicted the malignant transformation of leukoplakia with 100% sensitivity and 99.2% specificity (García-Pola et al. 2021).

Clinical Significance

- AI-assisted cytology can reduce the need for invasive biopsies.
- These models provide early risk assessment, guiding timely clinical referrals.

AI in Telemedicine and Mobile-Based Oral Cancer Screening

Telemedicine and mobile AI applications offer remote and accessible screening solutions, especially in underserved areas.

- AI models integrated with mobile phone-based telemedicine platforms demonstrated a positive predictive value of 100% in diagnosing suspicious oral lesions (García-Pola et al. 2021).
- AI-assisted smartphone-based autofluorescence imaging (AFI) and WLI showed enhanced lesion classification and referral accuracy.

Clinical Significance

- Telemedicine enables early detection in remote or low-resource settings.
- AI-powered mobile applications support frontline healthcare workers in triaging and referring patients with high-risk lesions.

AI in Risk Prediction and Early Diagnosis of Oral Cancer

AI models have been developed to predict oral cancer risk based on patient demographics, habits, and lesion characteristics.

- Machine learning-based predictive models incorporating demographics, smoking history, lesion characteristics, and biopsy data achieved 99.3% accuracy in predicting oral cancer risk (García-Pola et al. 2021).
- Fuzzy regression models performed similarly to expert clinicians in predicting high-risk oral lesions.

Clinical Significance

- AI-based risk models provide personalized risk assessment.
- They help in prioritizing high-risk patients for further clinical evaluation.

3.3 Oral Pathology

AI has emerged as a transformative tool in maxillofacial pathology, significantly enhancing the diagnosis of conditions such as odontogenic cysts, apical lesions, salivary gland diseases, and infections with image analysis, predictive modelling, and diagnostic support (Khanagar et al. 2022; Abdul et al. 2024; Ekert et al. 2019; Li et al. 2022).

AI in the Diagnosis of Odontogenic Cysts and Maxillofacial Cysts

Odontogenic cysts, such as dentigerous cysts, periapical cysts, and keratocystic odontogenic tumours (KCOTs), are commonly found in the jaw. AI, especially deep learning (DL) and convolutional neural networks (CNNs), has been applied in radiographic analysis for their detection.

- CNN models trained on panoramic radiographs and CBCT scans successfully differentiated benign odontogenic cysts from aggressive cystic lesions with high accuracy.
- AI-based image segmentation techniques improved the localization of cystic boundaries, aiding precise diagnosis.
- Deep learning models outperformed traditional radiographic interpretation, reducing observer variability.

Clinical Significance

- AI enhances early detection of odontogenic cysts, preventing unnecessary surgical interventions.
- AI-powered image analysis can assist in differentiating between benign and aggressive cysts, improving treatment planning.

AI in the Detection of Apical Lesions and Periapical Pathologies

Apical periodontitis and other periapical lesions can be difficult to detect using conventional radiographs. AI has been employed to improve detection accuracy and provide automated diagnoses.

- AI-assisted radiographic analysis using deep learning has shown high sensitivity and specificity in detecting periapical radiolucencies.
- AI models have been trained on cone-beam computed tomography (CBCT) images, achieving an accuracy of over 90% in detecting apical lesions (Ekert et al. 2019).
- AI also aids in monitoring healing post-endodontic treatment, predicting treatment outcomes.

Clinical Significance

- AI reduces diagnostic errors in detecting asymptomatic periapical infections.
- AI can predict lesion progression, allowing better treatment decisions and improved patient outcomes.

AI in the Diagnosis of Salivary Gland Diseases

Salivary gland disorders, including sialadenitis, salivary gland stones, and Sjögren's syndrome, pose diagnostic challenges due to their complex presentations. AI is being used to enhance imaging interpretation and predict disease progression (Khanagar et al. 2022).

- Machine learning (ML) models analysing ultrasound and magnetic resonance imaging (MRI) scans have been used to differentiate benign from inflammatory salivary gland diseases.
- AI-assisted pattern recognition models have improved the early detection of salivary gland dysfunctions such as Sjögren's syndrome.
- AI has been employed in sialography image analysis, detecting salivary gland stones with high precision.

Clinical Significance

- AI enhances diagnostic accuracy, reducing the need for invasive sialography or biopsy.
- AI models can predict glandular function loss, helping in early intervention and treatment.

AI in Predicting and Diagnosing Oral Infections

AI has been applied to detect bacterial and fungal infections affecting the oral cavity, such as candidiasis and bacterial bloodstream infections (Li et al. 2022).

- Machine learning models analysing clinical and microbiological data successfully predicted the risk of fungal and bacterial infections in patients.
- AI-assisted predictive models identified high-risk patients for invasive candidiasis, helping clinicians take preventive measures.
- AI has also been employed in detecting antibiotic-resistant bacterial infections, aiding in personalized antibiotic therapy.

Clinical Significance

- AI can predict oral infections before clinical symptoms appear, improving patient management.
- AI assists in preventing unnecessary antibiotic use, reducing the risk of antibiotic resistance.

3.4 TMJ Disorders

Artificial intelligence (AI) is revolutionizing the diagnosis of temporomandibular disorders (TMDs) by improving accuracy, automating medical imaging analysis, and assisting clinicians in decision-making. Based on multiple systematic reviews, AI applications in TMD diagnosis span across radiographic analysis, MRI-based detection, and predictive modelling (Almăşan et al. 2023; Jha et al. 2022; Zhang et al. 2024).

AI in Medical Imaging for TMD Diagnosis

Medical imaging is crucial for diagnosing TMD-related conditions such as disc displacement, osteoarthritis, and degenerative joint disease (DJD). AI, especially machine learning (ML) and deep learning (DL) models, has enhanced the detection and classification of TMD-related abnormalities in MRI, CBCT, and panoramic radiographs.

- MRI-based AI models have been highly effective in detecting articular disc displacement and joint effusions, with some models achieving accuracy levels above 83% (Almăşan et al. 2023).
- CBCT-based AI models showed a sensitivity of 0.76 (76%) and specificity of 0.79 (79%) in diagnosing TMJ osteoarthritis (Almăşan et al. 2023).
- Panoramic radiograph-based AI models using ResNet and CNN algorithms have also been effective in detecting degenerative changes in TMJ.

Clinical Significance

- AI-powered imaging analysis reduces diagnostic errors in detecting early-stage TMD conditions.
- AI can help automate the interpretation of MRI and CBCT scans, reducing the burden on radiologists and improving diagnostic consistency.

AI in Diagnosing TMJ Osteoarthritis (OA)

TMJ osteoarthritis is a degenerative condition affecting the temporomandibular joint. AI models have been used to analyse CBCT and panoramic radiographs for detecting condylar resorption, flattening, and osteophyte formation.

- AI models using machine learning algorithms such as XGBoost and Light Gradient-Boosting Machine (LightGBM) showed diagnostic accuracy above 75% (Almăşan et al. 2023; Jha et al. 2022).
- AI-based radiomics analysis identified TMJ OA using quantitative features from CBCT images, improving early detection rates.
- Transfer learning models (ResNet, MobileNet V2) achieved better performance metrics for detecting osteoarthritis changes.

Clinical Significance

- AI helps in early detection of degenerative joint changes, enabling timely interventions to slow disease progression.
- AI-based diagnostic tools reduce variability in human interpretation, ensuring consistent diagnoses across different clinicians.

AI in Detecting Disc Displacement in MRI

Disc displacement is one of the most common intra-articular TMD conditions. AI has been used to improve MRI-based detection of disc position.

- AI models have successfully automated the identification of disc displacement, achieving sensitivity values between 73.5% and 100% (Sankar et al. 2024b).
- Deep learning models (ResNet, MobileNet V2) outperformed traditional ML approaches in detecting abnormal disc positioning.

- AI can detect early signs of TMJ disorders, even before significant symptoms appear.

Clinical Significance

- AI reduces the need for manual MRI interpretation, which is time-consuming and requires expert radiologists.
- AI-based MRI analysis provides consistent, high-accuracy diagnostic results, improving treatment planning for disc-related disorders.

AI in Predicting TMD Risk and Progression

AI models have been developed to predict TMD risk and disease progression based on clinical, behavioural, and imaging data.

- AI models trained on demographic, behavioural, and imaging datasets predicted TMD onset with over 90% accuracy (Jha et al. 2022; Zhang et al. 2024).
- AI-based risk assessment models help in identifying high-risk individuals before clinical symptoms appear.

Clinical Significance

- AI can be used for preventive screening, helping patients adopt early interventions to manage TMD symptoms.
- AI-based predictive models improve personalized treatment planning, reducing disease severity over time.

3.5 Maxillofacial Trauma

Artificial intelligence (AI) is transforming maxillofacial trauma diagnosis and management by improving fracture detection, classification, and treatment planning. AI-powered algorithms, particularly deep learning (DL) and convolutional neural networks (CNNs), are being extensively used in radiographic analysis of maxillofacial fractures, especially mandibular fractures (Babu et al. 2024; Dashti et al. 2024).

AI in Detecting Mandibular Fractures

Mandibular fractures are among the most common facial injuries and require accurate and timely diagnosis. AI, particularly CNN-based models, has shown high accuracy in detecting mandibular fractures on panoramic radiographs.

- AI models analysing panoramic radiographs achieved a sensitivity of 97.1% and specificity of 81.3%, making them comparable to human experts in fracture detection (Babu et al. 2024; Dashti et al. 2024).
- AI-powered deep learning algorithms outperformed conventional radiographic interpretation, reducing misdiagnoses and false negatives.

- AI models were trained on large datasets of mandibular fractures, allowing them to detect various fracture types (symphysis, condyle, body, ramus, angle) with high precision.

Clinical Significance

- AI can improve early detection of fractures, leading to faster treatment initiation.
- AI-powered radiographic analysis helps reduce inter-observer variability, ensuring more consistent diagnoses.
- AI can assist junior clinicians or non-specialists in diagnosing mandibular fractures with higher confidence.

AI in CBCT-Based and 3D Analysis of Facial Trauma

AI is also being applied to CBCT and 3D imaging for complex fracture detection and classification.

- AI-enhanced CBCT analysis showed superior performance in assessing complex fractures, particularly midfacial fractures, orbital fractures, and zygomatic fractures.
- AI models could automatically segment fracture lines and predict displaced versus non-displaced fractures.
- Machine learning classifiers trained on 3D CBCT images provided automated fracture classification, improving decision-making for surgical versus non-surgical management.

Clinical Significance

- AI reduces the time required for fracture diagnosis in emergency settings.
- AI-powered 3D imaging provides precise anatomical reconstructions, aiding in surgical planning.
- AI improves treatment personalization by predicting fracture stability and prognosis.

AI in Automated Trauma Triage and Decision Support

AI models have been developed to triage facial trauma cases, identifying high-risk patients who need immediate intervention.

- AI-based trauma severity scoring models accurately identified patients requiring urgent surgery versus those needing conservative management.
- AI-assisted emergency room triage systems have been tested, helping prioritize facial trauma cases more efficiently.
- AI models integrating clinical history, radiographic findings, and fracture patterns provided automated treatment recommendations.

Clinical Significance

- AI reduces diagnostic delays in emergency settings.
- AI-powered triage ensures optimized resource allocation, reducing unnecessary hospital admissions.
- AI-based decision support improves treatment planning accuracy, particularly in multi-specialty trauma teams.

AI in Predicting Fracture Healing and Complications

AI models have also been employed to predict fracture healing outcomes and complications.

- AI-based predictive models assess fracture displacement, bone density, and patient factors to estimate healing time.
- AI-powered risk assessment models predict non-union, infection, and malocclusion risks, aiding in early intervention.

Clinical Significance

- AI helps personalize post-trauma care, ensuring better healing outcomes.
- AI can reduce complications by identifying high-risk patients early, leading to proactive interventions.

3.6 Exodontia

Artificial intelligence (AI) has revolutionized the diagnosis, treatment planning, and risk assessment of third molar surgery. AI-based models, particularly machine learning (ML) and deep learning (DL) algorithms, are being increasingly utilized to assist clinicians in predicting impaction, assessing nerve proximity, evaluating extraction difficulty, and managing post-operative complications (Assiri et al. 2024; Choi et al. 2022; Fukuda et al. 2020; Vinayahalingam et al. 2019).

AI in Diagnosing and Predicting Third Molar Impaction

Third molars (wisdom teeth) are the most commonly impacted teeth, often requiring surgical extraction. AI models have been applied to predict impaction risk and eruption patterns.

- CNN-based AI models have been trained on orthopantomograms (OPG) and CBCT scans to predict the likelihood of third molar impaction with high accuracy.
- Machine learning algorithms (YOLOv3, Faster R-CNN, ResNet-101) have been used to predict eruption potential, achieving up to 79% accuracy in molar angulation measurements (Assiri et al. 2024).
- AI models analysing age, gender, and anatomical measurements have been used to predict eruption patterns and future impaction risks, aiding preventive orthodontic decisions.

Clinical Significance

- AI can assist in early identification of impaction risk, enabling preventive orthodontic strategies.
- AI-based prediction tools help in treatment planning, allowing clinicians to decide whether early extraction is necessary.

AI in Determining the Position of Impacted Third Molars

The precise localization of an impacted third molar is crucial for planning extraction and avoiding surgical complications.

- AI models have been applied to CBCT and OPG scans to automatically classify third molar impaction based on Pell and Gregory and Winter's classification systems.
- AI models such as VGG-16, MobileNetV2, and ResNet50 have been used to predict mandibular third molar impaction positions, with higher accuracy than inexperienced clinicians.
- AI-assisted 3D segmentation models have been able to precisely locate the molar's orientation, angulation, and depth within the bone.

Clinical Significance

- AI-based automated classification of impaction improves treatment planning efficiency.
- AI helps in reducing surgical risks by providing precise localization of the tooth.

AI in Evaluating the Relationship Between the Inferior Alveolar Nerve (IAN) and Third Molar

One of the most critical concerns in third molar surgery is the risk of inferior alveolar nerve (IAN) injury, which can lead to permanent paraesthesia.

- AI-based deep learning segmentation models have been used to identify the relationship between impacted third molars and the mandibular canal on CBCT scans .
- Studies have found that CNN-based AI models achieved higher accuracy (83%) than human radiologists (76%) in determining the molar's proximity to the IAN (Assiri et al. 2024).
- YOLOv4 and MM3-IANnet AI models were highly effective in identifying high-risk cases, reducing the chances of surgical nerve damage.

Clinical Significance

- AI assists in preoperative risk assessment, reducing the likelihood of nerve injury.
- AI models can provide automated warnings for high-risk extractions, guiding clinicians in modifying surgical approaches.

AI in Predicting Extraction Difficulty and Surgical Planning

AI models have been developed to predict the difficulty of third molar extractions, helping surgeons plan safer and more efficient procedures.

- AI-assisted difficulty prediction models use variables such as tooth position, angulation, root morphology, and surrounding bone density.
- Machine learning models (YOLOv5, Laplace Net) have been used to predict surgical complexity, achieving accuracy above 80% (Assiri et al. 2024).
- AI-based automated scoring systems can classify extractions as simple, moderately difficult, or highly complex based on radiographic and clinical factors.

Clinical Significance

- AI helps optimize surgical planning by predicting difficult cases in advance.
- AI-guided decision-making enables minimally invasive techniques, reducing surgical complications.

AI in Post-Operative Management and Complication Prediction

AI has also been applied to predict post-operative complications, such as pain, swelling, and infection.

- AI models have been used to analyse preoperative imaging and patient data to predict post-extraction complications.
- AI-based models assessing bone healing patterns post-extraction can predict delayed healing or infection risks.
- Some studies have suggested that AI models can assist in personalized post-operative care, recommending analgesics, antibiotics, and follow-up schedules based on risk stratification.

Clinical Significance

- AI helps in proactive post-operative management, reducing complication rates.
- AI-based personalized patient care strategies improve recovery outcomes.

3.7 Dental Implants

Artificial intelligence (AI) is revolutionizing dental implantology by enhancing precision, efficiency, and patient-specific treatment planning. AI-driven machine learning (ML) and deep learning (DL) algorithms analyse CBCT scans, panoramic radiographs, and intraoral images, enabling highly accurate implant positioning, bone quality assessment, and nerve proximity evaluation (Kurt Bayrakdar et al. 2021).

Convolutional neural networks (CNNs) automate the segmentation of key anatomical structures, such as the inferior alveolar nerve, maxillary sinus, and cortical bone, significantly reducing the risk of nerve injury and sinus perforation during implant placement. AI-powered predictive analytics assist clinicians in selecting the optimal implant diameter, length, and angulation, based on bone density, occlusal forces, and biomechanical considerations, ensuring long-term implant success.

Beyond diagnostics, AI is revolutionizing surgical workflows, optimizing implant site preparation and drilling protocols to enhance primary stability and osseointegration. Advanced AI algorithms can even predict peri-implant disease risks, guiding clinicians in personalized post-operative care and long-term maintenance strategies.

The profound impact of AI on dental implantology is explored in greater depth in another chapter of this textbook.

4 Applications of Robotics in OMFS

Robotic surgery, often referred to as the 'third technological revolution' in the field of surgery, represents a ground breaking advancement, addressing many of the challenges associated with traditional surgical techniques. Nowadays, robotics offers lot of applications in OMFS (Fig. 2). Modern robotic surgical systems typically consist of multiple robotic arms designed to manipulate cameras and various surgical tools. The surgeon operates these arms remotely from a computer console situated away from the operating table. This console provides the surgeon with a high-definition, magnified, 3D visualization of the surgical site, ensuring exceptional clarity and precision during the procedure (Table 1). At present, the majority of robot-assisted head and neck surgeries are conducted using surgical systems such as the da Vinci robot. Originally designed for urological and abdominal procedures, the da Vinci system has emerged as the most widely utilized and successful platform in this domain (Ma et al. 2024).

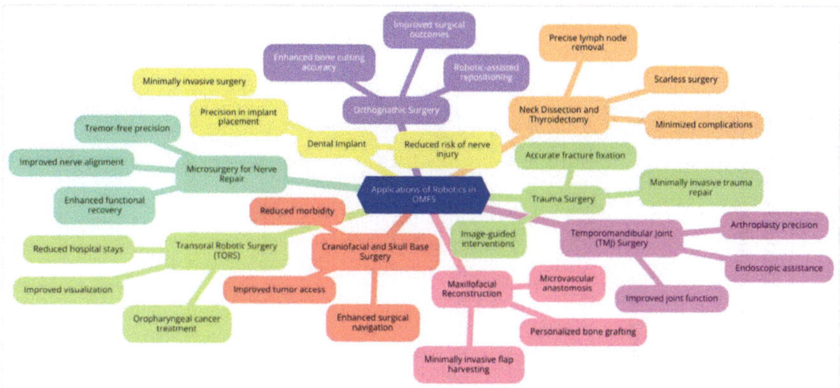

Fig. 2 Various application of robotics in OMFS

Table 1 Generations of robotic surgical systems

Generation	System	Manufacturer	FDA approval year	Key features	Limitations
Gen I	Automated endoscopic system for optimal positioning (AESOP)	CMI	1995	– First voice-controlled robotic camera platform – Provided stable camera positioning, replacing an extra surgical assistant	– Limited to camera stabilization – Lacked versatility and surgical instrument control
Gen II	Telerobot Zeus	Computer Motion	2000	– Master–slave teleoperation system – Allowed remote surgeries between hospitals – 3D visualization for improved accuracy – Tremor suppression for greater precision	– Discontinued after da Vinci system adoption – Less advanced than modern systems

(continued)

Table 1 (continued)

Generation	System	Manufacturer	FDA approval year	Key features	Limitations
Gen III	da Vinci surgical system	Intuitive Surgical	1999 (initial), 2009 (maxillofacial surgery)	– Surgeon's console with high-definition 3D real-time visualization – Multi-arm robotic cart with EndoWrist instruments for precise movements – Enhanced degrees of freedom, mimicking human hand dexterity – Applied in head, neck, urology, cardiology, and gynaecology surgeries	– Expensive – Large system footprint
Gen IV	da Vinci Xi and da Vinci X	Intuitive Surgical	2014 (Xi), 2017 (X)	da Vinci Xi: – Thinner, longer robotic arms for better manoeuvrability – Firefly fluorescent imaging for enhanced visualization – Overhead arm arrangement for better spatial orientation – Integration with a special operating table for repositioning without undocking da Vinci X: – Lower-cost alternative to Xi with similar features – Includes voice and laser guidance, lightweight endoscope	– Xi: High cost – X: Less versatile due to side cart

4.1 Dental Implant

Robotic technology enhances precision in dental implantology, particularly in challenging cases where freehand drilling is risky. It benefits patients with limited bone volume or proximity to critical structures by ensuring accurate osteotomy placement and reducing complications like nerve injury or sinus perforation. For full-arch rehabilitations and multiple implants (e.g. All-on-4), robotic assistance ensures parallel placement, optimizing prosthetic fit. It also enables minimally invasive, flapless surgery, reducing tissue trauma. Complex angulations, such as avoiding adjacent roots or angled ridgelines, are more precisely managed with robotic guidance.

For surgeons, robotics offer a flexible alternative to static guides, allowing real-time adjustments—especially in revision surgeries with tight anatomical constraints. In educational and clinical settings, it standardizes outcomes, aiding less experienced surgeons. Emerging applications include autonomous implant site preparation, particularly for zygomatic implants. Since the Food and Drug Administration's (FDA's) 2017 clearance of *Yomi* by Neocis, robotic-assisted implant surgery has seen widespread adoption, improving accuracy, safety, and efficiency.

Evolution of Robot-Assisted Dental Implant Surgery

Early Developments

- The first robot-assisted dental implant surgery was reported in 2001, using real-time visualization and a robotic guide for osteotomy site preparation.
- Dutreuil et al. introduced a 5-degree-of-freedom (DOF) robotic system for precise drilling.
- Sun et al. developed an image-guided robotic system (MELFA RV-3S), achieving a 1.42 ± 0.70 mm error margin but lacking tactile feedback.
- In 2019, Wu et al. highlighted the growing role of robotics in improving implant precision and efficiency.
- In 2017, the first FDA-approved robotic dental system marked a milestone in integrating robotics into dental care.
- Later in 2017, Zhao et al. in China developed the world's first autonomous dental implant system, capable of intraoperative adjustments with minimal human intervention.

Advancements in Tactile Feedback

- Kasahara et al. introduced a telerobotic system transmitting cutting forces via acceleration-based bilateral control.
- Syed et al. enhanced tactile capabilities with virtual force feedback, enabling remote robotic control using haptic devices.

Commercial and Autonomous Systems

- The first FDA-approved commercial dental robot (2017) was used in over 1,800 surgeries by 2020, offering:

  - Visual and physical guidance in preoperative and intraoperative phases
  - Haptic feedback for precise drill control

- In 2017, Beijing University and the Fourth Military Medical University developed the first autonomous dental implant robot, integrating an image-guided platform, mechanical robot, and Dental Navi software for minimal surgeon intervention.

Key Technologies in Robotic Dental Implant Systems

Advanced Technologies for Precision in Robotic Dental Implantology

Robotic dental implant systems integrate navigation, haptics, and automation to enhance placement accuracy. A system like *Yomi* consists of a lightweight robotic arm, an optical tracking system, and treatment planning software. Before surgery, a cone-beam CT (CBCT) scan generates a virtual implant plan, specifying sites, angles, and depths. The robot then ensures precise execution during the procedure.

Robotic Guidance Versus Robotic Autonomy

1. **Robotic Guidance (Semi-Active)**: The surgeon controls the drill, while the robotic arm constrains movement to the pre-planned trajectory. Systems like *Yomi* use haptic feedback, resisting deviations and stopping at the exact depth.
2. **Robotic Autonomy (Fully Active)**: Some experimental systems autonomously perform drilling with minimal human intervention, while the surgeon monitors.

Real-Time Tracking and Navigation

Robotic systems use ub millimetre tracking to align the virtual plan with the patient's anatomy. Optical tracking cameras monitor fiducial markers on the patient's jaw, allowing dynamic adjustments if movement occurs. Calibration is performed by referencing the drill tip to known landmarks or using a coordinate measuring machine (CMM) arm.

Haptic Feedback and Multi-Sensory Guidance

The robotic arm acts as a 'virtual cannula', restricting movement to the planned path while providing:

- **Tactile Feedback**: Resistance when deviating from the trajectory.
- **Visual Guidance**: On-screen tracking of the drill position.
- **Audio Alerts**: Beeps to confirm correct positioning or warn of deviations.

Automation and Workflow Integration

After calibration, the robotic arm guides the drill to the exact entry point and maintains the planned angle and depth. Some systems integrate intraoperative imaging or scanners to verify implant positioning in real time. For multiple implants, the robot follows the digital treatment plan sequentially.

Precision and Clinical Advantages

Robotic-assisted implant surgery provides:

- **0.3 mm accuracy in implant placement**
- **Less than 1° angulation error,** superior to freehand techniques
- Robots can adapt to intraoperative changes, allowing real-time adjustments in implant size—an advantage over static guides.

Common Pitfalls in Robotic Implant Surgery and Solutions

1. **Learning Curve and Workflow Efficiency**
    - **Pitfall**: Initial set-up and execution may prolong surgery.
    - **Solution**: Hands-on training and simulation before clinical use improve efficiency, reducing procedure times with experience.
2. **Registration Inaccuracy and Tracking Loss**
    - **Pitfall**: If tracking is lost due to movement or poor marker fixation, accuracy suffers.
    - **Solution**: Use rigid bone-anchored fiducial markers and verify registration before drilling. Re-register if discrepancies arise. Sedation can minimize patient movement.
3. **Limited Access in Certain Cases**
    - **Pitfall**: The robotic arm may struggle with posterior sites or limited mouth opening.
    - **Solution**: Select appropriate cases; for posterior implants, consider traditional guides or freehand techniques until smaller robotic arms are available.
4. **Soft Tissue Interference**
    - **Pitfall**: Robots do not retract soft tissue, potentially obstructing the drill.
    - **Solution**: Ensure adequate retraction with an assistant or use small incisions when necessary.
5. **Cost and Overuse**
    - **Pitfall**: High costs may lead to unnecessary use in simple cases.
    - **Solution**: Prioritize cases where robotic precision adds value, such as multiple implants, complex angulations, or limited bone availability.
6. **Lack of Tactile Feedback**
    - **Pitfall**: Surgeons may lose the sense of bone density.
    - **Solution**: Rely on auditory cues (drill pitch) and software indicators for resistance and depth. Maintain steady drilling pressure.
7. **System Failures or Software Errors**
    - **Pitfall**: Software malfunctions can disrupt surgery.

- **Solution**: Keep backup instruments ready. If issues arise, switch to freehand or a pre-planned surgical guide.

8. **Patient Anxiety and Gag Reflex**
   - **Pitfall**: The robotic arm near the face may cause discomfort or trigger gagging.
   - **Solution**: Communicate clearly with patients, offer sedation if needed, and use a throat pack for gag-prone individuals.
9. **Mid-Surgery Adjustments**
   - **Pitfall**: Reprogramming the robot for intraoperative changes can be time-consuming.
   - **Solution**: Pre-load alternative plans. If urgent, detach the robot and continue freehand.
10. **Limited Long-Term Data**
    - **Pitfall**: There is insufficient long-term research on robotic implant surgery outcomes.
    - **Solution**: Surgeons should document and track cases rigorously until more high-quality clinical data is available.

4.2 Transoral Robotic Surgery (TORS) for Head and Neck Cancer

Transoral robotic surgery (TORS) is a pivotal advancement in oral and maxillofacial surgery (OMFS) for addressing tumours of the oropharynx and adjacent areas. TORS employs a teleoperated robot, commonly the da Vinci system, to excise tumours via the oral cavity, therefore obviating the necessity for extensive exterior incisions like mandibulotomies. This approach was developed in the mid-2000s, with investigations including canine and cadaver models in 2005 culminating in the inaugural human TORS cases in 2006 (Shah et al. 2014).

In the earliest cases, surgeons effectively removed base-of-tongue tumours via a transoral approach. The robotic devices enhanced the visualization of essential structures such as cranial nerves IX and XII and the lingual artery, facilitating the avoidance of harm while ensuring clear margins. Since that time, TORS has been utilized treating several throat and laryngeal malignancies. The clinical effects of TORS have been quite promising. Numerous case series have indicated that TORS can attain oncological outcomes equivalent to open surgery while significantly decreasing morbidity (Bansal et al. 2016). In a cohort of 54 patients, the median duration of hospitalization following TORS was just 1–2 days, in contrast to standard open surgery, which often necessitates a recovery period of one week or longer in the hospital (Ansarin et al. 2014). **Iseli et al.** (54 patients) found that **72% were discharged after one night,** while **28% stayed two nights,** a major improvement compared to the **week-long stays of open surgery**. Even in **stages III–IV**, TORS combined with **adjuvant therapy** showed **promising disease-specific survival**, proving its viability for more complex cases. Only 9% of patients undergoing TORS required a temporary tracheostomy for airway protection, although such a procedure is routinely performed in many cases with open methods. A further investigation including 27 patients who had transoral robotic surgery (TORS) for tonsillar carcinoma attained negative tumour margins in 93% of instances (Cohen et al. 2011) and maintained exceptional swallowing function in 96% of participants; notably, none required a gastrostomy feeding tube post-operatively (Dziegielewski et al. 2013). These functional outcomes signify a substantial enhancement compared to conventional operations, which frequently compromise eating or speaking (Weinstein et al. 2010).

TORS has emerged as a common treatment for early to moderately advanced oropharyngeal tumours, particularly those associated with human papilloma virus (HPV), enabling several patients to circumvent disfiguring procedures or high-dose chemoradiation. In addition to malignancy, TORS is utilised for benign disorders such as obstructive sleep apnoea, where it robotically removes extra tissue from the tongue or throat, demonstrating encouraging outcomes in enhancing airway patency (Yin Tsang et al. 2012). TORS shows the transformative potential of robots in OMFS, offering a minimally invasive option that accelerates recovery while ensuring superior disease management (Genden et al. 2009).

For OPSCC, Aaronson et al. (Aaronson et al. 2015) studied the cost-effectiveness of transoral robotic surgery (TORS). TORS was cheaper than traditional surgery because to shorter hospital stays, fewer complications, and a higher chance of finding unknown cancers that may need fewer treatments. TORS patients had fewer gastrostomy tubes and tracheotomies, a shorter stay (1.5 to 11 days versus 6.8 to 19 days for standard surgery), and lower treatment costs. The investigation found issues such robotic equipment's high initial cost and cost calculation method unreliability. The study supports TORS as an effective therapy, but it calls for further studies with uniform cost assessments and long-term follow-up.

Challenges of Transoral Robotic Surgery (TORS)

1. **Access Limitations**
    - TORS requires sufficient mouth opening and favourable anatomy for optimal instrument manoeuvrability.
    - Tumours in areas beyond the reach of straight robotic instruments (e.g. high nasopharynx and deep hypopharynx) may be inaccessible.
    - Lesions with significant mandibular or deep tongue invasion often necessitate open surgery due to the inability to achieve bony exposure transorally.

- Inadequate visualization or instrumentation makes TORS contraindicated for certain tumour locations, increasing the risk of incomplete resection.

2. **Steep Learning Curve**
   - TORS is technically demanding, with longer operative times in early cases compared to open surgery.
   - Proper patient positioning (supine with head extension), robotic docking, and optimal port placement require experience to master.
   - Studies indicate that after 10–30 cases, operative time decreases, and margin status improves as surgeons gain proficiency.
   - Many institutions implement structured training programs, including simulations and cadaver labs, to credential surgeons for TORS.
3. **Bleeding Control Challenges**
   - The lack of direct tactile feedback complicates vessel management.
   - Major haemorrhage (e.g. from the lingual or carotid artery) can be difficult to control through the restricted oral aperture.
   - Ensuring an experienced bedside assistant and readiness for open conversion is crucial for patient safety.
4. **Equipment and Instrumentation Constraints**
   - The robotic set-up requires specialized mouth retractors, gags, and camera positioning, adding complexity.
   - The da Vinci system, originally designed for abdominal surgery, has limitations in the confined oropharyngeal space.
   - Newer 5-mm micro-instruments and flexible robotic lasers are being developed to improve transoral capabilities.
5. **Cost and Availability Issues**
   - TORS requires significant investment in robotic systems and specialized instruments, limiting access in some hospitals.
   - Many regions lack TORS programs, necessitating referrals to high-volume centres for treatment.

4.3 Robotic Applications in Orthognathic Surgery

Orthognathic surgery is the surgery and correction of the jaws to address skeletal abnormalities and malocclusions. These operations need meticulous accuracy to achieve the intended alignment of the teeth and facial bones. Robotic technology is advancing by facilitating the design and execution of osteotomies. Surgeons now use virtual surgical planning (VSP) software to model jaw motions and create cutting guides (Fig. 3). The subsequent phase involves using robots to implement such strategies in the operating room. Researchers have developed prototype systems in which

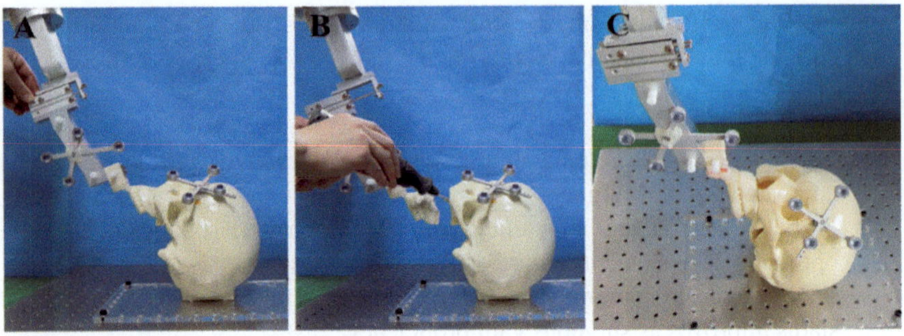

Fig. 3 Surgical planning and final position of maxilla by Lefort (Courtesy: Han et al. 2020)

a robotic arm, equipped with an optical navigation system, which aids in the repositioning of jaw bones in accordance with the digital blueprint. A research used phantom skulls demonstrated that a robotic arm equipped with a specialized end-effector could place a maxillary segment with sub-millimetre precision, achieving an average error of around 0.1–0.2 mm (Han et al. 2020).

This level of precision is beyond what is often attainable by manual placement and splints. The device might also assist in identifying and eliminating bone interferences during movement, activities that are laborious when performed manually. While completely robotic orthognathic surgery for humans has not yet materialized, these advancements suggest that robots may soon aid surgeons in executing jaw osteotomies and accurately arranging bone pieces. Expert surgeons assert that robotic-assisted jaw surgery offers potential for enhanced results by performing intricate bone incisions with precision beyond human capabilitiez (Theodossy and Bamber 2003).

For instance, a recent case report documented the world's first use of a robotic system to perform a Le Fort I osteotomy in orthognathic surgery. In this case, a robotic laser osteotome was programmed to cut the maxilla along a planned line, and it executed the midfacial osteotomy autonomously under the surgeon's supervision (Fig. 4). The motivation for such an approach is to overcome geometric limitations of conventional tools (like oscillating saws and reciprocating saws) which might not cut precisely along complex 3D trajectories (Ebeling et al. 2023). Additionally, surgeons have explored robot-assisted drilling of osteotomy guide holes in the mandible to aid in split osteotomies (Sun et al. 2021). Another indication in development is patient-specific bone shaping—for example, using a robot to mill a custom contour on a bone graft or resect a bony deformity very precisely according to a digital plan. While still largely experimental, these techniques could be indicated for patients with asymmetry or deformities where high precision is needed to achieve a symmetric result.

In 2003, Tamer Theodossy (Theodossy and Bamber 2003) conducted a comparative analysis of two orthognathic surgical models: one utilizing conventional techniques and the other employing robotic-assisted methods. The study revealed that the robot-assisted surgical model demonstrated greater accuracy in both the vertical

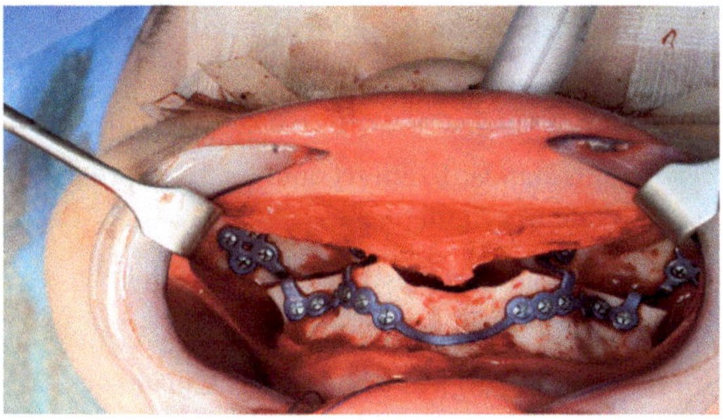

Fig. 4 Lefort I osteotomy fixation with PSI (Courtesy: Ebeling et al. 2023)

and anterior–posterior planes compared to conventional methods. This finding underscores the precision-enhancing capability of robotic systems in orthognathic surgery, potentially improving surgical outcomes and alignment accuracy.

It may also reduce variability—a robot will execute the same cut consistently, while human skill might fluctuate. Furthermore, robotic arms may enhance visualization by accommodating cameras or endoscopes, so providing surgeons with superior perspectives of concealed areas during jaw surgery. With the advancement of technology, we foresee the partial automation of duties such as drilling bone incisions for a Le Fort I osteotomy and placing the maxilla in three dimensions (Han et al. 2020). This would enable the surgeon to concentrate on decision-making and meticulous modifications, while the robot handles the repeated precision tasks. Initial clinical feasibility studies represent the subsequent phase; nonetheless, the ultimate objective is that robotic-assisted orthognathic operations will provide more reliable results, reduced surgical durations, and perhaps less invasive methods, such as endoscopically aided robotic jaw surgery.

Benefits

1. **Precision and Predictability**

   - Robotic systems execute pre-planned osteotomies with sub-millimetre accuracy, reducing variability between cases and surgeons.
   - For example, in a robot-assisted Le Fort I osteotomy, the system performed a straight-line maxillary cut as digitally planned, confirmed by post-operative imaging.
   - Improved bone segment fitting reduces manual adjustments and enhances surgical stability.

2. **Enhanced Safety and Protection of Vital Structures**

   - Robots can be programmed with ‘no-go’ zones to avoid critical structures such as the inferior alveolar nerve.
   - Haptic guidance systems (e.g. Yomi dental robot) prevent unintended deviation and reduce the risk of nerve damage, root injury, or soft tissue trauma.

3. **Consistency and Standardization**
   - Robots ensure identical cuts in repetitive procedures, enhancing predictability across cases.
   - This standardization could lead to more uniform surgical outcomes and better skeletal symmetry.
4. **Functional and Aesthetic Advantages**
   - More precise osteotomies improve occlusion fit, potentially reducing the need for post-surgical orthodontic adjustments.
   - Minimal periosteal stripping and controlled bone cutting may preserve vascular supply, promoting faster healing.
5. **Reduced Tissue Trauma and Faster Healing**
   - Precision cutting eliminates excessive force or bone fracturing, decreasing post-operative morbidity.
   - Laser osteotomy technology produces smooth, thin kerfs with minimal thermal damage, which may enhance healing.
6. **Expansion of Surgical Capabilities**
   - Robots can perform complex, multi-angle curved cuts that may be difficult manually.
   - Increased surgical precision may enable safer procedures in tumour resection and craniofacial trauma cases.
7. **Reduction in Radiation Exposure**
   - Future robotic integration with intraoperative imaging could minimize the need for frequent fluoroscopic verification, reducing surgeon radiation exposure.
8. **Enhanced Surgeon Performance**
   - Robots eliminate issues related to surgeon fatigue, hand tremors, or variability in manual dexterity.
   - They may facilitate longer or more intricate procedures without loss of precision.
9. **Integration with Digital Surgical Planning**
   - Direct translation of computer-aided design (CAD)/computer-aided manufacturing (CAM) surgical plans into robotic execution ensures high fidelity between planning and actual outcomes.

Challenges

1. **Workflow Integration and Digital Planning Compatibility**
   - Seamless transfer of virtual surgical plans to robotic execution is essential.
   - Registration errors (misalignment between patient anatomy and robotic coordinate system) can lead to inaccuracies.
   - Current methods require fiducial markers, CT scans, or optical trackers for calibration, adding complexity.
2. **Learning Curve and Training Requirements**
   - Operating robotic systems requires new technical skills and a shift from manual to automated osteotomy execution.
   - Surgeons must balance robotic precision with the ability to intervene if necessary.
   - Initial cases may take longer due to set-up and learning adjustments.
3. **Adaptation of Fixation and Splint Techniques**
   - Current robotic systems focus on bone cutting, but jaw positioning and fixation remain manual.
   - Future advancements may allow robotic-assisted repositioning of osteotomized segments.
4. **Safety and Regulatory Concerns**
   - Overheating risk in robotic laser osteotomy must be managed to prevent thermal damage.
   - Robots lack tactile feedback, making it difficult to detect subtle changes in resistance or deflections.
   - Semi-active systems (where the surgeon guides the robot) mitigate this risk but reintroduce human error.
5. **Limitations of Current Robotic Instruments**
   - Most surgical robots are designed for soft tissue, not high-torque bone cutting.
   - Dedicated robotic bone-cutting tools (e.g. CNC milling-type arms or laser cutters) are not yet widely available.
6. **High Cost and Justification of Investment**
   - Robotic systems are expensive, and the benefit in elective orthognathic procedures must be proven to justify hospital investments.
   - Cost-effectiveness remains a barrier to widespread adoption.
7. **Intraoperative Adaptability Challenges**
   - Robots follow pre-planned paths, making real-time adjustments difficult.
   - Surgeons may need to pause and reprogram or revert to manual methods if unexpected anatomical variations arise.

8. **Instrumentation and Working Envelope Constraints**
   - Robotic arms may have limited reach for complex osteotomy patterns (e.g. L-shaped cuts).
   - Some systems may only perform straight-line cuts, requiring manual completion of more intricate sections.
9. **Team Integration and Perioperative Adjustments**
   - Anaesthesiologists and surgical staff must adapt to robotic-assisted workflows.
   - Patient positioning may require modifications to accommodate robotic arms.
   - Longer operative times in early adoption phases can increase anaesthesia risks.

4.4 Role of Robotics in Temporomandibular Joint (TMJ) Surgery

Temporomandibular joint surgeries are delicate operations on the jaw joint, which is a small, complex, and functionally critical area. Traditional open TMJ surgery can be invasive, and arthroscopic procedures are technically demanding with limited manoeuvrability. Robotics offers a way to enhance precision in this domain. Although dedicated TMJ surgical robots are not yet in standard use, researchers and surgeons foresee several roles they could play. For instance, a robotic system could assist in TMJ arthroplasty (surgical repair of the joint) by accurately burring bone spurs or remodelling the joint surfaces with sub-millimetre control, reducing the risk of damaging adjacent structures like the ear canal or facial nerve. Robot-assisted endoscopes could potentially improve TMJ arthroscopy by stabilizing the camera and instruments within the tight joint space better than a human hand. According to some surgeons, robotic technology's fine control could allow more thorough debridement of diseased tissue and precise placement of TMJ implants or grafts. Early explorations have involved using the da Vinci system for TMJ procedures in cadavers, demonstrating that the robotic arms can indeed reach the joint through modified incisions and perform basic tasks. The enhanced 3D visualization and wristed instruments of a robot could help in suturing tiny TMJ tissues or navigating the narrow joint compartment.

Another potential application is in total TMJ replacement surgery, where patient-specific joints (often 3D-printed) are fitted. A robot could aid in drilling the screw holes in the skull and jaw bone with exact placement to match the custom prosthesis, ensuring a perfect fit—much like how robots are used in orthopaedic joint replacements. Additionally, by minimizing hand tremor, a robot could reduce the risk of inadvertent injury to the inner ear or skull base during TMJ surgery. While these ideas are still largely theoretical or in early research, the *benefits expected* are similar to other areas: more precise manipulation, reduced tissue trauma, and faster recovery. One day, a patient with a severe TMJ ankylosis (fused jaw joint) might have the joint released by an autonomous or semi-autonomous robot that can carefully carve away the bony fusion without harming the adjacent braincase—a level of precision difficult to achieve by freehand surgery. For now, the role of robotics in TMJ surgery is *emerging*, supported by the knowledge gained in other delicate surgeries, and it stands as a frontier for future innovation in OMFS.

4.5 Robotic in Complex Maxillofacial Reconstruction

Robotics in Free Flap Harvest

- **Minimally Invasive Flap Harvesting**:
  - Traditionally, **free flap surgery** requires **large incisions** (e.g. **fibula flap for mandible reconstruction** and **radial forearm flap for intraoral defects**).
  - Robotic systems allow **smaller incisions**, reducing donor-site morbidity (Lai et al. 2022).
- **Clinical Applications and Benefits**:
  - A **2023 systematic review** found robotic flap harvest improved **donor-site outcomes** in breast surgery without compromising flap success.
  - Robots enable **precise muscle or bone flap dissection**, **minimizing muscle injury and scarring**.
  - **For example,** a robotic-assisted **DIEP flap harvest** improved microsurgical precision and decreased donor-site morbidity.
- **Future in OMFS**:
  - A robotic arm could **dissect the fibula endoscopically**, preserving more muscle and avoiding large skin incisions.
  - **Potential application** to other donor sites (**scapula, iliac crest**) for improved **cosmetic and functional outcomes**.

Robotic Microvascular Anastomosis

- **Enhancing Vascular Suturing**:
  - Used for **joining small arteries and veins (1–3 mm diameter)** in **free flap reconstructions**.
  - Robots create **consistent, uniform vessel sutures**, reducing the risk of **flap thrombosis (clots)**.

- **Early Clinical Success**:
  - A **2018 clinical series from India** reported **good flap survival** with robotic microvascular suturing.
  - The **MUSA robot successfully revascularized eight free flaps**, showing improved **surgeon efficiency over time.**
- **Benefits for Surgeons and Patients**:
  - Robots reduce **fatigue** during long reconstructions, allowing for multiple anastomoses with **consistent precision.**
  - Expected to maintain or improve **functional outcomes** (e.g. **jaw movement after fibula flap and speech after tongue flap**).

Personalized Robotic-Assisted Bone Grafting

- **Advancing Digital Planning and Precision Cutting**:
  - Traditionally, **fibula grafts** for mandibular reconstruction are **manually shaped.**
  - Robotics enables **intricate osteotomy patterns** (e.g. **puzzle-like interlocking cuts**) for **better fit and stability.**
- **Key Robotic Innovations**:
  - **Cold Ablation Robot-Guided Laser Osteotome (CARLO) Robotic Laser System**: Allows **customized osteotomy shapes** beyond traditional straight-line cuts.
  - **Robotic-Assisted Screw Placement**: Ensures **high precision** in **implant positioning.**
- **Future Outlook**:
  - **CT-based preplanning** + robotic execution can optimize **bone segment placement.**
  - Robots may assist in **holding and aligning graft pieces** during fixation, **shortening ischemia time.**

Large-Scale Reconstructions and AI Integration

- **AI and Robotics in Surgical Planning**:
  - **AI algorithms** optimize **flap design**, **predict outcomes**, and guide robotic execution.
  - AI can **analyse defects**, suggest the best **flap donor site**, and **predefine robotic cutting paths.**
- **Emerging Technologies**:
  - **Mixed Reality and Robotic Navigation**:

    AR goggles overlay surgical plans on the patient, while robots **execute precise cuts.**

  - **Robotic Dental Implant Placement**:

    AI-driven planning ensures ideal implant positioning, executed by **robots like Yomi.**

- **Future Vision—AI as an Intelligent Co-Surgeon**:
  - **Automated Preoperative Planning**: AI designs the reconstruction, and the robot executes it.
  - **Adaptive Intraoperative Adjustments**: The robot can detect **variations via imaging** and suggest **real-time modifications**.
  - **AI-Assisted Safety Checks**: The system **prevents unsafe cuts**, enhancing surgical precision and safety.
- **Predictions for 2030 and Beyond**:
  - Robotics will evolve into **fully integrated fracture/reconstruction systems** with **automated planning** and **real-time AI-driven guidance**.
  - The surgeon will define **surgical goals**, and AI + robotics will **execute complex reconstructions** with **unprecedented accuracy**.

Robotic-Assisted Mandibular Reconstruction

- **Enhancing Bone Grafting Precision**:
  - Mandibular reconstruction often requires **fibula free flaps** to replace missing bone due to **tumours or trauma**.
  - Robotics is being applied to improve **accuracy in bone shaping and placement** over conventional methods (Fig. 5) (Boutray et al. 2024).
- **Pre-Programmed Robotic Osteotomies**:
  - **Robots perform bone cuts** based on **CT-based virtual surgical plans**.
  - A **2024 preclinical study** demonstrated **robot-guided osteotomy** for fibula flap mandibular reconstruction (Fig. 6).
  - The robot positioned a **custom cutting guide** with **0.5–1 mm precision** and ~ 2° deviation in laboratory tests.
- **Potential Clinical Benefits**:
  - **More precise and consistent osteotomies** than manual cutting.
  - **Better-fitting bone segments**, reducing the need for adjustments.
  - **Shorter operative times** due to reduced **intraoperative grinding**.
- **Expanding Robotic Applications**:
  - **Assistance in reconstruction plate placement** for improved fixation.
  - **Exploring robotic microvascular anastomoses**, though blood vessel suturing in OMFS remains rare.
- **Future Outlook**:
  - Early reports show feasibility in **robotic flap harvesting and graft in setting**.

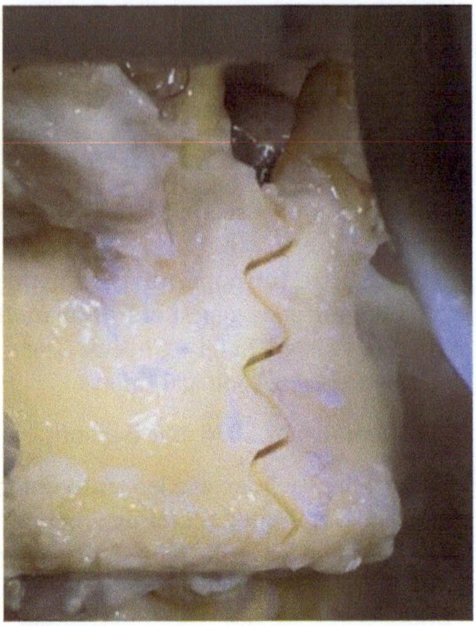

Fig. 5 Mandible osteotomy in cadaveric body (Augello et al. 2018)

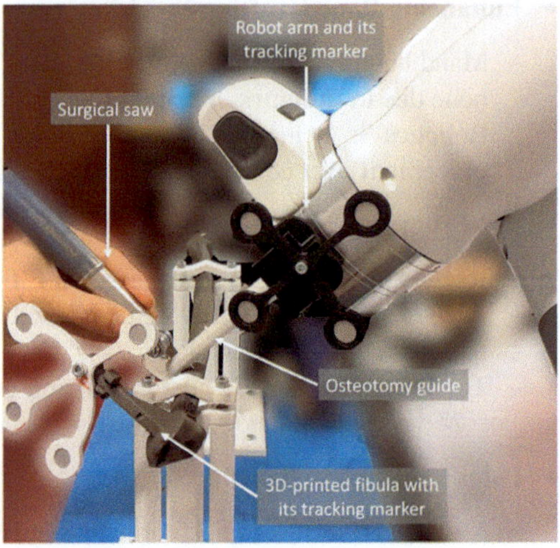

Fig. 6 Fibula osteotomy surgery with robotics (Boutray et al. 2024)

– As technology advances, **robot-assisted mandibular reconstruction** could become standard, allowing surgeons to execute **3D digital reconstructions with high precision**.

4.6 Robotic-Assisted Craniofacial and Skull Base Surgery

Robotic technology enhances visualization and access in confined anatomical spaces, making it applicable to select craniofacial and skull base procedures. It is particularly useful for tumours in the parapharyngeal space and infratemporal fossa, which are traditionally difficult to access (Augello et al. 2018). The University of Pennsylvania pioneered transoral robotic approaches (TORS) for such lesions, demonstrating feasibility in cadaveric and animal models before successfully performing the first human case in 2007. This approach allows for wide exposure, precise identification of neurovascular structures, and complete resection with minimal morbidity. Additional applications include robotic-assisted transoral access to the pituitary fossa in cases where trans-nasal routes are suboptimal (O'Malley and Weinstein 2007). Feasibility studies have shown that a transoral robotic approach, incorporating a palatal split, can provide access to the sphenoid sinus and sella turcica without external incisions (Chauvet et al. 2014). Robotic assistance has also been explored in craniofacial reconstructive procedures, particularly in microvascular free flap inset in confined spaces. However, robotic applications remain limited to relatively small, benign, or low-grade tumours without extensive neurovascular involvement (Fig. 7). Lesions with significant intracranial extension or those near the optic nerves, brainstem, or major intracranial vessels exceed the current capabilities of robotic surgery.

Successful robotic skull base surgery demands meticulous preoperative planning, including high-resolution imaging (CT, MRI, and angiography) to delineate tumour extent and its relationship to critical structures. Virtual surgical planning and 3D reconstructions enhance intraoperative navigation. A multidisciplinary approach—combining expertise from otolaryngologists, oral and maxillofacial surgeons, and neurosurgeons—optimizes outcomes. Intraoperative navigation can augment robotic surgery by integrating endoscopic views with preoperative imaging to ensure precise localization of key anatomical landmarks. Microdissection techniques leverage the robot's motion scaling to enhance precision while minimizing trauma to adjacent

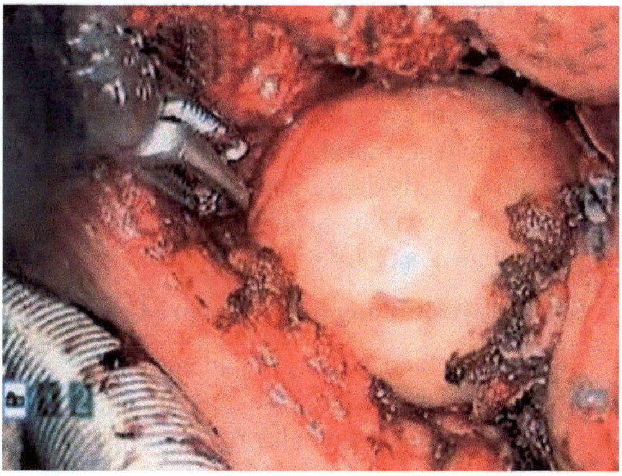

Fig. 7 The infratemporal fossa and parapharyngeal space neoplasm were dissected during surgery (Curtesy: Augello et al. 2018)

neurovascular structures. Additionally, patient positioning, such as slight Trendelenburg, may aid in reducing venous bleeding. Supplemental exposure techniques, such as palatal splitting or mandibular swing, may facilitate access to deep-seated lesions. Given the complex anatomy, contingency plans, including instruments for open conversion and predefined criteria for switching to an alternative approach, are essential for patient safety (Augello et al. 2018).

Best Practices

1. **Preoperative Imaging and Planning**
    - High-resolution imaging (CT, MRI, and angiography) is essential to delineate tumour extent and its relationship to vital structures (e.g. carotid arteries, cranial nerves, spinal cord).
    - 3D reconstructions and virtual surgical planning software aid in simulating the endoscopic view and instrument trajectories.
    - Given the confined surgical field, meticulous preoperative planning minimizes intraoperative risks.
2. **Multidisciplinary Team Approach**
    - Optimal outcomes require coordinated efforts among otolaryngologists, oral and maxillofacial surgeons (OMFS), and neurosurgeons.
    - The surgical approach may be handled by an OMFS or ENT specialist (e.g. creating a pharyngeal corridor or palatal split), while neurosurgeons perform intradural or bone drilling portions.
    - Collaborative robotic platform use ensures each aspect of the procedure is managed by the most specialized expert.
3. **Intraoperative Navigation and Image Guidance**
    - Image-guided systems integrated with TORS help surgeons correlate the endoscopic view with preoperative imaging.
    - Enhances safety in unfamiliar or high-risk areas, such as near the carotid canal or foramen ovale.
4. **Microdissection Techniques and Motion Scaling**
    - The robot's motion scaling allows large hand movements to translate into fine instrument control.
    - Slow, steady dissection minimizes trauma to nerves and vessels.
    - Gentle, layer-by-layer dissection with frequent bipolar cautery use helps maintain haemostasis.
5. **Patient Positioning and Exposure Optimization**
    - Slight Trendelenburg positioning (head-up) reduces venous pressure and intraoperative bleeding.
    - Adequate exposure may require adjunct manoeuvres, such as:
        - **Palatal split** for transoral pituitary access.

  - **Trans tonsillar approach with mandibular swing** to enhance lateral skull base access.

- These modifications can make robotic approaches feasible for otherwise inaccessible lesions.

6. **Backup Plans and Open Conversion Readiness**

   - Instruments for open conversion should be sterile and readily available.
   - Clear conversion criteria should be established (e.g. uncontrolled bleeding, inadequate visualization).

Common Pitfalls and Avoidance Strategies

1. **Limited Reach and Workspace Constraints**

   - **Pitfall**: The anatomical reach of robotic instruments is restricted, particularly in lateral or superior skull base areas. Beyond certain points (e.g. foramen ovale), instrument angles become too acute, limiting access.
   - **Avoidance**: Carefully assess tumour location relative to robotic reach; consider staging the procedure, utilizing adjunct incisions, or opting for an open approach when necessary.

2. **Risk to Neurovascular Structures**

   - **Pitfall**: The lack of haptic feedback in robotic surgery increases the risk of inadvertently injuring critical structures such as the internal carotid artery, jugular bulb, cranial nerves (IX–XII), and spinal cord.
   - **Avoidance**: Utilize high-definition visualization and meticulous anatomical mapping with neuro navigation. Employ fine-tip dissection techniques, visually skeletonizing key neurovascular structures before proceeding.

3. **Bleeding in a Confined Operative Space**

   - **Pitfall**: Even moderate bleeding can obscure visualization and complicate haemostasis in the narrow surgical corridor.
   - **Avoidance**: Maintain a low threshold for prophylactic cautery or vessel clipping. Use preoperative embolization for vascular tumours. Keep the patient slightly head-elevated to reduce venous pressure. Have a contingency plan for open conversion if bleeding becomes uncontrollable.

4. **Instrumentation and Access Limitations**

   - **Pitfall**: Rigid robotic instruments are not optimized for the intricate contours of the skull base, making navigation around tight angles difficult.
   - **Avoidance**: Improve access by performing adjunctive manoeuvres, such as soft palate splitting or limited tissue resection. Use the smallest available robotic instruments (e.g. 5 mm) and consider an auxiliary endoscope or suction for retraction in transoral cases.

5. **Patient Safety Considerations**
   - **Pitfall**: Prolonged retraction in the oral cavity may lead to tongue oedema, dental injury, or prolonged ischemia of soft tissues.
   - **Avoidance**: Periodically relieve retraction pressure, use adequate padding for the teeth, and minimize extended operative positioning.
6. **Lengthy Operative Time and Anaesthesia Risks**
   - **Pitfall**: Early in the learning curve, robotic skull base surgeries can be time-intensive, increasing patient exposure to anaesthesia risks.
   - **Avoidance**: Rehearse the set-up thoroughly and establish an experienced surgical team. As familiarity with robotic docking and dissection improves, operative time efficiency will increase.

4.7 Robotic-Assisted Neck Dissection and Thyroidectomy

Robotic-assisted neck surgery emerged primarily for improved cosmesis in thyroid and parathyroid procedures. Traditional thyroidectomy leaves a visible neck scar, prompting the development of remote-access approaches, such as trans-axillary or chest incisions, particularly in East Asia. Robotic systems facilitate these techniques, making them ideal for patients with thyroid tumours or benign nodules (<5 cm, no massive thyroiditis, no widespread metastases) seeking a scar-free neck.

A common technique is gasless trans-axillary thyroidectomy, using a 5- to 6-cm armpit incision to access the neck. The da Vinci robot enables lobectomy, total thyroidectomy, and central lymph node dissection while avoiding a neck incision. Indications include differentiated thyroid cancers (e.g. papillary carcinoma) in younger patients with limited disease and large benign goitres, especially in those prone to keloids or preferring a hidden scar.

Robotic surgery extends to neck dissection for thyroid cancer nodal metastases via trans-axillary, chest, or retro auricular ('facelift') approaches. Kang et al. first reported robotic lateral neck dissection (levels II–V) for thyroid cancer to avoid long scars. Select patients with nodal metastases from thyroid, cutaneous, or HPV-positive oropharyngeal cancers can benefit if disease distribution is suitable.

Another application is robotic-assisted parotid or submandibular gland surgery for benign tumours via a facelift incision, primarily for cosmetic reasons. Ideal candidates for robotic-assisted neck surgery include:

- Thyroid tumours (benign or low/intermediate-risk cancer) suitable for remote-access approaches.
- Nodal metastases in the lateral neck (levels I–V) from thyroid or HPV-positive oropharyngeal carcinoma in patients prioritizing aesthetics.

- Certain benign neck or salivary gland tumours where hidden incisions are preferred.

Robotic surgery is unsuitable for advanced thyroid cancer with tracheal/oesophageal invasion or extensive nodal disease requiring wide exposure. Extensive neck dissections with large nodes or extracapsular spread are best managed with open surgery. The optimal robotic candidates have small to moderate-volume disease within a well-defined surgical field.

Emerging Technique: Transoral Robotic Thyroidectomy

A newer approach, **transoral robotic thyroidectomy**, accesses the thyroid through the mouth (vestibular approach). Though less common in **oral and maxillofacial surgery (OMFS)**, it remains under evaluation. Robotic neck surgery relies on **remote incisions**—either in the axilla or behind the ear—to create a working space. Using robotic enhancements, surgeons perform **precise dissections** while avoiding visible neck scars. This technique aligns with the primary goal of **'invisible incision' surgery**, where incisions are strategically placed in natural creases or out of sight. These approaches often require a **larger skin flap dissection** compared to open surgery, as access must be tunnelled from a distance. **Mastery demands extensive practice**, and high-volume centres in **Asia** have refined these techniques to ensure safety and effectiveness.

Advantages

Cosmetic Benefits and Patient Satisfaction

Robotic neck and thyroid surgery have gained attention for its **superior cosmetic outcomes**, significantly improving **patient satisfaction**. Studies highlight that young patient, in particular, prefer robotic procedures due to the absence of a **visible anterior neck scar**, which helps preserve body image. Many centres emphasize the **'scarless thyroid surgery'** aspect in their marketing, as neck scars can impact confidence and serve as a lifelong reminder of surgery.

Oncologic and Surgical Efficacy

Multiple studies, including meta-analyses, confirm that **robotic neck procedures achieve outcomes comparable to open surgery**. **Complication rates** for thyroidectomy, such as recurrent nerve palsy and hypoparathyroidism, are similar when performed by experienced surgeons. A 2019 **systematic review** found that **lymph node yields in robotic neck dissection match those of traditional methods**, with no significant differences in recurrence rates. Additionally, **operative blood loss and overall complication rates** tend to be **comparable** between robotic and open approaches.

Post-Operative Recovery and Functional Benefits

Robotic surgery may offer **functional advantages beyond cosmetics**. Some studies suggest **reduced post-operative neck oedema and lymphedema**, possibly due to

more precise lymphatic handling and **avoiding long incisions** that disrupt drainage. Reports indicate that patients undergoing robotic neck dissection experience **less swelling** and **no significant increase in chyle leaks**. Furthermore, some patients report **less post-surgical discomfort** when incisions are placed in the **arm or behind the ear** instead of the neck.

Challenges and Economic Considerations

Despite its benefits, robotic surgery involves **longer operative times**—typically **45–60 min more than open surgery**—primarily due to **set-up and docking**. Additionally, robotic procedures require a **larger skin flap dissection**, which may cause **temporary tightness or numbness**. Proper **patient selection** is crucial; those with extensive disease or **unfavorable anatomy** may be better suited for conventional surgery to ensure **optimal oncologic and safety outcomes**.

From an economic standpoint, robotic thyroidectomy **has higher costs**, but patient demand and **marketability** help offset these expenses, especially in **Asia**, where **adoption is growing**. In **Western countries**, uptake has been slower due to **cost concerns and patient preferences**. However, as **technology evolves**, newer robotic systems and **streamlined instrumentation** may reduce costs and operative times, making the technique more widely accessible.

4.8 *Robotic-Assisted Trauma Surgery*

1 **Precision Fracture Reduction and Fixation**

- Robotic systems enhance **fracture alignment** and **hardware placement** with high precision.
- In **orthopaedic trauma**, robotic assistance improves alignment accuracy and reduces soft-tissue damage.
- Applied to **maxillofacial fractures**, robots can move bone fragments into place with **minimal incisions**, reducing scarring and aiding faster recovery (Muto et al. 2024).
- Early prototypes, such as **transoral robotic systems**, provide access to difficult jaw angles for **mandibular fracture reduction** (Kou et al. 2023).

2. **Minimally Invasive Trauma Surgery**

- Robotics enables **keyhole approaches** for facial fractures, reducing visible scars.
- **Articulated instruments** work in tight spaces, minimizing **soft-tissue dissection**, swelling, and drainage (Muto et al. 2024).
- Surgeons can use **multiple robotic arms** to reposition bone fragments with sub-millimetre precision, improving **occlusal outcomes** and reducing secondary corrections.

3. **Integration with Imaging for Real-Time Adjustments**

   - Advancement in Trauma Surgery: Image-guided robotic surgery is a significant development in trauma care.
   - Real-Time Imaging Input: The robotic system integrates intraoperative 3D imaging (e.g. cone-beam CT or fluoroscopy) for real-time fragment alignment feedback.
   - Surgeon Control and Live Feedback: The surgeon can move the robot or apply controlled forces while monitoring live images. Intraoperative CT detects shifts in zygomatic arch fragments, allowing the robot to adjust positioning or screw trajectories accordingly.
   - Closed-Loop Integration Benefits: Enhances fracture reduction accuracy and prevents malunions. Automates repetitive imaging adjustments, reducing radiation exposure for staff.
   - Surgeon–Robot Interaction: Imaging confirms bone alignment, and the surgeon can use a foot pedal to command the robot to tighten a plate.
   - Impact on Facial Trauma Surgery: The synergy of robotics, navigation, and imaging is expected to improve complex facial trauma outcomes (Kou et al. 2023).

4. **Clinical Benefits and Early Outcomes**

   - Experimental Stage: Dedicated maxillofacial trauma robots are still in the early research phase.
   - Anticipated Benefits:
     - Improved fracture alignment with high precision.
     - Shorter incisions, leading to less scarring and lower infection risk.
     - Reduced surgeon fatigue during long and complex reconstructions.
   - Enhanced Surgical Efficiency:
     - Robots can hold retraction and maintain reduction for extended periods, allowing surgeons to focus on other tasks.
     - Potential reduction in operative time due to robotic assistance.
   - Lower Complication Rates: Percutaneous or intraoral fixation minimizes large dissections, reducing risks like wound infections or nerve injuries.
   - Early Feasibility Studies:
     - Robotic fracture systems have shown reduction accuracy comparable to open surgery.
     - Achieves precise outcomes while using smaller incisions.

5. **Challenges and Limitations**

   - **Bone segment movement** complicates robotic navigation in facial trauma.
   - **Lack of haptic feedback** makes delicate bone manipulation difficult, increasing the risk of unintended damage.

- **Instrument size** is a limitation—existing surgical robots are too bulky for **small facial spaces**.
- **High cost and learning curve** hinder widespread adoption, but advancements in **compact, intelligent systems** are addressing these issues.

4.9 Robotic Microsurgery for Nerve Repair

Robotic microsurgery is revolutionizing how surgeons repair fine nerves by enabling tremor-free, scaled movements. Specialized microsurgical robots like the Micro-Sure's MUSA and the MMI Symani act as 'steady hands' to suture nerves that are only 1–3 mm in diameter. The surgeon operates from a console with joystick controls, and the robot filters out hand tremors and can downscale motions (e.g. a 5 mm hand movement might translate to a 1 mm instrument movement). This allows extremely delicate manoeuvres that far exceed human dexterity. In practical terms, a robotic system can precisely align nerve endings and place evenly spaced sutures with uniform tension, which is critical for optimal nerve healing. The anastomosis of a severed facial or trigeminal nerve (such as the infraorbital or inferior alveolar nerve) can be performed under high magnification with sub-millimetre accuracy. Early clinical reports confirm that robotic assistance yields safer and more precise peripheral nerve repair than manual techniques. The robot's precision helps avoid unintentional needle trauma to nerve fascicles and ensures a tension-free anastomosis by fine-tuning the approximation of nerve stumps (Fig. 8) (Dagnino et al. 2017).

Enhanced Outcomes for Facial and Trigeminal Nerve Injuries

- **Improved Functional Recovery**:
  - Robot-assisted **neurorrhaphy** enhances **nerve fascicle alignment** and reduces **fibrosis** at the repair site.
  - Patients may experience **better nerve recovery** (e.g. return of sensation or facial muscle function).

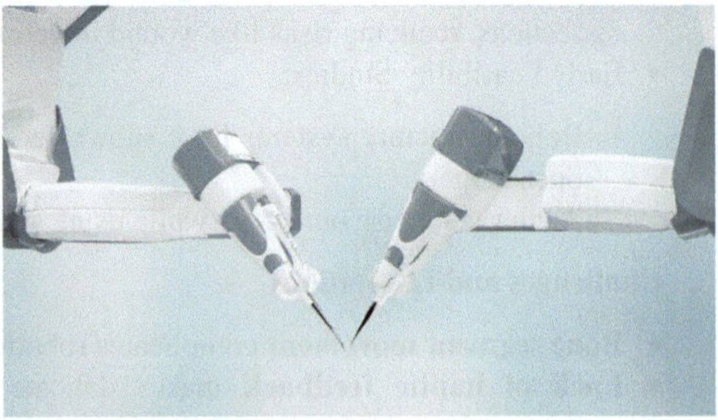

Fig. 8 Microsurgical robotic system (MUSA) with dual arms holding microsurgical instruments (Dagnino et al. 2017)

- **Early Clinical Evidence**:
  - A **review of robotic microsurgery** reported **high success rates** for nerve repairs, despite slightly longer operative times.
  - **MUSA robot** demonstrated **successful digital nerve repairs** in **nine cases**, with all rated at least 'satisfactory'.
  - Over time, surgeons **improved repair speed** without sacrificing accuracy.
- **Application in Facial Nerve Reconstruction**:
  - Used for **facial nerve grafting** after **parotid tumour resection**.
  - Allows nerve graft **placement under the jaw angle** through a **minimal incision**, preserving delicate branches.
  - Reduces **hand tremors**, minimizing **trauma to nerve fibres** and potentially leading to **faster recovery** (Coelho et al. 2024).

Robotic Neurorrhaphy Techniques and Technologies

- **Master–Slave Tele manipulator Design**:
  - The surgeon's movements at a **console** are replicated by **miniaturized robotic instruments**.
  - **Symani system** provides **3D microscope view** and micro instruments with **7 degrees of freedom** for complex suturing (Coelho et al. 2024).
- **Emerging Innovations**:
  - **Haptic Feedback Development**: Enables surgeons to **'feel' resistance** when passing a needle through nerve tissue (Dagnino et al. 2017).
  - **Super Microsurgical Robots**: Can **anastomose vessels or nerves under 0.5 mm**, allowing repair of **tiny nerve branches**.
  - **First Robotic Nerve Repair (2009, Nectoux et al.)** (Cannizzaro et al. 2024): Demonstrated safer and more precise suturing than manual techniques.
  - **Pilot studies** exploring:

    Brachial plexus surgery
    Nerve grafting

Clinical Trials and Early Results

- **Pilot Studies**:
  - A **2024 multicentre trial** reported **successful robotic digital nerve repairs** in **nine patients**, with no adverse events.
  - **Robotic facial nerve reanimation** being tested for cross-facial nerve grafting.
- **Comparative Analysis**:
  - Systematic reviews show robotic procedures initially take longer but **approach manual speed** with experience.
  - Robots provide **consistent suture quality** and reduce **surgeon fatigue**.

- A **super microsurgery trial** (lymphatic anastomosis) found robots performed **ultra-fine sutures reliably**, though clinical outcomes were similar to manual techniques (Coelho et al. 2024).

Challenges in Robotic Microsurgery

- **Time and Set-up Constraints**:
  - **Longer set-up and operative times** due to positioning, calibration, and instrument exchange.
  - **Need for dedicated microsurgical instruments** (now being developed by companies like **MicroSure** and **MMI**).
- **Technical Limitations**:
  - **Suturing fine nerves (1 mm) can be challenging**.
  - **Lack of tactile feedback** makes nerve manipulation less intuitive for surgeons.
- **Financial and Training Barriers**:
  - **High Costs**: Capital expenses and lack of insurance reimbursement for **robotic nerve repair**.
  - **Surgeon Learning Curve**: Requires adaptation to **foot pedals and scaled motion control**.

5 Applications of AR in OMFS

Virtual reality (VR) and augmented reality (AR) are rapidly transforming oral and maxillofacial surgery (OMFS) by enhancing surgical training, preoperative planning, intraoperative guidance, and patient education. These technologies allow realistic 3D visualization and interaction with anatomical structures, improving surgical accuracy and efficiency (Ayoub and Pulijala 2019; Stucki et al. 2024).

5.1 VR and AR in Surgical Training and Education

One of the most significant applications of VR and AR in OMFS is resident training and education. These technologies provide interactive, hands-on simulation environments where trainees can practice complex surgical procedures without patient risk.

- VR-based surgical simulations allow residents to perform procedures such as Le Fort I osteotomy, sagittal split ramus osteotomy, and orbital floor repair in a risk-free environment.

- Haptic feedback in VR simulators improves training by simulating bone cutting resistance, tissue elasticity, and needle insertion angles, making it a realistic alternative to cadaver-based training.
- Studies have shown that residents trained with VR-based models exhibit greater confidence, better performance, and improved surgical precision compared to those using traditional methods.

Clinical Significance

- Reduces dependency on cadaveric and animal models, making training more cost-effective and accessible.
- Allows repeated practice, helping residents refine their skills before real surgical cases.
- VR provides objective assessments of surgical performance, allowing instructors to measure speed, accuracy, and error rates.

5.2 VR and AR in Preoperative Planning

VR and AR have revolutionized preoperative planning in OMFS, allowing surgeons to visualize patient-specific anatomy in three dimensions before surgery (Stucki et al. 2024).

- VR-based surgical planning enables surgeons to simulate osteotomies, reposition bone segments, and assess outcomes before the actual procedure.
- AR overlays virtual anatomical structures onto real-world patient images, allowing precise alignment of osteotomies and implant placements.
- Facial transplantation planning has benefited from VR-based anthropometric analysis, ensuring better donor-recipient compatibility.

Clinical Significance

- VR improves surgical predictability, leading to better aesthetic and functional outcomes.
- AR reduces surgical errors by allowing real-time visualization of hidden anatomical structures.
- Enhances surgeon confidence and preparedness, especially for complex reconstructive procedures.

5.3 VR and AR for Intraoperative Guidance

AR is increasingly being used during surgery to provide real-time navigation and anatomical visualization (Ayoub and Pulijala 2019; Stucki et al. 2024).

- AR-assisted orthognathic surgery uses holographic overlays of planned osteotomy lines on the patient's face, improving precision and reducing surgical time.

- Wearable AR headsets provide real-time 3D guidance, eliminating the need for frequent CT/MRI reference during surgery.
- AR in TMJ surgery allows precise visualization of joint structures, reducing complications and improving prosthetic positioning.

Clinical Significance

- Improves surgical accuracy, reducing complications and revision surgeries.
- Decreases operative time by allowing surgeons to visualize anatomy without looking away from the surgical field.
- AR-assisted freehand surgeries improve bone graft positioning and reconstruction accuracy.

5.4 VR and AR in Trauma and Reconstruction Surgery

Maxillofacial trauma and reconstruction often require precise bone realignment and implant placement. VR and AR have enhanced surgical navigation and patient-specific reconstructions (Stucki et al. 2024).

- AR-guided navigation for orbito-zygomatic fractures has been shown to improve reduction accuracy and facial symmetry restoration.
- VR-based simulations allow preoperative testing of custom implants and bone grafts, reducing trial-and-error in reconstruction surgeries.
- AI-integrated AR predicts fracture stability and healing outcomes, optimizing fixation techniques and post-operative care.

Clinical Significance

- Minimizes surgical errors in complex maxillofacial fractures.
- Improves implant and graft positioning, reducing the need for secondary corrections.
- Reduces intraoperative decision-making time, leading to more efficient surgeries.

5.5 VR and AR in Patient Education and Anxiety Reduction

VR is being used to educate patients about their conditions and treatment plans, improving informed consent and reducing anxiety.

- VR simulations allow patients to visualize their surgical outcomes, leading to higher treatment acceptance rates.
- Studies have shown that patients who use VR relaxation techniques before oral surgery experience lower stress and anxiety levels.
- AR-based apps help patients understand complex procedures, improving their satisfaction and trust in their surgeons.

Clinical Significance

- Enhances patient engagement and understanding of surgical procedures.
- Reduces preoperative anxiety, leading to better cooperation during treatment.
- Improves doctor-patient communication, leading to higher satisfaction rates.

6 Role of Large Language Models in OMFS

Large language models (LLMs), such as ChatGPT, Google Bard, Bing AI, and Claude, are transforming oral and maxillofacial surgery (OMFS) by enhancing clinical decision-making, patient education, research assistance, and surgical planning. These AI-driven models leverage natural language processing (NLP) and deep learning to interpret complex clinical data, provide diagnostic support, and optimize communication between healthcare professionals and patients (Azadi et al. 2024; Johnson et al. 2024; Nectoux et al. 2009).

6.1 Large Language Models (LLM) in Clinical Decision-Making in OMFS

One of the most significant applications of LLMs in OMFS is assisting clinicians in decision-making for complex cases (Fig. 9).

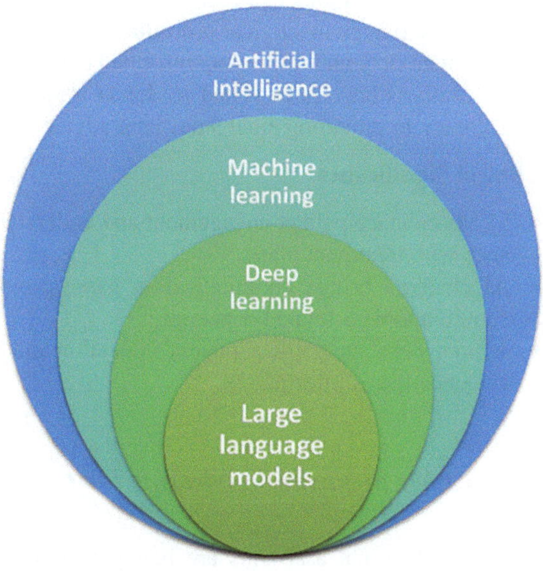

Fig. 9 Diagrammatic representation of large language models

- A study evaluating LLMs (ChatGPT, Google Bard, Bing AI, and Claude) on case-based clinical decision-making questions in OMFS found that GPT-4 and Claude-Instant performed best, with correct responses in 38% of cases (Azadi et al. 2024).
- Chatbots were particularly useful in diagnosing maxillofacial fractures, assessing surgical indications for orthognathic surgery, and predicting complications.
- However, chatbot-generated responses still contained inaccuracies, highlighting the need for human supervision in clinical decision-making.

Clinical Significance

- LLMs can serve as decision-support tools for junior surgeons or general dentists, improving diagnostic accuracy.
- They help in evaluating treatment options, especially in trauma, pathology, and reconstructive surgery.
- AI-assisted decision-making reduces cognitive workload, allowing clinicians to focus on patient-centred care.

6.2 LLMs in Patient Education and Preoperative Counselling

AI-driven chatbots are increasingly being used to educate patients about their conditions and upcoming surgical procedures.

- A multicentre study on ChatGPT's reliability in head and neck surgery found that 87.2% of AI-generated responses were accurate and provided useful explanations for patients (Nectoux et al. 2009).
- LLMs help explain surgical procedures, risks, and post-operative care, reducing patient anxiety and improving informed consent.
- AI chatbots have been tested in dental traumatology, demonstrating moderate accuracy in providing emergency care advice.

Clinical Significance

- LLMs enhance patient engagement and understanding, leading to better compliance with treatment plans.
- AI chatbots bridge communication gaps, providing 24/7 patient support for common OMFS-related concerns.
- AI can help standardize patient education materials, ensuring consistent and evidence-based information.

6.3 LLMs in Virtual Assistants for OMFS Clinics

AI-powered virtual assistants are being integrated into OMFS clinics to handle administrative and clinical queries.

- AI chatbots can manage appointment scheduling, follow-up reminders, and basic triage of OMFS emergencies.
- AI-driven preoperative and post-operative guidance can enhance patient adher ence to care protocols.
- Some virtual assistants are being tested for post-operative pain management recommendations, offering analgesic suggestions based on patient-reported pain levels.

Clinical Significance

- AI chatbots reduce administrative burdens, allowing staff to focus on direct patient care.
- Virtual assistants improve patient experience, ensuring timely access to pre- and post-surgical instructions.
- AI-driven triage systems help streamline urgent OMFS cases, optimizing emergency department efficiency.

6.4 Limitations of LLMs in OMFS

Despite their advantages, LLMs have certain limitations in clinical practice:

1. Potential for Misinformation: AI-generated responses can sometimes be inaccurate or misleading, requiring clinician validation.
2. Lack of Real-Time Data: Chatbots are trained on static datasets, which may lack the latest clinical guidelines.
3. Limited Case-Specific Decision-Making: AI models are not yet capable of handling complex, dynamic clinical scenarios requiring surgeon intuition and experience.
4. Ethical and Legal Concerns: Issues surrounding patient data privacy, liability, and informed decision-making must be addressed before widespread AI adoption.

7 Conclusion

Artificial intelligence (AI), robotics, and augmented reality (AR) have revolutionized the field of oral and maxillofacial surgery (OMFS), offering unprecedented advancements in diagnosis, treatment planning, and surgical execution. AI-driven technologies have enhanced imaging interpretation, virtual surgical planning, and real-time intraoperative guidance, significantly improving patient outcomes. Machine learning (ML) and deep learning (DL) models have demonstrated exceptional accuracy in diagnosing conditions such as skeletal malocclusions, oral malignancies, temporomandibular disorders (TMDs), and maxillofacial trauma, allowing for earlier interventions and personalized treatment strategies.

Furthermore, the integration of robotics and AR has enhanced precision in complex surgical procedures such as orthognathic surgery, dental implantology, and trauma reconstruction, reducing human error and improving surgical efficiency. Augmented reality has expanded its role beyond surgery into education, training, and patient communication, providing interactive 3D models that improve understanding and engagement. Additionally, the emergence of large language models and AI-driven virtual assistants has transformed patient interactions, streamlining clinical workflows and providing real-time support to both practitioners and patients. However, despite these advancements, challenges remain, including data standardization, ethical considerations, regulatory compliance, and AI explainability.

Looking ahead, continued advancements in AI, robotics, and AR will further refine the precision and efficiency of OMFS. Future research should focus on improving AI model transparency, integrating multimodal datasets, and expanding real-time intraoperative AI applications to maximize patient safety and outcomes. As these technologies continue to evolve, they will play an increasingly critical role in transforming OMFS into a data-driven, minimally invasive, and patient-centred specialty.

References

Aaronson NL, Neubauer PD, Judson BL (2015) Cost effectiveness of transoral robotic surgery for the treatment of oropharyngeal squamous cell carcinoma: a systematic review. Robot Surg Res Rev, 59–63

Abdul NS, Shivakumar GC, Sangappa SB, Di Blasio M, Crimi S, Cicciù M, Minervini G (2024) Applications of artificial intelligence in the field of oral and maxillofacial pathology: a systematic review and meta-analysis. BMC Oral Health 24:122

Almăşan O, Leucuţa DC, Hedeşiu M, Mureşanu S, Popa Ştefan L (2023) Temporomandibular joint osteoarthritis diagnosis employing artificial intelligence: systematic review and meta-analysis. J Clin Med 12

Ansarin M, Zorzi S, Massaro MA, Tagliabue M, Proh M, Giugliano G, Calabrese L, Chiesa F (2014) Transoral robotic surgery versus transoral laser microsurgery for resection of supraglottic cancer: a pilot surgery: Robotic surgery in supraglottic cancer. Int J Med Robot 10:107–112

Assiri HA, Hameed MS, Alqarni A, Dawasaz AA, Arem SA, Assiri KI (2024) Artificial intelligence application in a case of mandibular third molar impaction: a systematic review of the literature. J Clin Med 13:4431

Augello M, Baetscher C, Segesser M, Zeilhofer H-F, Cattin P, Juergens P (2018) Performing partial mandibular resection, fibula free flap reconstruction and midfacial osteotomies with a cold ablation and robot-guided Er:YAG laser osteotome (CARLO®)—a study on applicability and effectiveness in human cadavers. J Cranio-Maxillofac Surg 46:1850–1855

Ayoub A, Pulijala Y (2019) The application of virtual reality and augmented reality in oral and maxillofacial surgery. BMC Oral Health 19:1–8

Azadi A, Gorjinejad F, Mohammad-Rahimi H, Tabrizi R, Alam M, Golkar M (2024) Evaluation of AI-generated responses by different artificial intelligence chatbots to the clinical decision-making case-based questions in oral and maxillofacial surgery. Oral Surg Oral Med Oral Pathol Oral Radiol 137:587–593

Babu B, Vinayachandran D, Ganesh C, Shanthi M, Krithika C (2024) Bibliometric analysis of the role of artificial intelligence in detecting maxillofacial fractures. Cureus 16

Bansal A, Bansal V, Popli G, Keshri N, Khare G, Goel S (2016) Robots in head and neck surgery. J Appl Dent Med Sci 2:168–175

Bansal S, Managutti A, Babhulkar A, Patel N (1990) Artificial intelligence in oral and maxillofacial surgery: a road ahead. Learning 13:2–6

Birur PN, Sunny SP, Jena S, Kandasarma U, Raghavan S, Ramaswamy B, Shanmugam SP, Patrick S, Kuriakose R, Mallaiah J (2015) Mobile health application for remote oral cancer surveillance. J Am Dent Assoc 146:886–894

Cannizzaro D, Scalise M, Zancanella C, Paulli S, Peron S, Stefini R (2024) Comparative evaluation of major robotic systems in microanastomosis procedures: a systematic review of current capabilities and future potential. Brain Sci 14:1235

Chauvet D, Missistrano A, Hivelin M, Carpentier A, Cornu P, Hans S (2014) Transoral robotic-assisted skull base surgery to approach the sella turcica: cadaveric study. Neurosurg Rev 37:609–617

Choi E, Lee S, Jeong E, Shin S, Park H, Youm S, Son Y, Pang K (2022) Artificial intelligence in positioning between mandibular third molar and inferior alveolar nerve on panoramic radiography. Sci Rep 12:2456

Coelho M, Peltz T, Hunt J, Gianoutsos M (2024) Robotic surgery in plastic surgery: a review of its potential. Australas J Plast Surg 7:1–7

Cohen MA, Weinstein GS, O'Malley BW, Feldman M, Quon H (2011) Transoral robotic surgery and human papillomavirus status: oncologic results. Head Neck 33:573–580

Dagnino G, Georgilas I, Morad S, Gibbons P, Tarassoli P, Atkins R, Dogramadzi S (2017) Image-guided surgical robotic system for percutaneous reduction of joint fractures. Ann Biomed Eng 45:2648–2662

Dashti M, Ghaedsharaf S, Ghasemi S, Zare N, Constantin E-F, Fahimipour A, Tajbakhsh N, Ghadimi N (2024) Evaluation of deep learning and convolutional neural network algorithms for mandibular fracture detection using radiographic images: a systematic review and meta-analysis. Imaging Sci Dent 54:232

de Boutray M, Cuau L, Ohayon M, Garrel R, Poignet P, Zemiti N (2024) Robot-guided osteotomy in fibula free flap mandibular reconstruction: a preclinical study. Int J Oral Maxillofac Surg 53:343–346

Deng H, Liu Q, Chen A, Kuang T, Yuan P, Gateno J, Kim D, Barber J, Xiong K, Yu P (2023) Clinical feasibility of deep learning-based automatic head CBCT image segmentation and landmark detection in computer-aided surgical simulation for orthognathic surgery. Int J Oral Maxillofac Surg 52:793–800

Dot G, Schouman T, Dubois G, Rouch P, Gajny L (2022) Fully automatic segmentation of craniomaxillofacial CT scans for computer-assisted orthognathic surgery planning using the nnU-Net framework. Eur Radiol, 1–10

Dziegielewski PT, Teknos TN, Durmus K, Old M, Agrawal A, Kakarala K, Marcinow A, Ozer E (2013) Transoral robotic surgery for oropharyngeal cancer: long-term quality of life and functional outcomes. JAMA Otolaryngol Neck Surg 139:1099

Ebeling M, Scheurer M, Sakkas A, Wilde F, Schramm A (2023) First-Hand experience and result with new robot-assisted laser LeFort-I osteotomy in orthognathic surgery: a case report. J Pers Med. https://doi.org/10.3390/jpm13020287

Ekert T, Krois J, Meinhold L, Elhennawy K, Emara R, Golla T, Schwendicke F (2019) Deep learning for the radiographic detection of apical lesions. J Endod 45:917–922

Farajollahi M, Safarian MS, Hatami M, Esmaeil Nejad A, Peters OA (2023) Applying artificial intelligence to detect and analyse oral and maxillofacial bone loss—a scoping review. Aust Endod J 49:720–734

Fukuda M, Ariji Y, Kise Y, Nozawa M, Kuwada C, Funakoshi T, Muramatsu C, Fujita H, Katsumata A, Ariji E (2020) Comparison of 3 deep learning neural networks for classifying the relationship between the mandibular third molar and the mandibular canal on panoramic radiographs. Oral Surg Oral Med Oral Pathol Oral Radiol 130:336–343

García-Pola M, Pons-Fuster E, Suárez-Fernández C, Seoane-Romero J, Romero-Méndez A, López-Jornet P (2021) Role of artificial intelligence in the early diagnosis of oral cancer. a scoping review. Cancers 13:4600

Genden EM, Desai S, Sung C (2009) Transoral robotic surgery for the management of head and neck cancer: a preliminary experience. Head Neck 31:283–289

Han JJ, Woo S-Y, Yi W-J, Hwang SJ (2020) A robot arm and image-guided navigation assisted surgical system for maxillary repositioning in orthognathic surgery: a phantom skull-based trial. Appl Sci 10:1549

Jha N, Lee K-S, Kim Y-J (2022) Diagnosis of temporomandibular disorders using artificial intelligence technologies: a systematic review and meta-analysis. PLoS ONE 17:e0272715

Johnson AJ, Singh TK, Gupta A, Sankar H, Gill I, Shalini M, Mohan N (2024) Evaluation of validity and reliability of AI Chatbots as public sources of information on dental trauma. Dent, Traumatol

Kalan S, Chauhan S, Coelho RF, Orvieto MA, Camacho IR, Palmer KJ, Patel VR (2010) History of robotic surgery. J Robot Surg 4:141–147

Kato RM, Parizotto J de OL, Oliveira PHJ de, Gonçalves JR (2023) Artificial intelligence in orthognathic surgery–a narrative review of surgical digital tools and 3D orthognathic surgical planning. J Calif Dent Assoc 51:2202444

Kaul V, Enslin S, Gross SA (2020) History of artificial intelligence in medicine. Gastrointest Endosc 92:807–812

Kazimierczak W, Wajer R, Wajer A, Kiian V, Kloska A, Kazimierczak N, Janiszewska-Olszowska J, Serafin Z (2024) Periapical lesions in panoramic radiography and CBCT imaging—assessment of AI's diagnostic accuracy. J Clin Med 13:2709

Khanagar SB, Alfouzan K, Awawdeh M, Alkadi L, Albalawi F, Alghilan MA (2022) Performance of artificial intelligence models designed for diagnosis, treatment planning and predicting prognosis of orthognathic surgery (OGS)—a scoping review. Appl Sci 12:5581

Kou W, Zhou P, Lin J, Kuang S, Sun L (2023) Technologies evolution in robot-assisted fracture reduction systems: a comprehensive review. Front Robot AI 10:1315250

Kurt Bayrakdar S, Orhan K, Bayrakdar IS, Bilgir E, Ezhov M, Gusarev M, Shumilov E (2021) A deep learning approach for dental implant planning in cone-beam computed tomography images. BMC Med Imaging 21:86

Lai Y, Wang C, Mao C, Lu M, Ouyang Q, Fang Y, Cai Z, Chen W (2022) Mandible reconstruction with free fibula flaps: accuracy of a cost-effective modified semicomputer-assisted surgery compared with computer-assisted surgery—a retrospective study. J Cranio-Maxillofac Surg 50:274–280

Li Y, Wu Y, Gao Y, Niu X, Li J, Tang M, Fu C, Qi R, Song B, Chen H (2022) Machine-learning based prediction of prognostic risk factors in patients with invasive candidiasis infection and bacterial bloodstream infection: a singled centered retrospective study. BMC Infect Dis 22:150

Ma L, Kim D, Lian C et al (2021) Deep simulation of facial appearance changes following craniomaxillofacial bony movements in orthognathic surgical planning. Med Image Comput Comput-Assist Interv MICCAI Int Conf Med Image Comput Comput-Assist Interv 12904:459–468

Ma Z, Guo Z, Ding Z, Cao C, He J, Tang H, Hua Y, Hong J, Shen Q, Lubamba GP (2024) Evaluation of a newly developed oral and maxillofacial surgical robotic platform (KD-SR-01) in head and neck surgery: a preclinical trial in porcine models. Int J Oral Sci 16:51

Mashhadi Akbar Boojar F, Ziaei H (2021) Future of the oral surgery. Innov Perspect Oral Maxillofac Surg 483–489

Muto J, Tateya I, Nakatomi H, Uyama I, Hirose Y (2024) Transoral robotic-assisted neurosurgery for skull base and upper spine lesions. Neurospine 21:106–115

Nectoux E, Taleb C, Liverneaux P (2009) Nerve repair in telemicrosurgery: an experimental study. J Reconstr Microsurg 25:261–265

O'Malley BW, Weinstein GS (2007) Robotic skull base surgery: preclinical investigations to human clinical application. Arch Otolaryngol Neck Surg 133:1215

Paro MR, Hersh DS, Bulsara KR (2022) History of virtual reality and augmented reality in neurosurgical training. World Neurosurg 167:37–43
Salazar D, Rossouw PE, Javed F, Michelogiannakis D (2024) Artificial intelligence for treatment planning and soft tissue outcome prediction of orthognathic treatment: a systematic review. J Orthod 51:107–119
Sankar H, Shalini M, Rajagopalan A, Gupta S, Kumar A, Shouket R (2025) Dental implant placement accuracy with robotic surgery compared to free-hand, static and dynamic computer assisted techniques: systematic review and meta-analysis. J Oral Biol Craniofacial Res 15:69–76
Sankar H, Alagarsamy R, Lal B, Rana SS, Roychoudhury A, Agrawal A, Wankhar S (2024) Role of artificial intelligence in treatment planning and outcome prediction of jaw corrective surgeries by using 3-D imaging-A systematic review. Oral Surg Oral Med Oral Pathol Oral Radiol
Sankar H, Alagarsamy R, Lal B, Rana SS, Roychoudhury A, Barathi A, Ankush A (2024) Role of Artificial intelligence in magnetic resonance imaging based detection of temporomandibular joint disorder-a systematic review. Br. Oral Maxillofac Surg
Schwendicke F, Chaurasia A, Arsiwala L, Lee J-H, Elhennawy K, Jost-Brinkmann P-G, Demarco F, Krois J (2021) Deep learning for cephalometric landmark detection: systematic review and meta-analysis. Clin Oral Investig 25:4299–4309
Serafin M, Baldini B, Cabitza F, Carrafiello G, Baselli G, Del Fabbro M, Sforza C, Caprioglio A, Tartaglia GM (2023) Accuracy of automated 3D cephalometric landmarks by deep learning algorithms: systematic review and meta-analysis. Radiol Med (Torino) 128:544–555
Shah J, Vyas A, Vyas D (2014) The history of robotics in surgical specialties. Am J Robot Surg 1:12
Stucki J, Dastgir R, Baur DA, Quereshy FA (2024) The use of virtual reality and augmented reality in oral and maxillofacial surgery: a narrative review. Oral Surg Oral Med Oral Pathol Oral Radiol 137:12–18
Sun M, Lin L, Chen X, Xu C, Zin MA, Han W, Chai G (2021) Robot-assisted mandibular angle osteotomy using electromagnetic navigation. Ann Transl Med 9
Takeshita WM, Silva TP, de Souza LLT, Tenorio JM (2024) State of the art and prospects for artificial intelligence in orthognathic surgery: a systematic review with meta-analysis. J Stomatol Oral Maxillofac Surg 125:101787
Ter Horst R, van Weert H, Loonen T, Bergé S, Vinayahalingam S, Baan F, Maal T, de Jong G, Xi T (2021) Three-dimensional virtual planning in mandibular advancement surgery: soft tissue prediction based on deep learning. J Cranio-Maxillofac Surg 49:775–782
Theodossy T, Bamber MA (2003) Model surgery with a passive robot arm for orthognathic surgery planning. J Oral Maxillofac Surg off J Am Assoc Oral Maxillofac Surg 61:1310–1317
Uthoff RD, Song B, Birur P, Kuriakose MA, Sunny S, Suresh A, Patrick S, Anbarani A, Spires O, Wilder-Smith P (2018) Development of a dual-modality, dual-view smartphone-based imaging system for oral cancer detection. SPIE, pp 106–112
Vaira LA, Lechien JR, Abbate V, Allevi F, Audino G, Beltramini GA, Bergonzani M, Bolzoni A, Committeri U, Crimi S (2024) Accuracy of ChatGPT-generated information on head and neck and oromaxillofacial surgery: a multicenter collaborative analysis. Otolaryngol Neck Surg 170:1492–1503
Vertucci R, D'Onofrio S, Ricciardi S, De Nino M (2023) History of augmented reality. In: Springer Handb. Augment. Real. Springer, pp 35–50
Vinayahalingam S, Xi T, Bergé S, Maal T, De Jong G (2019) Automated detection of third molars and mandibular nerve by deep learning. Sci Rep 9:9007
Weinstein GS, O'Malley BW, Cohen MA, Quon H (2010) Transoral robotic surgery for advanced oropharyngeal carcinoma. Arch Otolaryngol Neck Surg 136:1079–1085
Welikala RA, Remagnino P, Lim JH, Chan CS, Rajendran S, Kallarakkal TG, Zain RB, Jayasinghe RD, Rimal J, Kerr AR (2020) Automated detection and classification of oral lesions using deep learning for early detection of oral cancer. IEEE Access 8:132677–132693
Wu Y, Wang F, Fan S, Chow J (2019) Robotics in dental implantology. Oral Maxillofac Surg Clin N Am 31:513–518

Xu L, Chen J, Qiu K, Yang F, Wu W (2023b) Artificial intelligence for detecting temporomandibular joint osteoarthritis using radiographic image data: a systematic review and meta-analysis of diagnostic test accuracy. PLoS ONE 18:e0288631

Xu Z, Xiao Y, Zhou L, Lin Y, Su E, Chen J, Wu D (2023c) Accuracy and efficiency of robotic dental implant surgery with different human-robot interactions: an in vitro study. J Dent 137:104642

Xu M, Liu B, Luo Z, Ma H, Sun M, Wang Y, Yin N, Tang X, Song T (2023) Using a new deep learning method for 3D cephalometry in patients with cleft lip and palate. J Craniofac Surg, 10–1097

Yin Tsang RK, Ho WK, Wei WI (2012) Combined transnasal endoscopic and transoral robotic resection of recurrent nasopharyngeal carcinoma. Head Neck 34:1190–1193

Zhang Y, Zhu T, Zheng Y, Xiong Y, Liu W, Zeng W, Tang W, Liu C (2024) Machine learning-based medical imaging diagnosis in patients with temporomandibular disorders: a diagnostic test accuracy systematic review and meta-analysis. Clin Oral Investig 28:186

Application of AI in Pedodontics

Faizal C, Tarun Kumar Singh, and Aakash Gupta

1 Introduction

The application of various applications of artificial intelligence (AI) in pedodontics is driven by several factors resulting from the surge in data collection. A branch of artificial intelligence called machine learning (ML) employs statistical models and algorithms to find patterns in big datasets, so that the data may be used for predictive analysis and decision-making to extract sound clinical perceptions from these data. Based on this model, ML can assist in identifying children who are most likely to experience specific dental disorders (Academy and of Pediatric Dentistry 2024).

Deep learning (DL), another model of artificial intelligence, uses artificial neural networks (ANNs), which are made up of layers of linked nodes that collaborate to evaluate data and identify patterns, whereas a specific type of deep learning uses convolutional neural networks (CNNs) to simulate how the human brain processes information such as to analyze two-dimensional (2D) and three-dimensional (3D) images. Due to their capacity to automatically extract features through repeated convolution and pooling, CNNs are the recommended option for picture categorization (Academy and of Pediatric Dentistry 2024). Therefore, artificial intelligence can be used by pediatric dentists to develop specialized preventive and treatment programs that address each child's particular requirements.

Applications of AI in Pedodontics

1. Early diagnosis
2. Predictive analysis

Faizal C (✉)
Department of Pediatric & Preventive Dentistry, Kannur Dental College, Anjarakandy, Kannur, Kerala, India
e-mail: drfaizalcp@gmail.com

T. K. Singh · A. Gupta
Division of Conservative Dentistry and Endodontics, Department of Dentistry, All India Institute of Medical Sciences, Bathinda, India

A. Gupta et al. (eds.), *Application of Robotics in Dentistry*, Lecture Notes in Bioengineering, https://doi.org/10.1007/978-981-95-1470-0_14

3. Treatment planning and decision support
4. Behavior management
5. Patient engagement
6. Preventive care

2 AI in Oral Disease Diagnosis in Children

Children are often more difficult to manage, and they are more likely to be recalcitrant during dental operations. AI-powered augmented reality (AR) and virtual reality (Fig. 1) help the clinician to regulate children behavior and lessen their dental anxiety. Augmented reality (AR) technologies are now being investigated to offer more entertaining and approachable dental experiences. American Academy of Pediatric Dentistry (AAPD) recommends frequent dental checkups, that is, once in 6 months for kids to avoid dental issues like caries, which may not initially manifest any symptoms. One of the most significant challenges in pediatric dentistry is the early detection of dental diseases especially caries in young children who may not be able to articulate pain or discomfort (Acharya et al. 2024). Early diagnosis is essential for effective intervention and prevention of further damage. Traditional diagnostic methods such as visual inspection, X-rays, and probing can sometimes miss early-stage caries, leading to delayed treatment.

Dental caries is a major global public health problem in children, and one of the most prevalent preventable noncommunicable diseases worldwide. The three main causes of dental caries are acid-producing microbes, dietary carbohydrates, and host factors including eating habits. For patients to receive the proper prevention and treatment for dental caries, early detection is essential. AI models are especially helpful in early carious lesion prediction, which reduces the need for further therapy. Caries on various tooth surfaces may be identified and categorized with the use of machine learning. Data mining techniques can be used to create a model for predicting dental caries with high specificity and sensitivity by using a number of input variables, such as salivary pH, the frequency of intake of sugary snacks, and the amounts of Streptococci mutans and other microorganisms in the saliva. The growth

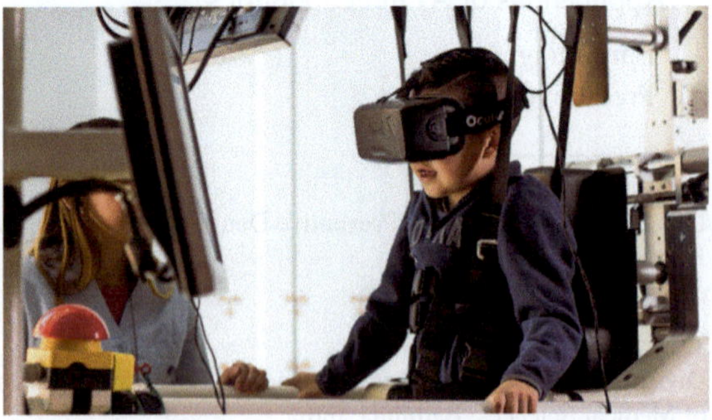

Fig. 1 Young patients use virtual reality to know about the procedure, thus decreasing their dental anxiety

and development of permanent teeth may be negatively impacted by the diseases like early childhood caries, which can be brought on by untreated dental plaque on primary teeth. The recent areas of focus for ML implementation include early childhood caries. Plaque accumulation is considered as important factor for development of caries. It is often difficult to detect plaque on primary teeth. It necessitates a clinical evaluation, and it gets much more difficult when a youngster is uncooperative. Using intraoral images taken with a digital camera AI model that could detect plaque on primary teeth with a sufficient degree of accuracy, allowing parents to utilize it at home (Ahmed et al. 2021).

Investigations such as intraoral radiographs pose challenges while doing clinical examinations and investigations. AI-powered tools, particularly those using machine learning and deep learning algorithms, have the potential to enhance early detection. AI systems can be trained on large datasets of dental images, including X-rays, photographs, and 3D scans, to recognize patterns indicative of caries that may be overlooked by the human eye. These systems can assess the severity of the caries and even predict its progression, providing dentists with more accurate and timely information. For example, deep learning models can detect microfractures or demineralization that are not immediately visible, allowing for earlier interventions that may prevent the need for more invasive treatments. Machine learning (ML) is making remarkable contributions to clinical diagnosis and investigations due to its reasonable predictive accuracy (Ahmad et al. 2021). It has the ability to reduce the repeated requirement for recurrent operations by assisting practitioners in diagnosis. These clinical examinations can be improved, and early oral condition diagnosis made easier by leveraging AI software's computational power. Neural networks and image processing techniques were used to detect caries on proximal and occlusal surfaces of teeth. A deep learning model (mask region-based convolutional neural network [Mask R-CNN]) has shown high specificity to detect and classify caries specifically inside the pits and fissures (Fig. 2a) and on the occlusal surfaces of teeth (Fig. 2b), where caries is most commonly found.

AI technologies are significantly enhancing the diagnostic process in dentofacial orthopedics by increasing precision, automating tasks, and offering advanced predictive capabilities (Alanazi et al. 2023). Here are the main ways AI is contributing: automated cephalometric analysis, 3D imaging and cone-bean computed tomography (CBCT) analysis, predictive growth modeling, facial aesthetic and symmetry analysis, AI-assisted diagnosis of temporomandibular joint (TMJ) disorders and functional issues, and AI-powered decision-support systems. For children with malocclusion and in the need of dentofacial orthopedic treatment, the timing of treatment is crucial. The peak growth period is considered as ideal time for commencing the treatment. For this purpose, usually the assessment of skeletal maturation and bone age are considered in growing children. By using CNN algorithms, high level of accuracy can be achieved (Kunz et al. 2020). Treatment objectives and planning for treatment especially for orthodontic extractions also can be computed with AI algorithms. Researchers have developed an ML model with ANN algorithm, to determine growth by cervical vertebrae maturation stages with good accuracy.

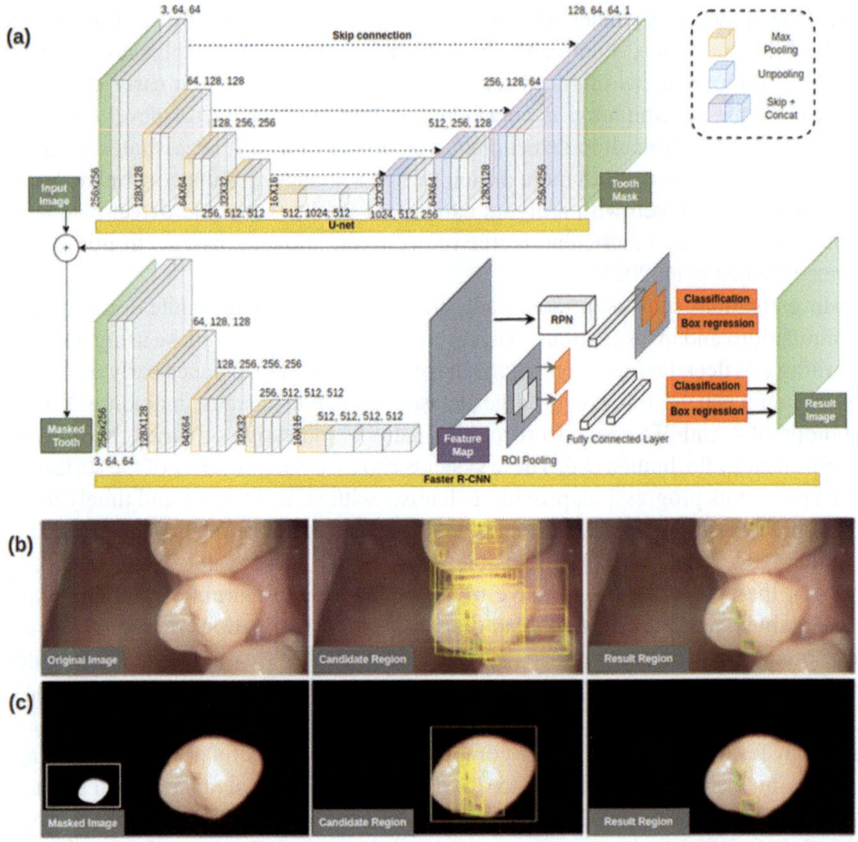

Fig. 2 Mask R-CCN model (**a**) used for the detection of pit and fissure caries on occlusal surface (**b**)

Gingival diseases, such as gingivitis and periodontitis, are often overlooked in children due to the misconception that such conditions primarily affect adults. However, poor oral hygiene and other factors can contribute to the early development of gingival issues in children. AI-powered systems can aid in the early diagnosis of gingival diseases by analyzing the images of the gingiva, evaluating for signs of inflammation, bleeding, and other indicators of gingival health (Albano et al. 2024). AI can also support the monitoring of disease progression, allowing for better management of treatments and interventions. For instance, AI algorithms can track the effectiveness of oral hygiene habits by comparing serial images over time, helping pediatric dentists tailor individualized care plans.

AI-powered diagnostic tools are capable of analyzing dental images with a high degree of precision, often detecting oral lesions or conditions that may be overlooked by the human eye. This increased accuracy leads to earlier detection, which is essential for preventing complications such as tooth impaction or misalignment.

Advanced imaging technologies, such as CBCT scans, provide detailed 3D views of the dental structures and surrounding tissues. AI-powered tools can assist in interpreting 3D data by isolating supernumerary teeth, mapping their exact location, and evaluating their impact on adjacent teeth. This comprehensive analysis helps pediatric dentists plan interventions, whether surgical removal or orthodontic treatment, with a greater degree of accuracy (Alessa 2024). Three-dimensional imaging and AI can also simulate the progression of supernumerary teeth, allowing dentists to make predictions about future dental development. This is particularly helpful when planning for interventions in younger children, where timing is critical for optimal outcomes.

3 AI in Early Childhood Caries

Early childhood caries (ECC) is a prevalent and serious dental condition affecting children, often leading to severe pain, tooth loss, and even systemic health issues. This dental disease, characterized by the rapid decay of teeth in children under the age of six, is largely preventable but remains widespread due to various factors including poor oral hygiene, diet, socioeconomic disparities, and lack of early interventions. Recent advances in healthcare and technology have led to the development of innovative tools, and one of the most promising is the application of artificial intelligence (AI) in the prevention, detection, and management of ECC (Academy and of Pediatric Dentistry 2024).

AI offers an exciting potential to revolutionize pediatric dentistry, addressing several challenges that have traditionally hindered the effective management of ECC. Early detection of ECC is crucial for successful intervention and management. Traditional diagnostic methods, such as visual examination and X-rays, can be subjective and require significant expertise. However, AI systems, particularly those utilizing machine learning algorithms, have the potential to improve diagnostic accuracy and speed. In ECC, AI can be used to analyze dental images, such as X-rays and intraoral photographs, to detect early signs of caries that may be invisible to the naked eye. Deep learning, a subset of AI, has been particularly effective in recognizing patterns in large datasets of dental images. By feeding these AI systems thousands of annotated images, they can learn to identify minute changes in tooth structure that indicate the presence of early-stage caries. AI's ability to analyze and interpret these images quickly and accurately can lead to earlier detection, allowing for more timely and effective interventions. AI-powered software has been shown to outperform human clinicians in the detection of dental caries in both primary and permanent teeth, especially in challenging areas such as the interproximal spaces, where cavities are often hard to spot (Anil et al. 2023). This enhanced diagnostic capability is particularly beneficial in resource-limited settings, where access to skilled dentists and advanced diagnostic tools may be limited.

AI can also play a significant role in developing personalized treatment plans for children with ECC. By analyzing a child's medical history, oral health data, dietary habits, and even genetic factors, AI can assist in creating tailored strategies for preventing and managing caries. For example, AI systems can recommend specific preventive measures, such as dietary modifications or fluoride treatments, based on an individual's unique risk factors. In addition, AI can help in predicting the progression of dental caries over time. By analyzing patterns in data from previous patients, AI models can estimate the likelihood of caries development and suggest appropriate interventions. This predictive capability allows for more proactive dental care, focusing on prevention rather than reactive treatment (Azhari et al. 202).

Early childhood caries, particularly in its mild-to-moderate stages, is often treatable with minimally invasive techniques. AI tools can help identify the extent of decay and recommend treatments that preserve as much of the natural tooth structure as possible. For instance, AI can guide decisions about the use of fluoride varnishes or dental sealants, which can help prevent the progression of caries without resorting to traditional restorative procedures like fillings.

In more advanced cases of ECC, AI can assist in the management of carious lesions by providing detailed guidance on the optimal approach to treatment. AI systems can assist dentists in planning restorative treatments, taking into account factors such as the child's age, the severity of the caries, and the child's medical and behavioral history (Barros Padilha et al. 2023). This results in more efficient and effective treatment, with fewer complications and better long-term outcomes.

AI can also assist in assessing the risk of early caries development in children by analyzing various factors that contribute to the condition. These factors may include the child's dietary habits, oral hygiene practices, fluoride exposure, genetic predisposition, and socioeconomic status. AI algorithms can process and analyze these data to create personalized risk profiles for individual patients.

AI can also estimate the likelihood of a child developing caries in the future. This helps dentists implement more effective preventive strategies, such as recommending lifestyle changes, tailored oral hygiene instructions, or fluoride treatments. Predictive analytics can also identify high-risk groups within a population, allowing public health initiatives to focus on children who are most vulnerable to dental decay.

1. Machine Learning Models for Caries Prediction
   - Predictive Analytics: Machine learning algorithms like decision trees, random forests, support vector machines (SVM), and gradient boosting are widely used to predict the risk of dental caries based on patient data (age, dietary habits, medical history, etc.).
   - Data Sources: These models often use clinical data (such as X-rays, intraoral photographs, and dental health records), combined with lifestyle and demographic data (diet, oral hygiene, and socioeconomic status), to generate risk assessments.
   - Examples: Tools like caries risk assessment tool (Fig. 3) or caries management systems use patient data to provide personalized caries risk assessments.

CARIES RISK ASSESSMENT TOOL

FACTOR	LOW	MODERATE	HIGH
Caries Activity	None	Within 24 months	Within 12 months
Demineralized areas	No white spots	1 white spot	> 1 white spot
Family History – Mother	No decay	Low caries rate	High caries rate
Family History – Father	No decay	Low caries rate	High caries rate
Family History – Siblings	No caries activity	Low caries rate	High caries rate
Presence of plaque, gingivitis	None	Moderate	Visible plaque on anterior teeth
Fluoride exposure	Optimal	Low to optimal	Low
Sugar consumption (including bottle or sippy cup use)	With meals only	1-2 between meals	> 3 between meals
Dental home	Established	Irregular use	None
Special conditions			Enamel hypoplasia Special needs patient Impaired salivary flow

Fig. 3 Caries risk assessment tool

2. Deep Learning Models (CNNs for Dental Images)

   - Convolutional Neural Networks (CNNs): CNNs are increasingly being used for image-based caries detection and risk assessment. By analyzing dental X-rays, intraoral photographs, or CBCT scans, these models can automatically detect carious lesions or predict the likelihood of future caries development (Bonny et al. 2023).
   - Dental X-ray Analysis: AI tools can detect early-stage dental caries, classify severity, and even predict how the caries might progress.
   - Examples: Products like VivaDx and DentAI utilize deep learning algorithms to analyze radiographs and identify areas of concern related to caries formation.

3. Risk Assessment Algorithms Based on Clinical Data

   - Caries Risk Prediction Models (CRPMs): These tools evaluate caries risk based on clinical examinations and data such as salivary flow rate, plaque index, and bacterial counts (e.g., Streptococcus mutans).
   - Statistical Models: Tools like caries risk and caries assessment tool use logistic regression or other statistical techniques to predict a patient's caries risk by processing various clinical variables.

4. Natural Language Processing (NLP) for Medical Records

   - Extracting Data from Electronic Health Records (EHRs): AI models using NLP can analyze unstructured data in patient records, such as notes from dental professionals, to gather insights about risk factors (e.g., medical history, medications that may influence oral health, or previous dental treatments). Example: Caries risk algorithm can analyze EHR data for factors like frequent dry mouth, history of restorative procedures, and medication use to predict caries susceptibility.

5. AI-Based Decision-Support Systems (DSSs)

   - Clinical Decision-Support Systems (CDSSs): These tools assist dentists in diagnosing and predicting caries risk by integrating various patient data points and providing evidence-based suggestions for preventive care or treatment.
   - Personalized Recommendations: Based on the caries risk prediction, AI can help recommend tailored preventive strategies, such as fluoride varnishes, sealants, diet modification, or enhanced oral hygiene practices.

6. Artificial Intelligence for Salivary Analysis

   - Salivary Biomarkers: AI tools can analyze biomarkers in saliva to predict the risk of caries. Features such as pH level, bacterial composition, and calcium phosphate balance are analyzed using AI algorithms to assess the risk of future caries formation.
   - AI Integration: Tools like Saliva Check integrate machine learning algorithms with saliva testing devices to provide real-time caries risk analysis.

7. AI-Driven Oral Health Apps

   - Mobile and Wearable Devices: AI-powered apps like "My Caries Risk or Cariogram" (Fig. 4) use smartphone-based diagnostics or integrations with oral health devices (such as electric toothbrushes) to monitor oral hygiene habits and predict the likelihood of caries risk.

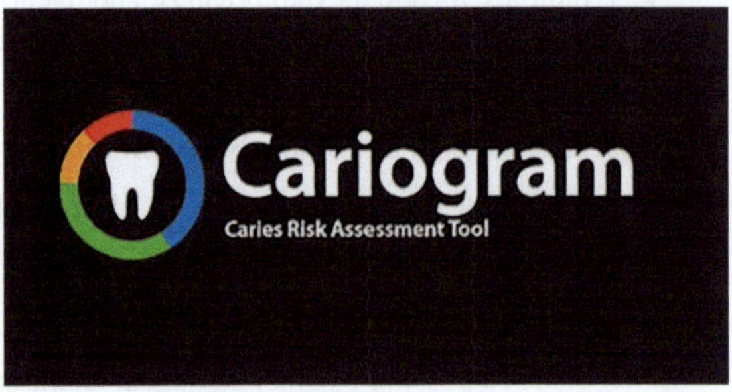

Fig. 4 Cariogram—caries risk assessment Google app

- Behavioral Prediction: These apps may provide real-time feedback on brushing habits, diet, and frequency of dental visits and offer personalized advice to lower caries risk.

8. AI for Prognostic Analysis and Treatment Planning

   - Predicting Caries Progression: AI models can analyze the progression of carious lesions over time and predict how the disease will develop. This helps clinicians prioritize which patients need immediate interventions.
   - Treatment Outcome Prediction: AI can also help predict the outcomes of various treatment plans, such as preventive or restorative interventions, to guide clinicians in offering the most effective treatment for caries management.

9. AI-Based Population Health and Epidemiological Studies

   - Population-Level Risk Assessment: AI tools are also used in large-scale studies to assess population-level trends in caries risk, enabling better public health strategies and preventive programs.
   - Analysis of Social Determinants: AI can be used to examine the role of social determinants like income, education, and access to healthcare, identifying higher-risk populations and guiding resource allocation.

10. Integration with Electronic Health Records (EHR)

   - Seamless Integration: AI tools integrated with EHRs can provide real-time risk assessment during dental appointments (Table 1). The model assesses the patient's historical data and real-time clinical findings to generate personalized caries risk profiles, which can be updated as new data are collected.

4 Plaque and AI

Dental plaque is a complex biofilm composed primarily of bacteria. Saliva, rich in proteins and carbohydrates, provides a nutrient-rich environment for bacteria to adhere to tooth surfaces. As bacteria multiply, they form a sticky matrix, known as an extracellular polymeric substance (EPS), which further facilitates biofilm development. One of the primary challenges in managing dental plaque is its early detection (Can Demirbaş et al. 2024). Plaque can often go unnoticed until it causes noticeable symptoms like tooth decay or gum irritation. Early detection is crucial in preventing more severe conditions. AI-powered tools are now being employed to improve plaque detection, offering quicker, more accurate, and less invasive methods than traditional techniques (Chau et al. 2023). AI applications in dental plaque detection generally revolve around the analysis of dental images, such as X-rays or photographs. Deep learning algorithms, particularly convolutional neural networks (CNNs), are trained on large datasets of dental images to identify the subtle early signs of plaque buildup.

Table 1 Examples of AI tools and platforms for dental caries risk prediction

• Caries Risk: A tool that predicts caries risk using clinical and demographic data • VivaDx: Uses deep learning to detect caries from dental X-rays • Caries Assessment Tool (CAT): A platform that evaluates risk factors and provides a risk score • DentAI: An AI-driven platform that analyzes X-rays and clinical data for caries risk prediction • Saliva Check: A diagnostic tool combining AI with saliva biomarker analysis for caries risk assessment • Second Opinion: FDA-approved software that uses high-resolution images to detect dental issues like tooth decay, abscesses, and calculus. It is designed to provide accurate, instantaneous results and reduce missed diagnoses • Overjet: FDA-cleared tool that provides measurements of decay and bone loss and highlights problem areas on X-rays • Dental Xrai Pro: Program that uses artificial neural networks to analyze X-rays and identify dental anomalies like caries, infections, and root canal fillings. It is designed to help dentists analyze radiographs more accurately and consistently • Pearl AI: Software that uses AI to analyze dental images and provide accurate diagnoses • Dentrix: Detect AI to focus on early detections of nearly all restorative, periodontal, and endodontic concerns identifiable on X-rays, including tooth decay not only in adults but also in pediatric patients ages 3 and above • Assist Dent: AI preventive dental software from Manchester Imaging. Recent upgrades include tooth labeling and a dentine caries detection function

These systems can recognize patterns that may be invisible to the human eye, enabling dentists to detect plaque earlier and with greater accuracy.

Some AI-based systems use intraoral cameras that capture high-resolution images of the teeth. These images are then processed by AI algorithms, which can identify the presence of plaque or even the early stages of tartar buildup. The AI can quantify the amount of plaque present, locate its precise location, and provide a detailed report for the dentist (DaSilva et al. 2022). This technology not only enhances the diagnosis but also helps in planning more personalized treatment strategies.

AI's role in plaque management goes beyond initial detection. Plaque accumulation is a dynamic process that requires continuous monitoring to prevent it from causing long-term damage to the teeth and gums. AI can be employed to monitor the progress of plaque removal or the effectiveness of oral hygiene routines. One example is AI-powered apps that track brushing habits. These apps use sensors embedded in toothbrushes or smart oral hygiene devices to record brushing duration, pressure, and technique. AI algorithms analyze these data to provide feedback to users, helping them improve their brushing technique and better manage plaque buildup. Over time, these apps can track the effectiveness of a patient's oral hygiene routine and offer personalized recommendations for improvement (Ezzat et al. 2022).

Moreover, AI can integrate data from multiple sources, such as dental visits, X-rays, and user inputs (like diet and health status), to create a comprehensive, dynamic profile of a patient's oral health. This allows for personalized plaque management plans that evolve with the patient's needs, optimizing care and potentially preventing the recurrence of plaque-related oral health issues.

The use of AI in preventive dentistry has the potential to greatly reduce the incidence of plaque-related diseases. By analyzing patient data, AI can predict an individual's risk for plaque accumulation and related dental diseases, such as gingivitis or periodontitis. Early interventions can be made based on these predictions, helping to prevent the progression of plaque buildup into more severe conditions (Feher et al. 2024).

AI algorithms can process complex data from multiple sources to predict when a person is at risk of developing plaque-related problems. For example, it can analyze a combination of genetic data, oral hygiene habits, diet, lifestyle, and even environmental factors. With this information, AI can generate personalized risk profiles and offer targeted preventive recommendations, such as changes in diet, adjustments in brushing technique, or the use of specific oral care products. In addition, AI can assist in the development of more effective plaque-control products. By analyzing patterns of plaque buildup in various populations, AI can help researchers design better oral hygiene products that are specifically tailored to combat plaque for particular groups, such as children with systemic conditions and those with certain genetic predispositions (Kazimierczak et al. 2024).

When plaque accumulates and hardens into calculus, it can lead to gingival disease and other oral health issues that may require medical intervention. Traditionally, this is treated through professional cleaning or scaling and root planing by a dentist or hygienist. However, AI has the potential to enhance treatment by offering more precise and tailored approaches to care. For instance, AI can analyze the progression of gingival disease and plaque buildup, helping clinicians to identify which areas of the mouth require more intensive treatment (Table 2). In some cases, AI could even help guide robotic-assisted dental tools during plaque removal, making the process faster, more efficient, and less invasive. Additionally, AI can be used to create 3D models of a patient's mouth, which can aid in designing custom-fit solutions like dental aligners, mouthguards, or even personalized oral care devices (Kuo and Wei 2019).

Furthermore, AI can assist in posttreatment care by monitoring patients' recovery progress. By analyzing images or data from sensors, AI can detect early signs of

Table 2 AI apps and technologies that can help with plaque detection and analysis

- Test my teeth: A smartphone app that uses AI to scan teeth and measure plaque levels. It can identify areas that need more brushing and track plaque on the inner, outer, and biting surfaces of teeth
- One Petri: An app that uses AI to automate plaque counts and assay calculations. It is available for download on the Apple App Store
- Artificial intelligence-enabled computed tomography (CT)-based quantitative coronary topography (AI-QCT): A technology that uses AI to analyze plaque in coronary CT scans. It can help with plaque volume and composition analysis and may help guide clinical decision-making
- AI in computed tomography plaque characterization: An AI technology that can help with plaque analysis in computed tomography angiography (CTA) scans. It can automatically assess stenosis and characterize plaque morphology

complications, such as infection or improper healing, and alert the dentist, ensuring that the patient receives timely follow-up care.

While AI has already demonstrated its effectiveness in dental plaque management, its full potential is yet to be realized. In the future, AI could integrate more advanced technologies, such as genomics, real-time data collection, and even wearable devices, to create a truly personalized approach to oral healthcare. For example, AI could use genetic data to identify individuals at higher risk of plaque-related diseases and suggest tailored preventive strategies. Additionally, real-time monitoring tools, such as smart toothbrushes, could offer instant feedback on plaque buildup and provide immediate suggestions for improvement.

As AI systems continue to evolve, they could also play a role in educating patients about the importance of plaque control. AI-powered virtual assistants could guide patients through proper brushing techniques, dietary choices, and other oral hygiene practices, making oral health education more accessible and interactive (Rosa et al. 2024).

5 AI in Behavior Management

One of the most challenging aspects of pediatric dentistry is managing a child's behavior during dental procedures. Children, especially those under the age of 12, are often more susceptible to stress and anxiety in medical environments. Fear, anxiety, and resistance to treatment are common, especially in younger children or those with special needs. AI can play a pivotal role in improving behavior management by creating a more comfortable and predictable environment for young patients (Maganur et al. 2024). AI-powered virtual assistants or chatbots can be used before appointments to educate children about dental procedures in an engaging and interactive way. These virtual assistants can use child-friendly language, visual aids, and gamification techniques to help children understand what will happen during their visit. This approach can reduce anxiety by familiarizing children with the process and giving them a sense of control over their experience (Mestre et al. 2024).

AI-driven facial recognition technology can assess a child's emotional state during dental visits by analyzing facial expressions and physiological responses, such as heart rate or skin temperature. This real-time analysis can help dental professionals understand a child's anxiety levels and adjust their approach accordingly. For instance, if AI detects that a child is becoming fearful or distressed, the dentist may opt to slow down the procedure, offer reassurance, or introduce calming techniques such as virtual reality (VR) distractions, which have been shown to reduce anxiety in pediatric patients (Nabavizadeh and Khosravani 2022).

Children with special needs, including those with autism spectrum disorder (Fig. 5), intellectual disabilities, or sensory processing disorders, often require a more tailored approach to dental care. AI has the potential to enhance care for these children by personalizing treatment strategies based on the child's individual needs and preferences.

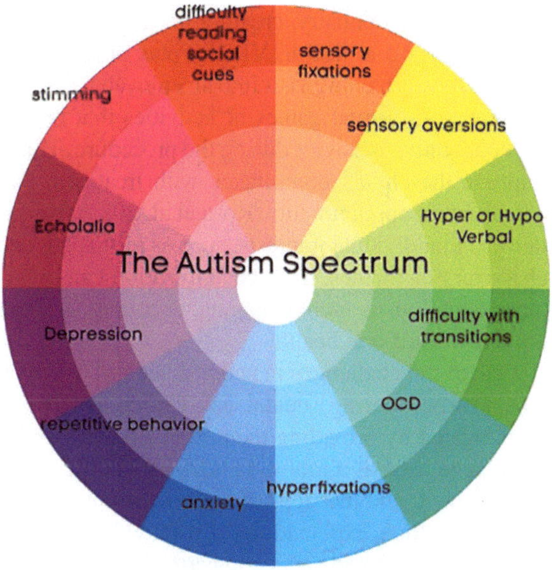

Fig. 5 Autism spectrum disorder

For instance, AI can assist in creating individualized treatment plans that take into account a child's sensory sensitivities, communication difficulties, and other factors that might affect their dental experience. AI-powered systems could suggest alternative techniques for behavior management, such as the use of sedation, music therapy, or sensory accommodations (Naeimi et al. 2024). Additionally, AI can help schedule appointments at times when the child is most likely to be calm, such as during nonpeak hours, to avoid sensory overload in busy dental clinics.

In children with autism spectrum disorder (ASD), AI-powered systems may use speech recognition and natural language processing to facilitate communication between the child and the dental team. These systems could be programmed to recognize the child's unique communication style, whether verbal or nonverbal, and provide real-time assistance to dental professionals in understanding the child's needs (Rahim et al. 2024).

One of the most significant advantages of artificial intelligence in pediatric dentistry is its ability to reduce dental anxiety, a common issue in children undergoing dental treatments. Dental anxiety can lead to avoidance of dental visits, which in turn can contribute to poor oral health. Studies have shown that fear of dental procedures is one of the primary reasons children avoid or delay dental appointments, leading to the development of dental phobia in adulthood (Riet et al. 2023).

By immersing children in a virtual world during dental procedures, virtual reality (VR) helps divert their attention away from the discomfort and sounds of dental tools. This distraction not only reduces anxiety but also helps in pain management. The immersive experience can transport children to a relaxing or engaging virtual environment, such as a beach or a forest, effectively "distracting" them from the reality of the dental procedure (Rokhshad et al. 2024).

In pediatric dentistry, creating positive associations with dental visits is crucial for long-term oral health. VR can play an essential role in this by transforming a potentially frightening visit into an enjoyable experience. For example, children can participate in virtual games or activities that reward them with points or rewards for cooperative behavior during the procedure. This positive reinforcement can help improve the child's compliance with treatment and increase their willingness to attend future appointments (Rosa et al. 2023). Additionally, VR experiences can be tailored to individual interests, such as virtual adventures based on a child's favorite characters or themes. This customization can enhance the overall experience and make dental visits more engaging, encouraging children to develop a more positive attitude toward oral health.

One of the challenges in pediatric dentistry is helping young patients understand what to expect during a dental visit. Children often fear the unknown, and this fear can be mitigated by providing them with a clearer understanding of dental procedures. VR can be used as a tool to familiarize children with dental instruments, the dental environment, and the steps of a procedure in a nonthreatening way. Virtual tours of the dental office, explanations of what will happen during the visit, and simulations of the procedure can reduce uncertainty and help children feel more prepared and less (Sayed et al. 2020).

By presenting dental procedures in a virtual space before the actual appointment, children can feel more in control of the situation, potentially leading to reduced anxiety and more cooperative behavior during treatment. VR offers several psychological benefits that can help alleviate these emotional challenges:

a. Distraction from Pain and Anxiety

The primary psychological benefit of VR is its ability to act as a distraction. The child's attention is redirected away from the potentially stressful aspects of the dental procedure and focused on an engaging, interactive virtual environment. Research has shown that immersive VR can reduce perceived pain and anxiety by shifting the child's attention to a more pleasant and captivating experience. VR headsets can be used during routine dental procedures like cleanings, fillings, or even more invasive treatments like root canals or extractions. By wearing VR headsets, children can be transported to a virtual world that takes their attention away from the dentist's tools and the sounds of the procedure (Schwendicke et al. 2022). This method has been shown to effectively reduce the perception of pain, the need for sedatives, and the overall stress of the procedure. This distraction is particularly effective during potentially painful procedures such as fillings, extractions, or cleanings.

b. Reduction of Fear of the Dentist

For children who experience extreme fear of the dentist, known as odontophobia, VR can serve as a therapeutic tool. By making dental procedures less intimidating through virtual scenarios, children may begin to associate dental visits with more positive emotions. Over time, this can reduce the overall fear of the dentist and increase cooperation during visits.

Before starting treatment, children can experience a virtual walkthrough of the procedure they will undergo. This preparation helps demystify the process, offering reassurance and minimizing fear. By experiencing the procedure in a virtual environment beforehand, children feel more prepared and less anxious when it is time for the real treatment (Semerci and Yardımcı 2024).

c. Stress Reduction

Stress is a common response among children when faced with unfamiliar or uncomfortable situations. Playrooms specially designed for children help in reducing anxiety of patients before dental treatment (Fig. 6). VR has been shown to induce a calming effect by engaging the senses and promoting relaxation. Interactive virtual environments designed to reduce stress can include soothing visuals, gentle sounds, and calming movements (Table 3). VR can also be used to educate children about oral health in a fun and interactive way. Through virtual games and experiences, children can learn about proper brushing techniques, the importance of flossing, and the role of good nutrition in maintaining healthy teeth. These educational tools can be integrated into the waiting room, where children can interact with the virtual content while they wait for their appointment, reinforcing positive oral health habits.

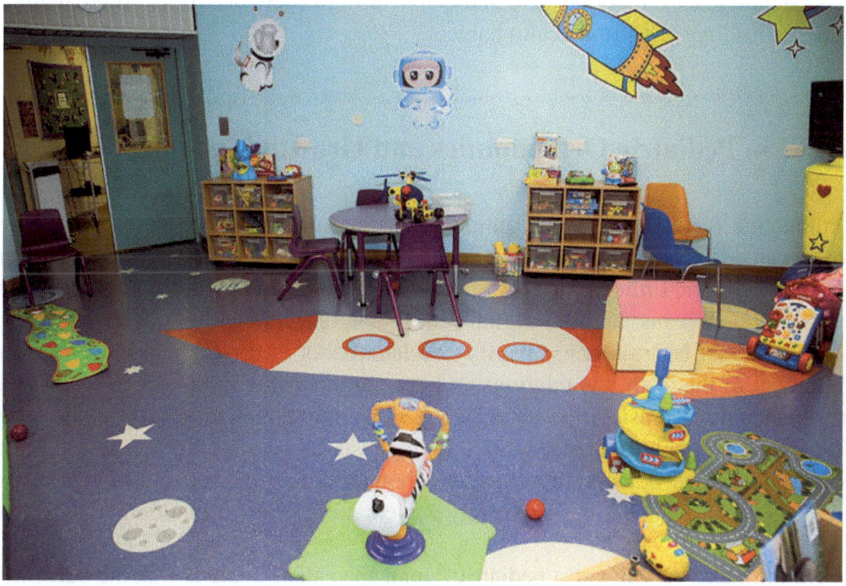

Fig. 6 Playroom designed for pediatric patients

Table 3 Practical applications of virtual reality in pediatric dentistry

1. VR as a distraction during procedures
2. Preoperative VR exposure
3. Educational VR games

While the use of VR in pediatric dentistry shows great promise, there are some challenges and limitations to consider. The cost of acquiring VR equipment can be prohibitive for some dental practices, particularly those in low-resource areas. Additionally, some children may experience discomfort or nausea while using VR headsets, although these issues can be mitigated with proper setup and guidance.

Another limitation is the potential for over-reliance on VR as a distraction, which may delay addressing the root causes of dental anxiety. Although VR can alleviate symptoms of fear and discomfort, it is important that dental professionals also work to build trust with their young patients and create a supportive and empathetic environment (Sharma et al. 2024).

VR offers an engaging and immersive experience, effectively diverting patients' attention away from the clinical environment, fostering a positive and enjoyable treatment experience. Virtual reality has the potential to revolutionize pediatric dentistry by addressing key challenges such as dental anxiety, fear, and pain management. By offering immersive and engaging experiences, VR can transform a traditionally stressful and intimidating environment into one that is fun, educational, and stress-free. As technology continues to evolve, it is likely that VR will become an increasingly common tool in pediatric dental practices, improving both the experience and outcomes for young patients. With careful implementation, VR has the capacity to make dental visits a more positive and empowering experience for children, helping to foster lifelong good oral health habits.

6 AI in Pediatric Orthodontics and Growth Modeling

Orthodontic methods often rely on manual assessments and radiographic imaging, which can be time-consuming and prone to human error. One significant contribution of AI in pediatric orthodontics is the ability to analyze radiographic images—such as X-rays, CT scans, and 3D digital models—more efficiently. Machine learning algorithms can be trained to identify key landmarks in these images, such as the alignment of the teeth, the relationship between the upper and lower jaws, and the presence of malocclusions (Sivari et al. 2023). By automating these tasks, AI reduces the risk of oversight and speeds up the diagnosis process. Moreover, AI-powered image analysis can detect subtle changes in bone structure or dental eruption patterns, allowing for early intervention that may prevent more severe orthodontic issues later on.

Additionally, AI can assist pediatric dental specialists in predicting the outcomes of different treatment approaches. By inputting data from a child's growth stage, medical history, and dental condition, AI algorithms can simulate various treatment scenarios and provide evidence-based recommendations. This predictive capability enables orthodontists to offer more personalized treatment plans, optimizing the use of orthodontic and orthopedic appliances expanders or retainers.

Monitoring the growth and development of children is a critical aspect of pediatric orthodontics, as early intervention can greatly influence the success of treatment.

Traditional methods of growth monitoring often rely on clinical observations, skeletal radiographs, and physical measurements. However, these methods may lack precision and may not capture subtle changes in a child's development. AI offers a more accurate and consistent way to track growth, enabling orthodontists to intervene earlier and more effectively (Surlari et al. 2023). AI-based growth monitoring systems use machine learning algorithms to analyze data from multiple sources, including digital impressions, 3D facial scans, and even wearable devices. By collecting data over time, these systems can create dynamic growth models that predict future development and identify any abnormalities in real time. For example, AI can detect patterns in the growth of the maxilla and mandible and predict when a child may be at risk for developing bite issues or other orthodontic concerns.

Moreover, AI can integrate genetic, environmental, and behavioral factors into its analysis, allowing for a more comprehensive understanding of how a child's growth may progress. This holistic approach is particularly useful in predicting growth spurts or determining the ideal time for orthodontic intervention. In turn, this reduces the need for frequent, uncomfortable visits to the orthodontist, as AI can monitor a child's growth remotely through periodic scans or data uploads.

The integration of AI in pediatric orthodontics and growth monitoring offers several advantages:

1. Improved Diagnostic Accuracy: AI algorithms can analyze complex datasets more efficiently than human clinicians, identifying potential issues that may not be immediately visible to the naked eye. This can lead to earlier and more accurate diagnoses of orthodontic problems.
2. Personalized Treatment Plans: AI's ability to analyze a child's unique growth patterns, medical history, and dental structure allows for more tailored treatment recommendations. This ensures that each child receives the most effective and least invasive treatment.
3. Enhanced Monitoring: AI-powered growth monitoring systems allow orthodontists to track a child's development over time without the need for constant physical examinations or radiographs. This reduces the radiation exposure for children and streamlines the monitoring process.
4. Predictive Capabilities: AI can predict future dental and facial development, enabling orthodontists to proactively address potential problems before they worsen. This reduces the need for emergency treatments and enhances long-term outcomes.
5. Efficiency and Cost-Effectiveness: Automating certain diagnostic and monitoring tasks can reduce the amount of time orthodontists spend on routine assessments, ultimately lowering the cost of treatment. In some cases, this could make orthodontic care more accessible to children who might not otherwise have the resources for it.

AI is transforming pediatric orthodontics by improving diagnostic accuracy, streamlining treatment planning, and enabling more effective growth monitoring (Fig. 7). By leveraging machine learning algorithms and advanced data analytics,

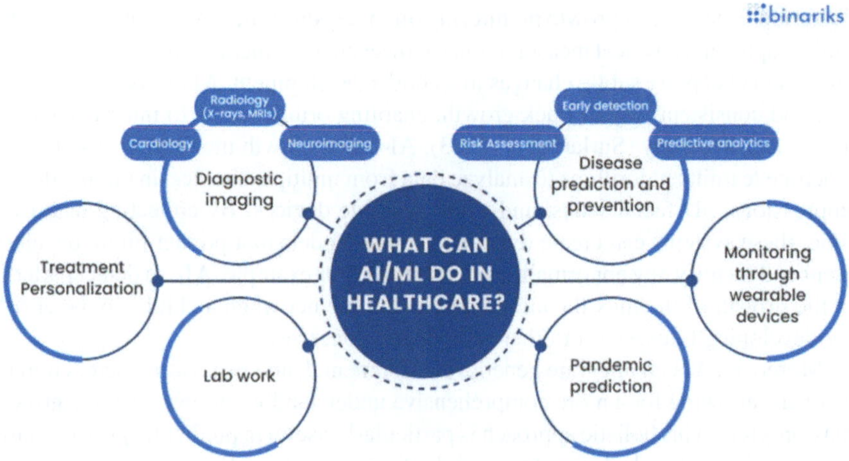

Fig. 7 Role of artificial intelligence (AI) and machine learning (ML) in healthcare

pediatric dental specialists can provide more personalized care for children and intervene earlier to prevent or correct orthodontic issues. AI tools, such as SmileMate and Fastbraces, use machine learning algorithms to predict how teeth will move in response to different types of orthodontic treatment (Thurzo et al. 2022). As AI continues to evolve, it is crucial to balance its use with human expertise to ensure the best outcomes for pediatric patients.

7 The Role of Robotics in Pediatric Dentistry

In recent years, the integration of robotics into healthcare has sparked significant advancements across various fields, including pediatric dentistry. Pediatric dentistry is a specialized branch that focuses on the oral health of children, from infancy through adolescence. This area of healthcare has seen notable improvements due to technological innovations, and robotics is playing an increasingly important role in transforming pediatric dental practices. From improving treatment outcomes to enhancing patient experiences, robotic technologies in pediatric dentistry promise to revolutionize how dental care is delivered to young patients (Tomášik et al. 2024).

Robotic systems in pediatric dentistry primarily aim to enhance precision, reduce human error, and improve efficiency in procedures. These systems combine mechanical devices with artificial intelligence (AI), sensors, and machine learning algorithms to support or directly perform various tasks. The two main areas where robotics are making an impact in pediatric dentistry include the following:

(a) Improving precision and minimizing human error
(b) Enhancing diagnosis and preventive care

In pediatric dentistry, children's teeth and oral structures present unique challenges due to their smaller size, developing anatomy, and the potential for anxiety during treatment. Robotic systems are able to assist dentists by offering highly precise movements during complex procedures. For example, robotic arms equipped with specialized tools can aid in dental restorations, implant placements, or cavity fillings, ensuring that treatment is delivered with a higher degree of accuracy. This precision reduces the risk of complications, such as inadvertent injury to surrounding tissues or unnecessary discomfort.

In addition, robotic systems equipped with sensors can continuously monitor treatment progress and adjust instruments in real time, helping pediatric dentists achieve optimal results with minimal intervention. The combination of automation and expert oversight makes robotic systems highly effective in delivering consistent, reliable care (Vishwanathaiah et al. 2023).

One of the most significant advantages of robotics in pediatric dentistry is its ability to assist in early diagnosis and preventive care. Robotic systems, integrated with advanced imaging technologies such as 3D scanning and digital radiography, can provide detailed and accurate images of a child's oral health. These systems can detect dental anomalies, cavities, or signs of early dental decay before they are visible to the naked eye.

AI-powered diagnostic robots can analyze vast amounts of dental data from X-rays, patient histories, and clinical examinations to detect subtle signs of tooth decay, malocclusions (misalignment of teeth), or even genetic predispositions to certain dental conditions. With this early detection, pediatric dentists can intervene sooner, thereby reducing the risk of long-term dental issues and ensuring that children receive timely treatment (Vodanović et al. 2023).

Robotic technologies in pediatric dentistry are also playing an important role in improving the overall patient experience, particularly for children who experience dental anxiety. The sight of intimidating dental instruments and the noise of dental drills often cause stress and fear in young patients, making it difficult for them to sit through appointments. Robotic systems, designed with child-friendly features, can ease some of this anxiety.

Robots, particularly in the form of robotic assistants, can engage with children during the procedure, providing reassurance, explaining the treatment in simple terms, and even offering interactive features such as games or storytelling. By creating a more comfortable and less intimidating environment, robotic technologies can help children feel more relaxed and cooperative, leading to a more positive dental experience. This, in turn, helps to foster a lifetime of positive dental habits and reduces the likelihood of future dental anxiety.

Minimally invasive dentistry (MID) is another area where robotics can make a significant contribution. Traditional dental procedures often involve the removal of a significant amount of healthy tissue, which can be both painful and distressing, especially for young children. Robotics, however, allows for more precise, minimally invasive techniques that conserve healthy tooth structures while treating dental issues.

For instance, robotic systems can be used in laser dentistry, where laser technology is used to treat cavities or soft tissue issues without the need for traditional drills. The high precision of robotic lasers minimizes damage to surrounding tissues, reduces bleeding, and shortens recovery time. This is particularly important for pediatric patients, as these treatments result in less discomfort and quicker healing, making it easier for children to undergo dental procedures.

While robotics in pediatric dentistry offers numerous advantages, there are also challenges and considerations that need to be addressed before these technologies can become mainstream in dental practices, which include a) cost and accessibility, b) training and adaptation, and c) ethical and practical concerns.

One of the primary barriers to the widespread adoption of robotic systems in pediatric dentistry is the cost. Robotic dental systems and their accompanying technology require significant investment, which can make them inaccessible to smaller or budget-conscious dental practices. While prices may decrease as the technology matures, the initial costs may limit the ability of some clinics to integrate these advanced systems into their practices.

Pediatric dentists and dental staff will need specialized training to effectively operate and maintain robotic systems. Dentists may require time to adapt to new workflows and develop the necessary skills to use these systems safely and efficiently. As with any new technology, there may be a learning curve before robotic systems can be fully integrated into daily practice.

The use of robotics raises ethical concerns regarding the balance between human expertise and machine involvement in healthcare. Some critics argue that excessive reliance on robotics might reduce the human element in patient care, potentially affecting the dentist–patient relationship. Furthermore, while robotic systems can assist with precision, they cannot replicate the nuanced judgment and empathy that an experienced pediatric dentist brings to a patient's care.

Looking ahead, the future of robotics in pediatric dentistry is promising. Continued advancements in AI, machine learning, and robotics will likely result in even more sophisticated systems capable of handling a broader range of procedures. The integration of robotics with other emerging technologies, such as virtual reality (VR) for patient education and remote monitoring, could further enhance the pediatric dental experience. As these technologies evolve, it is essential to ensure that their implementation aligns with ethical standards, prioritizes patient safety, and remains accessible to all socioeconomic groups. With ongoing research, innovation, and thoughtful integration, robotics can significantly improve pediatric dental care by increasing precision, reducing discomfort, and making dental visits a more positive experience for children.

8 AI in Pediatric Preventive Dentistry

One of the most crucial aspects of preventive dentistry is early detection and intervention. AI has a significant role in preventing future dental problems in children. AI has shown great promise in identifying potential dental problems before they become more serious, thus minimizing the need for complex treatments. AI algorithms, particularly those based on machine learning (ML) and deep learning (DL), are increasingly being used to analyze dental images such as X-rays, 3D scans, and photographs. These algorithms are trained to detect signs of cavities, misalignment, enamel demineralization, and early stages of gum disease—conditions that may not be immediately visible to the human eye. By analyzing a child's dental history and environmental factors (e.g., diet and oral hygiene habits), AI can predict the likelihood of issues like caries, gingivitis, or orthodontic concerns. This predictive capability allows dental professionals to take proactive measures, such as recommending specific oral care products or scheduling more frequent checkups for children at higher risk of dental problems. Additionally, AI can assist in educating both children and their parents about proper oral hygiene practices. AI-powered apps can deliver personalized reminders and tips for brushing and flossing, and some apps even gamify the process to make it more engaging for young users. With early intervention and better preventive care, the long-term oral health of children can be significantly improved.

AI-powered diagnostic tools can identify issues that may go unnoticed in routine checkups, allowing pediatric dentists to intervene at the earliest possible stage. This is especially beneficial for children who may be anxious or reluctant to undergo traditional diagnostic procedures. The use of AI can help reduce the frequency of invasive examinations and increase comfort for young patients.

The use of AI in preventive dentistry has the potential to greatly reduce the incidence of plaque-related diseases. By analyzing patient data, AI can predict an individual's risk for plaque accumulation and related dental diseases. Early interventions can be made based on predictions, which helps to prevent the progression of plaque buildup into more severe conditions. AI algorithms can process complex data from multiple sources to predict when a person is at risk of developing plaque-related problems. For example, it can analyze a combination of genetic data, oral hygiene habits, diet, lifestyle, and even environmental factors. With this information, AI can generate personalized risk profiles and offer targeted preventive recommendations, such as changes in diet, adjustments in brushing technique, or the use of specific oral care products.

In addition, AI can assist in the development of more effective plaque-control products. By analyzing patterns of plaque buildup in various populations, AI can help researchers design better oral hygiene products that are specifically tailored to combat plaque for particular groups, such as with certain genetic predispositions.

AI can also aid in preventive measures at a population level. With the integration of AI and digital health tools, dental professionals can monitor the oral health of large populations of children more effectively. For example, AI systems can analyze data from regular dental checkups to identify trends in caries incidence across different demographic groups, enabling targeted public health interventions. In communities where access to regular dental care is limited, AI-based applications can empower parents and caregivers to monitor and manage their children's oral health at home. Mobile apps powered by AI can provide reminders for brushing and offer educational content tailored to the child's age and dental risk factors. These apps can also offer virtual consultations or screen for early signs of caries, offering valuable support to caregivers who might not otherwise be able to visit a dentist regularly.

AI has the potential to revolutionize preventive care by enabling personalized treatment plans tailored to the unique needs of each child. By analyzing a child's medical history, dental records, genetic factors, and lifestyle habits, AI algorithms can help pediatric dentists create highly individualized preventive care strategies. For instance, AI can predict a child's risk of developing cavities based on factors like diet, oral hygiene habits, and previous dental history. This personalized approach can help ensure that children receive the most appropriate preventive care, such as fluoride treatments, sealants, or education on brushing techniques. AI can also track a child's oral health over time, identifying patterns and making real-time adjustments to their care plan. For example, if a child shows signs of developing caries at an earlier stage, AI can recommend more frequent checkups or targeted treatments to prevent further damage.

Another vital aspect of preventive dentistry is patient education. Many dental problems in children arise due to poor oral hygiene habits and a lack of understanding about the importance of regular care. AI can play a key role in improving patient education and engagement, especially by using interactive and visually engaging tools. AI-powered applications and chatbots can provide children and their parents with personalized tips on oral hygiene, recommend age-appropriate dental care routines, and even offer reminders for brushing and flossing. For example, AI-based mobile apps or virtual assistants can analyze a child's brushing technique using smartphone cameras and provide feedback on areas that need improvement. These tools can be gamified, making oral health education fun and engaging for children. The use of AI to enhance patient education not only empowers children to take charge of their oral health but also helps reduce anxiety associated with dental visits, as they become more informed about the procedures and their benefits (You et al. 2020).

AI can significantly enhance risk assessment in pediatric dentistry by providing more accurate predictions of a child's likelihood of developing oral diseases. AI algorithms can process vast amounts of data, including genetic information, family medical history, dietary habits, and environmental factors, to create more precise risk profiles. For instance, children who have a family history of dental issues and abnormal growth patterns can be flagged as higher-risk patients. Through these AI-driven risk assessments, pediatric dentists can prioritize preventive interventions and closely monitor at-risk children. This could include more frequent dental checkups, dietary recommendations, or the use of additional preventive treatments, such as fluoride varnishes or dental sealants. AI can also track the progress of high-risk children, adjusting preventive care plans as necessary to ensure optimal outcomes.

9 Challenges of Integration of AI in Pediatric Dentistry

The implementation of AI technologies in dental practices comes with significant upfront costs, which may include the purchase of AI software, training for staff, and integrating the technology into existing practice workflows. For small dental practices or those in lower-income areas, these costs could be prohibitively high, leading to disparities in access to advanced care.

While AI has the potential to reduce long-term costs by improving efficiency and reducing human error, its initial cost may limit its widespread adoption. Additionally, the accessibility of AI in dentistry must be considered from a global perspective, as countries with fewer resources may be unable to adopt cutting-edge technologies, exacerbating healthcare inequalities.

The use of AI in pediatric dentistry raises significant ethical and privacy concerns. Children are considered a vulnerable population, and their dental health data are highly sensitive. As AI systems depend on the collection and analysis of vast amounts of personal data, there is a risk that these systems may not always adhere to the strict privacy laws governing pediatric health information. There is also the issue of consent. Children, particularly those who are very young, cannot provide informed consent for their data to be used in AI training. Parental or guardian consent is required, but the process of ensuring that parents fully understand how AI works and how their child's data will be used is complex. Ethical concerns also arise when AI systems are involved in diagnosing and recommending treatments, as these systems may not always fully replicate the expertise and empathy that a human pediatric dentist brings to the table.

AI systems in pediatric dentistry may struggle with the emotional and psychological needs of young patients. Children often experience fear and anxiety when visiting the dentist, and a key component of pediatric dentistry is the ability of the dentist to engage with children in a comforting and empathetic manner. While AI can assist in diagnosis and treatment planning, it lacks the human touch that is often essential to making children feel comfortable in the dental chair. Dentists specializing in pediatric care are trained to read emotional cues, respond to children's needs, and engage with them in a playful and reassuring manner. AI systems, however, may not have the capability to understand or respond to emotional cues in the same way a human can. This lack of emotional intelligence could undermine the trust children and their parents place in dental professionals, ultimately affecting treatment outcomes.

Implementing AI in pediatric dentistry requires significant integration with existing workflows and systems. Pediatric dental practices, especially smaller ones, may lack the technological infrastructure needed to adopt AI tools. This includes not only the hardware and software requirements but also the need for specialized training for dental professionals to effectively use AI systems.

For AI to be effective in pediatric dentistry, it must seamlessly integrate with electronic health records (EHR) systems (Fig. 8), imaging software, and other digital tools already in use in the practice. However, many practices still rely on older technologies or paper-based systems, which can make the transition to AI adoption

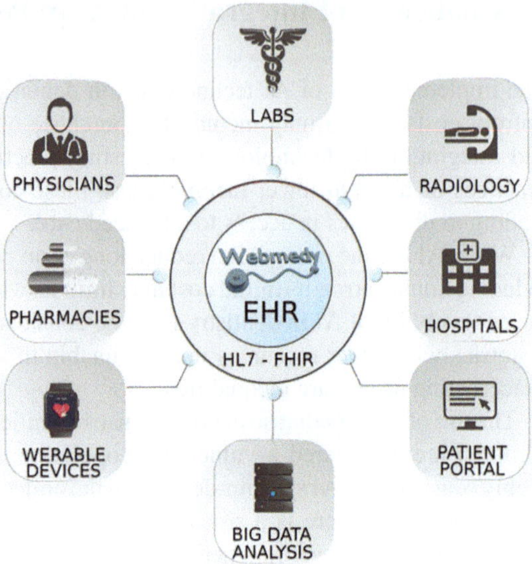

Fig. 8 Electronic health record system providing data regarding patients

more difficult. Additionally, there is a need for continued professional development, as pediatric dentists must learn how to work with AI tools without allowing them to replace the clinical judgment and hands-on experience that are central to effective patient care (Zhao and Xu 2020).

Another challenge is the acceptance of AI by both patients and dental professionals. Parents may be apprehensive about AI systems making decisions about their children's dental care. Dental professionals, too, may be resistant to adopting AI technology, particularly if they fear that it may diminish their role or undermine their expertise. Establishing trust in AI systems in pediatric dentistry will require transparent communication about how the technology works, its benefits, and its limitations.

References

American Academy of Pediatric Dentistry. Policy on early childhood caries (ECC): Consequences and preventive strategies. The reference manual of pediatric dentistry. Chicago, Ill.: American Academy of Pediatric Dentistry; 2024:89–92

American Academy of Pediatric Dentistry. The American Academy of Pediatric Dentistry research agenda. The reference manual of pediatric dentistry. Chicago, Ill.: American Academy of Pediatric Dentistry; 2024:12

Acharya S, Godhi BS, Saxena V, Assiry AA, Alessa NA, Dawasaz AA, Alqarni A, Karobari MI (2024) Role of artificial intelligence in behavior management of pediatric dental patients—a mini review. J Clin Pediatr Dent 48(3):24–30

Ahmad P, Alam MK, Aldajani A, Alahmari A, Alanazi A, Stoddart M, Sghaireen MG (2021) Dental robotics: a disruptive technology. Sensors (Basel) 21(10):3308

Ahmed N, Abbasi MS, Zuberi F, Qamar W, Halim MS, Maqsood A, Alam MK (2021) Artificial intelligence techniques: analysis, application, and outcome in dentistry—a systematic review. Biomed Res Int 2021(1):9751564

Alanazi A, Alghamdi G, Aldosari B (2023) Informational needs for dental-oriented electronic health records from dentists' perspectives. Healthcare (Basel). 11(2):266

Albano D, Galiano V, Basile M, Di Luca F, Gitto S, Messina C, Cagetti MG, Del Fabbro M, Tartaglia GM, Sconfienza LM (2024) Artificial intelligence for radiographic imaging detection of caries lesions: a systematic review. BMC Oral Health 24(1):274

Alessa N (2024) Application of artificial intelligence in pediatric dentistry: a literature review. J Pharm Bioallied Sci 16(Suppl 3):S1938–S1940

Anil S, Porwal P, Porwal A (2023) Transforming dental caries diagnosis through artificial intelligence-based techniques. Cureus 15(7):e41694

Azhari AA, Helal N, Sabri LM, Abduljawad A (2023) Artificial intelligence (AI) in restorative dentistry: performance of AI models designed for detection of interproximal carious lesions on primary and permanent dentition. Digit Health 30(9):20552076231216680

Barros Padilha DX, Veiga NJ, Mello-Moura ACV, Nunes CP (2023) Virtual reality and behaviour management in paediatric dentistry: a systematic review. BMC Oral Health 23(1):995. https://doi.org/10.1186/s12903-023-03595-7

Bonny T, Al Nassan W, Obaideen K, Al Mallahi MN, Mohammad Y, El-Damanhoury HM (2023) Contemporary role and applications of artificial intelligence in dentistry. F1000Res 12:1179

Can Demirbaş K, Yıldız M, Saygılı S, Canpolat N, Kasapçopur Ö (2024) Artificial intelligence in pediatrics: learning to walk together. Turk Arch Pediatr 59(2):121–130. https://doi.org/10.5152/TurkArchPediatr.2024.24002

Chau RCW, Li GH, Tew IM et al (2023) Accuracy of artificial intelligence-based photographic detection of gingivitis. Int Dent J 73:724–730

DaSilva AF, Robinson MA, Shi W, McCauley LK (2022) The forefront of dentistry-promising tech-innovations and new treatments. JDR Clin Trans Res 7(1_suppl):16S-24S

Ezzat H et al (2022) Predictive analytics for pediatric dental health: machine learning and AI approaches. J Med Syst 46(9):74

Feher B, Tussie C, Giannobile WV (2024) Applied artificial intelligence in dentistry: emerging data modalities and modeling approaches. Front Artif Intell 23(7):1427517

Kazimierczak N, Kazimierczak W, Serafin Z, Nowicki P, Nożewski J, Janiszewska-Olszowska J (2024) AI in orthodontics: Revolutionizing diagnostics and treatment planning—a comprehensive review. J Clin Med 13(2):344

Kunz F, Stellzig-Eisenhauer A, Zeman F, Boldt J (2020) Artificial intelligence in orthodontics. J Orofac Orthop 81:52–68

Kuo C, Wei S (2019) Artificial intelligence in pediatric dentistry: current and future perspectives. CRC Press

La Rosa S, Quinzi V, Palazzo G, Ronsivalle V, Lo GA (2024) The Implications of artificial intelligence in pedodontics: a scoping review of evidence-based literature. Healthcare (Basel) 12(13):1311. https://doi.org/10.3390/healthcare12131311

Maganur PC, Vishwanathaiah S, Mashyakhy M, Abumelha AS, Robaian A, Almohareb T, Almutairi B, Alzahrani KM, Binalrimal S, Marwah N, Khanagar SB, Manoharan V (2024) Development of artificial intelligence models for tooth numbering and detection: a systematic review. Int Dent J 74(5):917–929

Mestre R, Astobiza AM, Webster-Wood VA, Ryan M, Saif MTA (2024) Ethics and responsibility in biohybrid robotics research. Proc Natl Acad Sci USA 121(31):e2310458121

Nabavizadeh N, Khosravani A (2022) The role of AI in early detection of dental caries in pediatric patients. Int J Pediatr Dent 32(6):905–912

Naeimi SM, Darvish S, Salman BN, Luchian I (2024) Artificial intelligence in adult and pediatric dentistry: a narrative review. Bioengineering (Basel) 11(5):431

Rahim A, Khatoon R, Khan TA, Syed K, Khan I, Khalid T, Khalid B (2024) Artificial intelligence-powered dentistry: Probing the potential, challenges, and ethicality of artificial intelligence in dentistry. Digit Health 11(10):20552076241291344

Riet TV, Graaf W, Lange J, Kober J (2023) Analysis of movements in tooth removal procedures using robot technology. PLoS ONE 18(5):e0285503

Rokhshad R, Zhang P, Mohammad-Rahimi H, Shobeiri P, Schwendicke F (2024) Current applications of artificial intelligence for pediatric dentistry: a systematic review and meta-analysis. Pediatr Dent 46(1):27–35

Rosa A, Pujia AM, Docimo R, Arcuri C (2023) Managing dental phobia in children with the use of virtual reality: a systematic review of the current literature. Children (Basel) 10(11):1763. https://doi.org/10.3390/children10111763

Sayed D et al (2020) AI and deep learning for pediatric oral health diagnostics: a review of applications and prospects. BMC Oral Health 20(1):5

Schwendicke F, Cejudo Grano de Oro J, Garcia Cantu A, Meyer-Lueckel H, Chaurasia A, Krois J (2022) Artificial intelligence for caries detection: value of data and information. J Dent Res 101(11):1350–1356. https://doi.org/10.1177/00220345221113756. Epub 2022 Aug 22

Semerci ZM, Yardımcı S (2024) Empowering modern dentistry: the impact of artificial intelligence on patient care and clinical decision making. Diagnostics (Basel) 14(12):1260. https://doi.org/10.3390/diagnostics14121260

Sharma S, Kumari P, Sabira K, Parihar AS, Divya Rani P, Roy A, Surana P (2024) Revolutionizing dentistry: the applications of artificial intelligence in dental health care. J Pharm Bioallied Sci 16(Suppl 3):S1910–S1912

Sivari E, Senirkentli GB, Bostanci E, Guzel MS, Acici K, Asuroglu T (2023) Deep learning in diagnosis of dental anomalies and diseases: a systematic review. Diagnostics (Basel) 13(15):2512. https://doi.org/10.3390/diagnostics13152512./bioengineering11050431

Surlari Z, Budală DG, Lupu CI, Stelea CG, Butnaru OM, Luchian I (2023) Current progress and challenges of using artificial intelligence in clinical dentistry-a narrative review. J Clin Med 12(23):7378. https://doi.org/10.3390/jcm12237378

Thurzo A, Urbanová W, Novák B, Czako L, Siebert T, Stano P, Mareková S, Fountoulaki G, Kosnáčová H, Varga I (2022) Where Is the artificial intelligence applied in dentistry? Systematic review and literature analysis. Healthcare (Basel) 10(7):1269

Tomášik J, Zsoldos M, Oravcová Ľ, Lifková M, Pavleová G, Strunga M, Thurzo A (2024) AI and face-driven orthodontics: a scoping review of digital advances in diagnosis and treatment planning. AI 5(1):158–176

Vishwanathaiah S, Fageeh HN, Khanagar SB, Maganur PC (2023) Artificial intelligence its uses and application in pediatric dentistry: a review. Biomedicines 11(3):788. https://doi.org/10.3390/biomedicines11030788

Vodanović M, Subašić M, Milošević D, Savić PI (2023) Artificial intelligence in medicine and dentistry. Acta Stomatol Croat 57(1):70–84. https://doi.org/10.15644/asc57/1/8

You W, Hao A, Li S, Wang Y, Xia B (2020) Deep learning-based dental plaque detection on primary teeth: a comparison with clinical assessments. BMC Oral Health 20(1):141

Zhao Z, Xu J (2020) Artificial intelligence in dental medicine: applications and advances in dentistry. Elsevier

Outcome of Artificial Intelligence-Based Treatment

Ikroop Gill, Tarun Kumar Singh, and Aakash Gupta

1 Impact of AI on Mankind

In a variety of fields, including dentistry, artificial intelligence (AI) has significantly expanded its presence and impact. It can make advanced predictions and decisions in the medical field, especially in endodontics, by simulating human intelligence. Analysing the anatomy of the root canal system, predicting the viability of dental pulp stem cells, measuring working lengths, determining root fractures and periapical lesions, and predicting the success of retreatment procedures are merely some of the endodontic uses for AI models like convolutional neural networks and/or artificial neural networks (Ghaffari et al. 2024).

It is a remarkable creation that mimics human cognitive abilities and has drawn scrutiny from scientists worldwide. Neural networks, which are modeled after human brains and are capable of simulating human thought, are the fundamental building block of artificial intelligence technology. This kind of brain architecture is composed of highly interconnected neurones and serves mostly as a data processing system to solve a specific problem. This quickly developing technology enables robots to perform tasks that were previously limited to humans. Its usage in dentistry has only recently begun, and the results have been remarkable. An effective technique for evaluating clinical dental data is artificial intelligence (Dentistry Review 2024). Advances in AI raise the possibility of benefits for healthcare, such as reduced surgical complications, improved quality of life, improved decision-making, and a significant reduction in unnecessary treatments (Fig. 1).

As we know by now, AI is the ability of machines to perform tasks that normally require human intelligence. Although the concept of AI has been there since 1950, it has only come into practical use in the last two decades ago. In 1956, **John McCarthy**

I. Gill · T. K. Singh (✉) · A. Gupta
Division of Conservative Dentistry and Endodontics, Department of Dentistry, All India Institute of Medical Sciences, Bathinda, India
e-mail: drtarunkumarsingh@gmail.com

A. Gupta et al. (eds.), *Application of Robotics in Dentistry*, Lecture Notes in Bioengineering, https://doi.org/10.1007/978-981-95-1470-0_15

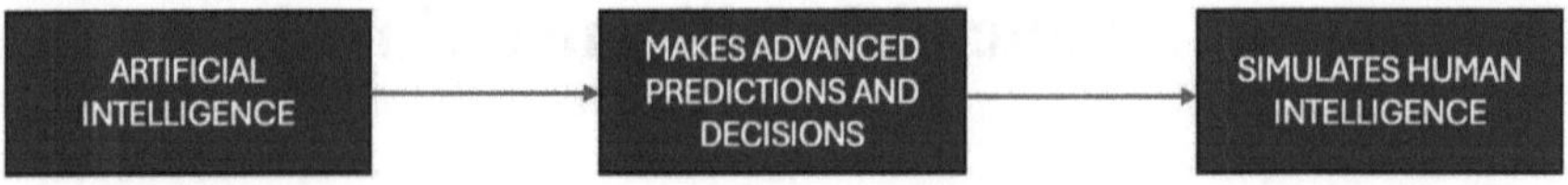

Fig. 1 Impact of AI on mankind

presented artificial intelligence as a branch of applied computer science (Ding et al. 2023). Some refer to it as the '**fourth industrial revolution**'.

When a computer emulates analytical processes that people commonly identify with other human brains, such as 'learning and problem-solving', the term 'artificial intelligence (AI)' is employed. The ability of AI techniques to identify significant patterns in data has led to a great deal of experimentation with them as clinical trial tools, particularly to help with prognostic and projection decision-making, as well as every stage of diagnosis and treatment. It has been shown that AI can more rapidly and economically improve accuracy, efficiency, and precision on par with medical expertise.

Although the majority of AI applications in dentistry are for diagnosis, there are still certain limitations because of data homogeneity, availability, and processing capacity for three-dimensional (3D) data. The aspects of oral health status and quality of life that are important to patients and their families, as well as the clinical or physiological metrics that are significant to medical experts, are referred to as oral health outcomes. Furthermore, results have several aspects, such as physiological and clinical components as well as those related to quality of life. Results are significant for a number of reasons, chief among them being their influence on public policy. The healthcare system is receiving increased public attention in an era of fiscal constraints, limited resources, and growing expenses (Agrawal et al. 2022).

Statistics also aid in identifying what works and what does not. They also enable us to evaluate the impact of dental care on a patient's life, as well as how well we prevent or cure diseases and restore function. The relative efficacy of several treatment approaches for the same ailment is also ascertained with the aid of outcomes.

2 Outcome Dimensions

Bader and Shugars defined four outcome dimensions associated with dental care: the physical/physiological, psychosocial, longevity/survival, and economic (Bader and Shugars 1995).

Presence of pathology, dental caries, deep periodontal pockets, malocclusion, discomfort, and functional ability are all included in the physical/physiological dimension. It has been usual practice to assess this outcome dimension using standard measures of oral health status. Radiographs and clinical tests may be used to determine objective measures of pathology (Edelstein 1998). Functional capability can be assessed objectively or by asking patients about their ability to speak or chew, for example. The patient's report must be used to assess whether pain is present.

Patients' self-perception, interpersonal relationships, perceived aesthetics, and level of oral health satisfaction are all represented in the psychosocial outcomes dimension of dental treatment.

The longevity and survival of dental restorations, tooth vitality, tooth retention, and similar factors are all included in the longevity/survival outcomes component of dental treatment.

Therefore, findings could be used to compare the relative efficacy of different treatment approaches or to evaluate how well a treatment is working for a particular clinical condition. Outcomes can be used to assist in developing clinical practice guidelines when more information about which treatments work becomes available. The guidelines are 'systematically developed statements to assist practitioner and patient decisions about appropriate health care for specific clinical circumstances'. Guidelines created by several dental associations, such as the **American Academy of Paediatric Dentistry (AAPD)**, have the potential to improve healthcare decision-making, improve methods for assessing and improving the quality of care, increase patient and public education regarding dental care for certain conditions, and direct the distribution of resources (Dhopte et al. 2023).

Not only may clinical guidelines and outcomes measurements help patients and practitioners make clinical decisions but they can also be used to create reimbursement policies that influence the behaviour of patients or practitioners. This chapter examines the different effects of AI in dentistry, emphasising how it affects clinical procedures, patient experiences, and the direction of dental treatment going forward (Fig. 2).

3 Enhanced Diagnostic Accuracy

An improvement in diagnostic precision is among the most crucial applications of artificial intelligence: disorders of the oral cavity, their diagnosis and treatment, and the identification and categorisation of abnormally altered mucosa exhibiting premalignant and malignant changes that are invisible to the naked eye. The genetic susceptibility of a large population to oral cancer may be accurately detected by artificial intelligence.

In Dental Radiology

Cone-beam computed tomography (CBCT) scans and panoramic radiographs are two examples of dental radiography pictures that AI algorithms may analyse to help identify and diagnose a variety of dental diseases. Dental caries (tooth decay), periodontal disorders, bone loss, and anatomical anomalies can all be detected and measured with the aid of AI-powered image analysis. The diagnosis of oral tumours, cysts, and other clinical diseases can also be aided by automated image analysis. Due

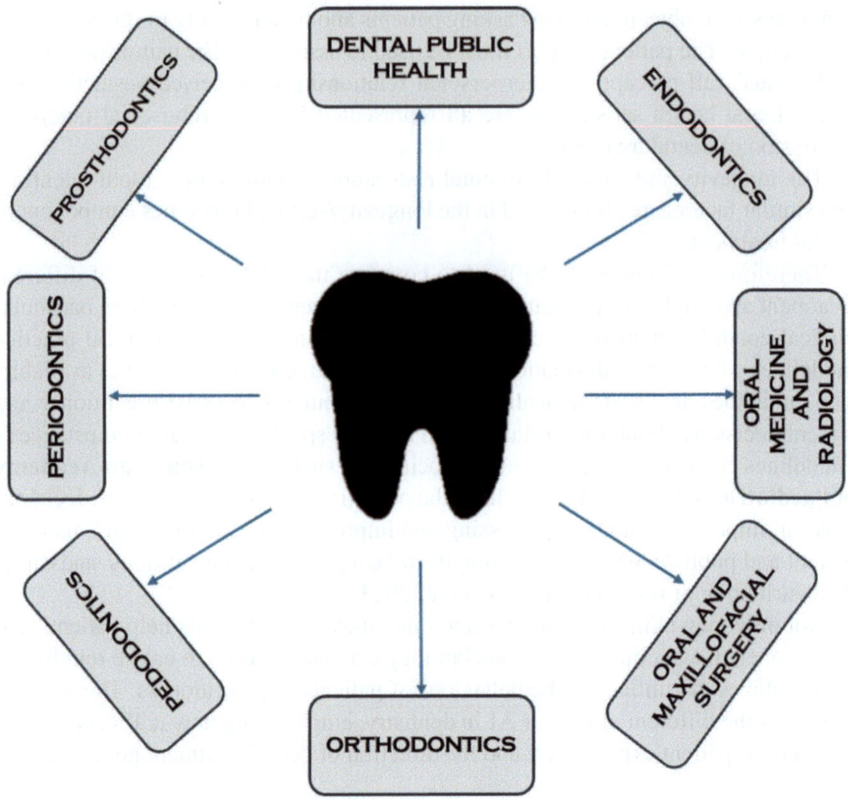

Fig. 2 Artificial intelligence in dental sectors

to the acquisition and processing of data from the usage of RVGs, CBCTs, and 3D images, artificial intelligence is assisting in diagnosis (Thomson and Kahler 2010).

Treatment Planning and Implant Placement

By evaluating CBCT scans, AI can assist with dental implant treatment planning. By simulating implant placement and providing dentists virtual treatment plans, artificial intelligence (AI) systems can optimise the insertion site and angulation for the best results. Artificial intelligence (AI) systems, for instance, can help detect dental irregularities including impacted teeth, supernumerary teeth, or developmental abnormalities. AI systems can identify any discrepancies and notify dentists of any problems by comparing patient data with preestablished standards and trends (Fatima et al. 2022). The detection of anomalies in the temporomandibular joint (TMJ) and its surrounding structures can also be aided by AI systems. AI systems may detect symptoms of TMJ diseases such disc displacement, osteoarthritis, and joint degeneration by examining radiographs and clinical data. This facilitates effective treatment planning and early intervention.

Fig. 3 Artificial intelligence outcome in dental radiology

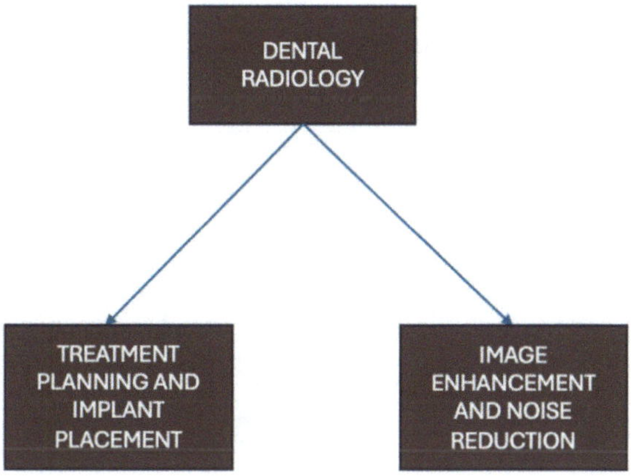

Image Enhancement and Noise Reduction

By minimising noise, increasing contrast, and enhancing resolution, artificial intelligence (AI) methods like deep learning can be used to improve the quality of dental radiography images. Better visualisation of dental structures can result from higher picture quality, which can help with diagnosis and interpretation of a variety of dental disorders (Fig. 3). AI technology has the ability to enhance early diagnosis and eventually save lives by helping dentists spot areas of risk (Babu et al. 2021).

4 Artificial Intelligence Outcome in Orthodontics

Cephalometric Analysis and Treatment Planning

Key anatomical features used in orthodontic diagnosis and treatment planning can be automatically identified and measured by AI algorithms that analyse cephalometric radiographs. In accordance with established treatment procedures, orthodontists can use AI-powered software to help generate cephalometric tracings, analyse face and dental measurements, and simulate treatment results.

Malocclusion Diagnosis and Classification

By evaluating a variety of diagnostic data, including radiography scans, facial photographs, and dental models, AI models can help with the diagnosis and classification of malocclusions. Artificial intelligence (AI) algorithms can recognise and classify various malocclusion types by training on enormous datasets, which aids orthodontists in treatment planning and selecting the best treatment modalities (Haidar 2023). Software driven by artificial intelligence (AI) may create virtual 3D models of patients' teeth and replicate the course and results of orthodontic therapy. By examining dental models and forecasting the best bracket locations based on the

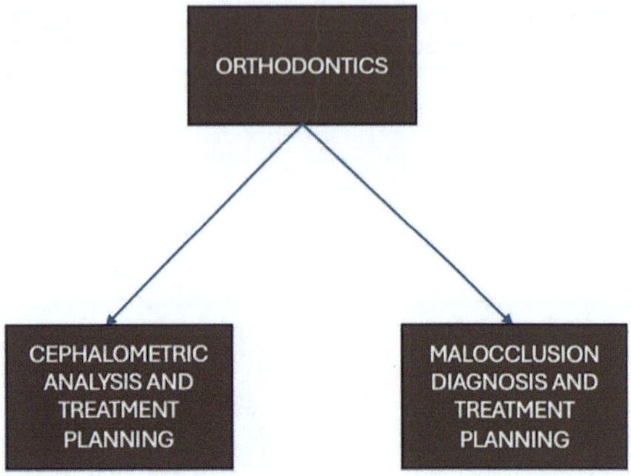

Fig. 4 Artificial intelligence outcome in orthodontics

unique structure of each tooth, artificial intelligence (AI) systems can automate the bracket placement procedure (Fig. 4).

5 Artificial Intelligence Outcome in Periodontology

AI systems can help with the diagnosis and categorisation of periodontal disorders by analysing a variety of diagnostic data, including radiographs, intraoral imaging, and clinical parameters. Early identification and customised treatment plans are made possible by AI models' ability to recognise patterns and markers of the severity of periodontal disease through learning from massive datasets. By evaluating clinical data taken from patient records, including bleeding scores, attachment levels, and probing depths, AI-based software can automate periodontal charting (Kalappanavar et al. 2018).

Automated charting can improve accuracy, minimise time and effort compared to manual charting, and offer a thorough visual depiction of periodontal health status. By evaluating patient-specific data and modeling treatment outcomes, artificial intelligence (AI)-powered software can help with implant placement and treatment planning for periodontal disorders. Artificial intelligence (AI) algorithms can help choose the best treatment options, optimise implant placement and angulation, and offer virtual simulations for assessing various therapy options. AI can improve implantology processes by helping with prosthetic rehabilitation, implant placement, and implant selection. In order to choose the ideal implant size and type, optimise implant location, and take into account variables like bone density and proximity to important structures, artificial intelligence (AI) algorithms can evaluate patient-specific anatomical data, such as CBCT scans (Afshari et al. 2024).

6 Artificial Intelligence Outcome in Endodontics

Endodontists may more precisely discover and examine intricate root canal systems with the aid of AI-powered technologies that can help detect and segment root canals within radiography images. Automated canal detection can increase productivity, reduce waiting times, and increase the accuracy of root canal therapy. Predictive models that assess the success or failure of endodontic treatments based on patient-specific data, including clinical factors, radiographic results, and treatment regimens, can be created using AI approaches, including machine learning (Fig. 5).

Instrumentation Techniques

By taking into account variables including canal form, anatomy, and mechanical properties, AI algorithms can evaluate and improve endodontic instrumentation approaches, such as rotary or reciprocating file systems. By examining the distribution and effectiveness of irrigants throughout the root canal system, artificial intelligence (AI) can also help optimise irrigation techniques, improving treatment results and disinfection (Bhatia and Tiwari 2019).

Root Fracture Detection

Root fractures can be challenging to diagnose clinically, but AI systems can identify them by analysing radiographic images. In order to make prompt treatment decisions and possibly avoid tooth extraction, automated fracture detection can help discover root fractures early.

Cari Screen AI

An AI tool called Cari Screen AI was created by engineers and dentists to help identify and diagnose dental caries or tooth decay. The device analyses dental images using complex algorithms to give dentists precise and effective evaluations of the potential risk of tooth decay (Mehrabanian and Artificial Intelligence in Dentistry 2024).

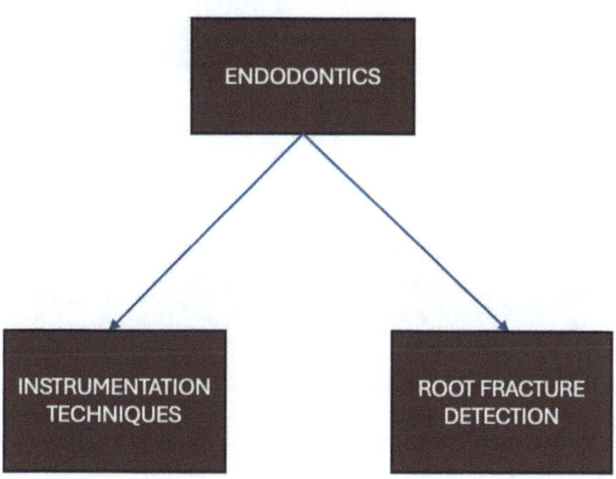

Fig. 5 Artificial intelligence outcome in endodontics

Dental clinics have observed a notable improvement in early caries identification through the use of Cari Screen AI, which enables prompt interventions and improves patient outcomes for oral health.

7 Artificial Intelligence Outcome in Prosthodontics

By evaluating patient data, including digital impressions, radiographs, and facial scans, artificial intelligence (AI) may aid in prosthodontic treatment planning through the creation of virtual three-dimensional (3D) models of the patient's oral anatomy. By optimising the shape, fit, and aesthetics of prosthodontic restorations—such dental crowns, bridges, and dentures—based on patient-specific factors and preferences, artificial intelligence (AI) algorithms can help in their design and fabrication (Rekow 2019).

Digital imprints and intraoral scans can be analysed by AI-powered software to precisely identify and define the edges of tooth preparations (Fig. 6). By enabling optimal fit and minimising the need for manual corrections, automated margin detection can increase the accuracy of prosthetic restorations.

Virtual Articulation and Occlusion Analysis

With the goal to evaluate functional dynamics, detect interferences, and assess occlusal relationships, artificial intelligence (AI) programmes can analyse digital models of the dentition and simulate virtual articulation. Prosthetic treatment planning can benefit from virtual articulation and occlusion analysis, which guarantees appropriate occlusal alignment and harmony for the best possible functional and aesthetically pleasing results (Liu et al. 2023).

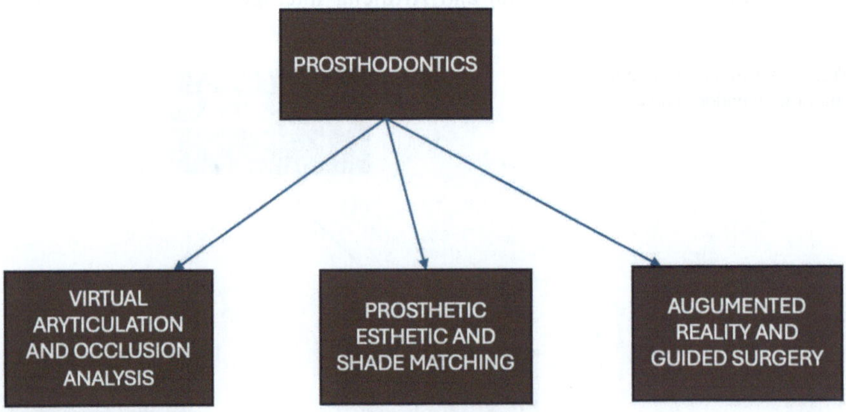

Fig. 6 Artificial intelligence outcome in prosthodontics

Prosthetic Aesthetic and Shade Matching

Artificial intelligence (AI) tools are able to evaluate digital images of patients' natural teeth and help with prosthetic aesthetics by proposing shade-matching and forecasting how prosthetic restorations may appear in various lighting scenarios.

Augmented Reality and Guided Surgery

By offering real-time navigation and visualisation of the implant placement procedure, AI-powered augmented reality platforms can help prosthodontists with guided implant surgery.

8 Artificial Intelligence Outcome in Oral Surgery

AI systems can diagnose oral and maxillofacial disorders, such as tumours, cysts, fractures, and impacted teeth, by analysing radiographic images, such as CBCT, magnetic resonance imaging (MRI), and panoramic radiographs. In order to facilitate precise diagnosis and treatment planning, AI-powered software can help with the identification, segmentation, and categorisation of anatomical structures and anomalies. Virtual surgical simulations can be produced using AI-based surgical planning systems using patient-specific data. Through the simulation of multiple scenarios and evaluation of the possible outcomes, surgeons can realistically plan intricate procedures like orthognathic surgery or tumour removal. Artificial intelligence (AI) algorithms can help in surgical simulation by offering insights into the best surgical strategy, implant placement, and reconstruction methods, improving surgical accuracy and patient safety (Toosi et al. 2014).

The precision and accuracy of surgical procedures can be improved by integrating AI into robotic-assisted operations and surgical navigation systems. Anatomical landmarks can be tracked by AI algorithms, which can also help with real-time navigation during surgery and give the surgeon feedback. In challenging circumstances with complicated anatomical structures or difficult access, this technique can be especially helpful in enhancing surgical results and lowering complications. By superimposing virtual models onto the surgical area, AR platforms can help with accurate tissue manipulation and incision placement while lowering the risk of intraoperative complications (Mitra and Tarnach 2022).

9 Artificial Intelligence Outcome in Oral Pathology

To help diagnose oral disorders like mouth cancer, precancerous lesions, and inflammatory conditions, artificial intelligence (AI) algorithms can examine histopathological images of oral tissue samples. AI-powered tools can help pathologists identify and categorise various histopathological patterns, increasing the precision and effectiveness of diagnosis (Sharma 2019).

Image Analysis and Feature Extraction

Digital histopathology images can be analysed using AI approaches like deep learning to extract pertinent aspects including tissue architecture, nuclear atypia, and cellular morphology. In order to help in disease diagnosis, grading, and prognosis, AI algorithms are able to quantify these characteristics and offer objective measurements.

Personalised Treatment Plans

By assessing each patient's distinct clinical data, such as genetics, lifestyle, and past dental history, artificial intelligence assists in creating individualised treatment regimens. Predictive analysis is used to help identify patients who are at risk of particular dental problems so that individualised preventive actions can be implemented. AI, for example, can identify patients who are at risk of developing periodontal disease by evaluating massive datasets, enabling early intervention and individualised treatment plans. Two artificial neural network (ANN) algorithms were used in a study by **Shankarapillai et al.** to predict periodontal risk (Shankarapillai et al. n.d.).

Improved Patient Experience

AI has been dramatically cutting down on healthcare inefficiencies, increasing patient flow and experience, and boosting patient safety and attendant experience throughout the care pathway. AI might be used, for instance, to remotely monitor patients in order to detect and treat them promptly.

AI-powered chatbots and virtual assistants give patients instant access to information and assistance. By providing answers to frequently asked questions, assisting with appointment scheduling, and even diagnosing dental issues, these technologies can greatly cut down on wait times and increase patient satisfaction (Nguyen et al. 2021).

AI-powered solutions also additionally boost patient education and engagement. Patients feel more engaged in their dental health journey when they are given personalised and interactive information. This helps people to make informed decisions, comply with treatment programmes, and actively engage in their dental care (Fig. 7). AI technology's accessibility and ease of use improve the overall satisfaction of patients. In order to improve convenience and lower obstacles to care, patients can obtain information, make appointments, and get help at the time and place of their choice. Furthermore, proactive AI-driven alerts and reminders guarantee that patients

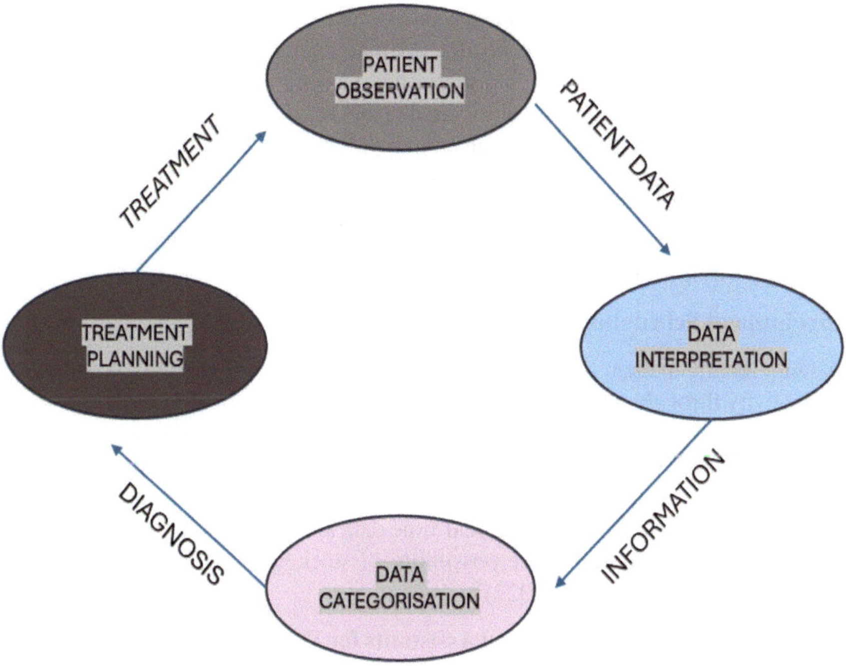

Fig. 7 Diagnostic cycle

maintain their dental care schedules, which improves treatment results (Chen et al. 2020).

10 Treatment Visualisation and Patient-Centric Approach

AI can produce lifelike models of suggested therapies, assisting patients in assessing how procedures like orthodontics or cosmetic dental work would turn out. Patients are encouraged to make educated decisions as a result of this transparency, which also fosters trust.

Data Analysis and Pattern Recognition for Evidence- Based Decision-Making

The capacity of AI to swiftly and precisely analyse vast volumes of data is one of its main benefits in the healthcare industry. Massive volumes of data have been generated by medical practices, including research articles, test findings, patient records, and medical photographs. These data can be processed and analysed by AI algorithms to find trends, connections, and insights that human healthcare professionals may overlook.

Medical practices can use evidence-based decision-making procedures by utilising AI. Based on past patient results, AI may evaluate patient data to find risk factors, forecast the course of a disease, and suggest suitable treatment options. Better patient outcomes and fewer medical errors result from doctors making better judgements thanks to this data-driven strategy (Secinaro et al. 2021).

Operational Efficiency

AI tools streamline various administrative tasks, improving overall operational efficiency within dental practices.

Appointment Scheduling and Resource Management

By anticipating patient cancellations and no-shows, AI systems can maximise productivity through appointment scheduling optimisation.

AI can also help with inventory management by forecasting dental supply demand, cutting waste, and guaranteeing that clinics have enough supplies on hand. Artificial intelligence (AI) systems can forecast inventory requirements, create buy orders, and optimise stock levels by examining real-time data and previous consumption trends. This reduces waste, removes the possibility of stockouts, and guarantees efficient practice operations (Qu et al. 2022).

AI-Powered Chatbots and Virtual Assistants for Patient Support and Guidance

Chatbots and virtual assistants with artificial intelligence (AI) features have become useful resources for patient support and direction. Throughout their dental journey, these AI technologies are intended to communicate with patients, respond to their enquiries, and offer support. Chatbots comprehend and react to patient questions instantly by using natural language processing algorithms. Information regarding dental procedures, oral health advice, instructions for after-treatment care, and other topics are available to patients. In an emergency, chatbots can also help patients by offering prompt assistance until they can get help from a specialist (Lee et al. 2018).

AI-powered virtual assistants offer patients individualised help and direction. They can help patients with follow-up treatment, appointment scheduling, and reminder messages. Because virtual assistants are available around the clock, patients can get care and information whenever it is convenient for them.

Financial Management

By examining billing trends and streamlining the reimbursement procedure, artificial intelligence (AI) solutions can contribute to financial management and can help dental offices increase their cash flow.

11 Research and Development

Beyond specific dental practices, AI has ramifications for the larger area of dental research. Large volumes of research data can be analysed by AI, which can spot patterns and connections that conventional analysis might miss.

Drug Discovery and Material Science

AI models are being used in fields like material science and drug research to forecast the effectiveness of novel dental materials or treatments, hastening the creation of cutting-edge dental care solutions.

Training and Education

Furthermore, dental practitioners must receive continual training in order to utilise AI technologies. To provide high-quality treatment, practitioners must be skilled at using these tools while retaining their capacity for critical thinking.

Virtual Simulations and Training

AI may be used to create training materials and virtual simulations that give dental students a realistic and engaging learning environment. Students can practise different dental procedures, develop their clinical skills, and strengthen their decision-making ability with the aid of these simulators. With the help of AI algorithms, students can receive individualised instruction and study at their own pace by receiving real-time feedback and advice (Putra et al. 2021).

Intelligent Tutoring Systems

Intelligent tutoring systems powered by AI are able to evaluate student performance, pinpoint areas of weakness, and offer recommendations and personalised learning resources. Students can receive specialised training and support because to these systems' ability to adjust to different learning styles and offer tailored feedback. The evaluation process can be streamlined by using AI algorithms to help with student work assessment and grading (Fukuda et al. 2019).

Adaptive Learning Platforms

Platforms for adaptive learning that customise course material to each student's unique requirements and skills can be powered by AI. To improve understanding and retention, these platforms can evaluate student performance data, spot knowledge gaps, and provide tailored learning resources. Additionally, by tracking students' progress over time, adaptive learning systems enable teachers to keep an eye on their growth and offer focused interventions as necessary.

12 Integration of AI with Other Emerging Technologies

The integration of AI with other emerging technologies holds immense potential in revolutionising dentistry.

Robotics and Automation

Dental operations can be made more accurate and automated by integrating AI with robotic technologies. Robots can precisely complete repetitive operations, such as placing dental implants and preparing teeth, which lowers human error and improves treatment results.

Augmented Reality (AR) and Virtual Reality (VR)

Dental training and patient education can benefit from the use of AI algorithms to improve AR and VR experiences. Dentists may more precisely visualise and plan treatments by combining real-time patient data with AI-generated dental models. Interactive simulations that help patients see possible outcomes and comprehend procedures can also be beneficial (Setzer et al. 2020).

Internet of Things (IOT)

AI algorithms can be used to improve AR and VR patient education and training experiences in dentistry. Real-time patient data combined with AI-generated dental models allow dentists to more precisely visualise and plan treatments. Interactive simulations can also help patients see possible outcomes and better understand operations.

13 Outcome of the Use of Robotics in Dentistry

The integration of robotics in dentistry represents a groundbreaking shift in how dental procedures are performed, enhancing precision, efficiency, and patient outcomes. As technological advances continue to emerge, robots are becoming increasingly sophisticated and are playing a significant role in various aspects of dental care. From aiding in surgeries to improving diagnostic capabilities, the incorporation of robotics is revolutionising the field. This chapter aims to explore the outcomes of robotics in dentistry, focusing on the key areas where robotic systems have made a significant impact, the benefits they offer, and the challenges that still need to be addressed for their widespread adoption (Lee et al. 2018).

Robotics in Dental Surgery

One of the most profound impacts of robotics in dentistry is in the field of dental surgery, particularly in procedures like dental implants, maxillofacial surgery, and periodontal surgeries (Fig. 8).

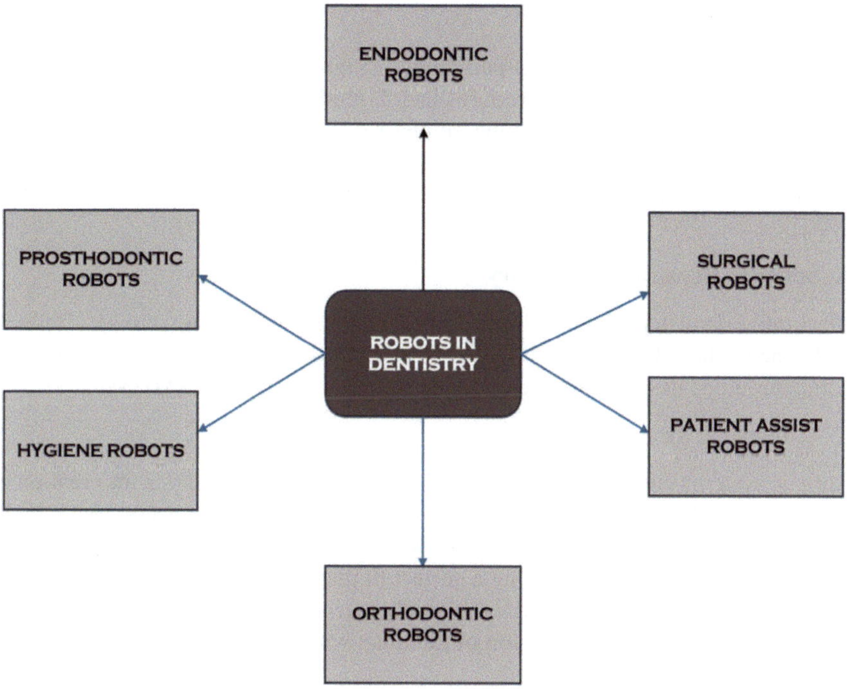

Fig. 8 Robots in dentistry

a. Dental Implantology

Robotic systems in dental implantology have brought about a new era of precision and predictability. Robots, such as the **Yomi** and **Navio**, have been used to assist in placing dental implants with enhanced accuracy. These robotic systems work in conjunction with 3D imaging to plan and guide the surgery. They can perform tasks such as determining the precise angle, depth, and location for implant placement (Alexander and John 2018).

The result is a reduction in human error, less invasiveness, and improved outcomes, including faster recovery times for patients. With robots, implant placement has become highly predictable, and complications such as nerve damage or incorrect angulation are significantly minimised.

b. Maxillofacial Surgery

Robots are also being used in maxillofacial surgeries to treat conditions such as jaw misalignments, tumours, and congenital deformities. Robotic-assisted systems allow for highly precise bone cuts, reducing damage to surrounding tissues. This precision leads to fewer complications, less blood loss, and shorter recovery times.

The flexibility and dexterity offered by robots enable surgeons to perform intricate procedures with greater control and less fatigue, which is particularly valuable in lengthy surgeries or cases that require repeated, fine movements (Aminoshariae et al. 2021).

c. Periodontal Surgery

Robots have made their mark in periodontal surgery by aiding in the treatment of gum diseases, particularly in procedures such as guided tissue regeneration or osseous surgery. The incorporation of robotics allows for precise removal of infected tissues, with minimal disruption to healthy gum tissues. This leads to enhanced recovery and better long-term outcomes for patients suffering from periodontal disease (Lee et al. 2022).

Robotics in Restorative Dentistry

Restorative dentistry, which includes procedures like cavity fillings, crowns, bridges, and veneers, has also benefited from robotic assistance, particularly in the fields of computer-aided design/computer-aided manufacturing (CAD/CAM) systems.

a. Automated Restorations

Robotic systems integrated with CAD/CAM technologies can help in the creation of custom-made dental restorations such as crowns, bridges, and veneers. Using high-precision milling machines, robotic arms can carve out restorations from materials like porcelain or zirconia, ensuring a perfect fit that aligns with the patient's natural teeth. This process, which would traditionally take a dental technician several hours, can now be completed in a fraction of the time, with greater consistency and fewer errors (Batra et al. 2023).

b. 3D Printing

The rise of 3D printing technology in conjunction with robotics has allowed for the creation of highly customised dental prostheses. Robots can manipulate printers to create precise dental models, dentures, and even full mouth restorations. The speed, accuracy, and customisation offered by robotic 3D printing are enabling dental practices to offer more personalised care, often with same-day service for certain restorative treatments (Reyes et al. 2022).

Robotics in Orthodontics

In orthodontics, robotic systems are being increasingly employed to improve treatment planning and outcome prediction, particularly in the creation of clear aligners and braces.

a. Clear Aligner Production

Robotic systems are now able to automate the process of creating clear aligners, ensuring that they are produced to precise specifications tailored to each patient's dental anatomy. Robotic precision ensures better fitting aligners, which results in improved treatment efficacy and a more comfortable experience for patients.

b. Braces and Wire Bending

Robots can also assist in the creation of custom braces and wire bending for orthodontic treatments. In traditional systems, wire bending is a manual task, often leading to slight variations in fit and function. Robotics enable more uniform bending of orthodontic wires, improving the final outcome and reducing the number of adjustments needed during treatment (Carrillo-Perez et al. 2021).

Robotics in Diagnostic Dentistry

Robotics has also had a significant impact on diagnostic dentistry, improving both the accuracy and efficiency of diagnostic procedures. Robotic systems are increasingly being used in conjunction with advanced imaging technologies such as cone-beam computed tomography (CBCT) and 3D scanning.

a. Enhanced Imaging Systems

In diagnostic imaging, robots are used to automate the positioning of patients and scanning equipment. Robotic arms ensure the precise alignment of imaging devices, eliminating human error in the positioning process. This leads to better-quality images that improve diagnostic accuracy for conditions such as tooth decay, bone loss, and tumours.

b. AI Integration

In combination with artificial intelligence (AI), robotic systems are able to interpret diagnostic images, identifying patterns and anomalies that might be difficult for the human eye to detect. This AI-enhanced robotic diagnosis allows for earlier detection of dental issues, which can be critical for effective treatment planning and better patient outcomes (Alzaid et al. 2023).

14 Benefits of Robotics in Dentistry

The introduction of robotics into dentistry has brought several significant benefits that have transformed the practice of modern dentistry.

a. Increased Precision and Accuracy

Robotic systems excel at performing repetitive, highly precise tasks, which has led to significant improvements in the accuracy of dental procedures. This has reduced the margin for error, leading to better outcomes, fewer complications, and a more predictable healing process.

b. Minimally Invasive Procedures

Many robotic systems are designed to carry out procedures with minimal disruption to surrounding tissues. This has resulted in less pain, smaller incisions, and faster recovery times for patients. Minimally invasive surgery also reduces the risk of infection and other postoperative complications (Sharma et al. 2024).

c. Improved Patient Experience

Patients benefit from the enhanced precision, shorter treatment times, and faster recovery rates associated with robotic procedures. Furthermore, some robotic systems enable more efficient procedures that reduce the number of visits a patient need, leading to less time off work and more convenience (Revilla-León et al. 2021).

d. Efficiency and Time Savings

Robots can reduce the time required for certain procedures, especially in the fields of implantology, restorative dentistry, and orthodontics. As robotic systems become more capable, dental professionals can perform procedures more efficiently, allowing them to see more patients and streamline operations within dental clinics (Khanagar et al. 2020).

15 Challenges and Limitations of Robotics in Dentistry

Despite the promising outcomes, there are still several challenges that limit the widespread adoption of robotics in dentistry.

a. High Initial Costs

One of the major barriers to adopting robotic systems in dental practices is the high upfront cost. Advanced robotic systems, along with their required maintenance, can be prohibitively expensive for smaller practices. This financial burden can limit accessibility for some dental practitioners and their patients (Ding et al. 2023b).

b. Learning Curve

Robotic systems require specialised training for dental professionals. The learning curve can be steep, and not all dental practitioners may be willing or able to invest the time and effort to master robotic technologies. This may slow down the integration of robotics into the broader dental community (Ossowska et al. 2022).

c. Limited Robotic Autonomy

While robots have advanced significantly, they are still limited by their need for human oversight. Robots in dentistry are not fully autonomous and require human input for certain steps of the procedure. This reliance on human operators can sometimes diminish the efficiency gains offered by robotic systems (Grischke et al. 2020).

d. Regulatory and Ethical Concerns

The use of robotics in healthcare is subject to stringent regulatory oversight. Dental robotics must comply with medical device regulations and undergo rigorous testing to ensure safety and efficacy. Additionally, there are ethical concerns related to the replacement of human practitioners with machines, particularly in areas where patient trust and rapport are essential (Ahmed et al. 2021).

16 Future Directions and Conclusion

The results of artificial intelligence in dentistry have the potential to profoundly influence the field's future. The advantages are extensive and range from better patient experiences and operational efficiency to increased diagnostic capabilities and individualised treatment regimens. Nonetheless, it is vital to manage the moral dilemmas and guarantee that the incorporation of AI is executed with consideration and inclusivity. AI has the potential to completely transform dental care as technology advances, paving the way for a time when oral health will be more widely available, effective, and efficient than ever (Pethani 2020).

The future of robotics with AI integration in dentistry holds tremendous promise. As technology continues to evolve, we can expect further improvements in the autonomy, precision, and affordability of dental robotic systems. Innovations such as advanced AI algorithms, greater integration with digital dental workflows, and more cost-effective systems are likely to pave the way for wider adoption (Meghil et al. 2022).

In conclusion, robotics in dentistry has led to significant improvements in clinical outcomes, patient satisfaction, and overall efficiency. While there are challenges to overcome, the potential benefits for both dental professionals and patients are immense. As the field continues to grow and evolve, robotics will undoubtedly play a central role in shaping the future of dental care.

References

Afshari Z, Khademi A, Iranmanesh P. Prospects of artificial intelligence in dentistry. Dental Res J [Internet] 21(1). Available from: https://doi.org/10.4103/drj.drj_30_24

Agrawal P, Nikhade P (2022) Artificial intelligence in dentistry: past, present, and future. Cureus [Internet]. Available from: https://doi.org/10.7759/cureus.27405

Ahmed N, Abbasi MS, Zuberi F, Qamar W, Halim MSB, Maqsood A et al (2021) Artificial intelligence techniques: analysis, application, and outcome in dentistry—a systematic review. BioMed Res Int [Internet], 1–15. Available from: https://doi.org/10.1155/2021/9751564

Alexander B, John S (2018) Artificial intelligence in dentistry: current concepts and a peep into the future. Int J Adv Res [Internet] 6(12):1105–8. Available from: https://doi.org/10.21474/ijar01/8242

Alzaid N, Ghulam O, Albani M, Alharbi R, Othman M, Taher H et al (2023) Revolutionizing dental care: a comprehensive review of artificial intelligence applications among various dental specialties. Cureus [Internet]. Available from: https://doi.org/10.7759/cureus.47033

Aminoshariae A, Kulild J, Nagendrababu V (2021) Artificial intelligence in Endodontics: current applications and future directions. J Endodontics [Internet] 47(9):1352–7. Available from: https://doi.org/10.1016/j.joen.2021.06.003

Babu A, Onesimu JA, Sagayam KM (2021) Artificial intelligence in dentistry: concepts, applications and research challenges. E3S web of conferences [Internet] 297:01074. Available from: https://doi.org/10.1051/e3sconf/202129701074

Bader JD, Shugars DA (1995) Variation, treatment outcomes, and practice guidelines in dental practice. J Dent Educ 59(1):61–95 PMID: 7884074

Batra AM, Reche A (2023) A new era of dental care: harnessing artificial intelligence for better diagnosis and treatment. Cureus [Internet]. Available from: https://doi.org/10.7759/cureus.49319

Bhatia AP, Tiwari S (2019) Artificial intelligence: an advancing front of dentistry. Acta Scientific Dental Scienecs [Internet] 3(12):135–8. Available from: https://doi.org/10.31080/asds.2019.03.0714

Carrillo-Perez F, Pecho OE, Morales JC, Paravina RD, Della Bona A, Ghinea R et al (2021) Applications of artificial intelligence in dentistry: a comprehensive review. J Esthetic Restorative Dentistry [Internet] 34(1):259–80. Available from: https://doi.org/10.1111/jerd.12844

Chen YW, Stanley K, Att W (2020) Artificial intelligence in dentistry: current applications and future perspectives. Quintessence Int [Internet] 51(3):248–57. Available from: https://europepmc.org/article/MED/32020135

Dhopte A, Bagde H (2023) Smart smile: revolutionizing dentistry with artificial intelligence. Cureus [Internet]. Available from: https://doi.org/10.7759/cureus.41227

Ding H, Wu J, Zhao W, Matinlinna JP, Burrow MF, Tsoi JKH (2023). Artificial intelligence in dentistry—a review. Front Dental Med [Internet] 4. Available from: https://doi.org/10.3389/fdmed.2023.1085251

Ding H, Wu J, Zhao W, Matinlinna JP, Burrow MF, Tsoi JKH (2023) Artificial intelligence in dentistry—a review. Front Dental Med [Internet] 4. Available from: https://doi.org/10.3389/fdmed.2023.1085251

Edelstein B, Oral Health Policy and Epidemiology, Harvard School of Dental Medicine, Boston, Massachusetts, White BA (1998) Oral health outcomes and evidence-based care [Internet]. American Academy of Pediatric Dentistry Pediatric Dentistry. Available from: https://www.aapd.org/globalassets/media/publications/archives/white-20-03-3.pdf

Fatima A, Shafi I, Afzal H, De La Torre Díez I, Lourdes DRSM, Breñosa J et al (2022) Advancements in dentistry with artificial intelligence: current clinical applications and future perspectives. Healthcare [Internet] 10(11):2188. Available from: https://doi.org/10.3390/healthcare10112188

Fukuda M, Inamoto K, Shibata N, Ariji Y, Yanashita Y, Kutsuna S et al (2019) Evaluation of an artificial intelligence system for detecting vertical root fracture on panoramic radiography. Oral Radiol [Internet] 36(4):337–43. Available from: https://doi.org/10.1007/s11282-019-00409-x

Ghaffari M, Zhu Y, Shrestha A (2024) A review of advancements of artificial intelligence in dentistry. Dentistry Rev [Internet] 4(2):100081. Available from: https://doi.org/10.1016/j.dentre.2024.100081

Grischke J, Johannsmeier L, Eich L, Griga L, Haddadin S (2020) Dentronics: towards robotics and artificial intelligence in dentistry. Dental Mater [Internet] 36(6):765–78. Available from: https://doi.org/10.1016/j.dental.2020.03.021

Haidar ZS (2023) Digital Dentistry: past, present, and future. Digital medicine and healthcare technology [Internet] 2. Available from: https://doi.org/10.5772/dmht.17

Kalappanavar A, Sneha S, Annigeri RG (2018) Artificial intelligence: a dentist's perspective. J Med Radiol Pathol Surgery [Internet] 5(2):2–4. Available from: https://doi.org/10.15713/ins.jmrps.123

Khanagar SB, Al-Ehaideb A, Maganur PC, Vishwanathaiah S, Patil S, Baeshen HA et al (2020) Developments, application, and performance of artificial intelligence in dentistry—a systematic review. J Dental Sci [Internet] 16(1):508–22. Available from: https://doi.org/10.1016/j.jds.2020.06.019

Lee JH, Kim DH, Jeong SN, Choi SH (2018a) Detection and diagnosis of dental caries using a deep learning-based convolutional neural network algorithm. J Dentistry [Internet] 77:106–11. Available from: https://doi.org/10.1016/j.jdent.2018.07.015

Lee SJ, Chung D, Asano A, Sasaki D, Maeno M, Ishida Y et al (2022) Diagnosis of tooth prognosis using artificial intelligence. Diagnostics [Internet] 12(6):1422. Available from: https://doi.org/10.3390/diagnostics12061422

Liu L, Watanabe M, Ichikawa T (2023) Robotics in dentistry: a narrative review. Dentistry J [Internet] 11(3):62. Available from: https://doi.org/10.3390/dj11030062

Meghil MM, Rajpurohit P, Awad ME, McKee J, Shahoumi LA, Ghaly M (2022) Artificial intelligence in dentistry. Dentistry Rev [Internet] 2(1):100009. Available from: https://doi.org/10.1016/j.dentre.2021.100009

Mehrabanian M (2024) Artificial intelligence in dentistry. BDJ [Internet] 236(7):522. Available from: https://doi.org/10.1038/s41415-024-7281-3

Mitra R, Tarnach G (2022) Artificial intelligence—a boon for dentistry. Int Dental J Student Res [Internet] 10(2):37–42. Available from: https://doi.org/10.18231/j.idjsr.2022.009

Nguyen TT, Larrivée N, Lee A (2021) Use of artificial intelligence in dentistry: current clinical trends and research advances. Dental News [Internet] 28(2):50–7. Available from: https://doi.org/10.12816/0059360

Ossowska A, Kusiak A, Świetlik D (2022) Artificial intelligence in dentistry—narrative review. Int J Environ Res Public Health [Internet] 19(6):3449. Available from: https://doi.org/10.3390/ijerph19063449

Pethani F (2020) Promises and perils of artificial intelligence in dentistry. Australian Dental J [Internet] 66(2):124–35. Available from: https://doi.org/10.1111/adj.12812

Putra RH, Doi C, Yoda N, Astuti ER, Sasaki K (2021) Current applications and development of artificial intelligence for digital dental radiography. Dentomaxillofacial Radiol [Internet] 51(1). Available from. https://doi.org/10.1259/dmfr.20210197

Qu Y, Lin Z, Yang Z, Lin H, Huang X, Gu L (2022) Machine learning models for prognosis prediction in endodontic microsurgery. J Dentistry [Internet] 118:103947. Available from: https://doi.org/10.1016/j.jdent.2022.103947

Rekow ED (2019) Digital dentistry: The new state of the art—Is it disruptive or destructive? Dental Mater [Internet] 36(1):9–24. Available from: https://doi.org/10.1016/j.dental.2019.08.103

Review of Advancements of Artificial Intelligence in Dentistry (2024) Dentistry Rev [Internet] 4(2):100081. Available from: https://doi.org/10.1016/j.dentre.2024.100081

Revilla-León M, Gómez-Polo M, Vyas S, Barmak AB, Özcan M, Att W et al (2021) Artificial intelligence applications in restorative dentistry: a systematic review. J Prosthetic Dentistry [Internet] 128(5):867–75. Available from: https://doi.org/10.1016/j.prosdent.2021.02.010

Reyes LT, Knorst JK, Ortiz FR, Ardenghi TM (2022) Machine learning in the diagnosis and prognostic prediction of dental caries: a systematic review. Caries Res [Internet] 56(3):161–70. Available from: https://doi.org/10.1159/000524167

Secinaro S, Calandra D, Secinaro A, Muthurangu V, Biancone P (2021) The role of artificial intelligence in healthcare: a structured literature review. BMC Med Inf Decision-Mak [Internet] 21(1). Available from: https://doi.org/10.1186/s12911-021-01488-9

Setzer FC, Shi KJ, Zhang Z, Yan H, Yoon H, Mupparapu M et al (2020) Artificial intelligence for the computer-aided detection of periapical lesions in cone-beam computed tomographic images. J Endodontics [Internet] 46(7):987–93. Available from: https://doi.org/10.1016/j.joen.2020.03.025

Shankarapillai R, Mathur LK, Nair MA, Rai N, Mathur A (2010) Periodontitis risk assessment using two artificial neural networks-a pilot study. Int J Dental Clinics 2(4)

Sharma S, Kumari P, Sabira K, Parihar AS, Rani PD, Roy A et al (2024) Revolutionizing dentistry: the applications of artificial intelligence in dental health care. J Pharmacy Bioallied Sci [Internet] 16(Suppl 3): S1910–2. Available from: https://doi.org/10.4103/jpbs.jpbs_1290_23

Sharma S (2019) Artificial intelligence in dentistry: the current concepts and a peek into the future. Inte J Contemp Med Res [IJCMR] [Internet] 6(12). Available from: https://doi.org/10.21276/ijcmr.2019.6.12.7

Thomson A, Kahler B (2010) Regenerative endodontics—biologically-based treatment for immature permanent teeth: a case report and review of the literature. Australian Dental J [Internet] 55(4):446–52. Available from: https://doi.org/10.1111/j.1834-7819.2010.01268.x

Toosi A, Arbabtafti M, Richardson B (2014) Virtual reality haptic simulation of root canal therapy. Appl Mech Mater [Internet] 666:388–92. Available from: https://doi.org/10.4028/www.scientific.net/amm.666.388

Use of Artificial intelligence in dentistry: current clinical trends and research advances | JCDA (2021)

Advancements in Dentistry

Tarun Kumar Singh, Aakash Gupta, and Ikroop Gill

1 Stem Cell Research and Regenerative Dentistry

Stem cells possess the unique ability to undergo self-renewal and differentiate into various cell types, thereby offering innovative approaches for the regeneration of absent tissues and the treatment of diseases. Stem cells are undifferentiated, immature cells characterized by their ability to differentiate into various specialized cell types (Thalakiriyawa and Dissanayaka 2024). According to the standard definition, these cells possess the capacity for unlimited self-renewal, allowing them to replicate indefinitely. Their characteristics and potential vary based on their anatomical location within the body and the specific types of cells they are capable of generating (Tirez and Pedano 2022).

The human species typically undergoes two phases of dentition throughout their lifetime. However, the possibility of a third set of teeth developing in the human mouth raises intriguing questions. It may be surprising to learn that extensive research is currently being conducted in this area (Butterfield 2023). There is only drug in the world that can regrow your teeth is "Toregem BioPharma."

Teeth are so much more important than you think; yes, you eat with your teeth but having unhealthy teeth actually can increase your chances of heart disease, diabetes, dementia, and many more. Sixty-nine percentage of adults lose at least one tooth because of tooth decay or disease but not anymore, because three doctors in Japan have discovered something life changing. They discovered a protein in our bodies called "USAG-1," synthesized by the gene which limits the growth of teeth. In other words, blocking the action of that protein could allow more teeth to grow in your mouth in the exact place you lost your old tooth (Tollemar et al. 2016).

T. K. Singh · A. Gupta (✉) · I. Gill
Division of Conservative Dentistry and Endodontics, Department of Dentistry, All India Institute of Medical Sciences, Bathinda, Punjab, India
e-mail: guptaaakash95@gmail.com

A. Gupta et al. (eds.), *Application of Robotics in Dentistry*, Lecture Notes in Bioengineering, https://doi.org/10.1007/978-981-95-1470-0_16

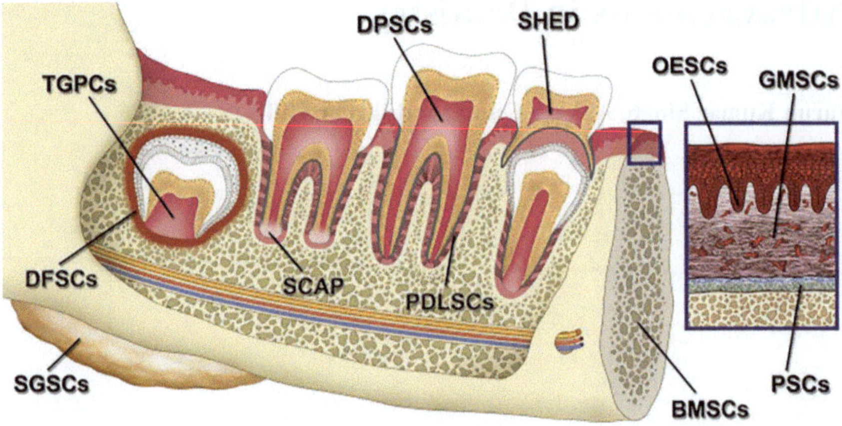

Fig. 1 Source of stem cells from different tissues

They first tested on mice, and it worked, and now humans are using it too. All it takes is one injection in your vein of an antibody that blocks the USAG-1 protein and your new teeth begin to grow.

Mesenchymal stem cells (MSCs) are among the most promising adult stem cells for clinical applications; they were originally found in the bone marrow, but similar subsets of MSCs have also been isolated from many other adult tissues, including skin, adipose tissue, and various dental tissues (Fig. 1).

In 2006, the International Society for Cellular Therapy (ISCT) established fundamental criteria for the identification of human multipotent mesenchymal stem cells (MSCs), designating them as mesenchymal stromal cells irrespective of their tissue origin. According to the ISCT guidelines, MSCs are required to adhere to tissue-culture-treated plastic under standard culture conditions. Furthermore, these cells must express specific surface markers, namely CD105, CD73, and CD90, while lacking the expression of CD45, CD34, CD14, CD11b, CD79α, CD19, and HLA-DR. Additionally, MSCs should demonstrate the capability to differentiate into osteoblasts, adipocytes, and chondroblasts in vitro. Recent studies have identified other distinctive cell surface markers for human MSCs, including CD271 and MSC antigen-1. Moreover, there has been a proposal to enhance the selection of MSCs through the use of stable mRNA markers that are specifically expressed in these cells (Granz et al. 2020; Morita et al. 2025).

Stem cells intended for use in regenerative medicine and dentistry must be meticulously regulated in terms of their fate within the body to guarantee patient safety. At present, only adult mesenchymal stem cells (MSCs) demonstrate feasible clinical applicability. The capacity of MSCs to regenerate bone and periodontal tissues has been thoroughly investigated (Soudi et al. 2021). Furthermore, ideal stem cells for dental tissue engineering should possess the ability to differentiate into the desired tissue or organ, be readily obtainable and processable, and exhibit potential immunomodulatory characteristics that could offer additional advantages.

Stem cells are being explored for their potential to regenerate teeth and tissues, leading to new possibilities for repairing damaged teeth or even regrowing lost teeth in the future. Biomarkers and different growth factors are also opening different frontiers in assessing tissue inflammation and regenerative potential (Cirillo 2024).

2 Smart Toothbrushes and Oral Health Tech

In recent years, advancements in technology have revolutionized the way we approach oral healthcare. One of the most notable innovations is the development of **smart toothbrushes** and other **oral health technologies**. These tools are designed to help users maintain better oral hygiene by providing real-time feedback, personalized guidance, and improved tracking of brushing habits. As technology becomes more integrated into daily life, these devices are making a significant impact on dental health outcomes and overall hygiene practices (Maini et al. 2025a).

Smart Toothbrushes: Revolutionizing Oral Care

Smart toothbrushes are electronic toothbrushes that connect to a smartphone or tablet, offering more than just vibration and brushing motions. They come with integrated sensors, Bluetooth capabilities, and apps that monitor and analyze brushing habits to provide personalized feedback and recommendations. These toothbrushes have features that can significantly enhance the efficiency and effectiveness of daily oral care routines (Pithpornchaiyakul et al. 2022).

How Smart Toothbrushes Work

At the core of a smart toothbrush is its ability to connect to a smartphone app, which gathers data from sensors embedded in the toothbrush (Maini et al. 2025b). These sensors track various aspects of brushing, such as the following:

- **Brushing Time**: The duration of each brushing session.
- **Brushing Pressure**: Whether the user is brushing too hard or too softly, which can damage gums and teeth.
- **Brushing Coverage**: Ensuring that all areas of the mouth are brushed, including the back teeth, gum line, and tongue.
- **Brushing Technique**: The motion of brushing, whether it is up and down, side to side, or circular, which affects the cleaning effectiveness.

Through the app, users can track their progress, set reminders, and even receive feedback about areas they may be neglecting. Some smart toothbrushes also offer real-time guidance through vibrations or visual cues to help improve brushing habits on the spot.

Key Features of Smart Toothbrushes

1. **Real-Time Feedback**: Many smart toothbrushes provide feedback as you brush, such as gentle vibrations when you are pressing too hard or notifications when you have spent enough time on a particular area of your mouth.
2. **Personalized Coaching**: With the help of connected apps, smart toothbrushes can provide personalized recommendations based on your brushing behavior, such as how to improve technique or how much time to spend on each section of your mouth.
3. **Pressure Sensors**: Over-brushing can cause gum recession and enamel wear. Smart toothbrushes can detect the force you are using and alert you if you are brushing too aggressively, encouraging gentler brushing.
4. **Timers and Quad Pacers**: These built-in features ensure that you are brushing for the dentist-recommended two minutes. Some models break this into 30 s intervals for each quadrant of your mouth, ensuring that all areas receive equal attention.
5. **Data Tracking and Progress Reports**: The data collected by the toothbrush are stored in the associated app, giving users detailed reports on their brushing habits over time. This can be particularly useful for individuals with braces, those undergoing dental treatments, or anyone wanting to improve their oral hygiene.

Benefits of Smart Toothbrushes

- **Improved Oral Hygiene**: Studies have shown that using a smart toothbrush can lead to better brushing habits, including improved plaque removal and gum health.
- **Enhanced Motivation**: Gamification elements in many smart toothbrush apps, such as tracking streaks, awarding badges, or offering challenges, can encourage better consistency in brushing routines.
- **Ease of Use**: The integration with smartphones and apps makes it easier for individuals to monitor their oral hygiene without needing to visit a dentist regularly.
- **Prevention of Common Dental Issues**: With features like pressure sensors and proper technique coaching, smart toothbrushes help prevent common issues like cavities, gum disease, and tooth sensitivity.

Popular Smart Toothbrush Brands

1. **Philips Sonicare** (Fig. 2): Known for its advanced sonic technology, Philips Sonicare offers several models with features like smart sensors, personalized feedback, and app connectivity to track progress.
2. **Oral-B Genius**: Oral-B's Genius line of smart toothbrushes includes features like real-time guidance, position detection to ensure thorough coverage, and integration with a smartphone app that tracks brushing habits.
3. **Colgate Hum**: Colgate's Hum toothbrush features an intuitive app that tracks brushing performance and provides personalized feedback. It also encourages proper brushing techniques and longer brushing times.

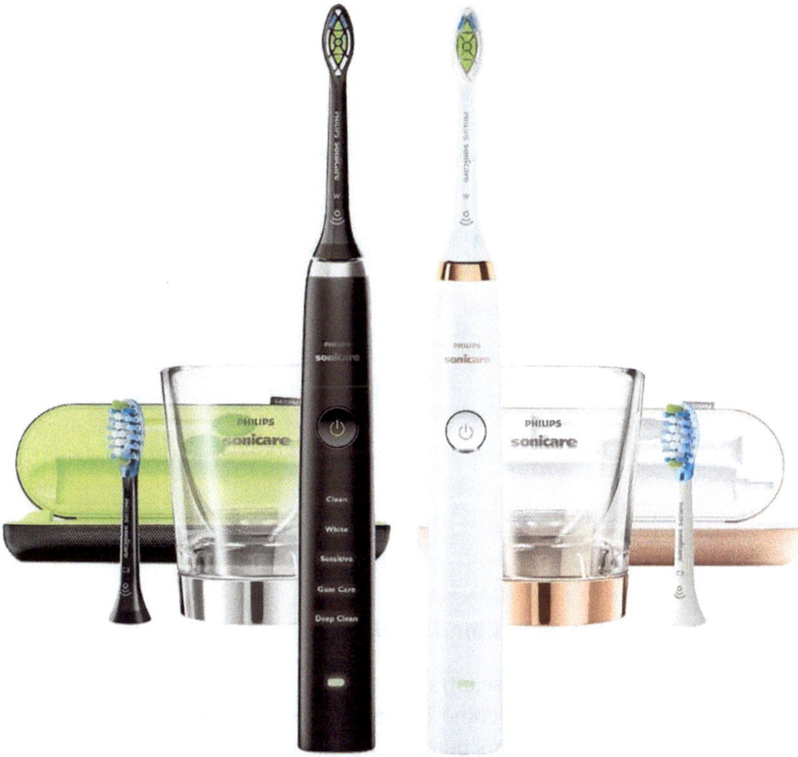

Fig. 2 Philips Sonicare smart toothbrush

Other Oral Health Technologies

While smart toothbrushes are a major breakthrough in oral hygiene, they are only part of the growing range of **oral health technologies**. Several other devices and innovations are helping individuals maintain better oral health from home, offering preventive care and improving dental habits.

1. **Smart Water Flossers**

Water flossers, like those offered by Waterpik (Fig. 3), use a high-pressure stream of pulsating water to remove food particles and plaque between teeth and below the gumline (Altalhi et al. 2023; Abdellatif et al. 2021). The addition of smart technology takes these devices a step further by offering features like the following:

- **Pressure Control**: Users can adjust the water pressure for a more comfortable experience.
- **Customizable Modes**: Different modes for gum care, plaque control, and other specific needs.
- **App Connectivity**: Some water flossers now connect to apps, providing real-time tracking and tips on improving flossing technique.

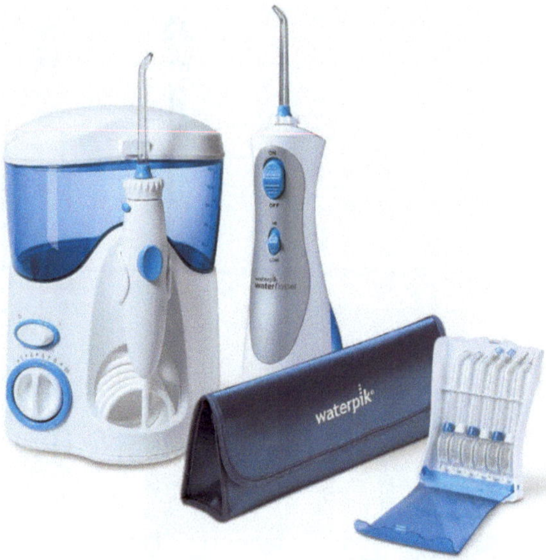

Fig. 3 Waterpik smart water flosser

2. **Ultraviolet (UV) Sterilizers for Toothbrushes**

UV sterilizers are devices that use ultraviolet light to kill bacteria and germs on your toothbrush. Since toothbrushes come into contact with the mouth, they can harbor bacteria and germs. UV sterilizers help ensure that toothbrushes stay clean and free of harmful pathogens. Some models even have built-in charging features for electric toothbrushes (Tomar et al. 2014; Gujjari et al. 2011).

3. **Smart Mouthguards and Sleep Apnea Devices**

Smart mouthguards are designed to monitor and protect against nighttime teeth grinding (bruxism). These devices can track the frequency and intensity of grinding, while providing real-time feedback to users. Some mouthguards even connect to apps that offer insights into patterns of teeth grinding and suggest preventive measures (Lemire 2024).

For individuals suffering from **sleep apnea**, there are now wearable devices that connect to mobile apps, helping to monitor breathing patterns during sleep and alerting users to issues. These devices can help manage mild sleep apnea by promoting better sleep posture or detecting irregularities that require further medical attention (McKinnon 2024).

4. **Artificial Intelligence (AI)-Powered Health Apps**

There are several human health apps that leverage **artificial intelligence (AI)** to help with everything from personalized oral care routines to detecting early signs of oral diseases. These apps often use images of a user's mouth to analyze for issues such as cavities, gum inflammation, or even early stages of oral cancer (Wang et al. 2025).

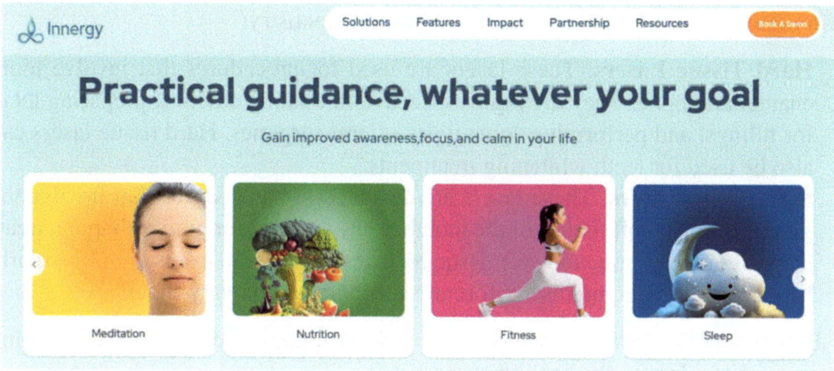

Fig. 4 Innergy: AI powered health app for holistic wellness

Apps like **Innergy** (Fig. 4) help you embrace holistic wellness with over 1000 + content items, personalized AI guide, and community support and provide detailed information on areas that require more attention, guiding users in improving their habits, diet planning, meditation, relieving stress, and many more.

5. **Electric Toothbrushes with Bluetooth Connectivity**

Some electric toothbrushes come with Bluetooth connectivity to allow users to sync their brushing data to a mobile app. These models can provide reports and reminders, track brushing progress over time, and help users stay on track with their oral hygiene goals. The app may also allow users to adjust the power or speed of the toothbrush, providing a more tailored cleaning experience.

3 Laser Dentistry

Laser dentistry represents a significant leap forward in the field of dental care, offering a minimally invasive alternative to traditional dental procedures. By using focused light energy, lasers can target and treat a wide range of dental conditions with precision, efficiency, and reduced discomfort. Since its introduction, laser dentistry has become increasingly popular, both for routine dental treatments and more complex procedures (Verma et al. 2012).

In this section, we will explore the types of lasers used in dentistry, how they work, their benefits, and the various dental procedures that can be improved or enhanced with laser technology.

How Laser Dentistry Works

Lasers in dentistry use a concentrated beam of light energy to perform specific tasks, such as cutting or reshaping tissues, removing decayed tooth material, or stimulating healing. The type of laser used depends on the procedure and the type of tissue being treated (Cobb 2006).

Two main types of lasers are commonly used in dentistry:

1. **Hard Tissue Lasers**: These lasers are used for procedures that involve tooth enamel and bone. They are highly effective in treating cavities, preparing teeth for fillings, and performing some types of oral surgeries. Hard tissue lasers can also be used for teeth whitening treatments.
2. **Soft Tissue Lasers**: These lasers are designed for procedures that involve the gums and other soft tissues of the mouth. They are used for gum reshaping, treatment of gum disease, and soft tissue biopsies. Soft tissue lasers are particularly beneficial for reducing discomfort and speeding up recovery times.

Both types of lasers offer great precision, which minimizes damage to surrounding tissues and accelerates the healing process.

Types of Lasers Used in Dentistry

1. **CO_2 Lasers (Carbon Dioxide)**:
   - These are commonly used for soft tissue procedures due to their ability to precisely vaporize tissue. CO_2 lasers are effective in treating gum disease, removing lesions, and reshaping the gumline.
2. **Erbium-Doped Yttrium–Aluminum-Garnet (Er: YAG) Lasers**:
   - Er: YAG lasers are versatile and can be used for both hard and soft tissue procedures. These lasers are particularly effective for cavity preparations, as well as treating gum diseases and performing dental surgeries.
3. **Diode Lasers**:
   - These lasers are used for soft tissue treatments, such as managing gum disease and performing biopsies and also for endodontic retreatment (Gupta et al. 2023). Diode lasers are compact, easy to use, and effective in coagulating tissue, which minimizes bleeding during procedures.
4. **Neodymium-Doped Yttrium–Aluminum-Garnet (Nd: YAG) Lasers**:
   - These lasers are primarily used for soft tissue procedures, including the treatment of infections, gum disease, and surgical procedures involving soft tissue. Nd: YAG lasers also have the ability to penetrate deeper into tissues, making them suitable for deeper surgeries.

Common Dental Procedures Using Laser Technology

Laser dentistry is used in a wide variety of dental procedures, including those related to cavity treatment, gum disease, oral surgeries, and cosmetic dentistry. Some of the most common applications include the following:

1. **Treatment of Cavities and Tooth Decay**
   - **Laser Cavity Removal**: Lasers can be used to remove decayed tissue from a tooth before placing a filling. The precision of the laser reduces the need for

traditional drills, which can be uncomfortable and sometimes painful. Laser treatment also eliminates the vibrations and sounds associated with traditional dental drills, making the procedure more comfortable for the patient (Hibst January 2002).

Advantages:

- Reduced discomfort compared to traditional drilling.
- Minimal need for anesthesia in many cases.
- Preservation of healthy tooth structure.

2. **Gum Disease Treatment**

 - **Gingivectomy**: Lasers are used to remove unhealthy gum tissue and treat gum disease, including gingivitis and periodontitis. The laser effectively targets infected areas without damaging surrounding healthy tissue. It also sterilizes the area, reducing the chances of further infection.
 - **Laser Bacterial Reduction**: Lasers can help reduce the bacteria in periodontal pockets during deep cleaning procedures (scaling and root planing). This improves the effectiveness of the treatment and speeds up healing (Afkhami et al. 2024).

Advantages:

- Minimally invasive and requires little to no suturing.
- Reduces bleeding and swelling.
- Faster recovery time compared to traditional methods.

3. **Soft Tissue Procedures**

 - **Crown Lengthening**: In this procedure, lasers are used to reshape the gum tissue around a tooth, either to expose more of the tooth's surface or to improve its appearance. It is commonly performed before placing a crown or to correct a "gummy smile."
 - **Frenectomy**: A frenectomy involves the removal or alteration of the frenulum, the small band of tissue that connects the upper lip to the gums or the tongue to the floor of the mouth. Lasers can be used to remove excess tissue with minimal discomfort and faster recovery (Elavarasu et al. 2012).
 - **Treatment of Lesions**: Soft tissue lasers can be used to remove benign oral lesions such as canker sores, fibromas, or papilloma. Lasers can also remove oral cancerous lesions in early stages with reduced bleeding and scarring.

Advantages:

- Little to no bleeding.
- Reduces discomfort and swelling.
- Quicker healing and recovery.

4. **Teeth Whitening**

- **Laser-Assisted Whitening**: Some teeth-whitening systems use lasers to activate the whitening agents applied to the teeth, speeding up the whitening process. The light energy from the laser helps break down stains and discoloration on the tooth surface (Anagnostaki et al. 2023).

Advantages:

- Faster results compared to traditional whitening methods.
- Often results in less tooth sensitivity posttreatment.
- Targeted activation of whitening agents ensures uniform results.

5. **Oral Surgery**

- **Biopsy and Tumor Removal**: Lasers can be used to remove or biopsy soft tissue tumors, including those found in the mouth and throat. Laser surgery is precise and minimizes trauma to surrounding tissues, making the process less painful for the patient.
- **Cyst Removal**: Lasers are effective in removing cysts in the oral cavity, as they can vaporize the cyst with minimal bleeding and faster healing.

Advantages:

- Reduced bleeding and swelling.
- Lower risk of infection.
- More precise cuts, leading to minimal damage to surrounding tissue.

6. **Vital Pulp Therapy**

Diode lasers can be used in vital pulp therapy as a hemostatic agent and time required for hemostasis is about 20–30 s. Hemostasis plays a critical role in vital pulp therapy for intraoperative evaluation and indicates level of inflammation in pulp. Less the time of hemostasis, more favorable will be the prognosis. It works on the principle of "photothermal coagulation" in which light emitted by laser is absorbed by Hb in blood, which leads to protein denaturation and coagulation (Fig. 5).

Benefits of Laser Dentistry

Laser dentistry offers a wide range of benefits over traditional dental methods, for both patients and dental professionals. Some of the key advantages include the following:

1. **Minimally Invasive**

Lasers are incredibly precise, which means that they can target only the area of concern, leaving surrounding tissues largely untouched. This makes many laser procedures less invasive than traditional methods, reducing the need for stitches and making recovery faster.

Fig. 5 Hemostasis achieved after complete pulpotomy using diode laser

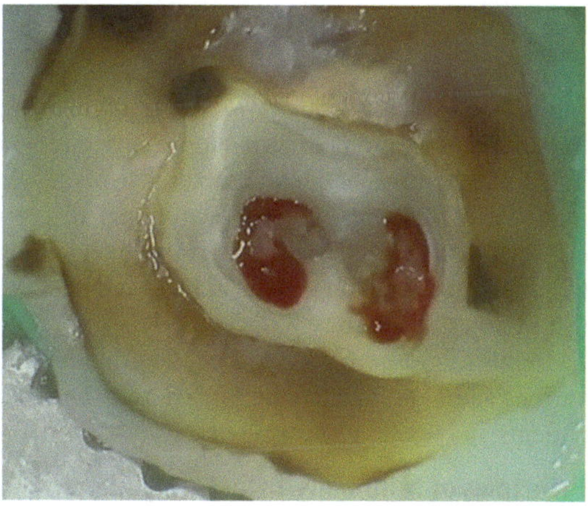

2. **Reduced Discomfort and Pain**

Laser dentistry generally requires less anesthesia because the procedures are less invasive. Patients often report less pain both during and after treatment, and many procedures can be completed without the need for numbing injections, which are a common source of anxiety for patients.

3. **Faster Recovery Times**

Because lasers promote faster healing by sterilizing the treated area and reducing tissue trauma, recovery times are often much shorter compared to traditional methods. This is especially beneficial for procedures like gum reshaping or cavity treatment.

4. **Less Bleeding**

Laser technology minimizes bleeding during procedures by coagulating the tissue as it cuts. This is particularly beneficial in soft tissue surgeries like gingivectomy or frenectomy, where traditional cutting methods would result in significant bleeding.

5. **Reduced Risk of Infection**

Laser procedures also minimize the risk of infection by sterilizing the treatment area during the procedure. The heat generated by the laser kills bacteria and reduces the chances of postoperative infections.

6. **Greater Precision**

Lasers offer superior accuracy compared to traditional dental tools, allowing for more precise removal of decay or tissue. This leads to better outcomes and a lower likelihood of the need for repeat procedures.

4 Minimally Invasive Dentistry

Minimally invasive dentistry (MID) is a modern approach to dental care that prioritizes the preservation of natural tooth structure while providing effective treatments. The goal is to prevent dental problems from developing or worsening by using techniques and materials that cause minimal disruption to the teeth and gums. MID emphasizes early intervention, advanced technology, and a conservative approach to treatment, focusing on the least invasive procedures that still deliver optimal results (Showkat et al. 2020).

In this section, we will explore the principles of minimally invasive dentistry, the various techniques and technologies used, and the benefits of this approach for both patients and dental professionals.

Principles of Minimally Invasive Dentistry

Minimally invasive dentistry is based on the concept of preserving as much healthy tooth structure as possible while providing necessary treatments (Par et al. 2024). The key principles include the following:

1. **Prevention**: MID emphasizes the prevention of dental issues before they require more invasive treatments. This can include regular checkups, early detection of cavities, and the use of preventive treatments like fluoride, dental sealants, and oral hygiene education.
2. **Conservation**: The approach aims to conserve as much of the natural tooth as possible. Instead of removing large portions of a tooth during procedures like fillings or root canals, MID focuses on more conservative treatments that target the problem area while leaving surrounding healthy tissue intact.
3. **Early Detection and Intervention**: With the help of advanced diagnostic tools, MID enables early identification of issues like cavities or gum disease, allowing for intervention before the problem becomes severe and requires extensive treatment.
4. **Use of Advanced Technology**: Modern technologies such as lasers, digital imaging, and air abrasion are integral to minimally invasive techniques, as they allow for more accurate diagnosis and treatment with less discomfort and faster healing times.

Techniques and Technologies in Minimally Invasive Dentistry

Several techniques and technologies are used in minimally invasive dentistry to help preserve the natural tooth and provide effective treatment while minimizing damage. Some of the most common methods include the following:

1. **Air Abrasion**

Air abrasion is a technique used to remove tooth decay without the need for drills or anesthesia. A stream of fine particles (usually aluminum oxide) is directed at the decayed area of the tooth, which gently removes the decay. This method is particularly effective for small cavities, allowing dentists to treat the affected area with minimal disruption to the surrounding healthy tooth structure (Hegde and Khatavkar 2010).

Advantages:

- No vibration or noise, which makes the procedure more comfortable.
- Requires little or no anesthesia.
- Precise removal of decay with minimal damage to surrounding tissue.

• **Applications**: Air abrasion is typically used for small-to-moderate cavities, surface stains, and certain fillings.

2. **Resin-Based Fillings**

In minimally invasive dentistry, resin-based composite fillings are preferred over traditional metal fillings, as they bond to the tooth structure more effectively and can be shaped to match the natural contours of the tooth. These fillings are ideal for small-to-medium cavities and can be placed with minimal removal of healthy tooth material.

Advantages:

- Matches the color of natural teeth, making them more aesthetically pleasing.
- Requires less removal of tooth structure compared to traditional fillings.
- Bonds to the tooth, providing additional strength and reducing the risk of breakage.

• **Applications**: Resin-based fillings are commonly used for cavities in the front and back teeth, where aesthetics and tooth preservation are important.

3. **Preventive Care with Dental Sealants**

Dental sealants are thin, plastic coatings applied to the chewing surfaces of the back teeth (molars) to prevent tooth decay. Sealants act as a barrier, protecting the tooth from bacteria and food particles that can lead to cavities. The procedure is noninvasive and can be performed quickly in a single visit.

Advantages:

- Helps prevent tooth decay by protecting vulnerable areas of the teeth.
- Simple, pain-free procedure with no drilling required.
- Long-lasting protection for children and adults at risk of cavities.

• **Applications**: Sealants are primarily used on children's molars, but they can also be applied to adult teeth that have deep grooves or pits.

4. **Microdentistry (Microinvasive Techniques)**

Microdentistry uses advanced technology such as microscopes and specialized instruments to perform extremely precise dental procedures (Prathima et al. 2015). This allows the dentist to target very small areas of decay or damage without affecting the surrounding healthy tooth structure.

Advantages:

- High degree of precision and accuracy
- Less invasive, preserving more natural tooth material
- Ideal for early-stage cavities and enamel defects.

- **Applications**: Microdentistry is used for treating very small cavities, enamel defects, and cracks.

5. **Minimally Invasive Gum Disease Treatment (Scaling and Root Planing)**

For the treatment of gum disease, minimally invasive techniques such as **scaling and root planing** are used. This procedure involves the gentle removal of plaque and tartar from the teeth and beneath the gum line using ultrasonic tools or laser technology. Scaling and root planing can often be done without the need for surgical intervention, reducing pain and recovery time (Rainey 2001).

Advantages:

- Nonsurgical, with minimal discomfort.
- Reduces gum inflammation and promotes gum healing.
- Faster recovery compared to traditional gum surgery.

- **Applications**: Scaling and root planing are used to treat mild-to-moderate gum disease (gingivitis and periodontitis).

Benefits of Minimally Invasive Dentistry

Minimally invasive dentistry offers numerous advantages for patients seeking both preventive care and restorative treatments. The primary benefits include the following:

1. **Preservation of Natural Tooth Structure**

The key benefit of minimally invasive dentistry is that it preserves as much of the natural tooth as possible. This not only improves the aesthetic outcome but also maintains the tooth's structural integrity, ensuring that the tooth remains strong and functional.

2. **Reduced Pain and Discomfort**

Minimally invasive techniques are generally less painful than traditional procedures, reducing the need for anesthesia and the discomfort associated with more invasive treatments. Many procedures can be performed without the use of drills or needles, making the experience more pleasant for patients.

3. **Faster Recovery Times**

Because minimally invasive techniques are less traumatic to the tissues, patients typically experience quicker healing and less posttreatment discomfort. Recovery times are significantly shorter compared to traditional procedures, allowing patients to return to their normal activities sooner.

4. **Lower Risk of Complications**

Minimally invasive dentistry reduces the risk of complications such as infection, nerve damage, or excessive tooth sensitivity. The focus on preserving healthy tissue and using less invasive techniques minimizes the chances of adverse reactions.

5. **Enhanced Aesthetics**

Many minimally invasive procedures, such as composite fillings or teeth whitening, deliver more aesthetically pleasing results than traditional methods. For example, resin-based fillings blend seamlessly with the natural tooth color, while in-office whitening can brighten teeth without causing damage.

6. **Long-Term Benefits**

By prioritizing prevention, early detection, and conservative treatments, minimally invasive dentistry helps patients maintain optimal oral health in the long term. This can lead to fewer dental issues over time, reducing the need for more extensive and costly procedures.

5 Advancements in Anesthesia in Dentistry

Anesthesia has always played a critical role in ensuring patient comfort and reducing pain during dental procedures. Over the years, significant advancements in dental anesthesia have revolutionized the way dentists manage pain, allowing for more effective, safer, and less stressful treatments for patients (Ruparel n.d.). These innovations aim to improve the patient experience, reduce recovery times, and minimize side effects.

In this section, we will explore the various advancements in dental anesthesia, ranging from local anesthetics to sedation techniques, and how they enhance dental care.

1. **Local Anesthesia: Refinements and Innovations**

Local anesthesia has been the cornerstone of pain management in dentistry for decades. It works by blocking nerve signals in a specific area of the mouth, allowing dental procedures to be performed without discomfort. Over the years, there have been notable improvements in both the types of anesthetics used and the methods of administration.

a. **New Local Anesthetic Agents**

In recent years, several new local anesthetic agents have been developed, providing better efficacy, faster onset, and fewer side effects than traditional options. Some of the advancements include the following:

- **Articaine**: Articaine is a local anesthetic that is gaining popularity in dentistry due to its enhanced potency and ability to penetrate bone tissue more effectively. It has a faster onset and a shorter duration of action, making it ideal for many dental procedures (Shah et al. 2018).

Advantages:

- More effective in achieving profound anesthesia.
- Less chance of post-procedure numbness or discomfort.
- Works well for both soft and hard tissues, making it a versatile choice for dental work.

- **Mepivacaine**: Mepivacaine is another commonly used local anesthetic, known for its relatively fast onset time and moderate duration. It is often preferred when a patient cannot tolerate the vasoconstrictors in other anesthetics (such as epinephrine) (Kaye et al. 2022).

Advantages:

- Works quickly, with a moderate duration of anesthesia.
- Preferred in patients with certain contraindications to epinephrine.
- Minimal side effects compared to other anesthetics.

- **Bupivacaine**: Bupivacaine is a long-acting anesthetic often used for procedures requiring extended numbness, such as surgeries that involve the gums or jawbone.

Advantages:

- Long-lasting effects, reducing the need for additional injections during lengthy procedures.
- Ideal for postoperative pain control.

b. **Topical Anesthetics**

Topical anesthetics have also improved in their formulations and delivery methods. Traditionally, it is used to numb the surface of the gums or mucous membranes before an injection; advancements have made these agents more effective and faster-acting (Jaan et al. 2020; Boyce et al. 2016).

- **Lidocaine**: Lidocaine-based gels are now commonly used to numb the surface of the gums before administering a local injection, making the procedure less painful.

Advantages:

- Improved formulations that allow for faster onset and longer duration of effect.
- Numbing agents are often combined with other substances to enhance their penetration and efficacy.

- **Pharmaceutical Innovations**: New topical anesthetic formulations, such as **Oraqix** (a combination of lidocaine and prilocaine), are designed for use in periodontal pockets and can be applied without the need for injections, making them ideal for treating gum disease.

2. **Sedation Techniques: More Comfortable and Relaxed Procedures**

For patients who experience dental anxiety, pain, or discomfort, sedation dentistry offers an effective way to enhance comfort during treatment. Advances in sedation techniques allow dentists to offer varying levels of sedation, from light relaxation to deep sedation, based on the needs of the patient and the complexity of the procedure (Jin et al. 2021).

a. **Nitrous Oxide (Laughing Gas)**

Nitrous oxide, also known as "laughing gas," has been a staple in dental sedation for many years (Liu et al. 2024). However, recent improvements have made its delivery safer and more effective:

- **New Delivery Systems**: Modern nitrous oxide systems now include more precise control over the concentration of gas, allowing for better adjustment to individual patient needs. These systems also ensure quicker recovery times, as the gas leaves the body almost immediately once the procedure is completed (Attri et al. 2017; Johnston and Rai 2013).

Advantages:

- Safe and noninvasive.
- Fast onset and quick recovery with no lingering effects.
- Ideal for patients with mild anxiety or those undergoing short procedures.

b. **Oral Sedation**

Oral sedation uses medication to help patients relax during dental procedures. Sedatives like **diazepam** and **triazolam (Halcion)** can be taken orally before a dental appointment, helping patients feel more at ease (Donaldson et al. 2007).

- **Advances in Oral Sedation**:

- **Selective Sedation**: Dentists now have access to more controlled oral sedatives, allowing them to fine-tune the level of sedation based on patient comfort and the procedure required.
- **Combination Therapies**: Oral sedatives can be combined with local anesthesia to achieve an optimal balance of relaxation and pain control.

Advantages:

- Easy administration; no needles involved.
- More suitable for patients with moderate anxiety.
- Provides a relaxed, drowsy state during longer dental procedures.

c. **Intravenous (IV) Sedation**

IV sedation, also known as "conscious sedation," involves the administration of sedatives through a vein, allowing the dentist to control the level of sedation throughout the procedure. This technique is commonly used for more invasive dental surgeries or for patients with severe anxiety (Donaldson et al. 2007).

- **Advancements in IV Sedation**:

- **Propofol**: Propofol, a popular sedative used in many medical and dental procedures, allows for rapid onset and precise control of sedation levels. It is typically used for deeper levels of sedation or general anesthesia.
- **Patient Monitoring**: Advancements in monitoring equipment provide real-time data on a patient's vital signs, ensuring their safety during IV sedation procedures.

Advantages:

- Deep level of relaxation while still maintaining consciousness.
- Ideal for longer, more complex procedures like dental implants or oral surgeries.
- Patients often forget the procedure entirely after the sedation wears off.
- **General Anesthesia**

In some cases, general anesthesia is required for dental patients, particularly those undergoing complex oral surgeries or those who have extreme dental anxiety or medical conditions that require total sedation (Radkowski et al. 2024; Hutt and Hudetz 2015; Tobias and Leder 2011).

- **Advancements in General Anesthesia**:

- **Safer Agents**: New anesthetic agents, such as **sevoflurane**, allow for faster recovery and better control of sedation depth. These agents provide a smooth induction and recovery, reducing the side effects associated with general anesthesia.

- **Personalized Anesthesia Plans**: Dentists now have the ability to customize general anesthesia protocols based on the patient's specific health needs and medical history.

Advantages:

- Ideal for complex surgeries or patients with extreme dental phobia.
- Provides complete unconsciousness, eliminating pain and anxiety.
- Enhanced safety measures and faster recovery times.

3. **Digital and Computer-Controlled Anesthesia Systems**

Advancements in **computer-controlled local anesthetic delivery** have enhanced the precision and comfort of injections. Devices like **The Wand** and **Comfort Control Syringe** have revolutionized the way local anesthetics are administered (Janik 2024).

- **How They Work**: These systems allow for a slow, steady delivery of anesthesia, which minimizes the discomfort and pain associated with traditional syringe-based injections. The controlled flow prevents the "painful rush" of anesthesia that can cause discomfort.

- **Advantages**:

- Precise control over the rate and amount of anesthesia delivered.
- Reduced discomfort and anxiety associated with injections.
- Suitable for patients with needle phobia or those who require multiple injections.

4. **The Role of Pharmacogenetics in Anesthesia**

As pharmacogenetics advances, we can expect to see more personalized approaches to dental anesthesia. Pharmacogenetics studies how a person's genetic makeup influences their response to drugs. In the context of dental anesthesia, this knowledge can help dentists predict how patients will respond to specific anesthetics, allowing for more customized treatment plans (Goudra and Mason 2021).

- **Potential Applications**:

- **Customized Dosing**: By understanding genetic differences in drug metabolism, anesthetics can be tailored to achieve the optimal effect with minimal side effects.
- **Reduced Adverse Reactions**: Pharmacogenetics may reduce the likelihood of allergic reactions or adverse effects, especially for patients with complex medical histories.

5. **Patient-Centered Anesthesia Techniques**

Advancements in anesthesia in dentistry have shifted toward a more patient-centered approach, focusing on personalized care and comfort. Dentists are now able to assess a patient's specific needs, such as their level of anxiety, medical history, and the complexity of the procedure, and select the most appropriate anesthetic or sedation method (Dolmans et al. 2025).

- **Multimodal Pain Management**: Dentists are increasingly using a combination of anesthetics, sedation methods, and pain relievers to ensure that patients remain comfortable throughout their treatment and recovery.
- **Better Communication**: With the advancements in anesthesia, there is a greater emphasis on informing patients about their options, helping them choose the best solution for their specific needs.

Challenges and Considerations

While the rise of smart toothbrushes and oral health tech presents exciting opportunities, there are a few challenges and considerations to keep in mind:

1. **Cost**: High-tech devices, particularly smart toothbrushes, can be more expensive than traditional manual or basic electric toothbrushes. While the benefits are significant, the initial investment may not be feasible for all consumers.
2. **Privacy Concerns**: Many smart oral health devices collect personal data, including brushing habits, location, and even photographs of your mouth. Ensuring that these data are securely stored and managed is essential to maintain user privacy.
3. **Device Reliability**: With so many tech-dependent features, users may encounter technical issues, such as app connectivity problems or sensor malfunctions, which could affect the overall experience.
4. **Over-Reliance on Technology**: While these devices can significantly enhance oral hygiene, they should not replace regular visits to the dentist. Technology is a supplement, not a substitute, for professional dental care.

References

Abdellatif H, Alnaeimi N, Alruwais H, Aldajan R, Hebbal MI (2021) Comparison between water flosser and regular floss in the efficacy of plaque removal in patients after single use. Saudi Dent J. 33(5):256–259. https://doi.org/10.1016/j.sdentj.2021.03.005

Afkhami F, Rostami G, Xu C, Peters OA (2024) The application of lasers in vital pulp therapy: clinical and radiographic outcomes. BMC Oral Health 24(1):333. https://doi.org/10.1186/s12903-024-04026-x

Altalhi AM, Alqahtani NS, Alareefi JA, Alamri SS, Almutairi KS, Bin Dous RA, Albaqami IA (2023) A comparative review of water flossers in periodontal therapy. Cureus 15(12):e50162. https://doi.org/10.7759/cureus.50162

Anagnostaki E, Mylona V, Parker S, Cronshaw M, Grootveld M (2023) Assessing the viability of laser-activated dental bleaching compared to conventional in-office bleaching methods: a systematic review of clinical and in vitro studies. Appl Sci 13(22):12459. https://doi.org/10.3390/app132212459

Attri JP, Sharan R, Makkar V, Gupta KK, Khetarpal R, Kataria AP (2017) Conscious sedation: emerging trends in pediatric dentistry. Anesth Essays Res 11(2):277–281. https://doi.org/10.4103/0259-1162.171458

Boyce RA, Kirpalani T, Mohan N (2016) Updates of topical and local anesthesia agents. Dent Clin North Am 60(2):445–71. https://doi.org/10.1016/j.cden.2015.12.001. Erratum in: Dent Clin North Am. 2017 Apr;61(2):xiii. xxx10.1016/j.cden.2017.01.002

Butterfield M (2023) World's 1st drug to regrow teeth enters clinical trials. Global News September 25, 2023 4:40 pm

Cirillo N (2024) A roadmap for the rational use of biomarkers in oral disease screening. Biomolecules 14(7):787. https://doi.org/10.3390/biom14070787

Cobb CM (2006) Lasers in periodontics: a review of the literature. J Periodontol 77(4):545–564. https://doi.org/10.1902/jop.2006.050417

Dolmans RGF, Russo G, Anstey J et al (2025) Comparative effectiveness of midazolam-based sedation on the need for intracranial pressure lowering therapies in traumatic brain injury. Neurotrauma Reports 6(1):242–250. https://doi.org/10.1089/neur.2024.0077

Donaldson M, Gizzarelli G, Chanpong B (2007) Oral sedation: a primer on anxiolysis for the adult patient. Anesth Prog Fall 54(3):118–28; quiz 129. https://doi.org/10.2344/0003-3006(2007)54[118:OSAPOA]2.0.CO;2

Elavarasu S, Naveen D, Thangavelu A (2012) Lasers in periodontics. J Pharm Bio Allied Sci. 4(Suppl 2):S260–S263. https://doi.org/10.4103/0975-7406.100245

Goudra B, Mason KP (2021) Emerging approaches in intravenous moderate and deep sedation. J Clin Med 10(8):1735. https://doi.org/10.3390/jcm10081735

Granz CL, Gorji A, Granz CL et al (2020) Dental stem cells: the role of biomaterials and scaffolds in developing novel therapeutic strategies. World J Stem Cells 12:897–922

Gujjari SK, Gujjari AK, Patel PV, Shubhashini PV (2011) Comparative evaluation of ultraviolet and microwave sanitization techniques for toothbrush decontamination. J Int Soc Prev Community Dent. 1:20–26. https://doi.org/10.4103/2231-0762.86383

Gupta A, Showkat R, Singh TK (2023) Innovative *ex vivo* exploration: a comparative study of novel approaches of root canal filling material removal efficiency. J Conserv Dent Endod 26(6):713–718. https://doi.org/10.4103/JCDE.JCDE_162_23

Hegde VS, Khatavkar RA (2010) A new dimension to conservative dentistry: air abrasion. J Conserv Dent 13(1):4–8. https://doi.org/10.4103/0972-0707.62632

Hibst R (2002) Lasers for caries removal and cavity preparation: state of the art and future directions. 2(4):203–212

Hutt A, Hudetz AG (2015) Editorial: general anesthesia: from theory to experiments. Front Syst Neurosci 22(9):105. https://doi.org/10.3389/fnsys.2015.00105

Jaan, A, Munshi, R, Sareen, K, Parmar, E, Thakur, P, Anindita, A (2020) Local anesthesia—solution to pain: an overview. J Curr Med Res Opin 3(07):537–548. https://doi.org/10.15520/jcmro.v3i07.317

Janik K (2024) Computer-controlled local anaesthesia delivery efficacy literature review. Saudi Dent J 36(8):1066–1071

Jin Z, Olivia D, Ali I, Ru L, Jun L (2021) Comparison of liposomal bupivacaine and conventional local anesthetic agents in regional anesthesia: a systematic review. Anesth & Analg 132(6):1626–16341. https://doi.org/10.1213/ANE.0000000000005406

Johnston KD, Rai MR (2013) Conscious sedation for awake fibreoptic intubation: a review of the literature. Can J Anaesth 60(6):584–599. https://doi.org/10.1007/s12630-013-9915-9

Kaye AD, Edinoff AN, Yan JY, Kaye AJ, Alvarado MA, Pham AD, Chami AA, Shah RJ, Dixon BM, Shafeinia A, Cornett EM, Fox C (2022) Novel local anesthetics in clinical practice: pharmacologic considerations and potential roles for the future. Anesth Pain Med 12(1):e123112. https://doi.org/10.5812/aapm.123112

Lemire J (2024) Orb sport smart mouthguard launches sensor-laden mouthguards to improve athlete performance. Sport Bus J

Liu S, Shen H, Yang F et al (2024) Local anaesthesia with conscious sedation in parotid gland tumour resection: a retrospective review. BMC Oral Health 24:1531. https://doi.org/10.1186/s12903-024-05318-y

Maini V, Roy R, Gandhi G, Chopra A, Bhat SG (2025a) Artificial-intelligence-based smart toothbrushes for oral health and patient education: a review. Hygiene 5(1):5. https://doi.org/10.3390/hygiene5010005

Maini V et al (2025b) Artificial-intelligence-based smart toothbrushes for oral health and patient education: a review. Hygiene 5:5. https://doi.org/10.3390/hygiene5010005

McKinnon J (2024) The future of mouth guards: smart guards with tracking features. Remi 2024

Morita K, Wang J, Okamoto K, Iwata T (2025) The next generation of regenerative dentistry: from tooth development biology to periodontal tissue, dental pulp, and whole tooth reconstruction in the clinical setting. Regenerative Therapy 28:333–344

Par M, Cheng L, Camilleri J, Lingstrom P (2024) Applications of smart materials in minimally invasive dentistry – some research and clinical perspectives. Dent Mater 40(11):2008–2016

Pithpornchaiyakul S, Naorungroj S, Pupong K, Hunsrisakhun J (2022) Using a chatbot as an alternative approach for in-person toothbrushing training during the COVID-19 pandemic: comparative study. J Med Internet Res 24:e39218

Prathima GS, Bhadrashetty D, Babu SB, Disha P (2015) Microdentistry with Lasers. J Int Oral Health 7(9):134–137

Radkowski P, Oniszczuk H, Fadrowska-Szleper M, Onichimowski D (2024) Decoding the neurological sequelae of general anesthesia: a review. Med Sci Monitor: Int Med J Experimental Clin Res. 30:e942740-942741

Rainey JT (2001) Understanding the applications of microdentistry. Compend Contin Educ Dent. 22(11A):1018–25; quiz 1044–5. PMID: 11915643

Ruparel NB (n.d.) Successful local anesthesia for restorative dentistry and endodontics. J Endod 38(2):259

Shah J, Votta-Velis EG, Borgeat A (2018) New local anesthetics. Best Pract Res Clin Anaesthesiol 32(2):179–185. https://doi.org/10.1016/j.bpa.2018.06.010

Showkat N et al (2020) Minimal invasive dentistry: literature review. J Curr Med Res Opin 3(09). https://doi.org/10.15520/jcmro.v3i09.340

Soudi A, Yazdanian M, Ranjbar R, Tebyanian H, Yazdanian A, Tahmasebi E, Keshvad A, Seifalian A (2021) Role and application of stem cells in dental regeneration: a comprehensive overview. EXCLI J 22(20):454–489. https://doi.org/10.17179/excli2021-3335

Thalakiriyawa DS, Dissanayaka WL (2024) Advances in regenerative dentistry approaches: an update. Int Dent J 74(1):25–34

E Tirez, MS. Pedano (2022) Regeneration of the pulp tissue: cell homing versus cell transplantation approach: a systematic review. Materials (Basel) 15(23):8603

Tobias JD, Leder M (2011) Procedural sedation: a review of sedative agents, monitoring, and management of complications. Saudi J Anaesth 5(4):395–410. https://doi.org/10.4103/1658-354X.87270

Tollemar V, Collier ZJ, Mohammed MK et al (2016) ScienceDirect stem cells, growth factors and scaffolds in craniofacial regenerative medicine. Genes Dis 3:56–71

Tomar P, Hongal S, Saxena V, Jain M, Rana K, Ganavadiya R (2014) Evaluating sanitization of toothbrushes using ultra violet rays and 0.2% chlorhexidine solution: a comparative clinical study. J Basic Clin Pharm 6(1):12–8. https://doi.org/10.4103/0976-0105.145769

Verma SK, Maheshwari S, Singh RK, Chaudhari PK (2012) Laser in dentistry: an innovative tool in modern dental practice. Natl J Maxillofac Surg 3(2):124–132. https://doi.org/10.4103/0975-5950.111342

Wang YJ, Choo WC, Ng KY et al (2025) Evolution of AI enabled healthcare systems using textual data with a pretrained BERT deep learning model. Sci Rep 15:7540. https://doi.org/10.1038/s41598-025-91622-8

Conclusion

Artificial intelligence (AI) integration with robotics has the potential to significantly enhance the quality of life for millions by advancing sectors such as healthcare, education, and agriculture, among others. It can facilitate the creation of a world where the pursuit of Sustainable Development Goals is more efficient and expedited. In order to achieve these objectives, it is essential to consolidate resources and expertise. The development of open-source systems that promote trust and transparency is crucial. Additionally, it is imperative to construct high-quality datasets that are devoid of biases. Technology must be democratized, leading to the creation of applications that prioritize the needs of individuals. Furthermore, it is vital to tackle issues associated with cybersecurity, misinformation, and deepfakes. Lastly, ensuring that technology is integrated within local ecosystems is necessary for its effectiveness and utility.

The potential for job displacement is one of the most significant concerns associated with the rise of artificial intelligence and robotics. However, historical evidence suggests that technology does not eliminate employment; rather, it transforms the nature of work and gives rise to new job categories. It is imperative that we prioritize investment in the training and retraining of our workforce to prepare for a future characterized by the integration of AI and robotics.

It has been emphasized that the need for ethical, inclusive, and people-centric AI applications is more critical than ever. We stand on the threshold of the artificial intelligence era, a period poised to significantly influence the trajectory of human civilization. While there are concerns regarding the potential for machines to surpass human intelligence, it is essential to recognize that the authority over our collective future and shared fate resides solely with humanity. This awareness of responsibility should serve as our guiding principle.

Robotics offers several benefits, such as enhancing precision, reducing human error, increasing the efficiency of procedures, and improving patient outcomes.

A. Gupta et al. (eds.), *Application of Robotics in Dentistry*, Lecture Notes in Bioengineering, https://doi.org/10.1007/978-981-95-1470-0

Robotic systems, like robotic-assisted surgery and advanced imaging, allow for minimally invasive treatments, which lead to faster recovery times and less discomfort for patients.

Moreover, the integration of artificial intelligence with robotics can assist dentists in making better diagnostic decisions and planning treatments more accurately. While the technology still requires high levels of expertise and may involve initial investment costs, it holds promise for revolutionizing dental procedures and improving overall healthcare delivery.

As advancements in robotics continue to evolve, we can expect more widespread adoption of these technologies, making dental treatments more accessible, efficient, and patient-friendly in the future.

Digital technology has had a profound impact on the dental profession, streamlining many aspects of treatment while increasing precision. The evidence indicates that although the promising capabilities of artificial intelligence are truly remarkable, there exist numerous biases that warrant careful consideration. As these technologies continue to evolve and become more accessible, they hold the potential to significantly reduce dental problems and improve the overall health of millions of people worldwide. However, like any technology, they should complement rather than replace traditional dental care practices, ensuring that oral health remains a holistic and ongoing priority.

MIX
Papier aus verantwortungsvollen Quellen
Paper from responsible sources
FSC® C105338

If you have any concerns about our products,
you can contact us on
ProductSafety@springernature.com

In case Publisher is established outside the EU,
the EU authorized representative is:
Springer Nature Customer Service Center GmbH
Europaplatz 3, 69115 Heidelberg, Germany

Printed by Libri Plureos GmbH
in Hamburg, Germany